Westmead
Anaesthetic Manual

This manual is dedicated to my beautiful, patient and long-suffering wife Tracey, who has supported me through all my laborious projects, especially these books. It is also dedicated to my adult sons Max, Angus and Hugo who, through my inspirational example, have never shown any interest in medicine whatsoever.

Westmead Anaesthetic Manual

Fifth Edition

Anthony P. Padley

MBBS (UNSW), FANZCA

This fifth edition published 2024
First edition published 2000, Second edition published 2004, Third edition published 2009, Fourth edition published 2015
Reprinted 2009, 2011
Copyright © 2024 McGraw Hill Education (Australia) Pty Ltd
Additional owners of copyright are acknowledged in on-page credits.

National Library of Australia Cataloguing-in-Publication Entry

 A catalogue record for this work is available from the National Library of Australia

Authors: Anthony P. Padley
Title: Westmead anaesthetic manual
Edition: 5th edition
ISBN: 9781760427283

Published in Australia by
McGraw Hill Education (Australia) Pty Ltd
Level 33, 680 George Street, Sydney NSW 2000
Publisher: Rochelle Deighton
Production manager: Martina Vascotto
Copyeditor: Paul Hines
Proofreader: Meredith Lewin
Permissions manager: Rachel Norton
Cover design: Simon Rattray, Squirt Creative
Internal design: Peta Nugent, Simon Rattray
Typeset by Straive
Printed in China by 1010 Printing International Ltd

Contents

B

C

M

N

O

Abbreviations

5-HT	5-hydroxytryptamine	**BiPAP**	bi-level positive airway pressure
ABG	arterial blood gas	**BIS**	bispectral index monitoring system
AC	assist control		
ACE	angiotensin-converting enzyme	**BLM**	bleomycin
ACV	assist control ventilation	**BLS**	basic life support
ADP	adenosine diphosphate	**BMS**	bare metal stents
AED	automated external defibrillator	**BNP**	brain natriuretic peptide
AF	atrial fibrillation	**BNP**	B-type natriuretic peptide
AFE	amniotic fluid embolism	**BPB**	brachial plexus block
AICD	automatic implantable cardioverter defibrillator	**BPF**	bronchopleural fistula
		BSA	body surface area
ALS	advanced life support, amyotrophic lateral sclerosis	**CABG**	coronary artery bypass graft(s)
		CAD	coronary artery disease
AML	amyotrophic lateral sclerosis	**CAS**	coronary artery stent
AP	accessory pathway	**CAVM**	cerebral arterio-venous malformation
APH	antepartum haemorrhage		
APO	acute pulmonary oedema	**CBD**	cannabidiol
APTT	or **aPTT** activated partial thromboplastin time	**CCA**	common carotid artery
		CCF	congestive cardiac failure
ARB	angiotensin II receptor blocker	**CF**	cystic fibrosis
ARDS	acute respiratory distress syndrome	**CHD**	congenital heart disease
		CICO	Can't intubate, can't oxygenate
ARM	artificial rupture of the membranes	**CK**	creatine kinase
		CMV	controlled mandatory ventilation
ARNI	angiotensin receptor-neprilysin inhibitor		
		CMV	cytomegalovirus
AS	aortic valve stenosis	**CN**	cyanide
ASD	atrial septal defect	**CO**	cardiac output
ASIS	anterior superior iliac spine	**COMT**	catechol-O-methyl transferase
AST	aspartate aminotransferase	**COPD**	chronic obstructive pulmonary disease
ATLS	advanced trauma life support		
AVM	arterio-venous malformation	**COX**	cyclo-oxygenase
AVNRT	atrioventricular nodal re-entrant tachycardia	**CP**	cervical plexus
		CPAP	continuous positive airway pressure
AVRT	atrioventricular re-entrant tachycardia		
		CPK	creatine phosphokinase
BAEPs	brainstem auditory evoked potentials	**CPP**	cerebral perfusion pressure
		CPP	coronary perfusion pressure
BBB	blood–brain barrier	**CrCl**	creatinine clearance
BE	base excess	**CRT**	cardiac resynchronisation therapy
BIH	benign intracranial hypertension		
		CS	Caesarean section

CSE	combined spinal epidural	**G6PD**	glucose-6-phosphate dehydrogenase
CSF	cerebrospinal fluid		
CSL	compound sodium lactate	**GA**	general anaesthesia
CUSA	Cavitron ultrasonic surgical aspirator	**GCS**	Glasgow coma score
		GFR	glomerular filtration rate
CVA	cerebrovascular accident	**GTN**	glyceryl trinitrate
CVP	central venous pressure	**h**	hour
CVS	cardiovascular system	**HAE**	hereditary angioedema
CVST	cerebral venous sinus thrombosis	**HB**	heart block
		HbC	haemoglobin C
DAPT	dual antiplatelet therapy	**HbE**	haemoglobin E
DCM	dilated cardiomyopathy	**HbH**	haemoglobin H
DES	drug-eluting stents	**HbS**	haemoglobin S
DIC	disseminated intravascular coagulation	**HCM**	hypertrophic cardiomyopathy
		HFNC	high-flow nasal cannula
DILV	double inlet left ventricle	**HFNO/**	high-flow nasal oxygen/
DKA	diabetic ketoacidosis	**HHS**	hyperosmolar hyperglycaemic state
DLCO	diffusing capacity of lungs for carbon monoxide		
		HIT	heparin-induced thrombocytopenia
DLT	double lumen tube		
DM	diabetes mellitus	**HOCM**	hypertrophic obstructive cardiomyopathy
DN	dibucaine number		
DORV	double outlet right ventricle	**IAP**	intra-abdominal pressure
DTI	direct thrombin inhibitor	**IBW**	ideal body weight
DVT/PE	deep venous thrombosis/ pulmonary embolus	**IC**	inspiratory capacity
		IHD	ischaemic heart disease
ECG	electrocardiography	**IJV**	internal jugular vein
ECMO	extra corporeal membrane oxygenation	**IM**	intramuscular
		INR	international normalised ratio
EDS	Ehlers–Danlos syndrome	**IO**	intraosseous
EEG	electroencephalograph	**IOP**	intraocular pressure
EJV	external jugular vein	**IR**	immediate release
ER	extended release	**IRV**	inspiratory reserve volume
ERS	emergency response system	**ITP**	immune thrombocytopenic purpura
ERV	expiratory reserve volume		
ESP	erector spinae plane	**IUFR**	intrauterine fetal resuscitation
ET	endotracheal	**IV**	intravenous
EXIT	ex utero intrapartum treatment	**IVC**	inferior vena cava
		IVIG	intravenous immunoglobulin
FDPs	fibrin degradation products	**IVT**	intracranial venous thrombosis
FEIBA-NF	factor VIII inhibitor bypassing activity	**JVP**	jugular venous pressure
		KCCT	kaolin-cephalin clotting time
FES	fat embolism syndrome	**LA**	left atrium
FFP	fresh frozen plasma	**LA**	local anaesthetic
FIB	fascia iliaca block	**LBBB**	left bundle branch block
FO	foramen ovale	**LDH**	lactate dehydrogenase
FOB	fibre-optic bronchoscope	**LFV**	liberation from ventilation
FONA	front of neck access	**LMA**	laryngeal mask airway
FRC	functional respiratory capacity	**LMWH**	low-molecular-weight heparin

LOC	level of consciousness	**NMBDs**	neuromuscular blocking drugs
LOR	loss of resistance	**NMDA**	N-methyl-D-aspartate
LP	lumbar puncture	**NMJ**	neuromuscular junction
LQTS	long QT syndrome	**NMS**	neuroleptic malignant
LRS	lactated Ringer's solution		syndrome
LSO	Laser Safety Officer	**NOAC**	non-vitamin K oral
LV	left ventricle		anticoagulant drug
LVEF	left ventricular ejection fraction	**NPPO**	negative pressure pulmonary
LVOT	left ventricular outflow tract		oedema
MAC	minimum alveolar concentration	**NSAID**	non-steroidal anti-
MAP	mean arterial pressure		inflammatory drug
MAT	multifocal atrial tachycardia	**NSTEMI**	non-ST segment elevation
max	maximum		myocardial infarction
MD	mitochondrial disease	**NT-proBNP**	N-terminal-pro b-type
MD	muscular dystrophy		natriuretic peptide
MELAS	mitochondrial	**OCP**	oral contraceptive pill
	encephalomyopathy, lactic	**OI**	osteogenesis imperfecta
	acidosis and stroke-like	**OLV**	one lung ventilation
	episodes syndrome	**OSA**	obstructive sleep apnoea
MEP	motor evoked potential	**PAF**	platelet activating factor
MET	metabolic equivalent of task	**PAI**	plasminogen activator inhibitor
MetHb	methaemoglobin,	**PCA**	patient-controlled analgesia
	methaemoglobinaemia	**PCC**	prothrombin complex
MG	myasthenia gravis		concentrate
MH	malignant hyperthermia	**PCEA**	patient-controlled epidural
MI	myocardial infarction		anaesthesia
min	minute	**PCI**	percutaneous coronary
MMR	masseter muscle rigidity		intervention
MMS	mediastinal mass syndrome	**PCV**	pressure-controlled ventilation
MND	motor neurone disease	**PD**	Parkinson's disease
MR	magnetic resonance	**PDA**	patent ductus arteriosus
MR	mitral valve regurgitation,	**PDE**	phosphodiesterase
	modified release (of drug)	**PDPH**	post-dural puncture headache
MRA	mineral corticoid receptor	**PE**	pulmonary embolism
	antagonist	**PEA**	pulseless electrical activity
MRI	magnetic resonance imaging	**PEEP**	peak end expiratory pressure
MS	mitral valve stenosis	**PEFR**	peak expiratory flow rate
MS	multiple sclerosis	**PFO**	patent foramen ovale
MTP	massive transfusion protocol	**PICC**	peripherally inserted central
MV	minute ventilation		catheter
MVP	mitral valve prolapse	**PIEB**	programmed intermittent
NA	noradrenaline		epidural bolus
NBCA	n-butyl cyanoacrylate	**PIP**	peak inspiratory pressure
NCTs	narrow complex tachycardias	**PONV**	postoperative nausea and
NDNMBD	non-depolarising neuromuscular		vomiting
	blocking drug	**POTS**	postural orthostatic
NGT	nasogastric tube		tachycardia syndrome
NIV	non-invasive ventilation	**PP**	placenta praevia
NK1	neurokinin-1	**PP**	pulse pressure

PPH	postpartum haemorrhage	**sGC**	soluble guanylate cyclase
Pplat	plateau pressure	**SGLT2**	sodium-glucose cotransporter-2
PRVC	pressure-regulated volume control mode ventilation	**SIADH**	syndrome of inappropriate anti-diuretic hormone secretion
PS	pressure support		
PS	pulmonary stenosis	**SIMV**	synchronous intermittent mandatory ventilation
PSVT	paroxysmal supraventricular tachycardia	**SIRS**	systemic inflammatory response syndrome
PT	prothrombin time		
PTT	partial thromboplastin time	**SNP**	sodium nitroprusside
PV	polycythaemia vera	**SPG**	sphenopalatine ganglion
PVD	pulmonary vascular disease or peripheral vascular disease, depending on context	**SQTS**	short QT syndrome
		SR	sarcoplasmic reticulum, sustained release (of drug)
PVR	peripheral vascular resistance	**SR**	sinus rhythm
PVR	pulmonary vascular resistance	**SR**	sustained-release tablet
		SSEPs	somatosensory evoked potentials
q	every		
RA	right atrium	**SSS**	sick sinus syndrome
RBBB	right bundle branch block	**STEMI**	ST segment elevation myocardial infarction
RBC	red blood cells		
RE	response entropy	**STIG**	steerable pre-curved intubating guide
Rh	Rhesus factor		
RIC	rapid infusion catheter	**subcut**	subcutaneous
ROSC	return of spontaneous circulation	**SV**	stroke volume
		SVC	superior vena cava
RR	respiratory rate	**SVCS**	superior vena cava syndrome
RSBI	rapid shallow breathing index	**SVR**	systemic vascular resistance
RSI	rapid sequence induction	**SVT**	supraventricular tachycardia
rtPA	recombinant tissue plasminogen activator	**TACO**	transfusion-associated circulatory overload
RV	residual volume	**TAP**	transversus abdominis plane
RV	right ventricle	**TAPVR**	total anomalous pulmonary vascular return
RVOT	right ventricular outflow tract		
s	second	**TAVI**	transcatheter aortic valve implantation
SA	sinoatrial node		
SAB	subarachnoid block	**TBSA**	total body surface area
SAH	subarachnoid haemorrhage	**TBV**	total blood volume
SANRT	sinoatrial nodal re-entrant tachycardia	**TCAR**	trans-carotid arterial revascularisation
		TCI	target-controlled infusion
SBP	systolic blood pressure	**TCR**	trigeminal cardiac reflex/ trigeminocardiac reflex
SBT	spontaneous breathing trial		
SCD	sickle cell disease		
SCM	sternocleidomastoid	**TF**	tissue factor
SCT	sickle cell trait	**TGA**	transposition of the great arteries
SE	state entropy		
SEM	systolic ejection murmur	**TGV**	transposition of the great vessels
SFA	superficial femoral artery		
SFV	superficial femoral vein	**THC**	tetrahydrocannabinol

THRIVE	transnasal humidified rapid-insufflation ventilatory exchange	**TTP**	thrombotic thrombocytopenic purpura
THRIVE	transnasal humidified rapid-insufflation ventilatory exchange	**TURP**	trans-urethral resection of prostate
TI	tricuspid incompetence	**TV**	tidal volume
TIVA	total intravenous anaesthesia	**TVE**	total vascular exclusion
TLC	total lung capacity	**TXA**	tranexamic acid
TOE	transoesophageal echocardiography	**UACR**	urine albumin-to-creatine ratio
ToF	Tetralogy of Fallot	**UO**	urine output
tPA	tissue plasminogen activator	**VCV**	volume-controlled ventilation
TR	therapeutic range	**VF**	ventricular fibrillation
TR	tricuspid regurgitation	**VSD**	ventricular septal defect
TRALI	transfusion-related acute lung injury	**VT**	ventricular tachycardia
TRIM	transfusion-related immunomodulation	**VTE**	venous thromboembolism
TS	tricuspid stenosis	**VVECMO**	veno-venous ECMO
TSH	thyroid-stimulating hormone	**VWD**	von Willebrand disease
TT	thrombin time	**VWF**	von Willebrand factor
		WCC	white cell count
		WPW	Wolff–Parkinson–White (syndrome)
		y	year(s)

Preface to the fifth edition

The *Westmead Anaesthetic Manual* has been of invaluable assistance to anaesthetists, emergency doctors and nurses for more than 20 years. In this edition, every topic has been completely revised and updated and many new topics have been added, including COVID-19, vaping, bariatric surgery, onco-anaesthesia and cannabinoids. There is extensive coverage of new drugs relevant to anaesthesia, including tapentadol and idarucizumab.

New innovations in this manual include adding European and American generic and trade names to help with international communication. In addition, to assist with ultrasound-guided blocks, NYSORA, the world's leading educator in this field, has allowed the use of many of their high-fidelity illustrations. This edition also examines the impact of anaesthetic drugs on global warming, with particular emphasis on the harmful effects of desflurane.

The *Westmead Anaesthetic Manual* remains the most compact and readily accessible source of essential anaesthetic information available on the Australian market, by an Australian author. With its alphabetic layout, almost any drug, crisis, rare medical condition, procedure or ultrasound-guided block can be accessed in seconds. The guidelines are clear, concise and comprehensive, and presented in a logical step-by-step format. This manual will not only enhance the safety of your daily anaesthetic practice but also help deal with those clinical situations that make our stress levels go 'off the scale'.

Acknowledgments

I would like to extend my sincerest thanks to NYSORA for allowing the use of their state-of-the-art illustrations and providing their online educational material. I would also like to thank four of my anaesthetic colleagues for their invaluable assistance with this manual.

First and foremost, I would like to thank Dr Elizabeth Lin (MBBS, FANZCA) for her hundreds of hours of proofreading, fact checking and suggestions for improvements. Her attention to medical detail, spelling and grammar is simultaneously astounding and humbling.

Secondly, I would like to thank Dr Adam Hastings (MBBS, FANZCA) for his advice on sections covering cardiac and neurosurgical issues. Adam has helped me with many actual life-threatening anaesthetic emergencies and is always cool-headed, effective and non-judgemental.

Thirdly, I extend my sincerest gratitude to Dr Sarah Wong (MBBS, FANZCA) for her invaluable assistance with the sections covering ultrasound-guided nerve blocks. Her help extended to scanning my spine and lungs to obtain photos for the manual. She is an inspiring and zealous teacher of all things ultrasound.

Finally, I would like to thank Dr Jane McDonald (MBBS (Hons), FANZCA) for her help with paediatric-related anaesthetic material. Jane is one of the smartest people I know, and I am very grateful to her for more than 20 years of friendship.

◗ A-a gradient

The A-a gradient is the difference between the partial pressure of oxygen in the alveolus (PAO_2) and the partial pressure of oxygen in the arterial blood (PaO_2). PAO_2 is the 'ideal' alveolar PO_2. The A-a gradient is helpful in diagnosing the cause of hypoxia. *See Hypoxia/hypoxaemia.*

PAO_2 is calculated from the alveolar gas equation:

$$PAO_2 = (PB - PH_2O) \times FiO_2 - PaCO_2/R$$

Where:
- PB = barometric pressure (760 mmHg at sea level).
- PH_2O = partial pressure of H_2O (47 mmHg). Gas in the lungs is fully saturated with water vapour.
- FiO_2 = fraction of inspired O_2.
- $PaCO_2$ = partial pressure of CO_2 in arterial blood (NR 35–45 mmHg).
- R = gas exchange ratio, also called the 'respiratory quotient' (0.8).

Therefore, for a normal person breathing air at 1 atmosphere and assuming a $PaCO_2$ of 40 mmHg:

$$PAO_2 = (760 - 47\,\text{mmHg}) \times 0.21 - 40/0.8 = 99.73\,\text{mmHg}$$

The simplified version of the equation is: $PAO_2 = FiO_2 \times 713 - PaCO_2/0.8$

Points to note

1 PAO_2 is normally about 105 mmHg.
2 PaO_2 is normally about 100 mmHg.
3 Normal A-a gradient is 5–15 mmHg. It is 5–10 mmHg for a normal young adult.
4 If the A-a gradient is normal and the patient is hypoxic, the problem is extrinsic to the lungs.
5 If the A-a gradient is abnormal and the patient is hypoxic, the problem is in the lungs.
6 A-a gradient increases with age. It should be $\leq 0.3 \times$ age.

Hypoxaemia with a normal A-a gradient

Can be due to:
1 decreased partial pressure of inspired O_2 e.g. at altitude
2 hypoventilation
3 haemoglobin defects or anaemia.

Hypoxaemia with a widened A-a gradient

Can be due to:
1 ventilation/perfusion mismatch
2 alveolar hypoventilation—pulmonary fibrosis, interstitial lung disease.

◗ ABCDE assessment

A rapid assessment tool for a non-arrested patient. The letters relate to:
A – **A**irway—patency; is the patient talking?
B – **B**reathing-rate; pulse oximetry; is air entry equal; is trachea midline?

C – **C**irculation—pulse rate and quality; blood pressure; capillary return; skin colour.

D – **D**isability—assess conscious state using GCS or AVPU. *See Glasgow coma score and AVPU.*

E – **E**xposure—examine patient's entire body for any concealed evidence of injury, haemorrhage etc.

◐ ABCDEFG (A–G) assessment

An extension of the ABCDE tool above. The letters relate to:

A – **A**irway—patency.

B – **B**reathing—respiratory rate; pulse oximetry.

C – **C**irculation—pulse quality and rate; blood pressure.

D – **D**isability—mental state; GCS.

E – **E**xposure—wounds; rash; external bleeding.

F – **F**luids—intake, output.

G – **G**lucose.

◐ Abciximab (ReoPro)

IgG antibody platelet glycoprotein IIb/IIIa receptor antagonist. It is used IV with aspirin and heparin after coronary artery angioplasty/stent to reduce the risk of re-occlusion. Platelet function takes 24–48 h to recover after the infusion is stopped. *See Anticoagulant and antiplatelet drugs and surgery/neuraxial anaesthesia.*

◐ Abdominal aortic aneurysm (AAA) surgery

Introduction

Aneurysms are permanent dilatations of the aorta, with an increase in aortic diameter of more than 50% of normal (normal being about 3 cm). AAA repair can be elective or an emergency and can be open or endovascular. Aortic stenting is termed 'endovascular aneurysm repair' (EVAR). AAA repair is complex, high-risk surgery in patients who frequently have significant co-morbidities. 65% of aortic aneurysms are abdominal, and 95% of these are below the renal arteries. The mortality of elective open repair ≈ 2–5%. Ruptured AAA has a mortality ≈ 65–90%. Elective EVAR mortality ≈ 1% in younger, robust patients, increasing to 9% in high-risk patients.[1] Overall mortality after six years is about the same for open and EVAR surgery due to the need for reintervention in the EVAR group. Metformin appears to offer some protection against aneurysm formation, enlargement and rupture.[2]

Aetiology

Aneurysms develop due to diseases of the aortic wall connective tissue (elastin and collagen). These cause degradation of elastin fibres, collagen disruption, inflammatory infiltrates and other pathological processes.

The most important risk factors are:

1 smoking
2 hypertension
3 hyperlipidaemia/atherosclerosis
4 family history (the strongest predictor)
5 increasing age
6 male preponderance 4:1
7 rarer causes such as inflammatory vasculitis, trauma, Marfan syndrome (defect in fibrin I), type IV Ehlers–Danlos syndrome.

Diagnosis

Usually diagnosed by abdominal ultrasound. Elective surgery should be offered when the aneurysm reaches 5.5 cm or becomes painful. Aneurysms tend to enlarge over time, and the rate of expansion is considered rapid if > 10 mm/year. Paradoxically, patients with diabetes mellitus have reduced expansion rates.[3]

Open repair vs EVAR

This is a surgical decision based on the following factors:

1 Suitability of AAA for grafting.
2 Surgeon's preference.
3 Patient's preference.
4 EVAR may be preferable in higher-risk patients.
   Up to 70–80% of patients with AAA are candidates for EVAR.

Complications of AAA surgery

The main complications in this high-risk group are:

1 myocardial ischaemia, infarction, cardiac arrest
2 renal impairment/failure
3 spinal cord damage
4 bowel ischaemia
5 abdominal compartment syndrome—elevated intra-abdominal pressure > 20 mmHg causing organ dysfunction or failure
6 general complications (respiratory failure, infection, bleeding etc).

Pre-anaesthetic assessment

In addition to a routine peri-operative workup, the following should be considered:

1 Underlying cardiac disease is highly likely and risk assessment is required. *See Cardiovascular peri-operative risk prediction for non-cardiac surgery.*
2 Many patients are current or ex-smokers and may have COPD.
3 Optimise medical therapy. All patients should be taking statins. Aspirin is recommended to reduce cardiac risk factors.[4] Hypertension needs to be controlled with antihypertensive drugs. Diabetes is also common in this patient group and management should be optimised.
4 Patients with renal impairment are at increased risk of postoperative renal failure.

Anaesthesia for open AAA repair

1 Prepare for potentially massive blood loss—large-bore IV access × 2, blood group and save.
2 Invasive monitoring (arterial line, central line).
3 Consider siting a thoracic epidural at T8–9 for postoperative analgesia.
4 Aim for normothermia. Warm the upper body but not the lower.
5 The anaesthetist should use their personal anaesthetic agents of choice e.g. fentanyl, propofol, rocuronium used in appropriate doses; sevoflurane or TCI propofol/remifentanil to maintain anaesthesia.
6 Give prophylactic antibiotics. *See Antibiotic prophylaxis for surgery.*
7 Consider preparing a glyceryl trinitrate infusion (GTN) to use as a vasodilator at the time of aortic cross-clamping. *See Glyceryl trinitrate (GTN).*
8 Give heparin 75–150 units/kg prior to aortic clamping.
9 Aortic cross-clamping results in increased SVR, increased MAP and increased LV wall stress. Preload may increase, decrease or be unchanged. CO may decrease. HR is usually unchanged. Renal blood flow is decreased, even with infrarenal cross-clamping.

10 Consider 'underfilling' the patient prior to clamp application.

11 To offset the increase in SVR and MAP, deepen anaesthesia/increase opioid dose. If this is insufficient, commence GTN infusion, which is also indicated if myocardial ischaemia occurs.

12 Aortic unclamping results in a massive sudden decrease in SVR (70–80%). This is multifactorial (clamp release, vasodilation of lower body, washout of vasodilator substances). MAP falls.

13 To offset these effects, fluid load the patient prior to unclamping and cease GTN. After unclamping, vasopressors/inotropes may be required to maintain MAP. If MAP becomes critical and refractory, consider reapplying the clamp and releasing it gradually when the patient is more stable.

14 Postoperative care should be in an HDU or ICU setting.

EVAR surgery

The surgical entry point is usually the common femoral artery but can be brachial or subclavian. Grafts can be standard (simple tube grafts) or complex (branched). The graft is positioned under fluoroscopic guidance, from normal artery above to normal artery below, and then the ends are attached to the aorta. This is achieved by expanding the graft ends (self-expanding or with a balloon), which imbeds hooks at either end of the graft. Blood flows through the stent and is excluded from the aneurysmal sac, which undergoes thrombosis. EVAR are intermediate-risk procedures, but complex graft repairs should be considered high risk.[1] Potential problems with EVAR are significant and include leaking around the stent (endoleak) and malposition or migration of the graft.

Anaesthesia for EVAR

Surgery can be performed with LA ± sedation, neuraxial anaesthesia or GA.

If the patient is awake, they need to be able to remain still for the period of digital subtraction angiography.

1 Insert large-bore IV access.

2 Insert an arterial line.

3 Give heparin 5000 units IV when requested by the surgeon.

4 Maintain haemodynamic stability.

5 A feared complication of EVAR (and open AAA repair) is spinal cord ischaemia due to occlusion of the artery of Adamkiewicz. This arises from the aorta anywhere between T5–L3 and supplies the lower two-thirds of the spinal cord via the anterior spinal artery. *See Anterior spinal artery syndrome*.

6 Peri-operative hypotension, prolonged aortic occlusion, prolonged procedure time and complex surgery all increase the risk of this complication. Strategies to reduce the risk of this in high-risk patients include CSF drainage, hypothermia, steroids, augmentation of MAP and femorofemoral bypass.[1]

7 Renal impairment/failure can result from IV contrast required for graft positioning.

8 Post-implantation syndrome imitates sepsis and is characterised by pyrexia, elevated WCC and elevated inflammatory markers. The condition is usually self-limiting.

Ruptured AAA

A time-critical surgical emergency. Free intraperitoneal rupture usually results in exsanguination and death. Retroperitoneal rupture is more likely to tamponade, allowing more time for treatment. Presentation may include:

1 catastrophic haemorrhage, hypovolaemic shock, collapse and cardiac arrest

2 lower abdominal or lumbar pain.

Initial management

1 If the patient has suffered a cardiac arrest, further management is usually futile.
2 Ensure a clear airway and adequate breathing. Give supplementary O_2.
3 Site two large-bore IV cannulas and an arterial line. Send bloods for FBC, UEC, coagulation studies and cross-match.
4 Give IV fluid resuscitation sufficient to maintain consciousness—aim for SBP of 50–70 mmHg. This is because aggressive fluid resuscitation may cause more bleeding by thrombus dislodgement and dilution of clotting factors.[5]
5 Consider not transfusing RBC in the initial resuscitation phase unless the patient is unconscious or has myocardial ischaemia.
6 Haemodynamically stable patients may benefit from emergency CT scan to confirm the diagnosis and assess suitability for endovascular repair.

Anaesthesia and subsequent management

Management is the same as for other surgical emergencies associated with massive blood loss. *See Blood loss—assessment, management and anaesthetic approach.* EVAR may be possible in certain patients after spiral CT scanning to determine the aortic aneurysm's size and shape and confirm the diagnosis of rupture. EVAR may be performed under LA or GA in this situation. If LA is used, conversion to GA is required in about 25% of cases.[6]

Postoperative management

1 Patients requiring open repair either electively or emergently will usually require postoperative management in ICU, particularly if ventilated.
2 Other patients can be monitored in HDU post procedure.
3 These patients are at particular risk of myocardial ischaemia/infarction and renal impairment/failure.

◗ Abdominal pregnancy

In this condition, fertilisation takes place outside the uterine adnexa or a tubal pregnancy ruptures and survives in the abdominal cavity. Implantation occurs on the external uterine wall or some other organ such as the liver. The incidence is 1:10 000 births, and the main risk is massive haemorrhage, with a 30% maternal mortality and a 40–90% fetal mortality.

Diagnosis

Only about 50% of cases are diagnosed prior to placental rupture from the host organ. Diagnosis is by ultrasound or clinical evaluation with:
1 persistent transverse or oblique lie
2 abdominal pain
3 palpable fetal parts.

Management

If diagnosed before 24 weeks' gestation, surgery to remove fetus and placenta is indicated. If diagnosed after 24 weeks' gestation and the fetus is viable, admit to a tertiary obstetric hospital and prepare for massive blood loss at any time. A planned surgical delivery should be arranged for an appropriate time (as decided by obstetrician, anaesthetist and mother), again with preparation for massive obstetric haemorrhage. If abdominal pregnancy is undiagnosed and placental rupture occurs, *see Blood loss—assessment, management and anaesthetic approach.*

❍ Abruptio placentae

See Placental abruption.

❍ ACE inhibitors

See Angiotensin-converting enzyme (ACE) inhibitors.

❍ Acetylcholine receptors (cholinergic receptors)

Acetylcholine receptors are membrane proteins that bind the neurotransmitter acetylcholine. There are two main types, muscarinic and nicotinic.

Muscarinic receptors

These receptors are involved in the parasympathetic nervous system (sweat glands have muscarinic receptors but are part of the sympathetic nervous system). There are different types of receptors situated in the brain (M1), atrium, sinoatrial node (M2), and smooth muscle of bronchi, GIT, pupil and blood vessels (M3). There are also M4 and M5 receptors in the CNS. The muscarinic receptors in the sweat glands are also of the M3 type. Stimulation of muscarinic receptors results in:

1 bradycardia
2 bronchial constriction
3 pupillary constriction
4 vasodilation of blood vessels
5 urinary bladder, gall bladder and gut contraction
6 lacrimation, salivation, defecation.

Atropine blocks muscarinic receptors competitively. *See Atropine.*

Nicotinic receptors

These are located on the skeletal muscle at the neuromuscular junction. They are blocked by suxamethonium and non-depolarising neuromuscular blocking drugs (NDNMBDs).

❍ Acidosis

Blood pH < 7.35. *See Arterial blood gas (ABG) interpretation.*

❍ Activated clotting time (ACT)

ACT tests intrinsic and common clotting pathways. *See Clotting pathways.* The test is performed by adding a clotting activator such as celite or kaolin to a blood sample and measuring the time to clot formation. Clot formation is detected either by optical or electromagnetic techniques. ACT is used for monitoring high-dose heparin therapy during cardiac surgery where APTT measurements are beyond the test range. *See Activated partial thromboplastin time (APTT).* ACT NR 90–120 s. For endovascular procedures, an ACT of 180–200 s may be desirable, and for cardiopulmonary bypass > 500 s may be targeted.

❍ Activated factor VIIa (NovoSeven)

See Recombinant activated factor VII/rFVIIa/Eptacog alfa-activated (NovoSeven RT).

❍ Activated factor X inhibitors

See Anticoagulant and antiplatelet drugs and surgery/neuraxial anaesthesia.

◑ Activated partial thromboplastin time (APTT)

APTT tests the intrinsic clotting pathway. It is used to monitor IV heparin therapy and is affected by deficiencies in the clotting factors of the intrinsic and common clotting pathways. The test is done by adding platelet substitute, factor XII activator and calcium chloride to a sample of citrated blood. The time to clot formation is then measured. **See** *Clotting pathways*. NR 25–36 s. Prolonged APTT occurs with heparin therapy and impairment/reduction of clotting factors V, X, XI, XII and fibrinogen.

◑ Acute cerebrovascular accident

See *Acute stroke*.

◑ Acute coronary syndrome

Acute coronary syndrome describes a condition in which there is a sudden reduction of blood flow to the heart. It can present as:

1 unstable angina—ST segment and T wave changes, which are usually transient
2 non-ST segment elevation myocardial infarction (NSTEMI)
3 ST segment elevation myocardial infarction (STEMI).

Unstable angina
This can present as exertional angina of **new onset** which stops with rest and reoccurs with the same amount of exercise. Angina is also considered unstable if it occurs with less exercise than previously and/or occurs with rest for > 20 min.

NSTEMI
A myocardial infarction has occurred without ST elevation, as diagnosed by history and troponin rise.

STEMI
Myocardial infarction with elevation of ST segments. This is a higher-risk group.

Coronary artery disease (CAD) risk factors
There are five main risk factors for CAD—hypertension, hyperlipidaemia, diabetes, obesity and smoking.
There are two mechanisms to consider:

1 Flow-limiting coronary artery stenosis preventing sufficient supply when higher demand is required.
2 Acute coronary syndromes due to atherosclerotic plaque rupture with associated vascular inflammation and haemostatic mechanisms.

Pathophysiology
Acute coronary syndrome can be precipitated by an atherosclerotic plaque rupturing in a coronary artery, causing an atherothrombotic event. Other causes are increased demand when diseased coronary arteries are unable to meet supply, coronary artery dissection, vasospasm, emboli and microvascular dysfunction.

Coronary artery supply territories

1 The right coronary artery supplies the right ventricle (RV) and right atrium (RA). The right marginal artery supplies the RV and septum.
2 The left coronary artery supplies the left atrium (LA) and left ventricle (LV). The left circumflex artery supplies parts of LA and LV. The left anterior descending

artery (LAD) supplies the RV, LV and septum. The LAD is the most common site of coronary artery blockage, resulting in damage to the anterior wall of the heart. Heart muscle deprived of blood supply will die after about 30 min.

Clinical presentation of acute coronary syndrome

1 Chest pain.
2 Dyspnoea.
3 Palpitations.
4 Anxiety.
5 Nausea/vomiting.
6 Diaphoresis.
7 Dysrhythmias.
8 Acute heart failure.
9 Sudden death.

Types of myocardial infarction

1 **Type 1** (or primary MI) is due to CAD and usually an acute plaque rupture with formation of a platelet thrombus.
2 **Type 2** (or secondary MI) is due to another condition such as sepsis, hypovolaemia or anaemia causing inadequate coronary blood flow.

Diagnosis

1 ECG—typically shows peaked T waves initially, then inverted T waves, ST elevation in the territory of the infarction and reciprocal changes in opposite leads. Q waves may develop. New onset LBBB may also occur. The site of the infarct can be implied by changes in the following leads:
   a) Anterior—divided into anteroseptal V1–V4, antero-apical (or mid-anterior) V3–V4, anterolateral V3–V6 (left anterior descending coronary artery territory).
   b) Inferior—II, III, aVF (right or left circumflex coronary artery occlusion).
   c) Posterior—ST depression and dominant R wave with upright T waves in V1–V3.
Note: there can be ST depression with an NSTEMI. NSTEMIs usually represent less myocardial muscle damage than a STEMI.
2 CXR—may identify pulmonary oedema, cardiac enlargement.
3 Cardiac enzymes—troponins are the most useful. Troponin has subunits of troponin C, I and T. Troponin C is not clinically useful. Troponin I and T are called 'high-sensitive troponins' and are very useful for detecting myocardial damage. Serial testing is done to detect a rise and fall in troponin levels over hours and days to be diagnostic of myocardial muscle damage. Significant troponin levels are lab dependent. Troponin I is significant if $\geq$ 0.035–0.04 ng/mL, depending on the lab. Cardiac damage is indicated by troponin I > 0.04 ng/ml and is severe if > 0.4 ng/mL. Troponin levels rise within 2–3 h of the onset of chest pain and peak at about 12–48 h. Levels will return to normal over 4–10 days. Normal values of troponin T are up to 14 ng/L. Myocardial infarction is consistent with a troponin T > 22 ng/L in males and > 14 ng/L in females.
4 The term 'troponin leak' suggests subacute myocardial damage due to such causes as viral myocarditis or sarcoidosis. Acute strokes and chronic kidney disease can cause elevated troponin levels.
5 Full blood screen for other abnormalities such as diabetes, anaemia, renal impairment, liver disease.
6 Cardiac echo—may show evidence of ventricular wall abnormalities due to ischaemia, infarction.
7 Emergency coronary angiography—may show a site of blockage.

Treatment

1 Give supplementary O_2 only if oxygen saturation < 94%.

2 Aspirin—300 mg chewed and swallowed.

3 Nitrates—sublingual nitroglycerin 0.4 mg every 5 min × 3 doses to relieve pain. Consider a GTN infusion if ongoing chest pain and/or hypertension. Do not use nitrates in patients with a SBP < 90 mmHg, severe bradycardia, suspected RV infarction or phosphodiesterase inhibitor use (e.g. Viagra) in the previous 24 h.

4 Analgesia—give IV morphine 5–10 mg.

5 Details of ongoing management protocols are complex, controversial, site specific and evolving. These details are beyond the scope of this manual. They may involve measures including:

    a) a second type of antiplatelet drug such as ticagrelor or prasugrel. *See Anticoagulant and antiplatelet drugs and surgery/neuraxial anaesthesia*

    b) heparin

    c) urgent percutaneous coronary intervention (PCI)

    d) fibrinolysis therapy if PCI not available with drugs such as tenecteplase, reteplase or alteplase

    e) urgent coronary artery bypass graft(s) (CABG).

6 Ongoing management will be determined by the cardiologist and may include:

    a) beta blockers

    b) dual antiplatelet therapy

    c) statins

    d) ACE inhibitors

    e) control of risk factors.

7 In the absence of coronary artery intervention, elective surgery should be delayed for at least 60 days after acute myocardial infarction.

Myocardial ischaemia intraoperatively

See Intraoperative myocardial ischaemia.

▶ Acute dystonic reaction

See Dystonic reaction, acute.

▶ Acute fatty liver of pregnancy (AFLP)

Description

A rare (1:7000–20 000) condition that occurs in the third trimester or early postpartum period. It is characterised by fatty infiltration of hepatocytes without inflammation or necrosis. The cause is unknown and the mortality is about 18%.

Clinical signs/symptoms

1 Anorexia, nausea, vomiting, abdominal pain.

2 Fatigue.

3 Headache.

4 Fever.

5 Jaundice.

6 Acute renal failure, oliguria.

7 Encephalopathy.

8 Coagulopathy.

9 GIT bleeding.

10 Pancreatitis.

11 Other pregnancy diseases such as preeclampsia/eclampsia.

Diagnosis

1 FBC may show haemolysis, thrombocytopenia, elevated WCC.
2 Coagulopathy with prolonged APPT. DIC may occur.
3 Deranged LFTs.
4 Elevated serum ammonia, hyperbilirubinaemia, hypoglycaemia.
5 Lactic acidosis.

Anaesthetic management

1 Stabilise the mother—ensure adequate airway and ventilation. If needed, provide circulatory support/treatment of hypertension.
2 Correct hypoglycaemia, electrolyte and coagulation abnormalities.
3 Prompt delivery of the fetus is required to reduce maternal and fetal mortality. The optimal timing for this is decided by a multidisciplinary team (obstetrician, feto-maternal specialist, anaesthetist and patient). Normal vaginal delivery is preferable, but if induction fails caesarean section is required.
4 Prepare for intraoperative haemorrhage if coagulopathy is present, which will also preclude neuraxial anaesthesia.

◑ Acute haemolytic reaction

Description

Most commonly due to an incompatible blood group transfusion, which in turn is usually due to human error. There is intravascular haemolysis.

Clinical effects

1 Fever, chills, rigors.
2 Anxiety.
3 Chest, abdominal, flank and/or back pain.
4 Nausea, vomiting.
5 Diffuse bleeding.

Diagnosis

1 Clinical context.
2 Haemoglobinuria.
3 Decreased haemoglobin and haptoglobin and elevated lactate dehydrogenase.
4 Positive direct antiglobulin test.

Treatment

1 Cease transfusion immediately.
2 Supportive measures e.g. analgesia, IV fluid replacement, management of coagulopathy.
3 Notify the blood bank.

◑ Acute haemorrhage

See Blood loss—assessment, management and anaesthetic approach.

◑ Acute heart failure

See Cardiogenic shock.

◑ Acute intermittent porphyria

See Porphyria.

▷ Acute pulmonary oedema (APO)

Description

A medical emergency requiring immediate management. It can be defined as the sudden accumulation of fluid in the interstitial or alveolar spaces, resulting in impaired gas exchange. APO can be cardiogenic or non-cardiogenic.

Cardiogenic pulmonary oedema

The most common type. It is due to left ventricular (LV) failure. That in turn can have many causes. *See Congestive cardiac failure (CCF)—chronic* and *Cardiogenic shock.*

Non-cardiogenic pulmonary oedema

Causes include:

1 hypervolaemia
2 changes to the permeability of the alveolar membrane to fluid as can occur with preeclampsia, sepsis
3 negative pressure pulmonary oedema—*see Negative pressure pulmonary oedema (NPPO)*
4 pulmonary embolus
5 neurogenic pulmonary oedema due to cerebral pathology such as subarachnoid haemorrhage leading to massive sympathetic discharge
6 vasoconstriction of the pulmonary circulation with constant or increased cardiac output, leading to increased capillary pressure. This is thought to be the cause of high-altitude pulmonary oedema.

Clinical effects

1 Dyspnoea/tachypnoea.
2 Hypoxia.
3 Frothy, blood-tinged sputum.
4 Increased inspiratory pressures in ventilated patients.
5 Lung crackles/wheezes on auscultation.

Diagnosis

1 Clinical presentation.
2 CXR—typical findings are bilateral alveolar opacities, fluffy shadowing, perihilar shadowing with bat wing appearance, Kerley B lines.
3 Echocardiography—may indicate the cause e.g. cardiomyopathy.

Treatment

Aims are to reverse the cause (if possible), maintain oxygenation, maintain perfusion of vital organs and reduce excess extracellular fluid in the lungs. Steps include:

1 Oxygen therapy if O_2 saturation < 92%. If still < 92% with a non-rebreather mask and 15 L/min of O_2, start CPAP with 10 cm H_2O or BiPAP at 10/4 cm H_2O.[7] If COPD, the target O_2 saturation is 88–92%. *See Non-invasive ventilation.*
2 Intubation and IPPV and PEEP may be required if the patient has ongoing hypoxia, acidosis or respiratory distress despite the above measures, or the patient becomes exhausted or has decreased level of consciousness.
3 Sit the patient up.

4 Frusemide 40–80 mg IV if there is fluid overload. A continuous infusion may be required, starting at a rate of 5–10 mg/h. **See Frusemide**. Monitor urine output with a urinary catheter.

5 Morphine is no longer recommended.[8] It may be beneficial for the treatment of ongoing chest pain resistant to nitrates.

6 If BP > 100 mmHg, give GTN spray (0.4 mg/2 puffs) or sublingual tablet 0.3–0.6 mg. Begin a GTN infusion at 5–10 mcg/min. Double the dose every 5 min until the desired clinical effect is achieved (max 200 mcg/min). **See Glyceryl trinitrate (GTN)**. Maintain SBP > 90 mmHg.

○ Acute respiratory distress syndrome (ARDS)

Description

A generalised inflammation of the lungs resulting in swelling of the interstitial space and filling of the alveoli with proteinaceous fluid/hyaline membrane. It can occur with any type of infection or conditions such as aspiration. The lungs become very stiff (compliance is reduced). Plateau pressures are elevated. **See Ventilation strategies and modes**.

Ventilation strategies

Aims are to:

1 optimise oxygenation

2 minimise shear stress on the alveoli.

Settings to consider are:

1 Tidal volume—start with 6 mL/kg ideal body weight (IBW), with a range of 4–8 mL/kg. **See Ideal body weight (IBW)**. Aim for a low tidal volume because the opening and closing of the alveoli leads to shear stress and worsens the inflammation.

2 Plateau pressures should be < 30 cm H_2O. **See Plateau pressure**.

3 Peak end expiratory pressure (PEEP) should be high (> 10 cm H_2O). Consider PEEP 5–10 cm H_2O for mild ARDS, 10–15 cm H_2O in moderate disease and 15–20 cm H_2O in severe disease. This is to splint open as many alveoli as possible.

4 Use recruitment manoeuvres if required. **See Recruitment manoeuvres**.

5 Consider prone ventilation.

6 Limit the driving pressure, which is the plateau pressure minus the PEEP. Not all patients are PEEP responsive. **See Driving pressure**. Driving pressure should be < 13–15 cm H_2O.[9]

7 Neuromuscular blocking drugs (NMBDs) may be required e.g. for ventilator dyssynchrony, high-dose sedation requirements. If an infusion of NMBDs is required, limit this to 48 h if possible.

8 Consider inhaled nitric oxide for hypoxaemia refractory to the above measures.

9 ECMO if all else fails. **See Extracorporeal membrane oxygenation (ECMO)**.

○ Acute stroke

Description

Acute stroke can be defined as the acute onset of focal or global neurological findings as a result of cerebrovascular disease or embolus to the cerebral circulation. Acute stroke can be classified as:

1 ischaemic stroke due to blockage of the blood supply to an area of brain—usually due to a blood clot from carotid artery disease or a paradoxical blood clot embolus via a patent foramen ovale. It can also be due to trauma to the arteries of the neck or dissection of a neck or cerebral artery

2 haemorrhagic stroke due to bleeding from an artery in the brain. Can be from an arterio-venous malformation (AVM) or cerebral aneurysm rupture.

Risk factors

1 Hypertension.
2 Heart disease.
3 High cholesterol.
4 Blood clotting disorders.
5 Smoking.
6 Diabetes.
7 Use of the oral contraceptive pill (OCP).
8 Age.

Clinical effects

1 Hemiparesis.
2 Facial droop.
3 Visual loss.
4 Dysarthria.
5 Vertigo, ataxia.
6 Headache.
7 Decreased level of consciousness (LOC).
8 Death.

Investigation

1 Urgent CT scan of the head is usually sufficient to guide initial management.
2 MRI scan.
3 CT or MR angiography.
4 Ultrasound of carotid arteries.
5 Blood screen including BSL.
6 ECG—looking for cardiac cause such as atrial fibrillation +/− cardiac echo.

Treatment of ischaemic stroke

1 IV thrombolysis with recombinant tissue plasminogen activator (rtPA), preferably within 3 h of stroke onset. Consider giving IV rtPA up to 4.5 h after stroke onset. It is the only effective treatment for acute ischaemic stroke. *See Recombinant tissue plasminogen activator (rtPA).*
2 Endovascular treatment—either intra-arterial thrombolysis or clot retrieval. Indicated for major stroke within 6 h due to occlusion of the middle cerebral artery, especially if there is a contraindication to rtPA.

Anaesthesia for endovascular intervention

1 Can use GA or conscious sedation, depending on patient factors e.g. level of cooperation.
2 Invasive arterial BP monitoring—keep SBP 140–179 mmHg, DBP < 110 mmHg. Do not delay procedure for arterial line access. Interventional neuroradiologist can place an arterial sheath with sidearm for arterial access and blood pressure measurement. Measure NIBP every 1–3 min if no arterial line.
3 Do not insert a central line in view of the need for thrombolysis.
4 Maintain SpO_2 > 92% and PaO_2 > 60 mmHg.

5 Maintain normocapnia—$PaCO_2$ 35–40 mmHg.
6 Maintain body temperature between 35–37°C.
7 Keep blood glucose level between 3.9–7.8 mmol/L. Check BSL hourly.
8 Maintain euvolaemia. Note that contrast material promotes diuresis. Do not insert a urinary catheter if the patient has received thrombolysis.
9 Manage in neurosurgery high-dependency unit or ICU post procedure.

Endovascular intervention for ischaemic stroke complicated by intracranial haemorrhage

1 May need neurosurgical evacuation.
2 Discontinue thrombolytic agent.
3 Reverse heparin with protamine (10 mg/1000 IU heparin). *See Protamine*.
4 Cryoprecipitate—initial dose of 10 units.
5 If cryoprecipitate delayed, contraindicated or not available, give tranexamic acid 10–50 mg/kg over 20 min. *See Tranexamic acid (TXA)*.
6 Check fibrinogen levels—if < 1.5 g/L (150 mg/100 mL), give more cryoprecipitate.

◐ Adductor canal block

Used for blocking the saphenous nerve, which is a branch of the femoral nerve. This block is also called the sub-sartorial saphenous nerve block. It blocks sensation from the medial side of the knee to the medial side of the foot. Unlike the infra-inguinal femoral nerve block, there is good preservation of quadriceps function. It is indicated for surgery to the knee and medial leg. It can be combined with a sciatic nerve block for any surgery on the leg below the lower thigh. Use a 5–10 cm (depending on patient size) short-bevelled block needle. In adults use 20 mL of 0.5% ropivacaine for the block plus 1% lignocaine at the site of needle insertion. Lower volumes (10–15 mL) may be sufficient and result in less motor block. See Figure A1.

Anatomy

1 The saphenous nerve arises from the femoral nerve in the upper thigh and travels with the superficial femoral artery (SFA).
2 The adductor canal is on the medial side of the leg and is formed by the sartorius muscle (the roof of the canal), which is boat shaped (flat deck on top, rounded hull sides below) on ultrasound, vastus medialis and adductor longus.
3 Beneath the sartorius muscle is the superficial femoral artery (SFA) which is pulsatile, the superficial femoral vein (SFV) which is deep to the (SFA) and the saphenous nerve (SaN) which is lateral to the SFA.

Technique

The sartorius muscle runs from the anterior superior iliac spine to the medial side of the knee. The point of entry into the adductor canal lies roughly at the midpoint of a line between these two points. The canal is at a depth of 4 cm in the average adult patient.

1 Obtain IV access.
2 Position the patient supine, with the block leg externally rotated.
3 Use aseptic technique.
4 The probe is oriented at right angles to the long axis of the leg (Figure A2). Start in the mid-medial thigh area.
5 Identify the boat-shaped sartorius muscle and the SFA immediately below the sartorius. The nerve is just lateral to the artery.

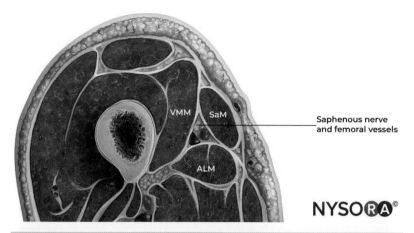

Figure A1 Cross-section of thigh showing the adductor canal. VMM = vastus medialis muscle, ALM = adductor longus muscle, SaM = sartorius muscle
Image courtesy of NYSORA

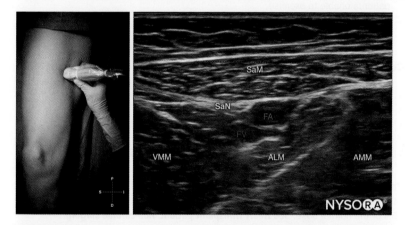

Figure A2 Probe position and sonoanatomy for adductor canal block. VMM = vastus medialis muscle, SaN = saphenous nerve, FV = femoral vein, FA = femoral artery, SaM = sartorius muscle, ALM = adductor longus muscle, AMM = adductor magnus muscle
Image courtesy of NYSORA

6 Insert the needle in-plane in the direction of the floor, through the vastus medialis, so the tip lies just deep to the nerve. A 'pop' may be felt as the canal is entered.
7 After negative aspiration and a 2 mL test dose, inject the remaining 18 mL.
8 If it is proving difficult to identify the adductor canal and the SFA, scan the femoral artery from the inguinal crease and follow the pulsations to the medial midthigh level.

▶ Adenosine (Adenocard, Adenoscan, Adenocor)

Description

Adenosine is a naturally occurring purine nucleoside that is essential for human life. Its use as a drug derives from its ability to depress conduction through the AV node and reduce automaticity of the SA node. It also decreases atrial contractility. It is short acting (minutes) and safe to use in patients on beta blockers.

Indications

Adenosine is useful for the following indications.

1 Reversion of paroxysmal SVT to sinus rhythm. *See Atrioventricular re-entrant tachycardia (AVRT), Atrioventricular nodal re-entrant tachycardia (AVNRT) and Wolff–Parkinson–White (WPW) syndrome.*
2 Helping to differentiate SVT from atrial flutter. It can be used to slow the atrial flutter down so that flutter waves can be seen on the ECG.
3 Helping to differentiate VT from SVT with aberrant conduction. Adenosine will have **no effect** on VT and will usually terminate SVT. In contrast, IV verapamil given to a patient in VT may cause cardiac arrest.
4 In radionuclide myocardial perfusion studies as an adjunct to thallium-201 in patients unable to exercise.
5 Producing transient flow arrest in situations such as intraoperative cerebral aneurysm rupture. This is to enable time for the surgeon to obtain haemorrhage control.

Contraindications

1 Sick sinus syndrome.
2 Second- and third-degree heart block.
3 Long QT syndrome.
4 Obstructive airway disease/asthma.
5 Decompensated heart failure.
6 Wolff–Parkinson–White syndrome with atrial flutter (AF). *See Wolff–Parkinson– White (WPW) syndrome*.

Precautions

The transplanted heart is extremely sensitive to the effects of adenosine. Use about 25% of the normal dose. *See Heart transplant patient, non-cardiac surgery*.

Dose

Adult

Give all doses over 1–2 s with an N/S flush. Initial dose 3 mg IV. If unsuccessful after 1–2 min, 6 mg IV. If not successful within 1–2 min, give 12 mg IV. Dose to produce flow arrest 0.3–0.6 mg/kg. Works for about 15–20 s.

Child

< 50 kg 0.05–0.1 mg/kg over 1 s with an IV saline flush. Repeat at incrementally higher doses (increasing by 0.05–0.1 mg/kg until a maximum dose of 0.3 mg/kg).

Side effects

1 Chest tightness.
2 Dyspnoea.
3 Bronchospasm.

4 Facial flushing.
5 Bradycardia unresponsive to atropine.
6 Feeling of impending doom.

● Adrenaline/epinephrine

Description
Catecholamine sympathomimetic drug that acts on all adrenergic receptors.
See Adrenergic receptors. It is used for its vasoconstrictive, positive inotropy, positive chronotropy, bronchodilation and mast cell stabilisation effects.

Indications
1 Cardiac arrest. *See Cardiac arrest.*
2 Anaphylaxis. *See Anaphylaxis.*
3 Inotropic support for low cardiac output states.
4 Chronotropic support for severe bradycardia. *See Bradycardia.*
5 As a vasoconstrictor to prolong the effects of some LA drugs and reduce bleeding.
6 Bronchospasm. *See Asthma.*
7 Nebulised adrenaline may reduce upper airway obstruction in situations such as anaphylaxis and inflammation.

Dose
See the relevant entries for the various conditions listed above. To make an infusion, mix 3 mg adrenaline with 50 mL N/S. The usual dose range for inotropic support is 0.01–0.1 mcg/kg/min. Start at 5 mL/h in adult patients and titrate to clinical effect. Can be used via a peripheral IV cannula in an emergency (e.g. anaphylaxis), until central venous access is established.

● Adrenergic receptors

These respond to adrenaline and noradrenaline and are located presynaptically, post-synaptically and on certain organs and tissues. Stimulation thus has a wide range of effects.
They are divided into two types, each with subtypes, as listed below.

Alpha receptors

Alpha-1 receptor stimulation causes:
- positive inotropy
- arterial and venous vasoconstriction.

Alpha-2 receptor stimulation causes:
- decreased noradrenaline release from sympathetic nerve endings by a presynaptic action
- decreased sympathetic outflow by a central action
- reduced spinal nociceptive transmission.

Beta receptors

Beta-1 receptor stimulation causes:
- positive inotropy, lusitropy (myocardial relaxation) and chronotropy
- increased renin release—*see Renin-angiotensin system.*

Beta-2 receptor stimulation causes:
- vasodilation of the vascular beds of skeletal muscle, heart and the splanchnic (abdominal gastrointestinal organs) circulation
- relaxation of bronchial smooth muscle
- insulin and glucagon secretion.

Beta-3 receptor stimulation causes:
- enhancement of lipolysis in adipose tissue
- thermogenesis in muscle
- breakdown of brown fat
- relaxation of the urinary bladder.

◗ Air embolism

See Gas embolism.

◗ Airway

See Difficult airway management.

◗ Airway bleeding

See Haemoptysis, life-threatening.

◗ Airway fire

See Laser surgery.

◗ Airway haemorrhage

See Haemoptysis, life-threatening.

◗ Albumin

Essential protein for the maintenance of plasma oncotic pressure, and with important binding functions. The normal level of albumin in plasma is 40 g/L or 4 g/dL, accounting for more than 50% of the total protein in plasma. Albumin has negatively charged binding sites. As pH increases, H^+ ions unbind from albumin, enabling more Ca^{2+} to bind to albumin. Measured Ca^{2+} levels will be the same but the ionised (free) form of Ca^{2+} will decrease. With acidosis the opposite occurs: ionised Ca^{2+} will increase. A low albumin level results in a falsely low Ca^{2+} measurement. For every 1 g/L decrease in serum albumin, measured Ca^{2+} will be falsely reduced by 0.02 mmol/L.

◗ Albumin solution

Description
Manufactured from pooled human albumin, albumin solution can be 4% (40 g/L) or 20% (200 g/L) (25% in the USA). The albumin is suspended in saline. Hypotension can occur in patients taking ACE inhibitors who receive albumin solution.

Indications
1 Albumin 4% is iso-oncotic, isotonic and has a pH of 6.7–7.3. It contains sodium 140 mmol/L, chloride 128 mmol/L and octanoate. It is used as a volume expander to treat shock associated with significant hypoalbuminaemia (< 25 g/L), as occurs with nephrotic syndrome, burns etc. It is also used during therapeutic plasmapheresis and cardiothoracic surgery.

2 Albumin 20% is hyper-oncotic and hypo-osmotic (130 mOsm/kg) and has a pH of 6.7–7.3. It is used for albumin replacement when patients may not be able to cope with a volume/electrolyte load. Examples include severe liver failure or renal failure and adult respiratory distress syndrome. It is used in haemodialysis and plasma exchange. Do not give faster than 2 mL/min.

◐ Aldosterone

See Renin-angiotensin system.

◐ Alfentanil

Description

Alfentanil is a fentanyl analogue. It has a faster onset than fentanyl and a shorter duration of action (about 10 min), making it highly suitable for procedures of short duration or for procedures that are intensely stimulating over a short period of time e.g. laryngoscopy. It is 5 × less potent than fentanyl.

Dose

IV bolus dose for adult

For short procedures in spontaneously breathing patients, 125–250 mcg boluses every 10–15 min. For reducing the hypertensive response to intubation, use 10–50 mcg/kg 1 min before intubation. Effects last 30–45 min. Muscle rigidity may occur.

Intrathecal dose

250 mcg.

Target-controlled infusion (TCI)

Using the Scott model, the recommended target effect site concentration is 40–60 ng/mL. Stop the infusion about 20 min before emergence time.

Advantages

1 Less PONV than fentanyl.
2 It is metabolised in the liver with no active metabolites.
3 It is safe to use in renal failure.

Disadvantages

1 Acute dystonia may occur in patients with untreated Parkinson's disease.
 See Parkinson's disease (PD).
2 Elimination half-life is increased in patients with liver disease.

◐ Allele

Each gene is made of alleles (sequences of nucleotides), which are inherited. Variation in alleles leads to variation in genes e.g. for eye colour. Alleles can be dominant or recessive. The blood group gene (ABO gene) is made up of six alleles. If two alleles are the same in an individual, the individual is a homozygote; if they are different, the individual is a heterozygote.

◐ Allergic reaction

See Anaphylaxis.

◖ Allergic reaction prevention

This can be required for patients requiring radiological contrast media when there is a history of allergic reaction to these substances. A suggested approach is:

Adult

1 Prednisone 50 mg PO 13 h, 7 h and 1 h before the procedure. Use methylprednisolone 40 mg IV at the same time intervals if oral administration is not feasible.
2 Diphenhydramine 50 mg PO 1 h before the procedure.

Child

1 Prednisone 0.5–0.7 mg/kg PO (max 50 mg) at same dosage intervals as above. If unable to take oral drugs, methylprednisolone 0.5 mg/kg IV (max 40 mg) at same dosage intervals.
2 Diphenhydramine 1.25 mg/kg (max 50 mg) PO 1 h before procedure.

◖ Alteplase/recombinant tissue plasminogen activator (rtPA) (Activase)

Description

Alteplase is a thrombolytic drug that acts by selectively binding to fibrin and converting plasminogen to plasmin, which dissolves the fibrin matrix of clots. It is used for the treatment of:

1 Myocardial infarction. **See *Acute coronary syndrome*.**
2 Pulmonary thromboembolism with haemodynamic instability. **See *Pulmonary embolism (PE)*.**
3 Ischaemic acute stroke. **See *Acute stroke*.**
4 Occlusive iliac venous thrombosis.

Contraindications

These are relative and include:

1 Bleeding disorder/thrombocytopenia.
2 Anticoagulation.
3 Prolonged CPR.
4 Recent surgery.
5 Rapid resolution of stroke symptoms.
6 SBP > 185 mmHg, DBP > 110 mmHg
7 Seizure.

Dose—adult

1 Myocardial infarction—bolus and infusion depending on timeframe.
2 PE—IV bolus 10 mg over 1–2 min then 90 mg IV infusion over 2 h. If patient is < 65 kg give a maximum total dose of 1.5 mg/kg.
3 Ischaemic stroke—0.9 mg/kg with 10% of this amount administered as a bolus and the rest IV over 60 min. Do not exceed a total dose of 90 mg.

◖ Alveolar gas equation

See *A-a gradient*.

◖ Alzheimer's disease medication and anaesthesia

Acetylcholinesterase inhibitor drugs such as galantamine (Razadyne), rivastigmine (Exelon) and donepezil (Aricept) can result in a considerably prolonged action of suxamethonium. The effects of NDNMBDs can be strongly inhibited. Donepezil has a very long half-life and should be stopped for two weeks before surgery.

American Society of Anesthesiologists (ASA) Physical Status Classification System

This grading system, which was first described in 1941, gives an approximate estimate of the patient's anaesthetic risk based on their preoperative health. The grades are:

- ASA I—normal, healthy patient
- ASA II—mild systemic disease (without functional limitation). BMI 30–40 and normal pregnancy are classified as ASA II
- ASA III—severe systemic disease that limits activity, BMI > 40
- ASA IV—severe systemic disease that is a constant threat to life
- ASA V—moribund patient, not expected to survive with or without surgery
- ASA VI—declared brain dead patient for organ harvest.
  The letter 'E' is added for emergency surgery.

Amiloride (Amizide)

Potassium-sparing hydrochlorothiazide diuretic drug used to treat hypertension, oedema of cardiac origin and hepatic cirrhosis with ascites.

Aminophylline

Methylated xanthine derivative used to treat bronchospasm. No longer recommended for acute severe asthma.

Dose

Do not give an LD if patient on oral xanthines. LD 5 mg/kg over 20 min then infusion of 0.5 mg/kg/h. Make sure oral xanthines are ceased. May cause tachycardia, ventricular arrhythmias or hypotension. Therapeutic level is 10–20 mcg/mL.

Amiodarone (Cardinorm, Cordarone)

Description

Class III iodinated benzofuran antiarrhythmic drug. *See Antiarrhythmic drug classes.* It prolongs the repolarisation of the cardiac action potential. It also has Class Ia, II and IV effects. It is structurally similar to thyroxine and has many side effects.

Indications

Due to its toxicity/side effects, amiodarone is indicated for serious, life-threatening tachydysrhythmias, including:

1 ventricular tachycardia (VT)
2 ventricular fibrillation (VF)—*see Cardiac arrest*
3 wide complex tachycardia
4 atrial fibrillation (AF), atrial flutter
5 paroxysmal supraventricular tachycardia (PSVT)
6 patients with AICDs with frequent appropriate shocks.

Dose

Adult

For shock-resistant VF, pulseless VT—*see Cardiac arrest*.

IV dose

Administer preferably through a central line with full monitoring. Mix amiodarone with 5% glucose in a glass bottle or polyolefin bag. Give a loading dose of 300 mg over 20 min–2 h, then 900 mg over 24 h. Switch to oral therapy as per cardiologist advice (normally after 24 h).

Oral dose- adult

200–400 mg q 8 h for 10–14 days. Maintenance 200–400 mg/day.

Side effects

1 Highly irritant to veins.
2 IV therapy can cause hypotension.
3 Corneal microdeposits may occur.
4 Blue-grey discoloration of the skin.
5 Peripheral neuropathy.
6 Thyroid dysfunction.
There are many other side effects.

Contraindications

1 Not for use in pregnancy unless cardiac arrest.
2 Cardiogenic shock.
3 Severe sinus node dysfunction.
4 Second- or third-degree AV block.
5 Bradycardia.
6 Iodine allergy (may not be an absolute contraindication).[10]
7 Pre-excitation (WPW syndrome) and concurrent AF. *See Wolff–Parkinson–White (WPW) syndrome.*

◐ Amlodipine

Dihydropyridine calcium channel-blocker drug used to treat hypertension and chronic stable angina. It acts by causing vasodilation of arteries, including the coronary arteries. It is not useful for acute angina. It should be used with caution (if at all) in patients with heart failure, renal impairment, hepatic impairment, pregnancy, lactation or aortic stenosis. *See Calcium channel blocker drugs.*

◐ Amniotic fluid embolism (AFE)

Description

AFE is an exceedingly rare syndrome that is unpredictable, unpreventable and often catastrophic. Occurring in about 4:100 000 live births, it is due to amniotic fluid, fetal cells, fetal hair and other debris entering the maternal circulation. This is theorised to cause:

1 physical obstruction to the pulmonary circulation (an outdated theory)
2 an anaphylactoid reaction. The term 'anaphylactoid syndrome of pregnancy' is suggested by some researchers.
3 activation of complement.

An AFE event is thought to result in a sudden increase in pulmonary vascular resistance (PVR), pulmonary hypertension and right heart failure. The maternal mortality is about 15–40%. Neonatal mortality is about 20–30%. Maternal survivors often have long-term neurological impairment. It can occur up to 48 h postpartum.

Causative event

AFE is thought to occur when there is a breach in the barrier between the maternal circulation and the amniotic fluid. It is most likely to occur:

1 during labour, especially if contractions are vigorous and frequent
2 soon after delivery or CS
3 second trimester termination
4 abdominal trauma
5 during amniocentesis
6 cervical suture removal.

Risk factors

These are many and include:

1 maternal age > 35 years
2 placental abnormalities (praevia, abruption)
3 eclampsia
4 induction/augmentation of labour.

Clinical signs/symptoms

The sudden rise in PVR and acute right heart failure leads to acute hypoxia and systemic hypotension. Some of the many other symptoms and signs are:

1 dyspnoea, cough, cyanosis
2 anxiety, agitation, LOC, seizures
3 fetal bradycardia
4 coagulopathy/DIC
5 uterine atony
6 cardiac arrest.

Diagnosis

AFE should be considered in any pregnant patient with sudden onset of dyspnoea, cyanosis, loss of consciousness, hypotension or fetal bradycardia. There is no specific test. Other causes of maternal collapse such as anaphylaxis and pulmonary embolus must be excluded if possible. Autopsy may provide a definitive diagnosis of AFE. Echocardiography may show a D-shaped septum, acute pulmonary hypertension and RV systolic dysfunction.

Treatment

The treatment of AFE is complicated because of its catastrophic, and often fatal, effects. It involves:

1 maintaining the patient's airway, intubating them if LOC has occurred
2 maintaining oxygenation. ARDS may develop, requiring complex ventilation strategies. *See Acute respiratory distress syndrome (ARDS)*
3 supporting the patient's circulation—IV fluids, pressor drugs, inotropic support. Insert an arterial line and central line
4 send urgent bloods for x-match, UEC, clotting studies
5 treat coagulopathy. *See Blood loss—assessment, management and anaesthetic approach*
6 expedite delivery of the fetus. Perimortem CS may be required. *See Resuscitative hysterotomy*.

If cardiac arrest occurs, *see Cardiac arrest management*. Specific treatments include nitric oxide, ECMO and plasmapheresis.

◖ AMPLE

This is an acronym for obtaining a quick relevant medical history for trauma patients.

A – **A**llergies
M – **M**edications
P – **P**ast medical history
L – **L**ast meal
E – **E**vents (of injury).

◖ Amrinone/inamrinone (Inocor)

Description
Bipyridine derivative phosphodiesterase III inhibitor useful for the treatment of cardiac failure. It has positive inotropic and vasodilator actions. *See Phosphodiesterase III inhibitors*. Its effects include:
1 increased contractility
2 arterial and venous vasodilation decreasing preload and afterload.

Dose
Mix 100 mg in 250 mL N/S (not glucose). Give an LD of 750 mcg/kg (for a 70 kg patient = 130 mL), then an infusion of 5–20 mcg/kg/min (50–200 mL/h for a 70 kg patient). The daily dose should not exceed 10 mg/kg.

Contraindications
1 Aortic stenosis.
2 Hypertrophic cardiomyopathy.

Advantages
1 Cardiac output is increased without a significant increase in myocardial O_2 demand.
2 Little increase in HR unless used at high doses.
3 Positive lusitropic effects improving ventricular compliance.
4 Has a pulmonary vasodilator effect that is useful in the setting of pulmonary hypertension with right heart failure.

Disadvantages
1 Vasodilation may cause hypotension.
2 May cause a transient thrombocytopenia due to the effects of N-acetyl amrinone, a metabolite.
3 May increase myocardial ischaemia, causing arrhythmias and CCF.

◖ Amyotrophic lateral sclerosis

See Motor neurone disease (MND).

◖ Anaemia

Definition
Anaemia is defined in adults as Hb < 130 g/L in males and < 120 g/L in females.

Types
1 Iron (Fe) deficiency anaemia—due to such causes as blood loss from menorrhagia. Diagnosed by low serum ferritin (< 30 mcg/L). Red cells show

microcytosis and hypochromia. Treatment is with oral Fe. This will increase Hb by 10 g/L/week. IV iron therapy e.g. ferric carboxymaltose works faster.

2 Anaemia due to the inability to utilise Fe. This occurs in chronic inflammatory states. It is due to the effects of the hepatic protein hepcidin, which blocks Fe absorption. Fe therapy is not effective.

3 B12 of folate deficiency in the diet or malabsorption. For example, pernicious anaemia is due to malabsorption of vitamin B12 resulting from a decreased production of intrinsic factor.

4 Renal failure—treat with erythropoietin (EPO).

5 Thalassaemia. *See Thalassaemia*.

6 Aplastic anaemia.

7 Haemolytic anaemia.

8 Sickle cell anaemia. *See Sickle cell disease (SCD)*.

▷ Anamorph

This a brand name of oral morphine. *See Morphine*.

▷ Anaphylaxis

Introduction

Anaphylaxis can be defined as a reaction to an antigen resulting in typical skin features (urticarial rash or erythema/flushing and/or angioedema) **plus** involvement of the respiratory and/or cardiovascular systems and/or persistent severe gastrointestinal symptoms. Skin manifestations may be absent. Anaphylaxis represents a life-threatening crisis, requiring prompt recognition, rapid administration of adrenaline in appropriate doses and aggressive fluid management.

Anaphylaxis is the most common cause of death that is primarily due to anaesthesia. Its incidence is about 1:6000–1:20 000 anaesthetics. The most common causes are:

1 neuromuscular blocking drugs ($\approx$ 60%), especially suxamethonium and rocuronium

2 antibiotics, especially cefazolin due to its frequency of use ($\approx$ 15%)

3 chlorhexidine.

There is no familial association of drug allergy. It is interesting to note that the rate of anaphylaxis from all causes (food, drugs, industrial, cosmetics) has increased by more than 300% in the last 10 years.[11]

Anaphylaxis box

To facilitate anaphylaxis management, an anaphylaxis box should be available and used. It should contain laminated cards from ANZAAG and ANZCA. These should include:

1 Immediate management adults 12+ card.

2 Immediate management paediatric 0–12 card.

3 Refractory management adult 12+ card.

4 Refractory management paediatric 0–12 card.

5 Differential diagnosis card.

6 Post-crisis management card.

The box should also include:

1 Local infusion protocols for adrenaline, noradrenaline, vasopressin and salbutamol.

2 Collection tubes for tryptase. Measure at 1, 4 and 24 h. Tryptase levels peak at 15–120 min. Rare conditions such as systemic macrocytosis can result in chronically elevated tryptase levels.

3 Patient form letters and referral forms, and information for the patient.

Pathophysiology of anaphylaxis

Anaphylaxis means 'attacking self'. It is a type 1 hypersensitivity reaction due to IgE antibody mediated degranulation of mast cells and basophils in response to a triggering agent such as a drug. Anaphylactoid reactions are clinically indistinguishable from anaphylaxis and also involve mast cell and basophil cell degranulation. However, this reaction is not IgE mediated (and is alternatively termed 'non-IgE mediated anaphylaxis').

The sequence of events in the anaphylaxis process is:

1 Exposure to a substance such as a drug may cause specific IgE antibodies to that substance being produced by plasma cells. This substance has become an antigen and the subsequent IgE antibodies produced are specific to that antigen.
2 These IgE antibodies bind to tissue mast cells and circulating basophils.
3 Re-exposure to the antigen results in the antigen binding two IgE antibodies, resulting in degranulation of the mast and basophil cells.
4 The granules contain vasoactive substances such as histamine, proteases, proteoglycans and leukotrienes. These substances cause profound vasodilation, increased vascular permeability and transudation of fluid into tissues.
5 These effects result in profound hypovolaemia, hypotension, decreased myocardial perfusion, exudation of fluid into the tissues and bronchospasm.

Anaphylaxis can occur despite no prior exposure to the causative agent due to cross-sensitisation with other drugs, cosmetics, food, industrial substances or other molecules with a similar structure. For example, anaphylaxis due to rocuronium is more common in countries with easy access to pholcodine in cough suppressants.

Clinical manifestations of anaphylaxis

1 Hypotension, tachycardia or bradycardia.
2 Bronchospasm.
3 Skin signs—rash, erythema, urticaria.
4 Soft tissue swelling (angioedema)—eyelids, lips, tongue, airway.
5 Cramping abdominal pain, vomiting.
6 Anxiety, dysphoria.
7 Runny nose, cough, dyspnoea, circumoral tingling, dysphagia.
8 Circulatory collapse, cardiac arrest.

Grades of anaphylaxis

Mild: Grade 1

Mucocutaneous signs—skin changes and/or angioedema.

Moderate: Grade 2

Multiorgan manifestations—mucocutaneous signs combined with hypotension and/or bronchospasm.

Life threatening: Grade 3

Life-threatening hypotension and/or bronchospasm/high airway pressure compromising oxygenation. Cutaneous signs are frequently absent.

Cardiac arrest: Grade 4

There is no effective cardiac output. Treat as for other causes of cardiac arrest in adults but give adrenaline 1–2 minutely instead of 3–5 minutely, elevate the legs and give 2 L of crystalloid.

Immediate management adults 12+ card

Inform the surgeon/obtain immediate skilled assistance. Manage as per the *Anaphylaxis during anaesthesia immediate management guideline (ANZAAG/ANZCA)*.

If cardiac arrest

Usually pulseless electrical activity (PEA). Treat as for non-shockable rhythm cardia arrest (*see Cardiac arrest*), but with the following caveats:

1 Give adrenaline 1 mg every 1–2 min instead of 3–5 minutely.
2 Give 2 L of crystalloid IV and elevate the legs.

If evolving anaphylaxis

DR: Danger and diagnosis/response to stimulus—unresponsive hypotension and/or bronchospasm. Remove triggers e.g. chlorhexidine, newly inserted urinary catheter. Stop procedure **if possible**. Use minimal volatile if GA.

S: Send for help and organise team—call for help and anaphylaxis box, assign a designated leader, scribe and card reader.

AB: Check/secure airway, breathing, give 100% oxygen—consider early intubation, administer 100% O_2.

C: Rapid fluid bolus, plan for large-volume resuscitation—if hypotensive, elevate the legs, give 2 L IV crystalloid and repeat fluid bolus as needed. Secure large-bore IV access. Warm IV fluids if possible.

D: Adrenaline bolus/repeat as needed. Prepare adrenaline infusion.

1 Give IM adrenaline if no IV access/monitoring. Give 0.5 mg adrenaline into lateral thigh, repeating every 5 min as needed.
2 If IV access and monitoring, give IV adrenaline **cautiously**. For moderate (Grade 2) reactions, give increments of 20 mcg. For more severe reactions (Grade 3), give 100–200 mcg.
3 If more than three bolus injections of adrenaline are required, start an adrenaline infusion—3 mg of adrenaline in 50 mL of N/S. Start at 3 mL/h and titrate to response to a maximum of 40 mL/h.

Immediate management paediatric 0–12 card

If paediatric cardiac arrest, give 0.1 mL/kg of 1:10 000 (10 mcg/kg) IV adrenaline repeated 1–4 min (e.g. 20 kg child, give 2 mL of 1:10 000 adrenaline). Provide CPR and give IV crystalloid 20 mL/kg.

DR: Danger and diagnosis/response to stimulus—as per adult card.

S: Send for help and organise team—as per adult card.

AB: Check/secure airway/breathing; 100% O_2—as per adult card.

C: Rapid fluid bolus, plan for large-volume resuscitation—if hypotensive, elevate legs, bolus 20 mL/kg crystalloid; repeat as needed. Insert large-bore IV access and warm IV fluids if possible.

D: Adrenaline bolus, repeat as needed and prepare adrenaline infusion:

- **IM adrenaline**—if no IV access or haemodynamic monitoring, give 1:1000 1 mg/mL lateral thigh: < 6 y 0.15 mL (150 mcg), 6–12 y 0.3 mL (300 mcg), repeat 5 min prn.
- **IV adrenaline**—dilute 1 mg of adrenaline into 50 mL N/S, resulting in a 20 mcg/mL concentration. Give boluses every 1–2 min. Moderate (Grade 2) reaction, give 0.1 mL/kg (2 mcg/kg). For a life-threatening (Grade 3) reaction, give 0.2–0.5 mL/kg (4–10 mcg/kg) boluses.

Adrenaline infusion

Add 1 mg of adrenaline to 50 mL N/S (20 mcg/mL). Commence infusion at 0.3 mL/kg/h to a maximum of 6 mL/kg/h.

Refractory management adults 12+ card

Request more help—consider calling arrest code, summoning more skilled assistance/staff.

Triggers removed—ensure all potential triggers are removed, including chlorhexidine, synthetic colloids, urinary catheter and latex.

Monitoring—consider arterial line and TOE/TEE.

Resistant hypotension—hypotension not responding to an adrenaline infusion (which must be continued) can be treated with:

1 additional IV fluid bolus 50 mL/kg
2 add a second vasopressor—noradrenaline (NA) infusion, 3–40 mcg/min (0.05–0.5 mcg/kg/min) and/or vasopressin bolus 1–2 units then 2 units per h
3 metaraminol or phenylephrine by infusion if NA or vasopressin are unavailable. **See _Metaraminol_** and **_Phenylephrine_**
4 glucagon 1–2 mg every 5 min until response (especially if patient is on beta blockers).

Resistant bronchospasm—continue the adrenaline infusion and consider any equipment malfunction and/or tension pneumothorax. Consider:

1 salbutamol; metered dose inhaler 12 puffs (1200 mcg), IV bolus 100–200 mcg +/− infusion 5–25 mcg/min
2 magnesium 2 g (8 mmol) over 20 min
3 inhalational anaesthetics or ketamine. **See _Asthma_**.

Pregnancy—use manual left uterine displacement. Caesarean section within 4 min if arrest or peri-arrest. **See _Resuscitative hysterotomy_**.

Consider other diagnoses—*see Differential diagnosis card*.

Refractory management paediatric 0–12 card

Request more help. Triggers removed? Monitoring as per adult.

Resistant hypotension—continue the adrenaline infusion and consider insertion of a central line.

1 Give an additional IV fluid bolus of 20–40 mL/kg.
2 Noradrenaline 0.1–2 mcg/kg/min (add 0.15 mg/kg of NA to 50 mL 5% glucose). Run at 2–40 mL/h.
3 Alternatively, use vasopressin. Mix 1 unit/kg in 50 mL N/S. Give a bolus of 2 mL then run infusion at 1–3 mL/h (equals 0.02–0.06 units/kg/min).
4 Glucagon 40 mcg/kg IV (max 1 mg).

Resistant bronchospasm—continue adrenaline infusion. Consider equipment malfunction, pneumothorax and alternative bronchodilators.

1 Salbutamol metered dose inhaler 100 mcg/puff; 6 puffs < 6 years; 12 puffs > 6 years.
2 Salbutamol bolus and infusion.
3 Magnesium—give 50 mg/kg IV to a maximum of 2 g over 20 min.
4 Aminophylline—10 mg/kg over 1 h (max 500 mg).
5 Hydrocortisone—2–4 mg/kg (max 200 mg).

Consider other diagnoses—*see Differential diagnosis card*.

Differential diagnosis card

Cardiac arrest—4Hs and 4Ts. *See Cardiac arrest*.

High airway pressure/airway compromise

Dyspnoea, wheeze, stridor, difficulty inflating lungs. Consider equipment malfunction—check using a self-inflating bag. Check ET tube—pass a suction catheter through the tube. Also consider:

1 tension pneumothorax
2 exacerbation of asthma
3 foreign body
4 acid aspiration.

Hypotension

Consider:

1 hypovolaemia
2 sepsis
3 drug overdose
4 vasodilation by drugs
5 neuraxial blockade
6 embolism (thrombotic, air, amniotic)
7 vasovagal.

Skin and mucosa

Hives, flushing, erythema, urticaria, swelling head and neck or peripheries. Consider:

1 direct histamine release
2 venous obstruction
3 head-down position
4 C1-esterase deficiency (angioedema only). *See Angioedema*
5 mastocytosis
6 cold-induced anaphylaxis.

Post crisis management card

Once situation is stabilised

1 Consider steroids—dexamethasone 0.1–0.4 mg/kg (paediatric max 12 mg) **or** hydrocortisone 2–4 mg/kg (paediatric max 200 mg).
2 Consider oral histamines e.g. loratadine (Claratyne) 10 mg. **Do not use IV or IM antihistamines.**
3 Consider whether to cancel surgery or proceed. Organise appropriate postoperative placement (ICU/HDU).

Investigations

1 Tryptase at 1 h, 4 h and > 24 h. Use serum (SST) tube (gold top) or plain tube. Refrigerate if > 1 h to lab.
2 Coagulation screening if proceeding with surgery.

Observations

1 Monitor closely for 6 h.
2 Consider 24 h ICU/HDU if moderate to severe reaction.

Follow-up

1 Patient informed of reaction and given letter stating what was given prior to reaction and treatment of reaction.
2 Referral for patient testing and allergy assessment. For nearest testing centre, go to www.anzaag.com

▶ Andexanet alfa (Andexxa)

Description

Antidote to apixaban and rivaroxaban. Also known as coagulation factor Xa (recombinant) inactivated-zhzo. Acts by binding to the factor Xa inhibitors apixaban and rivaroxaban. Acts in 2 min. It is expensive—about $25 000 for a low dose course.

Dose

1 Use the low dose if apixaban/rivaroxaban given more than 8 h ago. Use the high dose if < 8 h since last dose or severe bleeding.
2 Low dose 400 mg IV bolus over 15 min then infusion of 4 mg/min for 2 h.
3 High dose 800 mg IV bolus over 30 min then infusion of 8 mg/min for 2h.

▶ Angioedema

Description

A rapid swelling of the epidermis, dermis, subcutaneous tissue and/or mucus membranes. The main risk is to the airway, which can become obstructed.
Securing the airway is the most important treatment. Angioedema can be classified as:
1 mast cell mediated, as with anaphylaxis—*see Anaphylaxis*
2 bradykinin mediated. Adrenaline, antihistamines and steroids have no effect on this type of angioedema. Pruritis and urticaria are absent.

Bradykinin mediated angioedema

This can be divided into:
1 hereditary angioedema (HAE)
2 acquired—due to drugs such as angiotensin I-converting enzyme inhibitor or dipeptidyl peptidase-4 (DPP4) inhibitors e.g. sitagliptin, which is used to treat diabetes. *See Diabetes mellitus (DM)*
3 acquired C1-esterase inhibitor (C1-INH) deficiency. This can be due to consumption of C1-INH by immune complexes or anti C1-INH antibodies. This illness can be associated with lymphoproliferative diseases such as B-cell lymphoma and autoimmune disease such as SLE. C1-INH inhibits the complement system and thus bradykinin production. *See Complement system*
4 angioedema of unknown cause. This type of disorder may be associated with SLE and other autoimmune disorders
5 inducible angioedema—can be due to vibration or cold.

Hereditary angioedema (HAE)

An inherited disorder characterised by recurrent episodes of severe swelling of the limbs, face, gastrointestinal tract and airway. About one-third of sufferers also get a rash called erythema marginatum. This condition can be confused with anaphylaxis. *See Anaphylaxis*. It is also called C1 esterase inhibitor deficiency or C1 inhibitor deficiency. About 30% of cases are due to spontaneous mutations.

Pathophysiology

There is disruption to C1 inhibitor protein production. This leads to excessive amounts of bradykinin generation, which causes inflammation by dilating arterioles and constricting veins. This increases pressure in capillary vascular beds, causing fluid extravasation into tissues, resulting in tissue swelling.

There are three types of hereditary angioedema:

- **Type 1**—accounts for 85% of cases. A mutation blocks production of the gene responsible for the production of C1 inhibitor protein. In Type 1 disease, the C1 inhibitor protein is normal but present in reduced quantities.
- **Type 2**—accounts for 15% of cases. This mutation results in the production of abnormal C1 inhibitor protein.
- **Type 3**—is very rare. The cause is unknown.

Clinical features

An attack can occur every 1–2 weeks and lasts 3–4 days. Attacks can be brought on by minor trauma, stress and surgery, especially dental and airway surgery.

1 Severe abdominal pain, nausea, vomiting.
2 Airway swelling, which can be life threatening (larynx, tongue).

Prevention

1 Androgens such as danazol.
2 Tranexamic acid—mechanism for efficacy unknown.
3 A plasma-derived C1-esterase inhibitor.
4 A progestin such as norethisterone.
5 Lanadelumab.

Treatment

1 Analgesia/antiemetics for abdominal pain, nausea and vomiting.
2 C1-inhibitor concentrate IV (derived from donor blood plasma or recombinant). Berinert and Cinryze are examples. The dose of Berinert is 20 U/kg IV.
3 Plasma kallikrein inhibitor (ecallantide, lanadelumab, berotralstat).
4 Bradykinin receptor antagonist (icatibant). It has a similar structure to bradykinin and blocks the bradykinin receptor. The dose of icatibant is 30 mg subcut. For children 12–25 kg give 10 mg, 26–40 kg give 15 mg, 41–50 kg give 20 mg.
5 Solvent detergent treated plasma (SDP) if above not available.
6 Fresh frozen plasma (FFP) if above not available.

Prophylaxis for surgery

1 Preoperative infusion of C1-esterase inhibitor concentrate 20 units/kg up to 24 h before procedure.
2 If above unavailable, give 2 units of FFP.

◐ Angiotensin-converting enzyme (ACE) inhibitors

Introduction

These drugs inhibit the activity of angiotensin-converting enzyme which converts angiotensin I to angiotensin II. **See Renin-angiotensin system.** Angiotensin II is a potent vasoconstrictor, therefore reducing its production results in vasodilatation. They are useful in the treatment of hypertension and congestive cardiac failure (CCF). These drugs also increase bradykinin levels. **See Bradykinin.** Bradykinin causes arterioles to dilate, increasing the blood pressure-lowering effect.

ACE inhibitors are contraindicated in pregnancy. Examples include ramipril, perindopril, enalapril, lisinopril and captopril.

Anaesthesia and ACE inhibitors

Severe refractive hypotension may occur with GA in patients on ACE inhibitors. They should be withheld for 24 h prior to surgery.[12]

ACE inhibitors and angioedema

Recurrent angioedema episodes occur in about 0.1–0.7% of patients on ACE inhibitors, probably due to bradykinin accumulation. These episodes can involve the tongue, airway and gut, and can be life threatening. Icatibant (a bradykinin receptor blocker) and C1-inhibitor concentrate can be helpful treatments. ***See*** ***Angioedema***. A frequent cause of intolerance of ACE inhibitors is a persistent cough.

'Triple whammy' warning

The combination of ACE inhibitor or angiotensin II receptor blocker and a diuretic and an NSAID may cause renal failure in susceptible patients (advanced age, pre-existing renal disease, dehydration).

Note: ACE inhibitors are teratogenic and must be ceased during pregnancy.

Angiotensin II receptor blocker (ARB) drugs

Description

These drugs cause vasodilatation by preventing angiotensin II from attaching to its receptor (AT1 receptor) on vascular smooth muscle. ***See*** ***Renin-angiotensin system***. They are used to treat hypertension and/or congestive cardiac failure (CCF). They are effective in reducing left ventricular (LV) hypertrophy, improving diastolic function and decreasing the incidence of ventricular dysrhythmias. ARBs may inhibit the progress of diabetic nephropathy. Although angiotensin II levels are increased, bradykinin levels are **not** increased as occurs with ACE inhibitors. See entry above. Examples include candesartan, telmisartan and irbesartan. These drugs are contraindicated in pregnancy.

Anaesthesia and ARBs

Withhold ARBs for 24 h prior to elective surgery as severe refractory hypotension may occur under anaesthesia.[12]

Anion gap

See ***Arterial blood gas (ABG) interpretation for acidosis/alkalosis***.

Ankle block

Useful for surgery on the foot. The foot is innervated by the terminal branches of the sciatic nerve and the saphenous nerve (a branch of the femoral nerve). The saphenous nerve supplies the arch of the sole and medial foot. The sciatic branches are the deep and superficial peroneal nerves, the tibial nerve which branches into the medial and lateral plantar nerves, and the sural nerves (from the tibial and common peroneal nerves). These nerves supply the rest of the foot.

Preparation and positioning

Position the patient supine with a pillow under the calf. There are three injection sites. Use ropivacaine 1% (max 20 mL) and a short-bevelled block needle. Sterilise the injection site with chlorhexidine. Always aspirate prior to injection of LA.

Landmark technique

1 Block the tibial nerve by inserting the block needle posterior to the medial malleolus and posterior tibial artery (or half-way between the medial malleolus and Achilles tendon). Contact the underlying bone and then withdraw the needle 1 cm. Inject 5 mL of LA in a fan-like pattern.
2 Draw a line around the ankle just proximal to the malleoli and anterior to the Achilles tendon. The saphenous, superficial peroneal and sural nerves can be blocked with a superficial circumferential injection of 10–15 mL of LA along this line.
3 The deep peroneal nerve is blocked by an injection of 5 mL LA just lateral to the extensor hallucis longus tendon on the same line.

◐ Antepartum haemorrhage (APH)

APH is defined as bleeding from the birth canal after the 20th week of pregnancy up until labour begins. Bleeding during labour is intrapartum haemorrhage. The most common causes of antepartum/intrapartum haemorrhage are:

1 placental abruption—**see** *Placental abruption*
2 placenta praevia—**see** *Placenta praevia*
3 vasa praevia—**see** *Vasa praevia*
4 uterine rupture—**see** *Uterine rupture*
5 trauma
6 cervical lesions.

◐ Anterior spinal artery syndrome

Description

The anterior spinal artery is fed by branches from the aorta and supplies the anterior two-thirds of the spinal cord. Interruption to this supply leads to ischaemia or infarction of the anterior spinal cord. This part of the cord contains the descending corticospinal tract (motor) and the ascending spinothalamic tract (pain and temperature). Anterior spinal artery syndrome is also known as anterior spinal cord syndrome and Beck's syndrome.

Causes of anterior spinal artery injury

1 Aortic aneurysm/dissection/surgery/trauma.
2 Vasculitis.
3 Polycythaemia.
4 Decompression sickness.
5 Sickle cell disease.
6 Collagen and elastin abnormalities.
7 Spinal pathology such as ankylosing spondylitis.

Clinical diagnosis

1 Motor paralysis with loss of reflexes.
2 Loss of pain and temperature sensation.
3 Preservation of fine touch, proprioception and vibration sense.
4 Autonomic dysfunction such as hypotension, bladder and bowel dysfunction.

◐ Antiarrhythmic drug classes

These classes are the Vaughan-Williams classification system, which is based on the drugs' primary mechanism of action. Some agents fall into more than one class.

1 **Class I**—divided into Class Ia, Ib and Ic. Class Ia drugs block fast sodium channels and include quinidine, procainamide and disopyramide. Class Ib drugs

are sodium channel blockers which results in a shortened action potential (AP) duration. They include lignocaine, phenytoin and mexiletine. Class Ic drugs do not shorten the AP duration, and they include flecainide and propafenone.

2 **Class II**—beta-adrenergic receptor blocker drugs e.g. metoprolol. *See Beta-adrenergic receptor blocker drugs*.

3 **Class III**—potassium channel blockers, including sotalol (also a beta blocker), amiodarone and ibutilide.

4 **Class IV**—calcium channel blocker drugs e.g. verapamil, diltiazem. *See Calcium channel blocker drugs*.

5 **Class V**—work by another mechanism not listed above. These drugs include digoxin, atropine, magnesium and adenosine.

▶ Antibiotic prophylaxis for surgery

Introduction
The following guidelines are for adults only. They are based on the *Western Sydney Local Health District Guideline, Surgical Antibiotic Prophylaxis (Adult)*, WSLHD 7 June 2022. Antibiotics should be administered ideally 15–30 min before surgical incision, and prophylactic antibiotics should not be used for more than 24 h.

Doses of antibiotics (all given IV unless otherwise stated)
1 Cefazolin 2 g (3 g > 120 kg) repeated after 4 h
2 Ciprofloxacin 400 mg q 8 h (or 750 mg PO q 12 h)
3 Gentamicin 2 mg/kg
4 Metronidazole 500 mg
5 Clindamycin 600 mg
6 Vancomycin 15 mg/kg started 15–120 min before surgery run at 60 min/500 mg dose—*see Red man syndrome*
7 Amoxicillin/clavulanic acid 2.2 g stat then 2.2 g q 8 h for 24 h
8 Fluconazole 400 mg.

Colorectal surgery/appendicectomy
Metronidazole + cefazolin **or** clindamycin + gentamicin.

Routine upper GI surgery (including laparoscopic surgery)
Cefazolin **or** clindamycin.

Biliary tree/Whipple's/major hepatectomy
Amoxicillin/clavulanic acid + gentamicin **or** vancomycin + gentamicin. If special circumstances (prolonged antibiotic use, immunocompromised, chemotherapy etc), give fluconazole.

ERCP/sclerotherapy/oesophageal dilatation
Cefazolin **or** clindamycin + gentamicin.

Endoscopic ultrasound-guided fine needle aspiration of cystic lesion near gastrointestinal tract
Cefazolin + metronidazole **or** clindamycin + gentamicin.

Gastrostomy or jejunostomy tube insertion
Cefazolin **or** vancomycin + gentamicin (add metronidazole if risk of bowel entry or obstruction).

Hernia
Cefazolin (if bowel lumen entered, add metronidazole) **or** vancomycin + gentamicin + metronidazole.

Breast
Cefazolin (if MRSA colonised, add vancomycin) **or** vancomycin.

Cardiac
Cefazolin (add vancomycin if MRSA positive or unknown) **or** vancomycin + gentamicin.

ENT/head/neck/lung
Cefazolin (add metronidazole if incision through mucosal surfaces) **or** clindamycin + gentamicin.

Neurosurgery
Cefazolin **or** vancomycin.

Gynaecological
Cefazolin + metronidazole **or** clindamycin + gentamicin.

Termination of pregnancy
Doxycycline 100 mg PO 60 min prior to procedure then 200 mg PO 90 min post procedure.

Orthopaedic (elective)
Cefazolin (add vancomycin if known/suspected MRSA) **or** vancomycin.

Compound fractures
If MRSA negative, amoxicillin/clavulanic acid + vancomycin **or** ciprofloxacin + clindamycin (continue for 7 days).

Lower limb amputation
Cefazolin (add metronidazole if ischaemic limb, add vancomycin if MRSA) **or** vancomycin + gentamicin (add metronidazole if ischaemic limb).

Radical prostatectomy
Cefazolin + gentamicin **or** vancomycin + gentamicin.

Transrectal prostate biopsy
Ciprofloxacin 500 mg PO 2 h before procedure **or** cefazolin **or** gentamicin.

Percutaneous nephrolithotomy
Norfloxacin 400 mg PO q 12 h from 48 h before procedure **or** gentamicin **or** cefazolin.

TURP
Gentamicin **or** cefazolin.

Open or laparoscopic urological procedures
Cefazolin + gentamicin (vancomycin if MRSA) **or** vancomycin + gentamicin.

Urinary tract endoscopy
Cefazolin **or** gentamicin.

Cystectomy/ileal conduit
Cefazolin + metronidazole **or** gentamicin + clindamycin.

Vascular
Cefazolin (add metronidazole if ischaemic limb) **or** vancomycin + gentamicin (add metronidazole if ischaemic limb).

⊙ Anticholinergic crisis

See Myasthenia gravis.

⊙ Anticholinergic drugs

See Cholinergic receptors. Anticholinergic drugs are used for a variety of indications, including:

1 sinus bradycardia—atropine, glycopyrrolate
2 oral secretions, as a drying agent—atropine, glycopyrrolate
3 movement disorders due to antipsychotic/antidopaminergic medication. *See Dystonic reaction, acute.* Benztropine is an example of this type of agent. *See Benztropine.*
4 Parkinson's disease. Selective M1 muscarinic acetylcholine receptor blockers such as benztropine increase dopamine availability in the basal ganglia by blocking its reuptake and storage. *See Parkinson's disease (PD).*

⊙ Anticoagulant and antiplatelet drugs and surgery/neuraxial anaesthesia

Introduction

This section is concerned with types and indications for various anticoagulant and antiplatelet drugs. It also covers situations in which these drugs should be ceased or reversed. *See Anticoagulant/antiplatelet drug antidotes.* The main area of concern relates to the risk of surgical and/or neuraxial bleeding in patients requiring these drugs. Deep regional nerve blocks may also be of concern. These are defined as blocks where, if there is associated bleeding, such bleeding would be difficult to control e.g. supraclavicular brachial plexus block. For this section, advice about neuraxial block can also be applied to deep regional nerve blocks. However, as always, the potential risks of a deep nerve block must be balanced against the potential benefits.

Anticoagulant drugs

Used to reduce the risk of thromboembolic disease (DVT, PE, thromboembolism associated with AF and heart valve disease). They are also used to treat DVT/PE. Oral anticoagulants other than warfarin are known as 'NOACs' (**N**on-vitamin K **O**ral **A**nti**C**oagulant drugs). NOACs are mainly renally excreted, and creatinine clearance is used as a measure of renal function. *See Renal function tests.*
A creatinine clearance of > 50 mL/min results in a normal half-life, and a creatinine clearance of 30–60 mL/min generally doubles the NOACs' half-life. NOACs are not suitable for a patient with a creatinine clearance < 30 mL/min. Use warfarin instead. Surgery can, somewhat arbitrarily, be divided into low risk and high risk for bleeding. Neuraxial anaesthesia is best viewed as being in the high risk category.
The anticoagulant drugs include:

1 vitamin K antagonists—warfarin
2 activated factor Xa inhibitors e.g. rivaroxaban, apixaban, edoxaban, danaparoid
3 direct thrombin inhibitors e.g. dabigatran, hirudin, argatroban
4 fractionated and unfractionated heparin.

Warfarin and surgery (see *Warfarin*)

Warfarin does not need to be ceased when the bleeding risk from surgery is minimal. This includes cataract surgery, minor dental procedures including extractions and skin biopsy. If the bleeding risk is significant, for elective surgery:

1 take the last dose of warfarin 6 days before surgery
2 check INR on the day before surgery. If < 1.5, proceed with surgery. If INR ≥ 1.5, give vitamin K PO 1–2 mg or IV 5 mg. Recheck INR on day of surgery. If INR < 1.5, proceed with surgery.

Is bridging therapy required before surgery while the effects of warfarin are wearing off?

The risk of thrombotic stroke must be balanced against the risk of bleeding if bridging therapy is used. Expert advice from the patient's cardiologist/haematologist should be sought. The CHA_2DS_2-VASc Score is a useful tool to help make this decision. **See *Warfarin*.** In general:

Low risk of thrombotic stroke

1 Bi-leaflet aortic valve prosthesis without AF and no other risk factors.
2 AF with a CHA_2DS_2-VASc Score of 0–2. **See *Warfarin*.**
3 VTE > 12 months ago and no other risk factors.

Medium risk of thrombotic stroke

1 Bi-leaflet aortic valve and other risk factors such as AF, prior stroke.
2 VTE 3–12 months ago.
3 Recurrent VTE.
4 Active cancer.
5 Non-severe thrombophilia.

High risk of thrombotic stroke

1 Any mitral valve prosthesis.
2 Caged ball or tilting aortic valve.
3 Mechanical heart valve and stroke/TIA within 6 months.
4 AF and stroke/TIA within 3 months, CHA_2DS_2-VASc Score 5–6, rheumatic heart disease.
5 VTE within 3 months.
6 Severe thrombophilia.

Is bridging therapy required after surgery?

Some patients are at very high risk of thromboembolism e.g. those with a ball valve-type aortic valve. These patients should have a heparin infusion started 6–48 h after surgery (depending on the nature of the surgery and the surgeon's opinion). Alternatively, use LMWH in therapeutic doses. Restart warfarin on the evening of surgery. These patients are unsuitable for epidural catheters for postoperative pain relief.

Warfarin and neuraxial procedures

An INR < 1.5 is acceptable for neuraxial procedures and deep nerve blocks. Do not restart warfarin if an epidural catheter is in situ. Use heparin or Clexane in prophylactic doses if required.

Activated factor Xa inhibitors

There is a lack of published evidence on the safety of neuraxial anaesthesia in patients taking NOACs. The following are suggested conservative guidelines. Seek expert haematologist advice if in any doubt.

1 **Rivaroxaban, Apixaban and Edoxaban** (*see Rivaroxaban, Apixaban and Edoxaban*)
   a) Moderate bleeding risk surgery, creatinine clearance > 50 mL/min—cease drug for 24 h.
   b) Moderate bleeding risk surgery, creatinine clearance 30–50 mL/min—cease drug for 48 h.
   c) High bleeding risk surgery, neuraxial block, creatine clearance > 50 mL/min—cease drug for 48–72 h.
   d) High bleeding risk surgery, neuraxial block, creatinine clearance 30–50 mL/min—cease drug for 72 h.

Rivaroxaban and apixaban can be recommenced 48 h after high-risk procedures.
All 3 drugs can be reversed by andexanet alfa. *See Andexanet alfa (Andexxa).*

2 **Fondaparinux** (*see Fondaparinux*)
   a) Used as an alternative to heparin in patients with HIT type II. *See Heparin-induced thrombocytopenia (HIT).*
   b) Experience with neuraxial anaesthesia and fondaparinux is limited. Do not perform SAB within 3–4 days of the last dose. Do not use epidural catheters.

Direct thrombin inhibitors

1 **Dabigatran**
   a) Moderate bleeding risk surgery, creatinine clearance > 50 mL/min—cease drug for 24 h.
   b) Moderate bleeding risk surgery, creatinine clearance 30–50 mL/min—cease drug for 48–72 h.
   c) High bleeding risk surgery, neuraxial block, creatine clearance > 50 mL/min—cease drug for 48–72 h.
   d) High bleeding risk surgery, neuraxial block, creatinine clearance 30–50 mL/min—cease drug for 96 h.

2 **Argatroban**
   Administered IV. Surgery can be performed when APTT returns to baseline (2–4 h).

3 **Bivalirudin**
   Administered IV. Surgery can be performed when APTT returns to baseline (1–2 h).

4 **Desirudin (Iprivask)**
   First-generation direct thrombin inhibitor used as a substitute for heparin in patients with HIT type II. It is used subcut. Neuraxial anaesthesia can be performed 8–10 h after the last dose, but check that APTT has returned to normal. Usually does not require anticoagulation monitoring.

5 **Lepirudin** Used IV in patients with HIT type II. It is a recombinant form of hirudin from leeches. *See Lepirudin.* Needs to be monitored with APTT tests.

General comments about timing of elective surgery

1 Elective procedures requiring neuraxial anaesthesia should be delayed for at least 3 months after a thrombotic event or major haemorrhage.[13]
2 Elective procedures requiring neuraxial anaesthesia should be delayed for at least 6 weeks post-partum.[13]

NOACs and bridging therapy

As the onset and offset of these drugs is so fast, bridging therapy is usually not required.

Fractionated and unfractionated heparin and neuraxial anaesthesia/ epidural catheter removal

See Heparin (unfractionated and low-molecular-weight heparins).

1 Heparin subcut—wait at least 6 h before neuraxial anaesthesia. Do not remove an epidural catheter within 4–6 h of subcut heparin. Do not give subcut heparin until 1 h after epidural catheter removal or SAB block.

2 Heparin infusion—wait at least 6 h before neuraxial anaesthesia. Check APTT. Do not start a heparin infusion within 1 h of epidural catheter removal.

3 Prophylactic LMWH—wait 12 h (longer if renal impairment) before neuraxial block. Restart 12 h after neuraxial block. Do not remove an epidural catheter within 12 h of LMWH (longer if renal impairment). Do not give the next dose of LMWH until 4 h after epidural catheter removal.

4 Therapeutic LMWH—wait 24 h (longer if renal impairment) before neuraxial block. Do not remove an epidural catheter within 24 h of last dose (longer if renal impairment). Do not give next dose of LMWH within 12 h after epidural catheter removal.

Danaparoid

Classified as a heparinoid and used in patients with HIT type II requiring either prophylactic or full anticoagulation for DVT/PE. *See Danaparoid*. It has a very long half-life. It is unclear from the literature how long to withhold this drug before surgery. Cessation for at least 24 h before invasive procedures is suggested.[14] Neuraxial block recommendations are not available.

Antiplatelet drugs

Used to reduce the risk of coronary artery and cerebral artery thromboses due to platelet plugs. They include the following.

1 *Aspirin*—irreversibly inhibits cyclooxygenase 1 (COX-1) on the platelet, leading to reduced thromboxane A_2 production. This in turn inhibits platelet activation and causes vasodilatation. The effect lasts for the lifetime of the platelet. About 10% of the platelet population is replaced each day, so it takes 10 days for the aspirin effect to completely wear off. Aspirin does not preclude neuraxial anaesthesia. Ceasing aspirin for 5 days will usually be sufficient, but 7–10 days is commonly recommended for high-risk surgery e.g. brain surgery.

2 *Dipyridamole*—inhibits platelet aggregation and causes vasodilation by inhibiting the breakdown of cyclic adenosine monophosphate (cAMP) by phosphodiesterase in platelets. It also inhibits the uptake of adenosine into platelets and other cells. Adenosine acts on the platelet A2 receptor to increase intraplatelet cAMP levels. On its own, it should be stopped for 24 h before surgery. If combined with aspirin (Asasantin), it should be stopped 7–10 days before surgery.

3 *NSAIDs—see Non-steroidal anti-inflammatory drugs (NSAIDs)*. Easiest approach is to stop these drugs for 7–10 days before surgery. In practice, 3 days will be sufficient for most agents. Meloxicam and piroxicam should be stopped for 10 days. Selective (COX-2 inhibitor) NSAIDs such as Celebrex should be stopped for 2 days to be conservative.

4 *Platelet adenosine diphosphate (ADP) receptor antagonists, also called P2Y$_{12}$ receptor antagonists*—used for patients requiring strong platelet inhibition e.g. coronary artery stents. Their cessation should be discussed with the relevant specialist e.g. cardiologist. They include:
   - **clopidogrel (Plavix, Iscover)**—cease for at least 5 days before surgery (7 days for neuraxial block)
   - **ticlopidine (Ticlid)**—cease for 14 days before surgery/neuraxial block

- **prasugrel**—cease for at least 7 days before surgery/neuraxial block
- **ticagrelor (Brilinta)**—must be used with aspirin to treat acute coronary syndrome. It should be stopped for 5 days before elective surgery. **See Acute coronary syndrome.**

5 **Platelet glycoprotein IIb/IIIa receptor antagonists**—these drugs are used IV during percutaneous coronary artery interventions (angioplasty or stenting) to reduce the risk of thrombus formation. They act by blocking the glycoprotein receptor, preventing fibrinogen from binding to platelets. They include:

- **abciximab (ReoPro)**—cease for 48 h before surgery
- **tirofiban (Aggrastat)**—cease for 8 h before surgery
- **eptifibatide (Integrilin)**—cease for 8 h before surgery.

Fibrinolytic agents

1 **Alteplase (tPA)**—acts by catalysing the conversion of plasminogen to plasmin. Plasmin destroys blood clots by degrading fibrin. Ten days should elapse before major surgery or invasive procedures.

2 **Streptokinase**—acts by forming a complex with plasminogen with increased conversion to plasmin. It is unclear from the literature when major surgery or invasive procedures can be safely performed.

◖ Anticoagulant/antiplatelet drug antidotes

This section is a brief reference guide to antidotes for anticoagulant and antiplatelet drugs.

Abciximab (ReoPro)—platelet glycoprotein IIb/IIIa receptor antagonist (prevents binding of fibrinogen). Stop abciximab infusion and allow 10–30 min for clearance of the drug. Then give a platelet transfusion.

Apixaban (Eliquis)—factor Xa inhibitor, reversed by andexanet alfa. Alternatively use prothrombin complex concentrate 50 IU/kg.

Aspirin—COX-1 inhibitor, inhibits platelet aggregation irreversibly. Minor bleeding can be treated with desmopressin 0.3 mcg/kg. Treat major bleeding with platelet transfusion.

Edoxaban—factor Xa inhibitor; use prothrombin complex concentrate 50 IU/kg.

Enoxaparin (Clexane)—low-molecular-weight heparin. Acts by inhibiting factor Xa and enhances the action of antithrombin III. 60% reversed by protamine.

Clopidogrel (Plavix, Iscover)—platelet adenosine diphosphate (ADP) receptor antagonist, also called a $P2Y_{12}$ receptor antagonist. Minor bleeding can be reversed with desmopressin 0.3 mcg/kg. Treat major bleeding with platelet transfusion.

Dabigatran (Pradaxa)—direct thrombin inhibitor. Reversed by idarucizumab (Praxbind), a monoclonal antibody which binds to dabigatran. Inject 5 g IV as two consecutive infusions of 2.5 g over 5–10 min. **See Idarucizumab (Praxbind).** Prothrombin complex concentrate can also be used.

Edoxaban (Savaysa)—factor Xa inhibitor. Reversed by prothrombin complex concentrate.

Eptifibatide (Integrilin)—platelet glycoprotein IIb/IIIa receptor antagonist (prevents binding of fibrinogen). Reversal with desmopressin 0.3 mcg/kg is effective in healthy volunteers but is untested in actual patients.[15]

Fondaparinux—selective inhibitor of factor Xa. Can be reversed with FEIBA. **See FEIBA-NF (factor VIII inhibitor bypassing activity).** It is partially reversed with recombinant activated FVII.

Heparin (unfractionated)—antithrombin III activator. Reversed by protamine. **See** *Protamine*.

Prasugrel (Effient)—platelet adenosine diphosphate (ADP) receptor antagonist, also called a P2Y$_{12}$ receptor antagonist. Minor bleeding can be reversed with desmopressin 0.3 mcg/kg. Treat major bleeding with a platelet transfusion.

Rivaroxaban (Xarelto)—factor Xa inhibitor, reversed by andexanet alfa. If not available, use prothrombin complex concentrate 50 IU/kg.

Ticagrelor (Brilinta)—platelet adenosine diphosphate (ADP) receptor antagonist, also called a P2Y$_{12}$ receptor antagonist. Minor bleeding can be reversed with desmopressin 0.3 mcg/kg. Treat major bleeding with a platelet transfusion.

Tirofiban (Aggrastat)—platelet glycoprotein IIb/IIIa receptor antagonist (prevents binding of fibrinogen). Wears off quickly, usually within 2–4 h. Platelet transfusion is not usually necessary.

Warfarin—inhibits hepatic synthesis of vitamin K-dependent clotting factors II, VII, IX and X. Reversed by the administration of vitamin K and prothrombin complex concentrate, Prothrombinex-VF. If both are unavailable or ineffective, give FFP.

◑ Anticoagulation in pregnancy

Indications
1 Mechanical heart valves.
2 DVT/PE.
3 AF.

Drugs
1 Low-molecular-weight heparin up to 12 weeks of pregnancy.
2 Warfarin—although effective, warfarin is linked to fetal demise and teratogenicity if used in the first trimester. Use from 12–36 weeks is acceptable.
3 Low-molecular-weight heparin after 36 weeks.

◑ Anti-emetic drug classes

1 5-HT$_3$ antagonists—**see** *5-Hydroxytryptamine 3 (5-HT$_3$) antagonists.*
2 Neurokinin-1 (NK1) receptor antagonists such as aprepitant.
3 Dopamine antagonists—these include droperidol, maxolon and prochlorperazine.
4 Alpha-2 agonists—clonidine and dexmedetomidine.
5 Corticosteroids—dexamethasone is the most commonly used drug in this group.
6 Antihistamines e.g. cyclizine.
7 Anticholinergics e.g. scopolamine.
8 Gabapentinoids—gabapentin and pregabalin.

◑ Antiphospholipid antibodies/antiphospholipid antibody syndrome

These are antibodies against phosphorus-fat components of the lipid bilayer of cell membranes, and certain proteins in the blood. The presence of these antibodies is associated with thromboembolic events and increased risk of miscarriages. Complications such as these form part of the antiphospholipid antibody syndrome. The most common antiphospholipid antibodies are lupus anticoagulant and antibodies to cardiolipin and beta-2 glycoprotein. Antiphospholipid antibody syndrome may be caused by an underlying autoimmune disease such as lupus.

◗ Antithrombin deficiency

Antithrombin acts primarily by inactivating thrombin and FXa. Antithrombin also inactivates FVII, FIX and FXII. Deficiency leads to an increased tendency to thromboembolic disease. Normal levels of antithrombin are 70–132%. Less than 60% results in thrombosis.[13]

◗ Aortic aneurysm repair

See Abdominal aortic aneurysm (AAA) repair.

◗ Aortic dissection

Description

This is a catastrophic, potentially fatal event, in which the layers of the aortic wall are split apart by the egress of blood, producing a false lumen. The split is between the intima and the media. It is usually an ascending dissection within 10 cm of the aortic valve. Blood can re-enter the lumen at any point, making a communicating dissection. Side branches may be compromised (coronary, carotid, subclavian, coeliac and renal arteries).

Classification

Stanford classification

- Type A—any part of the aorta proximal to the origin of the left subclavian artery. These dissections require surgery. Mortality of ascending dissections is about 1–2% per hour for the first 48 h.[16]
- Type B—arises distal to the left subclavian artery. These dissections may be managed medically if uncomplicated.

DeBakey classification

- Type 1—involves the ascending and descending aorta.
- Type 2—involves the ascending aorta only.
- Type 3—involves the descending aorta only, commencing after the left subclavian artery (= Stanford B).
- Type 3a—as for 3 but dissection extends as far as the diaphragm.
- Type 3b—as for 3 but dissection extends below the diaphragm.

Risk factors

1 Hypertension.
2 Aortic dilatation/aneurysmal disease.
3 Advanced age.
4 Smoking.
5 Hypercholesterolaemia.
6 Cocaine use.
7 Connective tissue disorders such as Marfan syndrome, Ehlers–Danlos syndrome and Turner syndrome. *See Marfan syndrome, Ehlers–Danlos syndrome (EDS) and Turner syndrome.*
8 Pregnancy-related hypertension. *See Preeclampsia/eclampsia.*
9 Vascular inflammation such as giant cell arteritis and Takayasu's arteritis (also called TAK).
10 Trauma.

Presentation

1 Excruciating, tearing pain in the chest or back.
2 Tachycardia with hypertension or hypotension.
3 Acute aortic valve regurgitation.
4 Acute myocardial ischaemia. *See Acute coronary syndrome*.
5 Differential or absent pulses in the extremities, limb ischaemia.
6 Syncope/stroke.
7 Bleeding into mediastinum, pericardium or pleura.
8 Paraplegia.
9 Acute renal impairment.

Diagnosis

Due to the urgency of the situation and patient instability, time for investigations is limited. Tests may include:

1 ECG—may show ischaemia/infarction due to involvement of coronary artery ostia.
2 CXR—may show mediastinal widening, double aortic knob sign, tracheal displacement to the right, enlarged cardiac shadow due to pericardial effusion (blood), pleural effusion (blood).
3 Aortography—very sensitive but rarely performed due to time constraints.
4 CT with contrast angiography.
5 MRI.
6 Transoesophageal echocardiography (TOE).
7 Elevated smooth muscle myosin heavy chain protein.

Management

1 Ensure adequate airway and breathing. Give supplementary O_2 if needed.
2 Pain relief.
3 Intensive monitoring in an HDU or ICU environment—ECG, invasive blood pressure monitoring (using the left radial artery),[16] urine output. Obtain large-bore IV access, cross-match, FBC, UEC and coagulation studies.
4 Rapid blood pressure and heart rate control. *See Hypertension*. This is to decrease the risk of extension of the dissection. Aim for a HR < 60 bpm and SBP 110–120 mmHg. Beta-adrenergic receptor blockers are an excellent choice in this situation. *See Beta-adrenergic receptor blocker drugs* and *Hypertension*. Useful agents include esmolol, metoprolol and labetalol. *See Esmolol, Metoprolol* and *Labetalol*. Use calcium channel blocker drugs if beta blockers not tolerated or contraindicated. *See Calcium channel blocker drugs*.
5 Add sodium nitroprusside if more aggressive management required. *See Sodium nitroprusside (SNP)*.
6 Adequate hydration. Overhydration may worsen dissection.

Anaesthetic considerations

A cardiothoracic anaesthetic team is required with a sternotomy or left thoracotomy approach. Cardiothoracic anaesthesia is beyond the scope of this manual.

◗ Aortic valve incompetence/regurgitation (acute and chronic)

Acute aortic valve incompetence

This is usually due to a catastrophic event such as:

1 aortic dissection—*see Aortic dissection*
2 endocarditis.

The normal-sized left ventricle (LV) cannot compensate for the sudden increase in regurgitant volume and acute heart failure occurs. There is usually acute pulmonary oedema and hypotension. Immediate aortic valve replacement is required. Stabilisation of the patient may require:

1 sodium nitroprusside
2 dobutamine
3 milrinone.

Further management of this catastrophic condition is beyond the scope of this manual.

Chronic aortic valve incompetence/regurgitation

Pathophysiology

Results in chronic left ventricular (LV) volume overload, which in turn results in progressive LV dilation and eccentric hypertrophy. This maintains stroke volume (SV) until the LV begins to fail, leading to congestive cardiac failure. Forward flow is dependent on LV contractility, SVR and heart rate. This process usually occurs over many years. Aortic incompetence is much better tolerated than aortic stenosis.

Causes

1 Endocarditis.
2 Rheumatic heart disease.
3 Congenital.
4 Dilation of the aortic root due to causes such as Marfan syndrome (**see Marfan syndrome**), Ehlers–Danlos syndrome (**see Ehlers–Danlos syndrome (EDS)**) and ankylosing spondylitis.

Clinical effects

1 Dyspnoea, paroxysmal nocturnal dyspnoea, orthopnoea.
2 Palpitations.
3 Reduced exercise tolerance.
4 Widened pulse pressure (water-hammer pulse).
5 Diastolic decrescendo heart murmur at the left sternal border. The murmur intensity increases with a sustained hand grip due to increased SVR.

Investigations

1 ECG—shows LVH.
2 CXR—cardiomegaly with boot-shaped heart. The aortic root may be dilated.
3 Echocardiography.
4 Cardiac catheterisation.

Management

1 Augment forward flow by afterload (SVR) reduction and avoid/treat bradycardia.
2 Useful drugs include ACE inhibitors or ARBs (**see Angiotensin converting enzyme (ACE) inhibitors and Angiotensin II receptor blocker (ARB) drugs**) to reduce afterload.
3 Digoxin to increase LV contractility.
4 Valve replacement, especially if exercise capacity < 4 METS (unable to climb a flight of stairs or walk briskly on level ground). **See Cardiac risk for non-cardiac surgery**.
5 Non-cardiac surgery may need to be delayed for valve replacement.

Anaesthesia and aortic valve incompetence (non-cardiac surgery)

1 Asymptomatic patients usually tolerate anaesthetics well. Patients with an LVEF < 55% and atrial fibrillation have an increased risk of cardiac morbidity and mortality.

2 Provide adequate volume loading.

3 Maintain HR—a mild tachycardia is beneficial. Preserve sinus rhythm.

4 Decrease SVR—neuraxial anaesthesia is usually well tolerated.

5 Maintain contractility/avoid drugs which are myocardial depressants. If inotropes are needed, use dobutamine or milrinone.

6 Consider bacterial endocarditis prophylaxis—*see Bacterial endocarditis (BE) prophylaxis*.

▷ Aortic valve stenosis (AS)

Patients with moderate to severe AS having elective non-cardiac surgery have double the 30-day mortality of aged-matched controls.

Aetiology

The usual causes are:

1 rheumatic heart disease

2 calcification

3 bicuspid aortic valve (2%).

Pathophysiology

LV outflow obstruction leads to the following:

1 LV concentric hypertrophy.

2 The thickened ventricle has reduced compliance and there is reduced LV cavity volume. This leads to impaired ventricular filling with an increased reliance on atrial filling (atrial kick), which accounts for 40% of LV filling (compared with 20% in normal circumstances).

3 CO becomes 'fixed'.

4 The thickened LV walls have increased O_2 requirements, leading to ischaemia, even with normal coronary arteries. Maintenance of diastolic blood pressure is essential to maintain coronary artery perfusion.

5 Tachycardia can result in inadequate time for LV filling, leading to a fall in CO.

6 Loss of sinus rhythm can also result in a severe reduction in CO.

7 Bradycardia can result in LV distension.

Clinical signs/symptoms

1 Systolic ejection murmur second intercostal space right sternal edge, with a slow-rising pulse and reduced pulse pressure. A pulse pressure < 30 mmHg suggests severe disease.

2 Dyspnoea, angina, reduced exercise tolerance, syncope. Symptoms usually occur when valve area is < 1 cm². Normal valve area is 3–4 cm².

3 Sudden death can occur.

Investigations

1 ECG—LVH, LV strain pattern and LBBB. *See Electrocardiography (ECG) quick guide*.

2 CXR—may appear normal until LV begins to fail. Post-stenotic dilatation of the aorta and calcification of the aortic annulus may be seen.

3 Echocardiography will show valve area. The severity of AS can be classified as:

   a) mild > 1.5 cm²

   b) moderate 1–1.5 cm²

   c) severe < 1 cm²

   d) critical < 0.6 cm².

   A cardiac echo within 12 months of surgery does not need to be repeated unless the patient's condition has deteriorated.

4 Coronary angiography to assess for co-existent CAD and measure pressure gradient across the valve. The severity of AS based on valve gradient can be classified as:

a) mild 12–25 mmHg

b) moderate 25–40 mmHg

c) severe 40–50 mmHg

d) critical > 50 mmHg.

A low-pressure gradient across the valve may reflect heart failure rather than less severe AS.

AS and peri-operative risk for elective non-cardiac surgery

The main issue is whether aortic valve replacement should be undertaken before significant elective non-cardiac surgery. Patients should have AV replacement prior to major surgery if:

1 there is symptomatic AS

2 the pressure gradient across the valve > 50 mmHg, even if asymptomatic.

Consider percutaneous balloon valvotomy or transcatheter aortic valve implantation (TAVI) if the patient refuses AV surgery or is at very high risk for AV surgery.

Management aims during anaesthesia

Aim for preinduction haemodynamic parameters for pulse and BP. Use anaesthetic drugs very cautiously.

1 Maintain sinus rhythm and avoid bradycardia or tachycardia. Aim for HR 70–80 bpm.

2 Keep the patient euvolaemic. Replace fluid losses promptly. Preload must be maintained.

3 Defend SVR. A sudden fall in SVR may lead to hypotension, with a subsequent decrease in coronary artery perfusion. This can lead to myocardial ischaemia, impaired LV function and a vicious spiral. Treat a fall in SVR with vasoconstrictors such as metaraminol or phenylephrine. SAB is contraindicated in patients with significant AS.

4 A gradual, controlled reduction in SVR may improve CO if preload is maintained.

5 Use an arterial line.

6 Intraoperative TOE may be very helpful.

7 Consider SBE prophylaxis. *See Bacterial endocarditis (BE) prophylaxis.*

AS and neuraxial anaesthesia for obstetrics

Severe aortic stenosis in pregnancy is a high-risk lesion. During pregnancy the transvalvular gradient tends to increase in patients with AS due to increased blood volume and decreased SVR. In some cases of severe AS, the patient may benefit from percutaneous balloon valvotomy. Consider the need for antibiotic prophylaxis.

The important considerations are:

1 Keep the patient well hydrated to maintain preload. Both hyper- and hypovolaemia are detrimental.

2 Maintain SVR and HR in the normal range as explained above. Tachycardia and/or a fall in SVR are particularly undesirable.

3 Depending on severity of the AS, monitoring with pulse oximetry ± invasive arterial monitoring should be considered.

4 Carefully titrated epidural anaesthesia can be used for labour and delivery.

5 For a CS, a single-shot spinal is contraindicated but a CSE technique using a low-dose spinal component can be considered.

GA for CS

There are many concerns with GA in the presence of severe AS, as described above. Use invasive arterial monitoring. Drugs must be used thoughtfully and carefully in an attempt to maintain haemodynamic stability.

Oxytocin

A large IV bolus of oxytocin can cause hypotension and tachycardia. Give oxytocin 3 units slowly and carefully on delivery and a standard infusion of 40 IU in 1000 mL Hartmann's solution over 4 h.

◐ Aortopulmonary window (AP window)

This a rare congenital heart defect in which there is a connection between the ascending aorta and pulmonary artery. This results in aortic blood flow entering the pulmonary circulation, leading to pulmonary hypertension and CCF. It may occur in isolation or be associated with other congenital heart diseases such as Tetralogy of Fallot. It produces similar problems to a patent ductus arteriosus (PDA). It is repaired by closing the connection.

◐ Apixaban (Eliquis)

Description

This is a phenylpiperidine anticoagulant drug. Its mechanism of action is to prevent FXa from converting prothrombin to thrombin (factor Xa inhibitor). It is used for the prevention of thromboembolic disease due to non-valvular AF, prevention of DVT after elective hip and knee replacement and DVT/PE treatment.

Dose

Adult

- Prevention of VTE after elective hip replacement 2.5 mg q 12 h for 32–38 days. After elective knee replacement 2.5 mg q 12 h for 10–14 days. Start 12–24 h after surgery.
- Non-valvular AF stroke prevention 5 mg q 12 h. Reduce to 2.5 mg q 12 h in patients with renal impairment or ≥ 80 years old.
- DVT/PE treatment 10 mg q 12 h for 7 days, then 5 mg q 12 h.
- Prevention of DVT/PE 2.5 mg q 12 h.

Advantages

1 No testing required.
2 Reversed by andexanet alfa. *See Andexanet alfa (Andexxa).*

Disadvantages

Not suitable for patients with severe renal impairment.

Treatment of haemorrhage

The effects of apixaban can be measured by APTT. PT/INR may be affected. Thrombin time (TT) is not affected. Its effects can be reversed by andexanet alfa. Alternatively, use prothrombin complex concentrate 50 IU/kg.

◐ Aprepitant (Cinvanti)

Long-acting NK1 receptor antagonist used to treat/prevent nausea and vomiting, including PONV. It is more effective at treating vomiting than nausea. It can be used PO or IV.

Dose

The dose for adults for prevention of PONV is PO 40 mg within 3 h of induction. The IV dose is 150 mg over 20–30 min. Women using the OCP must use alternative contraception for 1 month after aprepitant.

◖ Argatroban (Acova)

See Anticoagulant and antiplatelet drugs and surgery/neuraxial anaesthesia.

Description

Direct thrombin inhibitor like dabigatran. It is used intravenously for the management of HIT type II and is eliminated by the liver. APTT normalises 2–4 h after cessation.

Dose

Adult

2 mcg/kg/min adjusted to keep APTT 1.5–3 × normal. Neuraxial anaesthesia can be performed when the APTT returns to normal, usually after about 4 h.

◖ Arm blocks in the elbow region

These blocks can be used to supplement a brachial plexus block or for surgery on the forearm, wrist and hand. Use 1% ropivacaine or 2% lignocaine with adrenaline. Use aseptic technique.

Innervation of forearm/hand

1 **Radial nerve**—innervates the posterior structures of the forearm and wrist.
2 **Median nerve**—innervates the lateral palm and palmar surface of thumb, index and middle fingers.
3 **Ulnar nerve**—supplies the medial hand and forearm.

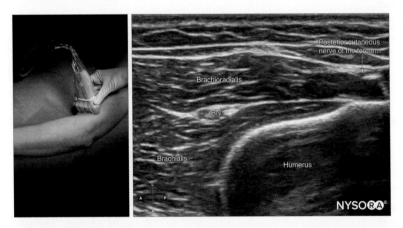

Figure A3 Probe position and sonoanatomy for radial nerve block in the elbow region
Image courtesy of NYSORA

Radial nerve block technique

1 Identify the lateral epicondyle of the elbow and place transducer 2–3 cm proximal to this in transverse orientation. The nerve is just lateral to the insertion of the biceps tendon.

2 Scan this area to identify the radial nerve near the humerus between the brachioradialis muscle and the brachialis muscle (Figure A3).

3 Insert the block needle in-plane from medial to lateral until the tip is near the nerve.

4 Inject 3–5 mL of LA to encircle the nerve.

Alternatively

1 Position the patient with the arm flexed across the upper abdomen.

2 Place the probe across the lateral side of the humerus, just proximal to the elbow crease.

3 The radial nerve is easily seen spiralling around the lateral humerus, in the fascial plane between the brachialis and brachioradialis muscles.

4 Insert the needle from lateral to medial, entering the fascial plane containing the nerve.

5 Inject 3–5 mL of LA in this plane near the nerve.

Median nerve block technique

1 Place the transducer in a transverse orientation in the antecubital fossa, just proximal to the elbow crease (Figure A4). Identify the brachial artery. The median nerve lies on the medial side of this structure.

2 Insert the needle in-plane from medial to lateral.

3 Inject 3–5 mL of LA to encircle the nerve.

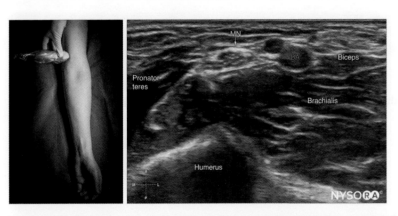

Figure A4 Probe position and sonoanatomy for median nerve block in the elbow region.
MN = median nerve
Image courtesy of NYSORA

Alternatively

1 Place the probe across the ventral/volar surface of the mid-forearm.

2 Identify the radius (it looks like a ski slope), the radial artery and, medial to this, the median nerve. Both structures lie in the fascial plane between the superficial and deep flexor muscles.

3 Insert the needle from lateral to medial, traversing under or over the radial artery. Enter the fascial plane containing the nerve then inject 3–5 mL of LA.

Ulnar nerve block technique

1 Position the transducer in a transverse orientation proximal to the medial epicondyle (Figure A5).
2 Find the ulnar nerve on the triceps muscle.
3 Use 3–5 mL of LA to block the nerve.

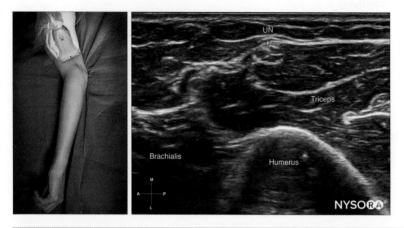

Figure A5 Probe position and sonoanatomy for ulnar nerve block in the elbow region.
UN = ulnar nerve
Image courtesy of NYSORA

Alternatively

1 Place the probe across the ventral/volar aspect of the mid-forearm. Identify the ulnar artery, which is on the medial side of the forearm. At the mid-forearm, the ulnar nerve and artery separate from each other, the nerve being medial to the artery.
2 Insert the needle from lateral to medial, avoiding the artery and entering the fascial plane containing the nerve.
3 Inject 3–5 mL of LA to bathe the nerve.

○ Arrhythmogenic cardiomyopathy (ACM)

Description

This disease is due to genetic defects in desmosomes in cardiac muscle cells leading to the muscle tissue dilating and weakening. Fibro-fatty tissue may replace the muscle cells. It was originally thought to be a disease of the RV (arrhythmogenic right ventricular cardiomyopathy/dysplasia), but it can be in both ventricles or just the LV. This results in:

1 hypokinetic areas
2 arrhythmias (including VF, VT), which can cause blackouts or sudden death
3 aneurysmal dilation of the ventricle(s).

Diagnosis

1 ECG abnormalities include T wave inversion in V1–V3, RBBB, an epsilon wave (a terminal notch in the QRS complex) and ectopic beats.

2 Echocardiography may show RV enlargement and hypokinesis. The RV wall may be thinned dramatically. There may be TR due to dilation of the tricuspid valve annulus.

3 Cardiac MRI—typical findings are fatty infiltration of the RV free wall.

4 Cardiac angiography may also show areas of hypokinesis.

5 Cardiac biopsy.

6 Genetic testing.

Management

1 Avoidance of competitive sports.

2 Antiarrhythmic drugs/beta blockers.

3 Treatment of heart failure. **See *Congestive cardiac failure (CCF)—non-acute*.**

4 Anticoagulants.

5 Catheter ablation.

6 AICD.

7 Heart transplant.

◗ Arterial blood gas (ABG) interpretation for acidosis/alkalosis

In addition to providing information about a patient's ventilation, the values for pH, $PaCO_2$ and bicarbonate (HCO_3^-) can be used to establish whether there is a metabolic or respiratory alkalosis or acidosis.

pH

Normal pH is 7.35–7.45. Less than 7.35 is an acidosis and greater than 7.45 is an alkalosis.

$PaCO_2$

Carbon dioxide levels are controlled by the lungs. The normal range for $PaCO_2$ is 35–45 mmHg. The higher the CO_2 in the blood, the more acidic the blood becomes. The lungs normally respond to acidosis by hyperventilation, and to alkalosis by hypoventilation.

HCO_3^-

Bicarbonate is controlled by the kidney, the normal range being 22–26 mmol/L. The higher the bicarbonate, the more alkaline the blood becomes. The kidney responds to acidosis by retaining bicarbonate and to alkalosis by reducing bicarbonate. These changes occur more slowly than respiratory compensatory mechanisms.

How to interpret ABG results

To interpret ABG results, ascertain whether the result for each of the three parameters above is normal or abnormal and whether it is compensatory or pathological. This is best shown by examples.

Example 1: pH 7.28, $PaCO_2$ 55 mmHg, HCO_3^- 50 mmol/L. There is a respiratory acidosis with partial metabolic compensation (the pH has not been returned to normal).

Example 2: pH 7.3, $PaCO_2$ 28 mmHg, HCO_3^- 18 mmol/L. There is an acidosis with an inappropriately low bicarbonate and an appropriate respiratory compensation. This is a metabolic acidosis with partial respiratory compensation. In an acidosis, if the pH numbers after the decimal point = the $PaCO_2$, this is termed a 'pure metabolic' acidosis.

Example 3: pH 7.55, $PaCO_2$ 28 mmHg, bicarbonate 22 mmol/L. There is an alkalosis with an inappropriate respiratory response and a normal bicarbonate. This is an uncompensated respiratory alkalosis.

Example 4: pH 7.35, $PaCO_2$ 30 mmHg, HCO_3^- 18. Although the pH is normal, a pH between 7.35–7.39 suggests an acidotic process. pH between 7.4–7.45 suggests an alkalotic process. Both the bicarbonate and CO_2 are abnormal, but it can be deduced that the low CO_2 is a response to a metabolic acidosis as the bicarbonate is also low. As the pH is in the normal range, this is a metabolic acidosis with full respiratory compensation.

Working out the type of metabolic acidosis

Calculate the anion gap, which is the positive ions (cations) minus the negative ions (anions), using the formula $Na^+ + K^+ - (HCO_3^- + Cl^-)$. The normal anion gap is 3–11 meq/L (lab specific). The anion gap is due to unmeasured cations (H^+) and anions (phosphates, sulphates, organic acids, albumin).

Metabolic acidosis with a normal anion gap

Also called hyperchloraemic acidosis, this is due to bicarbonate loss with increased reabsorption of chloride. This can occur with:

1 diarrhoea
2 type 2 renal tubular acidosis
3 acetazolamide
4 ureteral diversion
5 decreased renal excretion of H^+ as seen in renal failure and renal tubular acidosis types 1 and 4
6 hypoaldosteronism.

Metabolic acidosis with a high anion gap

Can be due to increased levels of organic acids in the blood such as:

1 Lactic acidosis—due to such causes as shock, salicylates.
2 Diabetic ketoacidosis.
3 Methanol poisoning—formic acid.
4 Ethylene glycol poisoning—oxalic acid.
5 Severe renal failure with reduced excretion of phosphates and sulphates.

Points to note

- With a respiratory acidosis, for every 10 mmHg rise in $PaCO_2$, bicarbonate increases by 1 mmol/L acutely and by 3–4 mmol/L chronically.
- With a metabolic acidosis, the $PaCO_2$ is usually within +/– 5 mmHg of the last 2 digits of the pH value down to a pH value of 7.15.

Metabolic alkalosis

See *Metabolic alkalosis*.

◖ Arterial injection of drugs (unintentional)

See *Intra-arterial injection of drugs (unintentional)*.

◖ Arterial switch procedure

See *Transposition of the great arteries (TGA)/transposition of the great vessels (TGV)*.

◖ ASA grade

See *American Society of Anesthesiologists (ASA) Physical Status Classification System*.

◗ Aspalgin

This is a trade name for a tablet combining aspirin 300 mg and codeine 8 mg.
See *Aspirin* and *Codeine*.

◗ Aspiration

Description

Aspiration is defined as the entry of solids or liquids from the patient's body into the respiratory system. It is the most significant cause of airway-related mortality due to anaesthesia. Aspiration may involve food, gastric acid, faeces (as can occur with a bowel obstruction) or pus from a pharyngeal abscess. Blood from oral haemorrhage (e.g. post-tonsillectomy) can also be aspirated. Aspiration can lead to a chemical pneumonitis and/or bacterial pneumonia. Aspiration more commonly affects the right lung in supine patients because the right main bronchus is more vertical. About 20% of patients who aspirate will require ventilation.

Prevention

1 Regional/neuraxial anaesthesia to avoid the use of GA.
2 Adequate fasting prior to anaesthesia. **See** *Fasting prior to anaesthesia*.
3 Appropriate choice of airway. Options range from none to cuffed ET tube. The choice will be based on experience and personal preferences. A second-generation supraglottic device is superior to a first-generation device in preventing aspiration.
4 Consider sodium citrate 0.3 M 30 mL to reduce gastric pH. This will make the effects of gastric acid aspiration less severe.
5 Metoclopramide can be administered to increase the rate of gastric emptying and increase lower oesophageal sphincter tone. The evidence for this is poor.
6 Rapid sequence induction (RSI)—**see** *Rapid sequence induction*. *Note:* RSI may make intubation more difficult, especially if inexpertly applied. It may need to be reduced or released to enable intubation.
7 Insertion of a naso-gastric tube (NGT) in patients with gastrointestinal obstruction and suctioning of gastric contents. This is **mandatory**. Do not remove an NGT already in situ for RSI but do suction out the stomach prior to RSI. Let the NGT vent to air during RSI.
8 Repeat suctioning of the NGT prior to extubation.
9 Extubate the patient awake and on their side at the end of surgery.

Patients most likely to aspirate

1 Inadequate fasting or unknown fasting status.
2 Gastrointestinal obstruction.
3 Injury soon after eating.
4 Acute abdomen.
5 Caesarean section (CS) under GA.
6 Severe reflux/hiatus hernia.
7 High BMI.
8 Surgery during pregnancy other than CS after 20 weeks' gestation.
9 Emergency surgery.
10 High ASA status. **See** *American Society of Anesthesiologists (ASA) Physical Status Classification System*.
11 Previous gastrointestinal surgery e.g. bariatric surgery.

12 Diabetes mellitus.

13 Renal failure.

14 Raised intracranial pressure.

15 Ascites.

Surgical factors increasing aspiration risk

1 Head-down positioning.

2 Laparoscopic surgery.

3 Pressure on the abdomen and/or supine positioning during colonoscopy.

Evidence of aspiration

1 Coughing/swallowing/straining.

2 Visible fluid in the mouth.

3 Desaturation.

4 Bronchospasm.

5 Stridor.

6 Laryngospasm.

Management

1 Prevention of ongoing aspiration—place the patient left lateral Trendelenburg (head-down) and suction out fluids/solids. Apply cricoid pressure if passive regurgitation **but not if active vomiting.** Bag mask ventilate with 100% O_2

2 Secure the airway with an ET tube if appropriate. Use a rapid sequence induction but cricoid pressure cannot be used if the patient is actively vomiting. If aspiration of clear oral secretions occurs at the end of the procedure, consider a 'wait and see' approach without intubation.

3 Elective surgery should be cancelled. Elective surgery in progress should be completed expeditiously.

Mild aspiration

This is aspiration of clear secretions. Patients can be extubated and observed for:

1 hypoxia—treat with supplementary O_2

2 CXR—to check for signs of aspiration

3 chest physiotherapy—encourage deep breathing and coughing.

If no symptoms or signs of hypoxia occur within 2 h of aspiration, respiratory complications are unlikely.

Moderate/severe aspiration

1 Intubate the patient using RSI.

2 Suctioning of the trachea and bronchi with a Y-cath suction catheter prior to ventilation unless the patient is critically hypoxic.

3 Consider urgent bronchoscopy to remove solids. Bronchial lavage may be helpful.

4 Insert a nasogastric tube to empty the stomach.

5 Obtain an urgent CXR and place an arterial line.

6 Supportive measures such as IPPV, PEEP.

7 If bronchospasm occurs, **see Asthma**.

8 Although experts advise not to start antibiotics unless there is evidence of infection, in practice all patients that have significant aspiration receive antibiotics.

9 Steroids have no role.

Aspiration pneumonia antibiotic selection[17]

1 For simple aspiration, consider ampicillin/sulbactam or amoxicillin and metronidazole. Use clindamycin in penicillin-allergic patients.
2 For more complex cases e.g. sick patient in hospital who has aspirated, consider vancomycin and piperacillin-tazobactam.
3 Antibiotic choice can be more focused if an infective organism is identified.

▶ Aspirin

Description
Aspirin (acetylsalicylic acid) is a non-steroidal anti-inflammatory drug (NSAID). It is a non-selective cyclo-oxygenase (COX) inhibitor. *See Cyclo-oxygenase*. It is used as an:
1 antiplatelet drug—antiplatelet effect lasts for the lifetime of the platelet (7–10 days)
2 analgesic
3 anti-pyretic
4 anti-inflammatory.

Dose
Antiplatelet: 75–100 mg daily PO.
Analgesia/anti-pyretic/anti-inflammatory: 300–900 mg PO up to every 4 h, max dose 3,600 mg per day.

Aspirin and surgery
1 Antiplatelet effect of aspirin does not preclude neuraxial anaesthesia (up to aspirin dose of 300 mg/daily).
2 Patients on aspirin for established cardiovascular disease/stents should continue aspirin unless closed space surgery (intracranial, spinal). Discuss with surgeon, cardiologist.
3 Aspirin should be stopped for 7 days before significant surgery in patients at low risk of a major cardiac event.

Points to note
1 Aspirin should not be used in children under 12 y due to the risk of Reye's syndrome, a life-threatening swelling of the brain and liver.
2 Some patients have aspirin-sensitive asthma.
3 Aspirin can cause adverse effects such as stomach discomfort, nausea, peptic ulcers, upper GIT bleeding.

▶ Asthma

Description
Asthma is a medical condition in which there is periodic constriction of the smooth muscle of the airways (bronchial hyperreactivity) and airway inflammation. There may also be mucus hypersecretion and mucus plugging. It can be mild to life-threatening.

Clinical manifestations
1 Wheezing, dyspnoea.
2 Coughing, chest tightness.

Investigations
See Lung function tests.
1 Spirometry—FEV_1 < 1 L and FEV_1 < 50% of FVC indicates severe disease.
2 Peak expiratory flow rate (PEFR) < 120 L/min suggests severe disease.

3 CXR—may show hyperinflation, flattened diaphragms and pulmonary infiltrate. Identify/exclude pneumothorax or complicating condition such as pneumonia.
4 Pulse oximetry < 90% and PaO_2 < 60 mmHg indicate respiratory failure.
5 FBC looking for elevated WCC, suggesting infection.

Treatment—mild to moderate

1 Avoidance of asthma triggers.
2 Inhaled short-acting beta-2 agonists e.g. salbutamol (Ventolin) and terbutaline (Bricanyl).
3 Inhaled corticosteroids (beclomethasone, budesonide).
4 Leukotriene modifiers—oral medications that include montelukast.
5 Long-acting beta-2 agonists such as salmeterol and formoterol, which may be used in combination inhalers e.g. budesonide-formoterol (Symbicort). Other long-acting beta-2 agonists include indacaterol and olodaterol.
6 Short-acting muscarinic antagonists e.g. ipratropium (Atrovent), tiotropium (Spiriva)—cause bronchodilatation by blocking muscarinic receptors. They are not systemically absorbed. Long-acting muscarinic antagonists include aclidinium and tiotropium.
7 Mast cell stabilising drugs e.g. disodium cromoglycate (Intal). These decrease airway inflammation.
8 Oral/IV steroids—for acute exacerbations of asthma.
9 Allergy shots (regular injections of triggering substances)—to reduce the immune system's reaction to specific antigens.
10 Biologics—used in severe asthma. These work in different ways. Omalizumab treats severe asthma triggered by allergies. Mepolizumab, reslizumab and benralizumab suppress eosinophils.
11 Theophylline (Theochron)—used as an add-on therapy in poorly controlled asthmatics
12 Bronchial thermoplasty—heat is used to reduce the smooth muscle in the airways.

Severe asthma attack/status asthmaticus

There may be air-trapping, dynamic hyperinflation, V/Q mismatch and RV overload. Pneumothorax may occur. Patients may go into acute respiratory failure. Clinical findings indicating severe asthma include:
1 tachypnoea > 30 breaths per min
2 tachycardia > 120 bpm
3 use of accessory muscles of inspiration
4 inability to talk in full sentences
5 inability to lie supine due to breathlessness
6 pulsus paradoxus (fall in SBP by at least 12 mmHg during inspiration)
7 PaO_2 < 60 mmHg, normal or elevated $PaCO_2$
8 auto-PEEP. This is due to breath stacking—failure to fully expire before the next inspiration.
   Investigations include pulse oximetry, ABGs and CXR.

Management strategies include:

1 oxygen therapy targeting an SpO_2 of 93–95%
2 nebulised beta-2 agonists such as salbutamol e.g. 2.5–5 mg every 20 min. Consider continuous nebulisation of 10–15 mg salbutamol over 1 h. Use of a metered dose inhaler and spacer may give similar results (six puffs equalling 1 nebulisation)

3 ipratropium 500 mcg by nebulisation or 4–8 puffs with a spacer 20 minutely × 3 doses

4 hydrocortisone 200 mg IV q 6 h (4 mg/kg q 6 h in children)

5 magnesium sulphate IV—administer 2 g over 20 min (40 mg/kg in children)

6 heliox-helium oxygen mixture—has a lower density than oxygen, decreasing airway resistance and work of breathing

7 high-flow humidified nasal cannula oxygen

8 non-invasive ventilation may be considered. Providing some PEEP may reduce the work of breathing

9 IV salbutamol. This is not recommended in current guidelines unless anaphylaxis is occurring.[18] In adults, give IV bolus 100–200 mcg +/− infusion of 5–25 mcg/min

10 adrenaline 0.3 mg intramuscularly. For IV boluses/infusion, *see Anaphylaxis*.

Invasive ventilation

Factors that suggest intubation is necessary include:

1 inappropriate slowing of respiratory rate

2 depressed mental status

3 inability to use inhaled therapy

4 hypercapnia

5 hypoxia

6 patient exhaustion.

Use ideal body weight for settings. Ventilation strategies include:

1 A volume-limited mode with reduced tidal volumes (5–7 mL/kg initially, reduce to 3–5 mL/kg if required).

2 Slow respiratory rate (start at 10 breaths/min but reduce to 6–8 breaths/min) with long expiratory times (I:E ratio 1:3–1:5) and an inspiratory flow rate of 80–100 L/min.

3 Low PEEP (e.g. 5 cm H_2O).

4 Breath stacking may occur due to patients being unable to fully exhale. This may cause severe hypotension/arrest. It may be noticed on the flow over time graph that expiratory flow does not return to baseline (full expiration does not occur). It may be necessary to disconnect the ventilator from the ET tube to enable full expiration and for auto-PEEP to dissipate. Physical pressure on the chest may also help exhalation.

5 Consider permissive hypercapnia but ensure blood pH > 7.2.

6 Note that peak inspiratory pressures may be high but check the plateau pressure— which is the pressure in the alveoli. This needs to be < 30 cm H_2O. **See Ventilation settings and modes**.

7 Barotrauma and pneumothorax are a constant risk.

Desperate measures

If all else has failed, consider:

1 ketamine 10–20 mg bolus IV then infusion 1–3 mg/kg/h

2 inhaled halothane, sevoflurane

3 GTN infusion

4 enoximone[18]

5 ECMO

6 aminophylline IV is **not recommended** for acute severe asthma.[19]

Anaesthesia and the asthmatic patient

The aims of anaesthesia in the asthmatic patient include avoiding drugs and procedures that may cause bronchoconstriction and to use drugs which cause bronchodilation.

1 Ensure the patient's asthma is optimally managed prior to anaesthesia. Preoperative pulmonary function testing may be required. *See Lung function tests*.

2 Consider regional/neuraxial anaesthesia to avoid the need for GA.

3 Propofol and ketamine produce bronchodilation and are preferred for induction. Thiopentone exacerbates bronchoconstriction through histamine release.

4 A laryngeal mask airway (LMA) is probably less likely to cause bronchospasm than endotracheal intubation.[20] If the patient is intubated, lignocaine 50–100 mg IV prior to intubation may reduce the risk of bronchospasm. Rocuronium is the preferred muscle relaxant.

5 Sevoflurane may or may not cause bronchodilatation. Desflurane is irritating to the airways and should not be used.

6 Avoid histamine-releasing opioids such as morphine. Use fentanyl.

7 If bronchospasm occurs, *see Severe asthma attack/status asthmaticus* above.

8 Sugammadex may be a safer reversal agent than neostigmine, which can cause excess secretions and muscarinic effects.

9 Patients with aspirin-sensitive asthma must not receive non-selective NSAIDs. *See Non-steroidal anti-inflammatory drugs (NSAIDs)*.

◗ Atenolol (Tenormin)

Selective beta-1 adrenoreceptor blocker drug used to treat hypertension, angina and tachydysrhythmias.

Dose for hypertension

Adult

2.5–10 mg IV. Give in 1 mg IV increments until desired response. PO 50–100 mg q 12-24 h.

Child

0.05 mg/kg IV every 5 min until desired response—maximum four doses. PO 1–2 mg/kg 12–24 h.

Dose for tachydysrhythmias

Adult

IV 2.5 mg over 2.5 min, repeat at 5 min intervals to achieve the desired effect. Maximum dose is 10 mg. PO dose 25–100 mg q 8–12 h.

◗ Atrial fibrillation (AF)

Introduction

AF is the most common pathological supraventricular tachyarrhythmia. In this condition, normal atrial contraction is lost, resulting in:

1 decreased ventricular filling (by up to 30%)

2 tachycardia, which can lead to cardiomyopathy or acute heart failure in the compromised heart

3 thromboembolic events

4 haemodynamic instability.

AF can be acute or chronic, asymptomatic or life threatening.

Diagnosis

The pulse is irregularly irregular. The ECG shows an absence of P waves, irregular R-R interval and a baseline between QRS complexes showing fibrillatory waves (S waves) or minute oscillations.

Causes

There are many causes of AF. It can be caused by almost any disease that affects the heart. Cardiac causes include:

1 ischaemic/valvular heart disease
2 cardiomyopathy/CCF
3 congenital heart disease
4 conduction abnormalities such as WPW
5 pericarditis/myocarditis
6 cardiac surgery.

Non-cardiac causes include:

1 thyrotoxicosis
2 electrolyte and acid/base disturbance
3 any acute severe illness
4 COPD
5 obesity/OSA
6 diabetes
7 alcohol
8 idiopathic (lone atrial fibrillation).

Aims of treatment

Always seek expert cardiologist advice urgently. Aims of treatment include:

1 conversion of AF to sinus rhythm (SR)
2 control of ventricular rate
3 prevention of thromboembolic events
4 identification and treatment of the cause.

Converting AF to SR

This can be by electrical and/or pharmacotherapy.

Emergency treatment

Patients require immediate treatment if:

1 ventricular rate > 150 bpm
2 chest pain
3 dyspnoea
4 haemodynamic compromise—SBP < 90 mmHg.

Administer synchronised biphasic cardioversion shocks 70–150 J utilising sedation or GA in the conscious patient. If cardioversion fails or AF reoccurs, give amiodarone 150–300 mg, ideally through a central line. Repeat cardioversion after amiodarone, and if this is not successful or AF reoccurs, give a second dose of amiodarone. A further 900 mg of amiodarone can be given by infusion over 24 h.

Non-emergency treatment

About 60% of cases will spontaneously revert within 16 hours of onset. Cardioversion must be done within 48 h of onset, otherwise a transoesophageal echo is required to exclude thrombus formation in the LA appendage.

Use sedation/GA and synchronised biphasic shocks 70–200 J. If this is unsuccessful or AF reoccurs, give amiodarone or flecainide. If the patient has atrial thrombus, heparinise the patient and commence warfarin. Anticoagulate the patient for 3–4 weeks. The thrombus must have resolved before cardioversion (electrical or drug treatment). If successful, continue to anticoagulate for 4 weeks.

For rate control while awaiting cardioversion consider:

1 beta blockers e.g. metoprolol 2.5–5 mg IV over 2–3 min, repeated at 5 min intervals as needed (maximum dose 15 mg). If using metoprolol PO, give 12.5–100 mg q 6–8 h.
2 digoxin. *See Digoxin*
3 calcium channel blockers e.g. diltiazem IV 0.25 mg/kg over 2 min then infusion of 5–15 mg/h for up to 24 h. A repeat bolus of 0.35 mg/kg may be needed. PO dose 30–120 mg q 6–8 h.

Persistent AF

This is treated with anticoagulation and rate control drugs. Catheter ablation therapy can be considered and has a high success rate.

⊙ Atrial flutter

Description

Re-entrant tachycardia that is usually due to a circuit between the orifice of the IVC and the tricuspid valve in the RA. This site is called the cavotricuspid isthmus (CTI). Typically, it is a regular, narrow complex tachycardia with an atrial rate of 300 bpm and a ventricular rate of 150 bpm. However, atrial flutter with variable block can be irregular.

Causes

1 Drugs used to treat AF e.g. amiodarone.
2 After ablation therapy for AF.
3 Any disorder that can cause AF can also cause atrial flutter—*see Atrial fibrillation (AF)*.

Diagnosis

The ECG shows a sawtooth atrial pattern (called F waves) at a rate of 300 (240–340) atrial complexes per minute. There is typically 2:1 block across the AV node so the ventricular rate is half the atrial rate. The patient requires a full cardiac workup, including cardiac echo.

Treatment

The treatment aims are the same as for AF—*see Atrial fibrillation (AF)*.

Rate control

1 Metoprolol or diltiazem.
2 Amiodarone—this may slow the flutter rate but also slow AV conduction with resultant 1:1 ratio between flutter waves and QRS complexes (slow atrial flutter).

Reversion to SR

1 Radiofrequency catheter ablation.
2 Cardioversion.
3 Ibutilide—available in the USA.

Prevention of thromboembolism

Treat as for AF.

◖ Atrial septal defect (ASD)

Description
An ASD is a congenital defect in which there is a hole in the septum between the left and right atria.

Types of ASD
1 Secundum ASD is a defect in the central part of the septum. It accounts for 75% of ASDs.
2 Primum ASD is close to the atrioventricular valves.
3 Sinus venosus defect—rare and occurs in the upper septum.
4 Coronary sinus defect—part of the wall between the left atrium and coronary sinus is missing.

Pathophysiology
Many ASDs spontaneously close, especially if they are < 3 mm in diameter. Due to the higher pressure in the left atrium compared with that in the right atrium, a left-to-right shunt occurs. A very small ASD may be of no clinical significance. However, a larger defect may cause the following.
1 Enlargement of the right ventricle (RV) due to RV volume overload.
2 Increased pulmonary blood flow, which can lead to the development of pulmonary hypertension and RV hypertrophy/failure.
3 Eventually RA pressure may exceed LA pressure and a right-to-left shunt occurs or the shunt can be bidirectional (Eisenmenger syndrome). *See Eisenmenger syndrome/Eisenmenger complex.*
4 Even if the shunt is predominantly left to right, some right-to-left shunting may also occur.[21]
5 Arrhythmias such as atrial fibrillation may occur.

Treatment
Although ASDs can usually be closed percutaneously with transcatheter techniques, open-heart surgery may be required.

Anaesthesia and ASD
The lesion may be repaired or unrepaired. Unrepaired ASDs may be trivial or have major clinical effects such as pulmonary hypertension or atrial fibrillation. (These complications are discussed under the relevant headings in this manual.) Cardiology consultation and advice is invaluable.
1 Ensure no air enters IV lines in case some right-to-left shunting is occurring and paradoxical embolism occurs.
2 Maintain adequate preload, normal heart rate and sinus rhythm.
3 Maintain balance between systemic vascular resistance (SVR) and pulmonary vascular resistance (PVR) to minimise shunt. An increase in SVR will increase left-to-right shunt and an increase in PVR will increase right-to-left shunt. Decreases in SVR or PVR will produce the opposite effect. *See Congenital heart disease (CHD) overview.*
4 Consider the need for bacterial endocarditis prophylaxis. *See Bacterial endocarditis (BE) prophylaxis.*

❏ Atrial switch procedure

See *Transposition of the great arteries (TGA)/transposition of the great vessels (TGV).*

❏ Atrioventricular block

See *Heart block (HB).*

❏ Atrioventricular nodal re-entrant tachycardia (AVNRT)

The most common form of SVT. There are episodes of tachycardia with abrupt onset and offset. It is due to a re-entrant circuit in or near the AV node. The circuit usually consists of a fast pathway and a slow pathway in the RA. The fast pathway is usually superior and posterior to the AV node, and the slow pathway is close to or within the AV node.

Usually antegrade conduction (atria to ventricles) is through the slow pathway, and retrograde conduction (ventricles to atria) occurs through the fast pathway (slow-fast AVNRT); but it can occur the other way around (fast-slow AVNRT).

Symptoms/signs

Usually occur in young females.
1 Palpitations.
2 Faintness.
3 Dyspnoea.
4 Hypotension.

Neck vein pulsations (cannon waves) may be prominent due to the atria and ventricles contracting at—or nearly at—the same time.

The ECG shows:
1 onset after a premature atrial beat
2 regular narrow complex tachycardia, usually between 140–280 bpm
3 inverted P waves which may be buried in the QRS complex or occur just after it (a secondary R wave). These are P waves travelling towards the SA node (like an echo). Often the P waves cannot be found but a hint is a rSr pattern in V1, which is not present when the patient is in sinus rhythm.
4 short RP distance (< 100 ms)
5 a wide QRS may occur due to bundle branch block.

Treatment

This arrhythmia is **not usually** life threatening. Treatment includes:
1 vagal manoeuvres—**see** *Vagal manoeuvres*
2 adenosine—**see** *Adenosine*
3 verapamil—this is preferred in patients with asthma
4 metoprolol
5 cardioversion
6 electrophysiological studies and radiofrequency ablation.

❏ Atrioventricular re-entrant tachycardia (AVRT)

This type of arrhythmia is due to an accessory pathway (AP) between the atria and ventricles (in addition to the AV node). This is a rapid tachyarrhythmia in which electricity travels in a circuit made up of atria, AP, AV node and ventricle. In orthodromic AVRT, electricity travels through the AV node in an antegrade direction (atria to ventricles). In an antidromic AVRT, electricity travels through the AV node in a retrograde direction (from ventricle to atria). The tachycardia is almost always induced by an atrial ectopic.

Orthodromic AVRT

On the ECG the QRS looks normal (unless there is bundle branch block). There is no delta wave and a P wave is seen after the QRS complex (a retrograde P wave). The rate is usually 150–250 bpm. It can be initiated by atrial or ventricular ectopics.

Antidromic AVRT

On the ECG there are widened QRS complexes with delta waves. It may be very difficult to distinguish this ECG appearance from VT. P waves are usually not visible but, if they are, they are seen before the QRS complex. HR is usually 150–250 bpm.

Treatment of orthodromic AVRT[22]

1 Urgent DC cardioversion if patient haemodynamically compromised.
2 Vagal manoeuvres. *See Vagal manoeuvres.*
3 Adenosine and/or verapamil.
4 Electrophysiological studies and radiofrequency ablation.

Treatment of antidromic AVRT[22]

1 Urgent DC cardioversion if patient haemodynamically compromised.
2 Procainamide.
3 Second-line antiarrhythmics—ibutilide, amiodarone.
4 Semi-urgent cardioversion.
5 Electrophysiological studies and radiofrequency ablation.

◘ Atrioventricular septal defect (AVSD)

Description

Only a brief description of this complex condition is offered. In this congenital heart disease (CHD) there are holes between the chambers of the right and left heart and abnormalities of the tricuspid and mitral valves. This is also called 'atrioventricular canal defect', 'endocardial cushion defect' or 'persistent AV ostium'. It is commonly associated with Down syndrome. *See Down syndrome.* It accounts for 4–5% of CHD.

Types of AVSD

1 Complete AVSD (CAVSD)—this is a large hole in the centre of the heart and all four chambers are connected to each other. There is one common valve between the atria and ventricles which is malformed. The CAVSD may be balanced or unbalanced. If balanced the ventricles are roughly equal in size and if unbalanced, one ventricle is hypoplastic. The single valve sits predominantly above the dominant ventricle.
2 Partial or incomplete AVSD—there is a hole in the upper ventricular septum or lower atrial septum or both and an abnormality of the mitral or, less commonly, the tricuspid valve.

Clinical effects of AVSD

AVSD may cause:
1 dysrhythmias
2 CCF
3 pulmonary hypertension.

Treatment

Surgical repair of the defect(s). Life-long follow-up is required. The most common complication is mitral incompetence.

◗ Atropine

Description
Atropine is an anticholinergic drug which acts competitively on muscarinic receptors. *See Acetylcholine receptors (cholinergic receptors)*. It is used to treat bradycardia by opposing vagal tone and to counteract the muscarinic-stimulating effects of acetylcholinesterase inhibitors such as neostigmine.
See Neostigmine. It is also used to treat organophosphate poisoning.

Dose

Adult
1   Bradycardia 0.4-1.2 mg IV up to 2 mg.
2   Counteract the side-effects of neostigmine used to reverse NMBDs—0.6 mg atropine IV.
3   Treatment of organophosphate poisoning—0.8 mg IM up to 2 mg IM every h.

Child
For bradycardia give 0.02 mg/kg up to 0.5 mg/dose. Repeat at 5 min intervals to a maximum dose of 1 mg.

Atropine effects on the brain
Atropine crosses the blood–brain barrier. It can result in confusion, hallucinations and excitation, especially in the elderly. *See Central anticholinergic syndrome.* The antidote is physostigmine. *See Physostigmine*.

◗ Autonomic hyperreflexia

See Spinal cord injury (pre-existing) and anaesthesia.

◗ AVPU

This is a neurological state assessment tool. The letters stand for:
A – **A**lert—eyes open spontaneously, aware and responsive to environment; obeys commands
V – **V**oice—eyes do not open spontaneously but will open to verbal stimuli; able to respond in some meaningful way to voice
P – **P**ain—responds to painful stimuli but not verbal stimuli
U – **U**nresponsive—patient does not respond to any stimuli
A person's score corresponds to what letter they are on the AVPU scale.

◗ Awake intubation

(Relative) indications
1   A patient that is known to be, or likely to be, very difficult/impossible to intubate.
2   Unstable cervical spine.
3   Threatened airway with pathology likely to make intubation difficult.
4   Inability to open the mouth more than 2.5–3 cm.

Options for awake intubation
1   Fibre-optic bronchoscope (FOB).
2   Non fibre-optic video-endoscope (VE).
3   Videolaryngoscope.
4   Oral or nasal route—the nasal route is easier.

Technique for awake nasal intubation using FOB or VE in the adult

There are many ways of topicalising the airway. This is one way. A second anaesthetist will be of great assistance. Use 2% lignocaine with 1:200 000 adrenaline for topicalisation. Do not use more than 20 mL in an adult. Decide which nostril is the most patent. Spray cophenylcaine into the selected nostril.

1 Give glycopyrrolate 200 mcg IV to dry oral secretions.
2 Administer 4 mL of LA via a nebuliser with an O_2 source of 5 L/min.
3 Using cotton swab sticks soaked in LA, anaesthetise the floor of the nose and the pathway the ET tube will take, by gradually advancing the swab sticks.
4 Ask the patient to gargle 4 mL LA and then swallow it.
5 Use a DeVilbiss-type nebuliser to spray the back of the mouth with LA, and swivel the nozzle downwards to spray the cords.
6 Smear a size 6.5 mm nasal airway with lignocaine jelly and pass this slowly through the chosen nostril.
7 When this is tolerated, spray LA through the lumen of the nasal airway with the DeVilbiss-type nebuliser.
8 The voice should become hoarse.
9 Provide O_2 with transnasal humidified rapid insufflation ventilatory exchange (the Fisher & Paykel Optiflow™ THRIVE system).
10 Give midazolam IV in incremental doses of 1–2 mg up to 5 mg.
11 Administer fentanyl IV in incremental doses of 25–50 mcg up to 100 mcg.
12 Start a propofol infusion TCI 1 mcg/mL—titrate up or down to desired level of sedation.
13 Suction oral secretions with a Yankauer sucker.
14 Prepare the FOB or VE. Apply anti-fog to the tip. Load an ET tube onto the scope. A Fastrach 6.5 mm for a female or 7.0 mm for a male works very well but may be too short. A Blue Line Nasal RAE tube is another good choice. If using a PVC non-reinforced tube, soften the tip in hot water. Make sure the ET tube is well lubricated.
15 Pass an epidural catheter through the working channel on the scope to give more LA.
16 The author's preference is to stand behind the patient with the bed ramped up in a semi-sitting position. Other anaesthetists stand facing the patient.
17 Ask an assistant to pull the jaw forward. Alternatively, the assistant can grasp the tongue with gauze and pull it forward.
18 Insert the FOB or VE through the nose and navigate to the vocal cords. Instil another 3–4 mL of LA onto the vocal cords via the epidural catheter.
19 Insert the scope through the cords and identify the carina.
20 Pass the ET tube so the tip is above the carina and then remove the scope.
21 Attach the anaesthetic circuit and confirm exhaled CO_2, then commence GA.

Awake oral intubation

1 Give IV glycopyrrolate and nebulised LA as described above.
2 Use a DeVilbiss-type nebuliser to spray the back of the mouth with LA, and swivel the nozzle downwards to spray the cords.
3 Place a layer of lignocaine jelly 2% on the upper tongue.
4 Sedate the patient as described above.
5 Provide O_2 with transnasal humidified rapid insufflation ventilatory exchange (the Fisher & Paykel Optiflow™ THRIVE system).

6 Prepare the intubating endoscope as described above. Consider blowing O_2 through the suction port to blow away secretions.

7 Insert a Berman or Ovassapian airway into the mouth. Make sure it is positioned in the midline.

8 Some intubating airways, such as the Ovassapian, have a tendency to allow the FOB or VE to fall out of the large rear slot. This can be mitigated by placing the ET tube into the Ovassapian airway, but not through it, to guide the FOB or VE.

9 Insert the intubating endoscope through the airway and into the larynx. Supplement topical anaesthesia with LA injected through the working channel of the FOB or VE.

10 Once the trachea is entered, remove the oral airway and intubate the patient. Confirm correct placement with $ETCO_2$.

11 Induce anaesthesia.

◗ Awareness monitoring

Introduction

The most common and effective types of awareness monitoring are Bispectral Index (BIS) and Entropy. Both systems use algorithmic analysis of highly processed electroencephalograph (EEG) brain waves.

BIS

A number between 0 and 100 is derived—0 corresponds to isoelectric EEG and 100 to wakefulness. Aim for a BIS 40–59 to reduce the risk of awareness while avoiding excessive anaesthesia.

Entropy

Two numbers are generated representing State Entropy (SE) and Response Entropy (RE).

State entropy (SE)

SE reflects the level of hypnosis of the patient. It is a stable indicator of the effect the anaesthetic is having on the brain, similar to BIS monitoring. It is measured between 0 and 91, and < 60 corresponds with anaesthesia.

Response entropy (RE)

This measurement is sensitive to the activation of facial muscles. It is designed to give a faster response than SE and give an early warning of arousal and potential consciousness (about 7 s faster than SE). RE is measured from 0–100 and, again, < 60 suggests anaesthesia.

◗ Axillary vein central venous access

See Subclavian vein central venous access.

REFERENCES

1 Kothandan H, Chieh GLH, Kan SA, Karthekeyan RB, Sharad SS. Anesthetic considerations for endovascular abdominal aortic aneurysm repair. *Ann Card Anesth* 2016; 19: 132–141.

2 Hinchliffe R. Editorial: Metformin and abdominal aortic aneurysm. *Eur J Vasc Endovasc Surg* 2017; 54: 679–680.

3 Thompson AR, Cooper JA, Ashton HA, Hafez H. Growth rates of small abdominal aortic aneurysms correlate with clinical events. *Br J Surg* 2010; 97: 37–44.

4   Metcalf D, Holt PJE, Thomson MM. The management of abdominal aortic aneurysms. *Br Med J* 2011; 342: 644–649.

5   Bickell WH, Wall MJ, Jr, Pepe PE et al. Immediate versus delayed fluid resuscitation for hypotensive patients with penetrating torso injuries. *New E J Med* 1994; 331: 1105–1109.

6   Leonard A, Thompson J. Anaesthesia for ruptured abdominal aortic aneurysm. *Cont Educ Anaesth Crit Care Pain* 2008; 8: 11–15.

7   Beasley R, Chien J, Douglas J et al. Thoracic Society of Australia and New Zealand oxygen guidelines for acute oxygen use in adults. *Respirology* 2015; 20: 1182–1191.

8   Purvey M, Allen G. Managing acute pulmonary oedema. *Australian Prescriber* 2017; 40: 59–63.

9   Aoyama H, Yamada Y, Fan E. The future of driving pressure: a goal for mechanical ventilation. *J Intens Care* 2018: 64. Accessed online: https://jintensivecare. biomedcentral.com/articles/10.1186/s40560-018-0334-4b04, December 2022.

10 Hamilton N, Nandkeolyar S, Lan H et al. Amiodarone: a comprehensive guide for clinicians. *Am J Cardiovasc Drugs* 2020; 20: 549–558.

11 Takazawa T, Mitsuhata H, Mertes PM. Sugammadex and rocuronium-induced anaphylaxis. *J of Anaesth* 2016; 20: 290–297.

12 Roshanov PS, Rochverg B, Patel A et al. Withholding versus continuing angiotensin-converting enzyme inhibitors or angiotensin II receptor blockers before noncardiac surgery: an analysis of vascular events in noncardiac surgery patients cohort evaluation prospective cohort. *Anesthesiol* 2017; 126: 16–27.

13 Douketis JD, Spyropoulos AC, Spencer FA et al. American College of Chest Physicians. Perioperative management of antithrombotic therapy: antithrombotic therapy and prevention of thrombosis, 9th ed: American College of Chest Physicians Evidence-Based Clinical Practice Guidelines. *Chest* 2012; 141 2 Suppl: e326–50S.

14 South Eastern Sydney Local Health District. *SESLHDPR/600 Protocol for the Safe Use of Danaparoid*. Version 2, October 2021. Accessed online: www.seslhd.health.nsw. gov.au/sites/default/files/documents/SESLHDPR%20600%20Danaparoid%20-%20 Prescibing%20Protocol.pdfline (nsw.gov.au), December 2022.

15 Parakh S, Naik N, Rohatgi N et al. Eptifibatide overdose. *Int J Cardiol* 2009; 131: 430–432.

16 Hebballi R, Swanevelder J. Diagnosis and management of aortic dissection. *Cont Edu Anaesth Crit Care Pain* 2009; 9: 14–18.

17 Sanivarapu RR, Gibson J. *Aspiration pneumonia*. StatPearls NCBI Bookshelf 2022, StatPearls Publishing. Accessed online: www.ncbi.nlm.nih.gov/books/NBK470459/, January 2023.

18 Fanta CH, Cahill KN. Acute exacerbations of asthma in adults: emergency department and inpatient management. *UpToDate* May 2022. Accessed online: www.uptodate.com/ contents/acute-exacerbations-of-asthma-in-adults-emergency-department-and-inpatient-management?search=asthma%20exacerbation%20adult&source=search_result&selecte dTitle=2~150&usage_type=default&display_rank=2, June 2022.

19 Barnes PJ. Theophylline. *Am J Resp Crit Care Med* 2013; 188: 901–906.

20 Burburan SM, Xisto DG, Rocco PRM. Anaesthetic management in asthma. *Minerva Anesthesiol* 2007; 73: 357–365.

21 Yen P. ASD and VSD flow dynamics and anesthetic management. *Anesth Prog* 2015; 62: 125–130.

22 Buttner R. Atrioventricular re-entry tachycardia (AVRT). *Life in the Fastlane—ECG Library* May 2020. Accessed online: https://litfl.com/atrioventricular-re-entry-tachycardia-avrt/#:~:text=Robert%20Buttner%20May%2020%2C%202022%20Home%20ECG%20 Library,circuit%20between%20the%20AV%20node%20and%20accessory%20pathway, December 2022.

B

○ Bacterial endocarditis (BE) prophylaxis

Description
Bacterial endocarditis is a life-threatening inflammation of the endocardium and valves caused by a bacterial infection. Certain lesions predispose to this infection, and antibiotic prophylaxis is recommended for some types of dental procedures or surgery. The evidence for this practice is sparse.

Patients predisposed to BE for whom prophylaxis is recommended[1]
1 History of BE.
2 Prosthetic heart valve.
3 Prosthetic material used for heart valve repair.
4 Congenital heart disease (CHD) involving unrepaired cyanotic heart defects, including shunts and conduits.
5 CHD with defects completely repaired with prosthetic material or device **for the first six months post repair**. After this time, the prosthetic material should be endothelialised.
6 CHD with repaired defects but with residual defects at, or adjacent to, the site of the prosthetic patch or device. The residual defect can inhibit endothelialisation.
7 Rheumatic heart disease in indigenous Australians or others at significant socio-economic risk.
8 Heart transplant patients (consult patient's cardiologist for specific recommendations). The usual indication is a structurally abnormal valve.

Procedures that require BE prophylaxis
Dental
1 Extractions.
2 Replanting avulsed teeth.
3 Periodontal procedures, including subgingival scaling and root planing.
4 Other invasive dental procedures.

Respiratory
1 Any procedure requiring incision into the respiratory mucosa, including tonsils, adenoids, bronchial, sinus, nasal or middle ear mucosa.
2 Nasotracheal intubation.

Genitourinary
1 Any procedure for which antibiotic prophylaxis is indicated for surgical reasons e.g. lithotripsy.
2 Any procedure where there is pre-existing infection unless the patient is already being treated with antibiotics targeting the infecting organism.

Gastrointestinal
1 Sclerotherapy for oesophageal varices.
2 Any procedure in the presence of intra-abdominal infection unless the patient is already being treated with antibiotics targeting the infecting organism.
3 Percutaneous endoscopic gastrostomy.

Other
1 Incision and drainage of abscesses (brain, epidural, lung, orbit, liver and other sites).
2 Surgery involving cutting through infected skin.

Antibiotics for BE prophylaxis[1]
1 Dental procedures—amoxicillin 2 g PO 1 h before procedure. If penicillin allergic, clindamycin 600 mg PO 1 h before procedure.
2 All other procedures—amoxicillin 2 g IV 30–60 min prior to procedure. If penicillin allergic, clindamycin 600 mg IV 30–60 min prior to the procedure or vancomycin 1 g IV over 1 h, started 30 min to 2 h before procedure. Give clindamycin over 20 min. Give vancomycin 1.5 g over 90 min if patient > 80 kg.
   Children's dosages are amoxicillin 50 mg/kg up to 2 g, clindamycin 20 mg/kg up to 600 mg, vancomycin 30 mg/kg.

◉ Ballantyne syndrome

See Mirror syndrome.

◉ Bariatric surgery

Introduction
Obese class 2 and 3 patients present a significant anaesthetic challenge. Some frequently associated co-morbidities are:
1 hypertension
2 NIDDM
3 OSA
4 elevated cholesterol.

Types of bariatric surgery
These can be divided into restrictive and malabsorptive procedures.

Restrictive surgery
1 Adjustable gastric band.
2 Sleeve gastrectomy—removes about 80% of the stomach.
3 Endoscopically placed gastric balloon.

Malabsorptive surgery
Roux-en-Y gastric bypass. Involves anastomosing a surgically formed gastric pouch to the proximal jejunum, bypassing the duodenum.

One anaesthetic approach
This section addresses pharmacological issues with bariatric surgery. Other issues such as intubation and positioning are not specific to bariatric surgery.

Induction
Many anaesthetists who provide a bariatric anaesthetic service minimise the use of opioids. Be prepared for a difficult intubation. Make sure the patient is well preoxygenated prior to induction.

QUICK FLICK B

1 Patient to walk into operating theatre and position themselves on the operating table. Both arms on arm-boards at right angles to the operating table. Wrap the arms. Under-arm cushions may be available.
2 Position the operating table with the upper body ramped and the head and neck in the ideal intubating position. **See *Difficult airway management*.**
3 Administer lignocaine 1–1.5 mg/kg IV.
4 Administer a loading dose of dexmedetomidine 0.5 mcg/kg over 10 min. For an 80 kg patient, this equals 40 mcg.
5 Induce anaesthesia with propofol and paralyse patient with rocuronium.
6 Spray the vocal cords with cophenylcaine prior to intubation.
7 Insert an orogastric tube to empty the stomach.
8 Do not insert a temperature probe as it might become sutured into the stomach.
9 Propofol infusion with entropy/BIS monitoring for induction and maintenance of anaesthesia.
10 Cefazolin 2 g (3 g > 120 kg).

Intraoperative medications
Use ideal body weight (IBW) for calculations. **See *Ideal body weight (IBW)*.**
1 Dexmedetomidine IV infusion—0.5 mcg/kg/h. For an 80 kg patient, this equals 40 mcg/h.
2 Ketamine—0.5 mg/kg/h. Aim for about 100 mg total dose by the end of the case.
3 Magnesium—2.5 g IV post induction then 2.5 g/h.
4 Lignocaine infusion—1 mg/kg/h.
5 Tramadol—200 mg over 2 h (load into first bag of IV fluids).
6 Ondansetron 4 mg + dexamethasone + droperidol 0.625 mg (all IV).
7 Boluses of IV metaraminol 0.5 mg for hypotension.
8 Oxycodone—2.5–5 mg IV.
9 Parecoxib—40 mg IV.
10 Buscopan—10 mg IV prior to head-up positioning and 10 mg IV prior to insertion of the bougie.
11 Sugammadex for reversal of muscle relaxation.
12 Hartmann's solution or Plasma-Lyte for IV fluids.

Postoperative instructions
1 Nurse semi-recumbent with supplementary O_2 via nasal prongs. Use CPAP/high-flow nasal O_2 as required.
2 Oxycodone 2.5 mg IV boluses to alleviate pain in recovery, to a maximum dose of 10 mg.
3 Tramadol—50–100 mg IV prn q 4 h to a maximum of 400 mg/day.
4 Cyclizine for nausea—50 mg IV q 8 h, maximum 150 mg/day.
5 Treat postoperative hypertension with hydralazine—10 mg q 10 min × 3 doses.
6 Oxycodone syrup PO for pain 5–10 mg q 3 h.
7 Buscopan—IV 10–20 mg q 6 h for 24 h.
8 Droperidol—0.625 mg IV q 8 h for 24 h.
9 Paracetamol—1 g IV q 6 h.
10 Pantoprazole—40 mg IV q 12 h.
11 DVT/PE prophylaxis (heparin or Clexane)—discuss with surgeon.

◖ Benign intracranial hypertension (BIH)

Description
BIH is characterised by raised intracranial pressure (> 20 cm CSF) in the absence of any identifiable cause. It is also called 'idiopathic intracranial hypertension' or

'pseudotumor cerebri'. BIH may be related to the oral contraceptive pill, vitamin A intake and the use of certain antibiotics such as tetracycline. Clinical effects include:

1 headaches
2 nausea and vomiting
3 vision disturbances
4 no enlargement of the brain's ventricles
5 no focal neurological signs except for papilloedema, and occasionally a VI nerve palsy
6 intracranial buzzing sounds
7 pulsatile tinnitus
8 normal CSF.

BIH is most commonly seen in overweight women between the ages of 20–50 years.

Diagnosis
1 Clinical history.
2 Papilloedema.
3 Brain imaging (CT, MRI) to exclude intracerebral pathology.
4 Lumbar puncture to measure CSF pressure and analyse the CSF, which should be normal.

Treatment
1 Weight loss.
2 Diuretics such as acetazolamide, frusemide.
3 Repeat lumbar punctures.
4 Steroids may provide temporary relief.
5 Surgery—lumbo-peritoneal shunting and optic nerve sheath fenestration.

BIH and obstetrics
1 BIH is not a contraindication to subarachnoid block.
2 Symptomatic patients with BIH may have an exacerbation of their symptoms with SAB. An epidural topped up slowly may be better tolerated.

◐ Benzatropine/benztropine (Cogentin)

Description
Anticholinergic and antihistamine drug that is useful for treating dystonic reactions, Parkinson's disease and dystonia. It is a centrally acting M1 muscarinic acetylcholine receptor blocker, which results in decreased reuptake and storage of dopamine.

Dose
For dystonic reaction, give 1–2 mg IV slowly. *See Dystonic reaction, acute.*

◐ Beta-adrenergic receptor blocker drugs

Types of beta blocker drugs
For a description of the function of beta receptors—*see Adrenergic receptors.*
There are two types of beta blocker drugs: selective and non-selective.

1 Selective beta blockers target mainly beta-1 receptors (also called 'cardio-selective drugs'). These are used to treat high blood pressure and heart failure by reducing the heart rate and force of contraction. They include atenolol, metoprolol and bisoprolol. These drugs are about 20 times more selective for beta-1 receptors than for beta-2 receptors.

2 Non-selective beta blockers are first-generation drugs and are more likely to have unwanted side effects such as bronchoconstriction. This group includes propranolol, timolol and pindolol. Sotalol, unlike other beta blockers, has type 3 antidysrhythmic properties.

Indications

1 Hypertension.
2 Angina control—by reducing heart rate, force of contraction and myocardial oxygen consumption.
3 Treatment of some tachydysrhythmias.
4 Heart failure.
5 Control of essential tremor.
6 Migraine.
7 Glaucoma.
8 Hyperthyroidism.
9 Alcohol withdrawal.

Side effects

1 Bronchoconstriction.
2 Inhibition of gluconeogenesis and glycogenolysis, which may result in hypoglycaemia.
3 Bradycardia.
4 Fatigue.

Contraindications

1 Asthma.
2 Severe conduction disorders.
3 Symptomatic bradycardia.
4 Symptomatic hypotension.

Beta blockers and pregnancy

Beta blockers should be avoided in pregnancy because they cause fetal bradycardia. Long-term use of atenolol can cause fetal growth restriction. However, labetalol and oxprenolol can be used in pregnancy.

Beta blocker overdose

This can result in profound bradycardia and hypotension. Atropine and isoprenaline may be ineffective. A suggested treatment is glucagon 50 mcg/kg LD then an infusion of 1–15 mg/h titrated to clinical effect (pulse rate, blood pressure). The mechanism of action of glucagon is unclear. **See *Glucagon*.**

◖ Betamethasone

This is a steroid drug given to the parturient to accelerate fetal lung maturity for threatened or anticipated premature birth. Give 12 mg IV repeated in 12 h. It reduces the risk of infant respiratory distress syndrome and decreases incidence of infant intracranial haemorrhage.

◖ Between the flags (BTF)

Description

This is a charting system (either hard copy or digital) that is used to identify the deteriorating patient in some hospitals. The chart is used to record vital signs. It has yellow zones indicating the need for escalation of care and red zones indicating the need for urgent escalation of care. This is a 'track and trigger' system. Observations 'between the flags' are satisfactory and do not 'trigger' a response. For observations in the yellow zone, the nurse in charge must be notified. If observations are in the red zone, a rapid response medical review must be initiated.

Vital signs recorded for adults are:

1 respiratory rate (breaths per min)—BTF 10–25; yellow zone lower rate 5–10 and yellow zone upper rate 25–30; red zone lower rate 0–5 and red zone upper rate 30+

2 heart rate—BTF 50–120 bpm; yellow zone lower rate 40–50 bpm and yellow zone upper rate 120–140 bpm; red zone lower rate < 40 bpm and red zone upper rate > 140 bpm

3 blood pressure (SBP is the trigger)—BTF 100–179 mmHg; yellow zone upper level 180–200 mmHg, yellow zone lower level 90–99 mmHg; red zone upper level > 200 mmHg, red zone lower level < 90 mmHg

4 oxygen saturation—BTF 95–100%; yellow zone 90–94%; red zone < 90%

5 disability/neurological state—use AVPU (*see AVPU*). Yellow zone, opens eyes to verbal stimuli; red zone, PU (relates to **P**ain or **U**nresponsive).

◗ Bidirectional Glenn shunt

Also known as a 'hemi-Fontan procedure', this is used in patients with congenital heart disease (CHD), resulting in a single functional ventricle. The superior vena cava (SVC) is connected to the pulmonary artery prior to bifurcation into the right and left pulmonary arteries. It is called 'bidirectional' because the SVC blood flows into both the right and left lungs. In the Glenn shunt, the SVC is connected to the right pulmonary artery. *See Glenn shunt*.

◗ Biostate

A lyophilised concentrate of human factor VIII (FVIII) and von Willebrand factor (VWF) from plasma. *See Von Willebrand disease (VWD)*. The ratio of FVIII to VWF is 1:2. It is useful for the prevention and treatment of bleeding associated with VWD. It can be used to treat haemophilia A, but factor VIII concentrate is preferred.
See Factor VIII concentrate.

Dose
Depends on the type of bleeding. Dose can be expressed as factor VIII units or VWF units.

Table B1 Dose of Biostate for different bleeding situations

Type of bleeding	Factor VIII units	VWF units
Epistaxis/menorrhagia	25 U/kg	50 U/kg
GIT bleeding	40 U/kg	80 U/kg
CNS bleeding	60 U/kg	120 U/kg
Trauma/surgery	60 U/kg	120 U/kg

◗ BIS monitoring

See Awareness monitoring.

⊙ Bisoprolol (Concor)

Beta-1 selective beta blocker drug. Used to treat stable, chronic, moderately severe heart failure (in addition to ACE inhibitors, diuretics ± cardiac glycosides).

⊙ Bivalirudin (Angiomax, Angiox)

Direct thrombin inhibitor similar to hirudin. It is used as an alternative to heparin for patients with HIT. *See Heparin-induced thrombocytopenia (HIT)*. Can be used as an alternative to heparin for percutaneous coronary intervention (with antiplatelet drugs). It increases APTT, PT and ACT.

Dose

Adult

0.75 mg/kg bolus IV, then infusion 1.75 mg/kg/h for the duration of the procedure and for up to 4 h afterwards. It has a fast onset (minutes) and offset (half-life 25 min).

⊙ Blalock–Taussig (BT) shunt

Procedure to connect the systemic and pulmonary circulations to improve pulmonary blood flow in congenital heart disease (CHD) causing impaired pulmonary blood flow. It is used as a palliative procedure for conditions such as Tetralogy of Fallot (TOF), pulmonary stenosis, hypoplastic left heart, tricuspid atresia and pulmonary atresia. Originally the surgery involved connecting the subclavian artery directly to the ipsilateral pulmonary artery. In the modified BT shunt, a synthetic graft is used for the connection. *See Tetralogy of Fallot (TOF)*. It functions in a similar way to the ductus arteriosus, but flow is in the opposite direction to that of the fetal circulation.

⊙ Bleomycin

See Immunosuppressive and chemotherapy drugs—anaesthetic implications.

⊙ Blood filters

There are several types of blood filters available. They include:
1 Standard 200 micron blood administration screen filter.
2 Leukocyte depletion filter—these have charged surfaces that attract negatively charged leukocytes. They are used in situations such as transplant surgery. *See Renal transplant*.
3 Lipid reduction filter—salvaged blood may contain a significant amount of lipid, as can occur with orthopaedic surgery. These filters minimise the infusion of lipid substances.

⊙ Blood groups

Blood groups are based on two factors: antigens on RBC and antibodies in the plasma. The blood groups are O, A, B and AB.
• AB has no antibodies in the plasma and is the universal recipient.
• O has anti-A and anti-B antibodies in the plasma.
• A has anti-B in the plasma.
• B has anti-A in the plasma.
  The Rhesus factor status (positive or negative) is included in the blood group. Rhesus (Rh) factor is a type of protein found on the surface of RBC of Rh-positive

individuals. 85% of the population is Rh positive. Blood groups have the following **approximate** population percentages:

1 O positive 42%, O negative 3%
2 A positive 31%, A negative 2.5%
3 B positive 15%, B negative 1%
4 AB positive 5%, AB negative 0.5%.

Table B2 Blood donor and recipient compatibility table

Recipient's blood group	Can have blood group	Can have FFP group
Rh positive	Rh negative or positive	Ignore Rh status
Rh negative	Rh negative	Ignore Rh status
O	O	O, A, B, or AB
A	A	A, AB
B	B	B, AB
AB	A, B, O, AB	AB

Blood loss—assessment, management and anaesthetic approach

Topics covered in this section
- Definitions of massive haemorrhage/transfusion and critical bleeding
- Classes of haemorrhagic shock (from the American College of Surgeons)
- Physiology of haemorrhagic shock
- Therapeutic aims
- Indicators of critical physiological derangement
- Resuscitation and anaesthesia in association with massive blood loss
- Massive transfusion protocol (MTP)
- Resuscitation targets
- Patient with unknown blood group
- Anaesthesia for patient with pre-induction massive blood loss
- Some practical aspects of transfusion

Definitions of massive haemorrhage/transfusion and critical bleeding
1 Transfusion of half of the patient's total blood volume (TBV) in 4 h, or more than patient's TBV transfused in 24 h. TBV in adults 17 mL/kg or about 10 units of packed cells. TBV in children older than 1 year is about 80 mL/kg.
2 Blood loss > 150 mL/min in the adult.
3 Critical bleeding is defined as bleeding that is life threatening or potentially life threatening.
4 In children, massive blood loss/critical bleeding can be defined as transfusion of more than 40 mL/kg of packed cells.

Classes of haemorrhagic shock (from the American College of Surgeons)
- TBV based on a 70 kg male—4.9–5 L
- Advanced trauma support (ATLS) classification

<15% or 0-750 mL of TBV lost (Class 1)
Little physiological effect—no resuscitation needed. Urine output (UO) > 30 mL/h. Systolic blood pressure (SBP) normal, pulse pressure (PP) normal or increased. *See Pulse pressure.* Normal capillary refill time (2 s or less).

15–30% TBV or 750–1500 mL (Class 2)

1 HR 100–120 bpm.
2 SBP normal, PP decreased. PP is considered low if it is < 25% of SBP.
3 Respiratory rate (RR) 20–30 breaths/min.
4 UO 20–30 mL/h.
5 Cool extremities.
6 Anxiety, light headedness, thirst.
7 Skin and capillary refill > 2 s, clammy skin.
IV fluid resuscitation required.

30–40% TBV or 1500–2000 mL (Class 3)

1 HR 120–140 bpm.
2 SBP decreased to 70–80 mmHg, PP decreased.
3 RR 30–40 breaths per min.
4 UO 5–15 mL/h.
5 Anxiety/confusion/weakness/fatigue—may feel nauseated.
6 Weak pulse, pale, cool and clammy skin.
7 Capillary refill > 3 s.
IV fluid resuscitation required +/− packed cells +/− other blood products.

More than 40% TBV or 2000 mL blood loss (Class 4)

1 HR > 140 bpm.
2 SBP/PP decreased (SBP 50–70 mmHg). Cardiopulmonary failure.
3 RR > 40 breaths/min.
4 UO negligible.
5 Confusion, lethargy, LOC.
6 Multisystem organ failure.
7 Cold, mottled skin.
8 Capillary refill > 3 s.
Critical blood loss. Provide packed cells +/− other blood products.

Physiology of haemorrhagic shock

The 'bloody lethal triad' of haemorrhage is acidosis, hypothermia and coagulopathy.

Acidosis

Acute blood loss leads to insufficient oxygen to the end organs/tissues, causing:
1 anaerobic metabolism
2 lactic acid production
3 acidosis.
   Acidosis can impair cardiac function, exacerbating tissue hypoperfusion.
It can also reduce coagulation factor activity and thrombin generation, and decrease clot stability. Acidosis can be worsened by the reduced pH in stored packed cells transfused in large quantities. Ischaemic tissues can also release inflammatory substances, producing the systemic inflammatory response syndrome (SIRS). This can result in exacerbation of hypotension and hypothermia, throwing, so to speak, more fuel on the fire.

Hypothermia (core temperature < 35°C)

The causes of hypothermia in haemorrhagic shock are many and include exposure, reduced metabolic activity of cells, impaired central thermoregulation (e.g. reduced shivering) and infusion of cold IV fluids. Hypothermia can cause reduced platelet activation, reduced enzyme activity (impairing thrombin generation) and increased fibrinolysis.

Coagulopathy

There are many causes of coagulopathy in haemorrhagic shock. They include loss of factors in shed blood, consumption of clotting factors and platelets, dilution of clotting factors by infused IV fluids/packed cells, the effects of acidosis and hypothermia and the effects of citrate in blood products. In severe trauma, 25% of patients develop a sudden acute coagulopathy called acute traumatic coagulopathy (ATC). This is most likely due to protein C activation, which in turn activates coagulation and fibrinolytic pathways. *See Protein C and protein S*.

Therapeutic aims

1 Identify the source(s) of blood loss. Bleeding may be concealed (long bone fractures—especially femur—chest, abdomen, pelvis) or revealed/external (on the floor, haematemesis/melaena/haematochezia).
2 **Stop the bleeding**—techniques include compression (including arterial compression); elevation of the bleeding site; tourniquet use; re-establishing correct anatomical position (splint, pelvic binder); rapid temporary closure of wounds; packing of wounds; intra-aortic balloon to reduce blood flow to bleeding site; surgery including damage control surgery; angiography with embolisation and topical haemostatic agents.
3 Maintain/achieve adequate blood volume and blood pressure. Consider permissive hypotension with minimal volume resuscitation while active bleeding is being controlled e.g. ruptured aortic aneurysm (termed 'damage control resuscitation'). A target SBP of 80–100 mmHg is suggested. Permissive hypotension is contraindicated in patients with traumatic brain injury and/or spinal injury. Use this approach with caution in the elderly. Colloids, especially albumin, should also not be used in the situation of critical brain injury.
4 Maintain/achieve a haemoglobin concentration sufficient to carry oxygen for the needs of the tissues.
5 Prevent/reverse coagulopathy, acidosis and hypothermia (the 'bloody lethal triad').
6 RBC salvage if appropriate e.g. blood not contaminated with bacteria, cancer cells, amniotic fluid. *See Blood salvage, intraoperative*.
7 Stabilise blood clots—in adults give tranexamic acid 1 g in 100 mL N/S IV over 10 min, followed by 1 g in 100 mL N/S infused over 8 h. *See Tranexamic acid (TXA) (Cyklokapron)*.

Indicators of critical physiological derangement

1 Temperature < 35°C.
2 pH < 7.2; base excess minus 6 or more negative; lactate > 4 mmol/L (all indicative of tissue hypoxia).
3 Ionised calcium < 1.1 mmol/L. *See Calcium*.
4 Platelet count < 50 000/mm³; PT > 1.5 × normal; APTT > 1.5 × normal; INR > 1.5; fibrinogen < 1.0 g/L (all associated with coagulopathy).
5 Deranged TEG or ROTEM. *See Thromboelastography/thromboelastometry*.

Resuscitation and anaesthesia in association with massive blood loss

Use the Advanced Trauma Life Support algorithm—ABCDE. The letters relate to:
A – **A**irway maintenance with cervical spine protection
B – **B**reathing and ventilation

C – **C**irculation with haemorrhage control
D – **D**isability: responsiveness/level of consciousness
E – **E**xposure/environment: expose patient, examine whole body (with cervical spine protection) but prevent hypothermia.

There are five trauma sites of blood loss—external, chest, abdomen, pelvis and long bones (especially femur). In other situations, gastrointestinal bleeding or obstetric bleeding may be the source of critical bleeding.

1 Insert two large-bore IV cannulas and send blood for FBC, cross-match, coagulation studies/fibrinogen and UEC. Also send blood for TEG/ROTEM.
2 Insert an arterial line and send ABGs.

Massive transfusion protocol (MTP)

Activate the MTP in the situation of massive haemorrhage or significant ongoing blood loss as described above. The laboratory involves the haematologist/transfusion specialist, who advises the anaesthetist on interpretation of results and appropriate blood component therapy. The transfusion laboratory will send packs containing (for adults):

1 RBC 4 units
2 FFP 2 units
3 platelets if platelet count is low or falling
4 cryoprecipitate if fibrinogen < 1 g/L.

The resuscitation team sends FBC and coagulation screen to the transfusion lab every 30–60 min.

Monitor arterial blood gases for pH, lactate and BE. Give tranexamic acid 1 g over 10 min.

Resuscitation targets

1 Temperature > 35°C—warm the patient; warm IV fluids.
2 pH > 7.2, BE less negative than minus 6, lactate < 4 mmol/L. Achieve these aims by ensuring adequate cardiac output (preload, contractility, afterload) oxygenation and Hb levels. Consider IV bicarbonate administration.
3 Ca^{2+} (ionised) > 1.1 mmol/L. Administer IV calcium chloride or calcium gluconate IV as required.
4 Platelets > 50 000/mm.[3] Give platelets as needed.
5 Aim for a platelet count > 100 000 mm³ if there is CNS injury or diffuse microvascular bleeding.
6 PT/APTT < 1.5 × normal, INR ≤ 1.5. Give FFP and more specialised clotting factor concentrates as needed.
7 Fibrinogen ≥ 1.5 g/L. Administer cryoprecipitate as needed.[3] For obstetric haemorrhage, keep fibrinogen > 2 g/L.[4]
8 Haemoglobin > 70 g/L. Transfuse RBC. Aim for a target Hb of 70–90 g/L.
9 Use cell salvage if appropriate. *See Blood salvage, intraoperative.*
10 If factor XIII deficiency, give factor XIII concentrate (30 IU/kg).
11 Urine output of at least 0.5 mL/kg/h (about 30 mL/h in adults).

Patient with unknown blood group

1 Ensure blood for cross-match has been taken before transfusion.
2 Give group O negative blood. It is acceptable to give O positive blood to males over the age of 16 years and females > 50 years from the outset. If an RhD negative female of child-bearing age receives RhD positive blood, give RhD immunoglobulin.
3 Once the blood group is known but before cross-match, use the same ABO/RhD blood group.

4 Platelets from any blood group can be used until the group is known. *See Platelet therapy.*

5 Use AB group FFP/cryoprecipitate (A is less preferred) until the patient's blood group is known. *See Fresh frozen plasma (FFP)* and *Cryoprecipitate.*

Anaesthesia for patient with pre-induction massive blood loss

In addition to the measures described above:

1 Insert 2 large-bore IV cannulas and an arterial line. Consider insertion of a Rapid Infusion Catheter (RIC). *See Rapid Infusion Catheter (RIC) exchange set.* A central line will be useful but can be delayed until the patient is stabilised.

2 Have two pump sets on warmers connected to the large-bore IV cannulas.

3 Consider having available a Belmont® rapid infuser or similar device.

4 Consider having an intraoperative blood collection (Cell Saver type) device available.

5 Prep and drape the patient prior to induction. Have blood available in the operating theatre.

6 Induce anaesthesia cautiously. Usually, a rapid sequence or modified rapid sequence induction is required. *See Rapid sequence induction.* A suggested approach in the adult:
  a) fentanyl 100–200 mcg
  b) propofol 50 mg
  c) suxamethonium 100 mg or rocuronium 70 mg.

7 Maintain anaesthesia with O_2, air and sevoflurane with entropy monitoring to detect awareness. Do not use N_2O.

8 The patient should be catheterised if this has not already been done.

9 Ensure adequate numbers of trained staff are in attendance. Place a team member on crowd control duties to invite unneeded staff to leave the operating room.

Some practical aspects of transfusion

1 If transfusing platelets through the same line, give platelets before the red cells.

2 Use a 170–200 micron filter.

3 If warming the blood, do not exceed 41°C.

4 If using a pressure bag, do not exceed 300 mmHg pressure.

◐ Blood patch

See Post dural puncture headache.

◐ Blood salvage, intraoperative

Introduction

Blood cell salvage devices consist of:

1 Sucker and suction tubing—handed to the surgeon.

2 Machine suction—the blood sucked from the surgical site is mixed with saline containing heparin 30 000 units/L to prevent clotting. Suction pressure should be < 200 mmHg to prevent RBC damage.

3 The blood is collected through a filter to remove non-blood debris.

4 Blood reservoir in which the blood is collected.

5 Washing bowl that is centrifuge driven. This washes away the heparin and separates the RBC from non-RBC fluids.

6 System for collecting the washed cells suspended in saline into a bag for transfusion to the patient. The haematocrit of the salvaged blood is 50–60%.
7 A waste bag for the heparin-containing fluid.

Indications
1 Expected blood loss > 1000 mL.
2 Expected blood loss > 20% of blood volume.
3 Rare/difficult to cross-match blood group.
4 Jehovah's Witnesses patients.
5 Unexpected severe blood loss.

Contraindications/precautions
1 Bowel surgery—not contraindicated if soiled abdominal contents are evacuated before salvage, additional cell washing is performed and broad-spectrum antibiotics are used.
2 Cancer surgery—not contraindicated if blood aspiration close to the tumour site is avoided and a leukodepletion filter is used.
3 Obstetrics—see below.
4 Sickle cell disease (but not trait).
5 Presence of infected material.
6 Do not allow any other substance to enter the blood salvage system such as water or hydrogen peroxide.

Obstetrics and blood salvage
The main concerns are amniotic fluid debris and Rh-negative fetal blood being infused into a Rh-positive mother. Once the amniotic fluid is suctioned away with a separate sucker, cell salvage is probably safe. Devices such as the Cell Saver should be considered when:
1 Massive blood loss may occur e.g. placenta accreta.
2 Significant blood loss is anticipated in a Jehovah's Witnesses patient.
3 Significant blood loss is anticipated in a patient who is difficult to cross-match.
   Transfuse salvaged blood through a leukocyte depletion filter to remove fetal cells and amniotic fluid debris.

◖ Blood transfusion (allogenic) reduction strategies

Preoperative
Preoperative strategies to avoid/minimise intraoperative allogenic blood transfusion include:
1 ceasing/reversing drugs that increase risk of bleeding. *See Anticoagulant and antiplatelet drugs and surgery/neuraxial anaesthesia*
2 autologous blood donation
3 pre-optimisation of the anaemic patient e.g. iron infusion for patient with iron deficiency anaemia.

Intraoperative
1 Restrictive Hb transfusion threshold (70–80 g/L).
2 Surgical factors—meticulous surgical technique, use of a tourniquet, use of thrombostatic pads or glues.
3 Permissive hypotension—to an MAP 60 mmHg. The benefits of decreased blood loss must be weighed against the risks of decreased cerebral and cardiac perfusion with hypotension.

4 Use of neuraxial anaesthesia.

5 Avoidance of hypothermia, hypocalcaemia, acidosis and haemodilution.

6 Intraoperative blood salvage using devices such as a Cell Saver. *See Blood salvage, intraoperative*.

7 Tranexamic acid—intraoperatively and postoperatively. *See Tranexamic acid*.

Postoperative

1 Postop blood recovery and reinfusion of the unwashed shed blood. An example is Stryker's ConstaVac™ Blood Conservation (CBC) System.

2 High-dose iron and/or erythropoietin therapy.

◗ Blood transfusion reactions/adverse events

Human error is the most common cause of serious transfusion reactions. Reactions/adverse events can be categorised as short term and long term.

Short-term reactions/adverse events

1 Febrile non-haemolytic reactions.

2 Allergy/anaphylaxis.

3 Acute and delayed haemolytic transfusion reactions—these can be due to ABO incompatibility, with a mortality of 5–10%.

4 Transfusion-associated circulatory overload (TACO)—defined as acute or worsening pulmonary oedema during or within 12 h of a blood transfusion.

5 Transfusion-related acute lung injury (TRALI)—occurs within 6 h of transfusion of plasma-containing products. Female donor plasma is less safe than male plasma. It commonly presents with acute dyspnoea, hypoxia, fever and hypotension. CXR shows bilateral pulmonary infiltration. Treatment is supportive, with ventilation if required. Patients usually recover in 72 h.[5]

6 Transfusion-related dyspnoea (dyspnoea not due to TRALI or TACO).[5]

7 Sepsis from bacterially contaminated blood.

8 Hyperkalaemia, hypocalcaemia.

9 Coagulopathy.

10 Post-transfusion purpura.

11 Hypotensive transfusion reactions—probably related to the generation of bradykinin.

Long-term reactions/adverse events

1 Viral infection.

2 Prion infection e.g. Creutzfeldt–Jakob disease.

3 Transfusion-related graft versus host disease. Occurs within 30 days of transfusion and is usually (if not always) fatal. It is due to lymphocytes from the donor engrafting in the recipient and then mounting an immune response against the recipient.

4 Increased risk of infection (other than pathogens in the donated blood).

5 Increased risk of cancer recurrence due to immunomodulation (termed 'transfusion-related immunomodulation' (TRIM)).

◗ Blunting haemodynamic response to intubation

See Intubation—minimising hypertensive response.

◗ Body mass index (BMI) and obesity

BMI = weight (kg)/height (m)^2.

Table B3 Weight description and BMI

Weight description	BMI
Very underweight	< 17
Underweight	17–18.4
Healthy weight range	18.5–25
Overweight but not obese	25.1–29.9
Obese class 1	30–34.9
Obese class 2	35–39.9
Obese class 3	≥ 40

BMI 30–40 is classified as ASA 2, and BMI > 40 is classified as ASA 3 (assuming there are no other co-morbidities).

See *American Society of Anesthesiologists (ASA) Physical Status Classification System*.

◗ Bone cement implantation syndrome

See *Fat embolism syndrome (FES) and bone cement implantation syndrome (BCIS)*.

◗ Bone marrow embolism

See *Fat embolism syndrome (FES) and bone cement implantation syndrome (BCIS)*.

◗ Brachial plexus block (BPB)

Four approaches to the brachial plexus using ultrasound will be described in this section. The following instructions apply to the performance of all these blocks.
1 Patients should be awake or lightly sedated.
2 Use strict aseptic technique.
3 Place an IV cannula in the non-block arm.
4 Place a bleb of LA in the skin at the needle insertion point and puncture the skin with a 19 G needle.
5 Always aspirate prior to injection, then inject a 2 mL test dose to check for pain (suggesting intraneural injection).
6 Inject the LA incrementally in 5 mL doses, checking the patient for any side effects.
7 If a patient is taking 1 or more anticoagulants, deep blocks are relatively contraindicated. An axillary brachial plexus block may be the safest option.

Interscalene BPB

This block is useful for surgery on the shoulder and clavicle. The brachial plexus is formed from the nerve roots of C5, C6, C7, C8 and T1 (Figure B1). These roots are sandwiched between the scalenus anterior and scalenus medius muscles, and fuse to form three trunks in the supraclavicular region. The fascia of scalenus anterior and medius form a sheath around the plexus. Phrenic nerve block is expected, so if the patient has impaired lung function, this block may not be appropriate. Use a 50 mm block needle, ropivacaine 0.75% 15 mL and a high-frequency linear transducer probe. Set the depth to 3 cm.

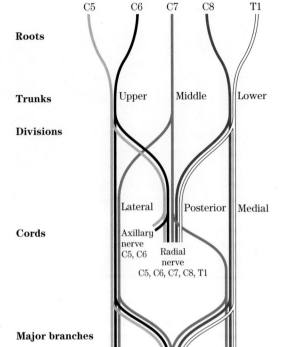

Figure B1 Brachial plexus illustrated schematically

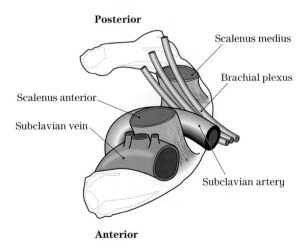

Figure B2 Anatomical relations of the brachial plexus in the region of the first rib

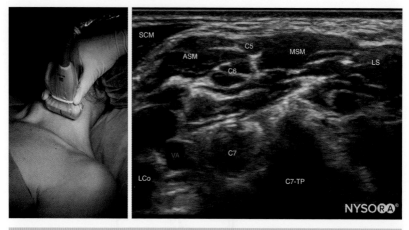

Figure B3 Probe position and sonoanatomy of the interscalene brachial plexus block.
SCM = sternocleidomastoid muscle, ASM = anterior scalene muscle, C5, 6, 7 = brachial
plexus nerve roots, MSM = middle scalene muscle, C7-TP = C7 transverse process
Image courtesy of NYSORA

Technique

1 Position the patient supine, with the upper body inclined at 30°. Arrange the pillow
   and a folded towel so there is good access to behind the lower neck for needling.
2 Orientate the probe transversely (Figure B3). The plexus can almost always be
   found under the external jugular vein in the lower neck, 2–3 cm above the clavicle
   and posterior to the carotid artery. Another approach is to identify the brachial
   plexus in the supraclavicular region (see below), then follow the plexus up the neck.
3 Look for the 'traffic light sign'—three or more circles lined up between the scaleni
   muscles. The plexus is very superficial (not deeper than 3 cm).
4 Insert the block needle with an in-plane approach from posterior to anterior, starting
   1 cm posterior to the probe. Aim to position the tip of the needle between the most
   cranial (C5) and the next root (C6). Consider using colour doppler to identify blood
   vessels that might be in the way. A click may be felt as the sheath is entered.
   After negative aspiration and a test dose of 1–2 mL, inject 13–14 mL of LA in 5 mL
   increments.
5 Only inject more LA if the spread looks inadequate.
6 Always aim between roots.
7 If using a catheter after a block dose, run an infusion of ropivacaine 0.2% at
   8–10 mL/h.

Supraclavicular BPB

This block is useful for all operations on the upper limb, except for the inner upper
arm, which is innervated by the intercostobrachial nerve (T2). The main risks with this
block are puncturing the pleura and phrenic nerve block. Use 20 mL of LA (10 mL
of lignocaine 2% with adrenaline mixed with 10 mL of 1% ropivacaine) and a short-
bevelled 10 cm needle.

Anatomy

The three trunks of the BP emerge from between scalenus anterior and scalenus medius muscles and cross the first rib (as divisions and trunks) latero-posterior and superficial to the subclavian artery. The BP lies only 2–3 cm or less below the skin. See Figure B4.

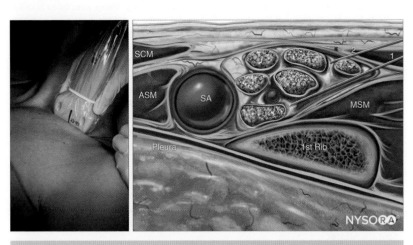

Figure B4 Probe position and anatomy for supraclavicular BPB. SCM = sternocleidomastoid muscle, ASM = anterior scalene muscle, SA = subclavian artery, MSM = middle scalene muscle
Image courtesy of NYSORA

Technique

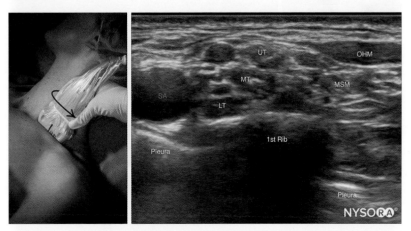

Figure B5 Probe position and sonoanatomy for supraclavicular BPB. SA = subclavian artery, UT, MT, LT = upper middle and lower trunk of the BP, MSM = middle scalene muscle, OHM = omohyoid muscle
Image courtesy of NYSORA

1 Position the patient supine with 30° head-up tilt of the upper body and a pillow and/or rolled-up towel giving good access to behind the supraclavicular region. The head is turned away from the block.

2 Place the transducer in the supraclavicular fossa in the same orientation as the clavicle and identify the subclavian artery (pulsatile) and the brachial plexus (hypoechoic oval structures) immediately behind the artery. These structures should be behind the midpoint of the clavicle. Rotate the probe to get the best plexus image. A bright white line will be seen deep to the plexus and artery. This will be either the pleura or the first rib. The needle **must not** go deeper than the white line. Use colour doppler to check if any blood vessels are in the needle path. See Figure B5.

3 Insert the needle in-plane from posterior to anterior, starting about 1 cm behind the probe, with a flat trajectory. The needle tip is positioned below the plexus and near the artery but above the white line (the 'corner pocket'). After aspiration and a test dose, inject 9.5 mL of LA. This will anaesthetise the median and ulnar nerves.

4 Redirect the needle to a position with the tip adjacent to the superior part of the plexus. After aspiration and a test dose, inject another 9.5 mL. This will anaesthetise the radial nerve.

Infraclavicular BPB

This block provides excellent coverage of the whole arm, except for the medial side of the upper arm. It is not suitable for shoulder surgery. Use 20–30 mL of LA (15 mL 1.5% lignocaine with adrenaline and 15 mL of 0.5 % ropivacaine) and a high-frequency linear transducer.

Anatomy

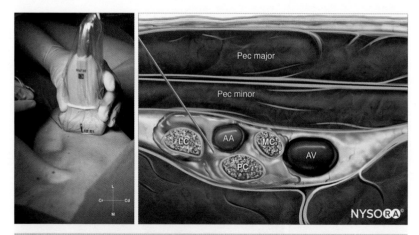

Figure B6 Probe position and anatomy for infraclavicular BPB. LC, PC, MC = lateral, posterior and medial cords of the BP, AA = axillary artery, AV = axillary vein
Image courtesy of NYSORA

The brachial plexus enters the axillary fossa through the costoclavicular space lateral to the axillary artery. It is arranged in three cords. The cords surround the axillary artery and are then called the 'lateral', 'posterior' and 'medial' cords, all under the pectoralis major and minor (Figure B6).

Technique

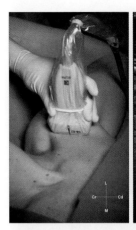
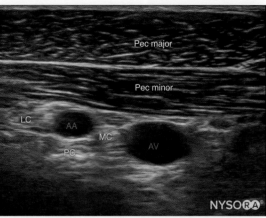

Figure B7 Probe position and sonoanatomy for infraclavicular BPB. LC, PC, MC = lateral, posterior and medial cords of the BP, AA = axillary artery, AV = axillary vein
Image courtesy of NYSORA

1 Position the patient supine, with upper body elevation of 30°. The arm to be blocked is abducted 90° and the elbow is flexed 90°.
2 The transducer is orientated para-sagittal, just below the clavicle, next to the coracoid process. If ribs are visible, you are too medial. The depth of the plexus is 3–5 cm.
3 Identify pectoralis major and minor, the axillary artery and axillary vein (Figure B7). The artery will be cranial to the vein. The plexus surrounds the artery.
4 Inset the block needle in-plane from cranial to caudal, just under the inferior edge of the clavicle.
5 Position the needle tip below the axillary artery, avoiding the cords. Reduce the downward pressure of the transducer when injecting to aid spread.
6 Using the precautions already described in preceding sections, inject 20–30 mL of LA very slowly as fast injection is painful. Aim to surround the axillary artery and cords.
7 If there is uneven spread of LA, reposition the needle.

Axillary BPB

This is the safest approach to the BP. There is no risk of pleural injury, and if the axillary artery is punctured, bleeding can be controlled with pressure. The phrenic nerve will not be blocked. It is suitable for surgery below the elbow. Use 20 mL of 0.5% ropivacaine.

Anatomy

See Figure B8. After crossing the first rib, the three trunks divide into six divisions which stream into the axilla. The divisions then re-join into three cords. These cords then divide into terminal branches. The median, radial and ulnar nerves are close to the artery and are contained in a fascial sheath. The musculocutaneous nerve is outside the sheath and must be blocked separately. It supplies sensation to the

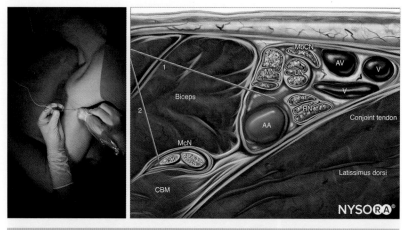

Figure B8 Probe position and anatomy of the axillary BPB. McN = musculocutaneous nerve, MN = median nerve, UN = ulnar nerve, MbCN = medial brachial cutaneous nerve, RN = radial nerve, AA = axillary artery
Image courtesy of NYSORA

radial side of the forearm and lies beneath the bulk of the biceps muscle and the coracobrachialis muscle.

Technique

1 Position the patient as described for the infraclavicular block (see above).
2 Place the ultrasound probe just distal to the axilla at right angles to the main axis of the arm, with one end in the groove between the pectoralis major and the biceps muscle. The image obtained will show the axillary artery (pulsatile) and axillary vein (compressible) above the artery. Also visible are the radial nerve (between the artery and the humerus), the ulna nerve (between the artery and the vein) and the median nerve (on the other side of the artery relative to the vein). Use a colour doppler to identify vascular structures in the needle path. The muscles that are visible are the biceps and the coracobrachialis on one side of the screen and the latissimus dorsi or triceps on the other side of the screen.
3 Insert the needle from the biceps side of the arm to position the tip below the artery, feeling a 'pop' as the fascial sheath is entered. After negative aspiration and a test dose, inject 8 mL of LA.
4 Redirect the needle to position the tip above the artery and, after negative aspiration and a test dose, inject another 8 mL of LA.
5 Reposition the needle tip to penetrate the fascia between the biceps and the coracobrachialis muscle, close to the musculocutaneous nerve. The musculocutaneous nerve is very bright on ultrasound and is in the biceps muscle. After a negative aspiration test, inject 4 mL of LA. The probe may need to be moved slightly distally.

◐ Bradycardia

Definition

A pulse rate < 60 bpm. Effects of bradycardia range from inconsequential to cardiac arrest.

Causes

1 Physiological—e.g. diving reflex, extreme fitness.
2 Vagally mediated—e.g. pneumoperitoneum, traction on eyeball.
3 Baroreceptor reflex—stimulation of the baroreceptors in the carotid sinus and aortic arch.
4 Pharmacological—e.g. suxamethonium, neostigmine.
5 Inadequate cardiac filling—elicits the Bezold–Jarisch reflex. This is due to mechano-receptors in the LV detecting inadequate LV filling and can occur with, for example, spinal anaesthesia or severe haemorrhage.
6 Intrinsic cardiac causes—conduction abnormalities, myocardial infarction.
7 Hypoxia.
8 Electrolyte disturbances.
9 Endocrine causes e.g. hypothyroidism.
10 Raised intracranial pressure.
11 Hypothermia.

Clinical effects

As with haemodynamic instability from all causes, the following may be seen:
1 altered mental state
2 hypotension (SBP < 90 mmHg)
3 chest pain
4 dyspnoea
5 evidence of shock—cool peripheries, pallor
6 cardiac arrest.

Treatment

If cardiac arrest, *see Cardiac arrest*. In other situations:
1 Treat the cause e.g. deflating pneumoperitoneum.
2 Atropine—600 mcg every 3–5 min to a maximum dose of 2 mg in adults. In children, use 0.02 mg/kg to a maximum dose of 0.5 mg/dose (maximum total dose 1 mg). This will not help complete heart block. *See Heart block (HB)*.
3 Pacing—this can be electrical or pharmacological pacing. Use isoprenaline by infusion—bolus of 1–10 mcg IV then infusion 1–8 mcg/min **or** adrenaline 2–10 mcg/min. *See Pacemakers*.
4 For adult patients with drug-induced bradycardia e.g. beta blockers or calcium channel blockers, consider glucagon 50 mcg/kg followed by an infusion of 1–15 mg/h. *See Glucagon*.

◐ Bradykinin

Bradykinin is a protein fragment of the kinin group of proteins. It is involved in promoting inflammation, and it causes arterioles to dilate and veins to constrict. This causes increased pressure in capillary beds, leading to leakage of intravascular fluid into the tissues. Increased bradykinin levels are a feature of hereditary angioedema. *See Angioedema*. Bradykinin is a potent dilator of cerebral arteries. ACE inhibitors increase bradykinin levels by inhibiting its degradation, increasing their antihypertensive effects. Bradykinin is also thought to cause the dry cough that affects some patients on ACE inhibitors.

◐ Brady tachy syndrome

See Sick sinus syndrome (SSS).

◐ Brainstem anaesthesia

Description

Occurs when there is an accidental spread of LA to the brainstem. It can occur with:

1 Peribulbar or retrobulbar eye block—the most common cause. This is due to injection into the dural sheath of the optic nerve enabling LA to enter the subdural space.
2 Neurosurgery—e.g. burr hole with LA leakage through a dura mater opening.[6]

Presentation

Effects usually begin about 5–10 min after LA injection.[7]

1 Restlessness, drowsiness, confusion, loss of consciousness, convulsions.
2 Apnoea.
3 Cranial nerve palsies.
4 Deafness.
5 Dysphagia.
6 Dysarthria.
7 Loss of pupillary light reflex and/or dilated pupils.
8 Hypotension/bradycardia. Sustained hypertension/tachycardia may also occur.[7]
9 Cardiac arrest.

Treatment

Supportive treatment until the LA wears off, including:

1 Optimise airway.
2 Ensure adequate ventilation.
3 Support the circulation—IV fluids, vasopressors.
4 Recovery should occur after about 10–60 min.[8]

◐ Breast feeding and maternal anaesthesia/postoperative care

General anaesthetic agents are excreted in such small quantities in breast milk that there is no need to discard it after GA. However, some drugs should be avoided for lactating mothers, including:[9]

1 Aspirin—can cause lactic acidosis in infant. NSAIDs and paracetamol are safe.
2 Codeine—due to rapid metabolism of codeine to morphine in some mothers.
3 Droperidol—can impair infant neurological status.
4 High-dose pethidine.
5 Diazepam—but it can be used as a one-off dose before a procedure. It has an active metabolite, desmethyldiazepam, which is transferred in breast milk in significant amounts.
6 Oxycodone—dosage should be limited to 40 mg/day.
7 Tramadol—use with caution. It has an active metabolite and can cause adverse effects in the infant.
8 Dexmedetomidine—no information on breast milk excretion available; use with caution.

The mother must be careful if co-sleeping with the baby in the first 24 h after GA. Observe the infant for any neurological changes, especially in infants < 6 weeks. If any occur, cease breast feeding and use formula feeds.

PCA use and breast feeding
Mother and baby should be observed closely for any adverse effects.
1 Morphine has been used safely.[q]
2 Hydromorphone—use with caution.
3 Fentanyl—use with caution.

⊙ Bronchopleural fistula (BPF)

Only a brief overview of this topic is provided. A detailed discussion of this complex pathological condition is beyond the scope of this manual.

Description
A BPF is a fistula between a major, lobar or segmental bronchus and the pleural space. Causes include:
1 thoracic surgery with breakdown of a suture line
2 ruptured lung abscess, bulla or cyst
3 erosion by malignancy, radiotherapy, chemotherapy
4 barotrauma
5 tuberculosis or other infection.

Clinical effects
1 Dyspnoea, cyanosis, coughing up blood or frothy pink fluid or pus.
2 Chest pain.
3 Subcutaneous emphysema.
4 Deviation of the trachea.
5 Tension pneumothorax.
6 Failure of a chest tube to drain a pneumothorax, often with a massive air leak.

Diagnosis
1 Chest X-ray—pneumothorax, fall in the post-pneumonectomy fluid level.
2 Chest CT scan—may show loculated cysts, empyema.
3 Bronchoscopy.

Treatment
1 Drain the fluid and air in the pleural cavity with a chest tube on minimal suction (5–10 cmH$_2$O).
2 Repair the fistula either surgically or via a bronchoscope.
3 In some cases, pleurodesis may be helpful.

Anaesthesia and BPF
Anaesthesia is challenging in these patients because positive pressure ventilation may be ineffective and/or cause a tension pneumothorax. A chest tube should be in situ. It is essential to avoid soiling of the healthy lung if infection is present. A double lumen tube (DLT) is usually required. *See One lung ventilation (OLV)*. In general:
1 Maintain spontaneous ventilation until DLT is sited if possible. Options are GA with spontaneous ventilation or awake intubation with airway topicalisation. *See Awake intubation*.
2 Apply IPPV to healthy lung. Use small tidal volumes or low CPAP to BPF lung.
3 Avoid high airway pressures on emergence if fistula has been repaired.

◗ Bronchospasm

See *Asthma*.

◗ Brown–Sequard syndrome

This condition results from hemi-section of the spinal cord from the side e.g. from a gunshot or stab wound. More rarely it is due to infection, inflammatory disease or spinal cord tumour. There is paralysis or weakness and loss of proprioception on the same side as the lesion and loss of pain and temperature sensation on the side opposite the lesion.

◗ Brugada syndrome

Description

This is a genetic disorder (inherited or mutation) affecting sodium channels of the right ventricular epicardium. The most common age of onset is 40 years, and it is more common in males. It causes 20% of sudden cardiac deaths in patients without structural heart disease.

Clinical features

1 Ventricular tachyarrhythmias or sudden cardiac arrest. These may be triggered by fever or drugs such as flecainide, amitriptyline and bupivacaine. Other triggers may include exercise, pregnancy and situations with high vagal tone such as sleep and recovery from exercise.
2 Palpitations.
3 Syncope.
4 Nocturnal agonal respiration.

Diagnosis

1 The typical ECG changes, seen in about 70% of patients, are RBBB and coved-type ST elevation in leads V1–V3. There is no structural heart disease.
2 A challenge with a powerful sodium channel blocker such as flecainide, procainamide or propafenone may reveal or accentuate the ECG changes.
3 Those patients with a normal resting ECG are probably at less risk of tachyarrhythmias than patients with typical ECG changes. Electrophysiological studies can quantify the risk of malignant tachyarrhythmias and the need for an implantable defibrillator.

Treatment

1 Implantable defibrillator (AICD).
2 Avoidance of precipitating drugs, including bupivacaine, calcium channel blockers, nitrates, selective serotonin re-uptake inhibitors and lithium.
3 Antiarrhythmic drugs (to avoid AICD shocks or if AICD refused) include amiodarone and quinidine.
4 If a ventricular tachycardia storm occurs, an isoprenaline infusion can be helpful.
5 Non-anaesthetic drugs to avoid are many and include lithium, cocaine, cannabis, heavy alcohol use, tricyclic antidepressants and ergonovine.

Anaesthetic implications

In patients with known Brugada syndrome:

1 take the necessary precautions for a patient with an AICD if this is present. ***See Pacemakers***
2 if ST elevation or VT occurs, consider an isoprenaline infusion
3 vagal stimulation can precipitate arrhythmia. Avoid any form of vagal stimulation and treat bradycardia promptly with atropine
4 propofol can be used for induction but a propofol infusion may not be safe
5 small doses of lignocaine with adrenaline are safe
6 ephedrine may be preferable to metaraminol as a vasoconstrictor
7 do not use a bupivacaine infusion by any route. Do not use procaine
8 bupivacaine for SAB is probably safe
9 avoid/treat hyperthermia, which can precipitate dysrhythmia
10 do not use beta blockers, alpha receptor agonists, nicorandil or neostigmine
11 use rocuronium with sugammadex as the reversal agent
12 do not use noradrenaline.

◑ B-type natriuretic peptide (BNP) and N-terminal-proBNP (NT-proBNP)

Pro-BNP is produced mainly in the left ventricle (LV). It is split by corin or furin to make BNP and NT-proBNP. The levels of these substances increase with LV stretch, hence these chemicals can be used as markers for congestive cardiac failure (CCF).

BNP

BNP can be elevated due to other illnesses such as renal failure and pulmonary hypertension. Trends in BNP levels are more helpful than one-off measurements.

Interpretation of BNP results

Normal = < 100 pg/mL
Mild/moderate heart failure = 100–300 pg/mL
Moderate/severe heart failure = 300–600 pg/mL
Severe/very severe heart failure = > 600 pg/mL.

NT-proBNP

NT-proBNP is the inactive fragment of pro-BNP.

Interpretation of NT-proBNP results

The NT-proBNP test is more standardised than BNP measurements. NT-proBNP levels rise with age. The levels should be < 125 pg/mL in patients < 75 years and < 450 pg/mL in patients > 75 years. Significant heart failure is suggested by NT-proBNP > 450 pg/mL in patients < 50 years old and > 900 pg/mL in patients > 50 years old.

◑ Bupivacaine (Marcain, Marcaine)

Description

Amide-type long-acting local anaesthetic drug. Can be used for all types of block except intravenous regional block and obstetric paracervical block. 0.5% bupivacaine is equivalent to 1% ropivacaine. Presented in strengths of 0.125%, 0.25% and 0.5%. Heavy Marcaine is used for spinal anaesthesia and contains glucose. It has increased baricity compared with plain bupivacaine. This results in a lower spinal block. EXPAREL is bupivacaine liposome injectable suspension and is very long acting (days).

Dose

The maximum dose should not exceed 2–2.5 mg/kg but do not exceed 175 mg. Maximum daily dose in adults is 400 mg.

Advantages

Longer acting than lignocaine. Adrenaline does not prolong its actions but may result in a drier surgical field.

Disadvantages

1 More cardiotoxic than lignocaine or ropivacaine, and CVS collapse is more difficult to treat.
2 Causes more motor block than ropivacaine when used epidurally.

Treatment of cardiotoxicity

See *Local anaesthetic (LA) toxicity* and *Intralipid for the treatment of ropivacaine/ bupivacaine toxicity*.

◗ Buprenorphine

Description

This drug is an agonist-antagonist opioid (mu receptor agonist, kappa receptor antagonist). It is 33–40 × more potent than morphine. It has a higher affinity for the mu receptor than any other opioid used clinically. The advantage of this type of drug is that, compared with morphine, analgesia occurs with less risk of ventilatory depression. There is also a lower addiction risk. However, these drugs can also antagonise stronger pure agonist opioids if they are needed for severe pain. Buprenorphine can cause withdrawal symptoms in opioid-addicted patients.

Buprenorphine is also used as an alternative to methadone when treating opioid addiction because it is safer (more difficult to overdose on due to ceiling effect), more convenient to use and the sublingual forms are harder to inject. It may be mixed with naloxone to further discourage IV use.

Dose

Adult

Acute pain in NBM patients—200–400 mcg sublingual q 4–6 h. Buprenorphine patches (Norspan) are used for chronic pain (often due to cancer) and are changed every seven days. Available strengths are 5 mcg/h, 10 mcg/h and 25 mcg/h. *Chronic pain in adult patients*—500 mcg–1 mg q 6 h.

Treatment of opioid addiction in adult patients

1 Short-acting opioids e.g. heroin, administer 4 mg sublingual ≥ 6 h after last opioid or when withdrawal signs begin. Repeat dose if needed. For maintenance, increase dose as needed incrementally to a maximum of 30 mg/day.
2 Long-acting opioids e.g. methadone, administer 4 mg sublingual ≥ 24 h after last opioid dose or when withdrawal signs begin. Maintenance as above. Maximum daily dose is 30 mg, above which there is a ceiling effect.

Buprenorphine and anaesthesia

These guidelines only apply to surgery that is associated with significant postoperative pain. Several approaches can be considered.
1 Patients taking ≤ 8 mg/day or transdermal patch (any dose) can continue treatment perioperatively.

2 Patients taking > 8 mg/day—consider changing to a traditional opioid such as hydromorphone PO. For example, if the patient is taking 8 mg buprenorphine q 8 h, substitute with hydromorphone PO 4 mg q 4–6 h. Methadone 30–40 mg/day could also be used. Conversion back to buprenorphine can occur after the period of acute pain has ended.

3 For patients on high-dose buprenorphine requiring emergency surgery—cease buprenorphine and use high doses of opioids plus supplementary analgesics (paracetamol, NSAIDs, gabapentin, alpha-2 agonists such as dexmedetomidine, ketamine). Consider regional anaesthesia options. Benzodiazepines (such as lorazepam and midazolam) and haloperidol may be required for delirium. Buprenorphine effects should have dissipated by the third postoperative day.

4 Patients with acute severe pain on buprenorphine may have no pain relief when given traditional opioids such as fentanyl or morphine.

◗ Burns

Description
Only a brief overview of this broad, complex topic can be provided in this manual. Burns can result from thermal energy, chemicals, electricity, radiation and friction.

The main considerations with burns are:
1 percentage of total body surface area (TBSA) burnt
2 depth of burns
3 airway burn injuries
4 inhalation of carbon monoxide, cyanide, smoke and other noxious substances
5 associated injuries.

Percentage of total body surface area (TBSA) burnt (adults)
Superficial burns are not counted.

Use the Lund–Browder chart or the 'rule of 9s'—head 9%; arm 9%; leg 18%; anterior/posterior trunk 18% each; palmar surface of whole hand 1%.

Major burns/burns requiring transfer to a burns centre
1 Greater than 10% TBSA.
2 Burns involving face, hands, feet, genitalia, perineum or major joints.
3 Any third-degree or fourth-degree burns.
4 Electrical, chemical burns.
5 Inhalational injury.

Depth of burns
The depth of a burn is classified as:
1 Superficial (first degree)—epidermis, red skin with pain e.g. sunburn.
2 Superficial partial thickness (second degree)—epidermis and dermis; blisters and moist, red, weeping skin.
3 Deep partial thickness (second degree)—blisters, variable colour (white to red); pain to deep pressure. Usually requires surgery.
4 Full thickness (third degree)—dermis and deeper structures involved. Waxy white to leathery grey or charred skin. No blanching with pressure, no pain in burn area. Requires surgery.
5 Deeper injury (fourth degree)—extends to deeper tissues such as muscle; no pain in burnt area. Requires surgery.

Treatment of minor burns

1 Remove non-adherent debris.
2 Run cool tap water over the burn area if possible, otherwise apply cool wet gauze.
3 Analgesia.
4 Clean burns with mild soap and water.
5 Debride sloughed or necrotic skin including ruptured blisters.
6 Moisturising cream e.g. aloe vera.
7 Tetanus prophylaxis.

Treatment of severe burns (first 24 h)

Obtain a relevant history of the injury: nature of burn, enclosed space or not, explosion etc. Obtain a relevant patient history. Use AMPLE, an acronym which stands for:

A – **A**llergies
M – **M**edications
P – **P**ast medical history
L – **L**ast meal
E – **E**vents surrounding injury.

Extinguish smouldering clothing. Remove burnt clothing unless adherent.

Priorities are as follows.

1 Stabilise airway, breathing and circulation—look for evidence of airway burn (singed nasal hair, soot). Provide supplementary O_2. The upper airway may be threatened by progressive swelling from head and neck burns. Flash burns to the face do not usually cause airway compromise.
2 Look for any evidence of lung injury; coughing, wheeze, carbonaceous sputum. This can be from smoke inhalation. The lower airway is not usually burnt unless there is inhalation of hot gases like superheated steam. With smoke inhalation, the patient can develop airway inflammation, mucosal sloughing, excess pulmonary secretions and bronchospasm. The full effects of smoke inhalation injury may take up to 48 h to manifest. The systemic inflammatory response syndrome (SIRS) and/or acute respiratory distress syndrome (ARDS) may occur.
3 Intubate the patient if head and/or neck burns, stridor, disorientation or combative, uncooperative patient. Suxamethonium can be used for the first 48 h after burn.[10]
4 Adequate analgesia.
5 Fluid resuscitation—use the modified Parkland formula: 3–4 mL/kg/TBSA% in the first 24 h. For a 70 kg patient with 35% TBSA deep burns administer 7.35–9.8 L. Give the first half over 8 h and the rest over 16 h.
6 Insert urinary catheter and aim for urine output of 0.5–1 mL/kg/h.
7 Insert arterial and central lines and send bloods for ABG, FBC, electrolytes, group and save, carboxyhaemoglobin (COHb) and coagulation studies. Perform ECG and CXR. Obtain cardiac enzymes if electrical burns.
8 Treat other injuries. Hypovolaemic shock in the first few hours after major burns is never due to the burns themselves.
9 Burns dressings—various types of dressings can be used, including foams, hydrogels and silver dressings. If the patient is to be transferred within 6 h to a burns centre, clean the burns with aqueous chlorhexidine 1% or N/S and cover the wounds with cling film.
10 Emergency escharotomy may be required for circumferential burns.

Carbon monoxide (CO) poisoning

1 Measure carboxyhaemoglobin levels with CO oximetry.
   COHb levels of:
   a) up to 12% may occur in smokers
   b) 15–20% significant toxicity
   c) > 30% COHb is associated with life-threatening hypoxia
   d) > 50% COHb is fatal.
2 Pulse oximetry and ABG are not helpful in the diagnosis of CO poisoning.
3 Symptoms include headache, dizziness, nausea, dyspnoea, weakness, chest pain, palpitations, confusion. Skin may have a cherry-red colour (severe or fatal poisoning).
4 COHb has a half-life in the blood of 3–4 h when breathing air.
5 Treatment is with high-concentration oxygen. Continue O_2 therapy until COHb < 10%. At 1 atm, 100% O_2 reduces COHb half-life to 30–90 min.
6 If COHb > 40% **or** there is evidence of cardiac or cerebral ischaemia **or** pregnant patient with COHb > 15%, use hyperbaric O_2. 100% O_2 at 2.5 atm reduces the COHb half-life to 15–23 min.
7 If cerebral oedema occurs, *See Intracranial pressure (ICP) and treatment of raised ICP.*
8 Permissive acidosis (pH > 7.15) shifts the oxygen-haemoglobin dissociation curve to the right (favours transfer of O_2 to the tissues).
9 Patients who survive can have brain damage, which can be delayed in manifesting (called 'delayed neurological sequelae' (DNS)).

Cyanide poisoning

Cyanide can be a toxic product of combustion and might be inhaled by the burns victim. Although hydrogen cyanide smells like bitter almonds, 20–40% of people are genetically unable to detect this odour. Cyanide binds to ferric ions in cytochrome c oxidase. This inhibits electron chain transport in the mitochondria, which blocks cellular aerobic metabolism. Levels of cyanide poisoning can be classified as:

• mild < 1 mcg/mL
• moderate 1–2 mcg/mL
• severe > 2 mcg/mL
• fatal > 3–5 mcg/mL.

Diagnosis of cyanide poisoning

1 Tachycardia, hypertension, palpitations.
2 Tachypnoea.
3 Nausea.
4 Headaches, anxiety, confusion, drowsiness, seizures, fixed pupils.
5 Cardiovascular collapse.
6 Death.
7 Lactic acidosis due to anaerobic metabolism. A plasma lactate > 10 mmol/L is a sensitive indicator of cyanide toxicity.[11]
8 Cyanide levels can be measured but the results will take too long to help acute management.

Treatment

1 Supportive measures.
2 Antidotes include hydroxycobalamin IV 5 g over 15 min **or** sodium thiosulphate 12.5 g IV over 10 min **or** dicobalt edetate 300 mg IV over 1 min (binds cyanide directly). Hydroxocobalamin is probably the most effective antidote.[11] *See Cyanide (CN) toxicity.*

Anaesthesia and burns patients

A highly specialised area, with innumerable challenges and controversies. A detailed discussion is beyond the scope of this manual. The following are points to note.

1 As stated above, suxamethonium can be used for the first 48 h after major burns, but after this life-threatening hyperkalaemia may occur. This risk persists until up to 12 months after burns have healed.[12]
2 Patients tend to be resistant to NDNMBDs.
3 Burns patients are prone to infections but prophylactic antibiotics are not recommended.
4 Acute kidney injury may occur in up to 25% of patients with major burns.
5 Maintain patient's body temperature perioperatively, including using a warmed operating theatre.

⊙ Buvidal

Buprenorphine is a modified-release formulation injected subcut once weekly or monthly. *See Buprenorphine*.

REFERENCES

1 Government of South Australia, SA Health. *Surgical Antibiotic Prophylaxis Guidelines. Prevention of Endocarditis or Infection in Prosthetic Implants or Grafts.* Endorsed by the South Australian expert Advisory Group on Antibiotic Resistance (SAAGAR) March 2012, last reviewed and amended August 2017. Accessed online: www.sahealth.sa.gov.au/ wps/wcm/connect/a39de780436f24c2b95cbff2cadc00ab/Surg-Ab-Prophylaxis-guideline-Appendix4%2BEndocarditis_v2.0-ics-cdcb-20171120.pdf?MOD=AJPERES, February 2023.

2 Peterson CD, Leeder JS, Sterner S. Glucagon therapy for beta blocker overdose. *Drug Intell Clin Pharm* 1984; 18: 394–398.

3 Joint United Kingdom (UK) Blood Transfusion and Tissue Transplantation Services Professional Advisory Committee (JPAC). *Transfusion Handbook.* Accessed online: www.transfusionguidelines.org, February 2023.

4 Matsunaga S, Takai Y, Seki H. Fibrinogen for the management of critical obstetric haemorrhage. *J Obstet Gynaecol Res* 2018; 45: 13–21.

5 Redding N, Plews D, Dodds A. Risks of perioperative blood transfusions. *Anaesth Intens Care Med* 2022; 23: 80–84.

6 Miyamoto S, Ikeda G, Akimoto K et al. Brainstem anaesthesia during removal operation for ventriculoperitoneal shunt-A case report. *Surg Neurol Int* 2022; 13: 1–4.

7 Tolesa K, Gebreal GW. Brainstem anesthesia after retrobulbar block: a case report of literature. *Ethiop J Health Sci* 2016; 26: 589–594.

8 Kostadinov I, Hostnic A, Cvenkel B, Potočnik I. Brainstem anaesthesia from retrobulbar block. *Open Med (Wars)* 2019; 14: 287–291.

9 Mitchell J, Jones W, Winkley E, Kinsella SM. Guideline to anaesthesia and sedation in breastfeeding women 2020. *Anaesth, Periop Med, Crit Care Pain* 2020; 75: 1482–1493.

10 Bishop S, Maguire S. Anaesthesia and intensive care for major burns. *Cont Edu Anaesth Crit Care & Pain* 2012; 12: 118–122.

11 McLennan L, Moiemen N. Management of cyanide toxicity in patients with burns. *Burns* 2015; 41: 18–24.

12 Stapelberg F. Challenges in anaesthesia and pain management for burns injuries. *Anaesth Intens Care* 2020; 48: 101–113.

C

C1-esterase inhibitor deficiency/C1-inhibitor deficiency

C1-esterase inhibitor controls a protein called C1, which is part of the complement system. **See Complement system.** A C1-esterase inhibitor deficiency can result in an acquired recurrent angioedema without urticaria. It can be caused by B cell lymphoproliferative disorders. This condition can be treated with icatibant. **See Angioedema.**

Caesarean section (CS)

See Physiology of term pregnancy.

Classification codes for CS urgency

1 Code critical/Class 1—delivery in under 15 min e.g. cord prolapse.
2 Class 2—within 1 h e.g. failed instrumental delivery.
3 Class 3—required within hours e.g. failure of labour to progress.
4 Class 4—CS can be arranged at a time to suit patient and staff.

Code critical CS pre-anaesthetic fetal/maternal resuscitation

1 Resuscitate the mother adequately if required.
2 Position the mother full left lateral.
3 Increase IV fluids if already in progress.
4 Turn off oxytocin infusion.
5 Continue fetal CTG monitoring. **See Intrauterine fetal resuscitation (IUFR).**

Preoperative assessment/preparation for elective/semi-elective CS

In addition to routine history, examination and preparation (e.g. fasting), the following are important considerations.

1 Carefully assess the airway, as there is an increased incidence of difficult airway in the pregnant patient. **See Difficult airway management.**
2 Consider acid aspiration prophylaxis with sodium citrate 0.3 M 30 mL, especially if GA likely.
3 A group and hold is not needed in an uncomplicated pregnancy. A FBC and group and hold should be performed for all non-elective CS, and any pregnancy with complications or increased risk e.g. previous PPH, multiple pregnancy.
4 Calf compressors and compression stockings are not necessary unless thromboprophylaxis is contraindicated or a patient is at an especially high risk for DVT/PE.
5 Diabetes in pregnancy is very common. **See Diabetes mellitus (DM).**
6 Neuraxial anaesthesia is preferred for safety and the parental birthing experience.

Subarachnoid block (SAB)

For insertion technique, **see Subarachnoid block (SAB).** Load the patient with 1 L IV fluid while preparing and administering the block.

1 Consider 4 mg ondansetron IV prior to SAB. This may reduce the incidence of maternal hypotension and nausea with SAB.[1]

2   Give prophylactic antibiotics e.g. cefazolin 2 g (unless cephalosporin or penicillin allergy).

3   Use a 27 G Sprotte spinal needle. Suggested drugs for SAB are heavy bupivacaine 0.5% 2.2–2.4 mL, fentanyl 20–25 mcg and preservative-free morphine 100 mcg.

4   Immediately after SAB injection, commence an IV infusion of metaraminol (10 mg in 20 mL N/S) or phenylephrine (2 mg in 20 mL N/S), run at 10–15 mL/h titrated to blood pressure readings.

5   Place the patient supine with left lateral tilt 15°. Recent studies suggest left lateral tilt is possibly unnecessary.[2]

6   A block to T4 is ideal for CS.

7   Treat hypotension (SBP < 100 mmHg) promptly with boluses of metaraminol (0.5–1 mg), phenylephrine (100 mcg) or ephedrine (9 mg). Treat bradycardia with atropine.

8   After delivery of the baby, administer oxytocin 3 units (or carbetocin 100 mcg over 1 min for elective CS).

9   Return the bed to the supine position if left lateral tilt used.

10 Run an infusion of oxytocin 40 units in 1000 mL Hartmann's solution over 4 h (**unless carbetocin was used**).

11 Wean the vasopressor infusion with the aim of ceasing it at the end of the surgery.

12 If the spinal block is obviously inadequate prior to surgery commencing, consider providing epidural anaesthesia as described below. Do not attempt a second SAB, as a very high block may result.

13 If the block is inadequate during surgery, convert to a GA.

14 Administer paracetamol 1 g IV and parecoxib 40 mg IV intraoperatively.

Epidural anaesthesia (*see Epidural anaesthesia/analgesia*)

1   Preload the patient with 500–1000 mL IV Hartmann's solution.

2   Insert the epidural at L3–4 interspace.

3   Use lignocaine 2% with adrenaline 1:200 000 + fentanyl 5 mcg/mL injected epidurally. Inject 10 mL then 5 mL boluses to a total of 20–25 mL. Aim for a block to T4. Consider left lateral tilt as described above.

4   If lignocaine 2% with adrenaline is not available, use ropivacaine 0.75% in the same volumes as lignocaine 2%.

5   Treat hypotension as described above. It is not necessary to run a vasopressor infusion. Administer oxytocin/carbetocin bolus as described above. Follow this with an oxytocin infusion as described above (**unless carbetocin was used**).

6   At the end of surgery, inject 3 mg of preservative-free morphine epidurally and remove the epidural catheter.

7   If the epidural is obviously inadequate prior to surgery, consider resiting the epidural. Another option is a combined spinal epidural (CSE) technique with a low-dose spinal component e.g. 1.5 mL heavy bupivacaine 0.5%. Do not perform a SAB on top of a partially working epidural as a very high block may result.

Combined spinal epidural (CSE) anaesthesia (*see Subarachnoid block (SAB)*)

1   The comments above regarding SAB anaesthesia also apply to CSE.

2   Use 2 mL heavy bupivacaine 0.5% + fentanyl 20–25 mcg + morphine 100 mcg for the spinal component.

3   Supplement the block with epidural 2% lignocaine with adrenaline if required.

General anaesthesia

1   For elective GA CS, some anaesthetists/obstetricians fully prep and drape the patient prior to GA; others do not. If it is an emergency CS, prep and drape and insert a urinary catheter prior to induction.

2 Consider tilting the operating table 15° left lateral (though, as noted above, it may be that left lateral tilt is unnecessary).
3 Preoxygenate the patient and perform a rapid (or modified rapid) sequence induction with propofol and suxamethonium or rocuronium and cricoid pressure. Do not give opioids or midazolam. If opioids are used, consider short-acting drugs such as remifentanil or alfentanil.
4 Maintain anaesthesia with oxygen, nitrous oxide (if available) and sevoflurane.
5 Administer oxytocin 3 units after delivery of the fetus, followed by an oxytocin infusion as described above.
6 Consider bilateral TAP blocks prior to emergence. ***See Transversus abdominis plane (TAP) block/subcostal TAP block.***

QUICK FLICK C

Postoperative management

1 SAB morphine (100 mcg) or epidural morphine (3 mg) provides excellent postoperative analgesia, which can be supplemented by oxycodone 10 mg up to every 4 h to a maximum of 40 mg/day. ***See Breast feeding and maternal anaesthesia/postoperative care.***
2 For patients who have had a GA, PCA fentanyl +/− TAP blocks can be very useful.
3 Regular paracetamol and diclofenac.

RBC cell salvage in obstetrics

See *Blood salvage, intraoperative*.

Calcium

Introduction

Calcium is an essential ion for body metabolism, including nerve conduction, muscle contraction and hundreds of enzymatic processes such as coagulation. It is the fifth-most abundant element in the human body and has a key role in bone metabolism. A 70 kg patient contains about 1.2 kg of calcium, 98% of which is in bone. NR 2.25–2.6 mmol/L.

Importance of ionised calcium

Around 50% of calcium in the plasma is free ionised Ca^{2+}, which is the clinically important form. NR for ionised calcium is 1–1.25 mmol/L. The other 50% is bound to albumin and anions (e.g. bicarbonate, citrate) and is inactive. The NR for albumin is 34–54 g/L.

1 If albumin is low and measured Ca^{2+} is also low, the ionised Ca^{2+} level may be normal.
2 If unable to read the ionised Ca^{2+} levels directly, the measured total Ca^{2+} can be 'corrected' by the following formula—for every 1 g/L reduction in serum albumin, increase the measured Ca^{2+} by 0.02 mmol/L. For example, if the measured Ca^{2+} is 2 mmol/L and the serum albumin is 30 g/L, the corrected Ca^{++} is 10×0.02 added to the measured Ca^{2+} ($10 \times 0.02 = 0.2$). Therefore, the corrected Ca^{2+} is 2.2 mmol/L.
3 Acidosis increases ionised (free) Ca^{2+} levels because there are more H^+ ions available to bind to albumin, resulting in fewer binding sites for Ca^{2+}. Total serum Ca^{2+} is unaffected.

Hypercalcaemia

Severe if $Ca^{2+} > 3.2$ mmol/L. Causes include:

1 hyperparathyroidism
2 malignancy e.g. bone metastases
3 iatrogenic e.g. TPN, vitamin D intoxication

4 endocrine disorders e.g. phaeochromocytoma, acromegaly
5 sarcoidosis, thyrotoxicosis
6 milk-alkali syndrome
7 Paget's disease of bone
8 immobilisation
9 thiazide diuretics
10 myeloproliferative disorders e.g. chronic myelogenous leukaemia, polycythaemia rubra vera, chronic neutrophilic leukaemia, multiple myeloma.

Clinical effects
1 Drowsiness, lethargy, anxiety, depression, psychosis, coma, headache.
2 Muscle weakness, hypotonia, hypoactive reflexes, tongue fasciculations.
3 Abdominal pain, nausea, vomiting, constipation, peptic ulceration.
4 Acute/chronic pancreatitis.
5 Hypertension.
6 ECG changes include shortened ST segment, reduced QT interval, arrhythmias, digitalis sensitivity, cardiac arrest. *See Electrocardiography (ECG)—a brief guide.*
7 Polyuria, dehydration, thirst, renal stones.
8 Thrombosis.

Treatment
1 Treat the cause if known.
2 Rehydrate with N/S and encourage early mobilisation if appropriate.
3 Establish forced saline diuresis with 1000 mL N/S over 4 h, then 1000 mL N/S + 20 mEq KCl + 20 mg frusemide every 4 h. Monitor K^+, Mg^{2+} and Ca^{2+} levels. Keep patient euvolaemic. Monitor urine output and keep urinary $Na^+ >$ 100 mmol/L.
4 If hypercalcaemia is due to a myeloproliferative disorder, give plicamycin 25 mcg/kg by infusion over 3 h (one dose only). IV etidronate is also effective.
5 Calcitonin is useful for hypercalcaemia associated with cancer. Give 3–4 u/kg IV then 4 u/kg subcut q 12–24 h.
6 Hydrocortisone 200–400 mg/day IV is useful in patients with lymphoproliferative diseases and diseases associated with elevated calcitriol levels e.g. sarcoidosis.
7 IV phosphate—this has potential for acute toxicity.
8 EDTA 15–50 mg/kg.
9 Dialysis.

Hypocalcaemia
Clinical manifestations occur if $Ca^{2+} < 2$ mmol/L or the ionised Ca^{2+} is < 0.8 mmol/L. Ionised $Ca^{2+} < 0.5$ mmol/L is life threatening. Causes include:
1 chronic and acute renal failure
2 pancreatitis
3 hypoparathyroidism, post parathyroidectomy, post thyroidectomy
4 lack of vitamin D
5 elderly/cachexia/malnutrition
6 drugs e.g. phenytoin, cis-platinum, bisphosphonates, loop diuretics e.g. frusemide
7 citrate toxicity from massive blood and/or blood product transfusion
8 massive soft tissue infection, sepsis
9 magnesium deficiency or excess
10 radiographic contrast with calcium chelators.

Clinical effects

1 Tetany, cramps, carpopedal spasm, positive Chvostek's and Trousseau's signs. Chvostek's sign is twitching of the facial muscles produced by tapping on the facial nerve. Trousseau's sign is carpopedal spasm in response to inflation of a blood pressure cuff above SBP.
2 Hyperactive reflexes.
3 Mental changes.
4 Reduced cardiac output, heart failure, hypotension, decreased efficacy of vasopressors.
5 Perioral and peripheral paraesthesia.
6 Laryngeal stridor, laryngospasm, bronchospasm.
7 ECG may show prolonged QT interval, T wave inversion and heart block. *See Electrocardiography (ECG)—a brief guide*.
8 Cardiac arrest.

Treatment

1 Identify and treat the cause.
2 Oral calcium supplements can be given for mild hypocalcaemia.
3 Resuscitate the patient if required (ABC).
4 Correct any co-existing respiratory or metabolic alkalosis.
5 Give 10 mL of calcium chloride 10% over 10 min via a central line or large-bore IV cannula (to reduce the risk of extravasation). Repeat as necessary. Each dose lasts 2–3 h. Max dose 3 mmol/kg/day. For a 70 kg patient, this equals 31 mL of calcium chloride 10%. If an infusion is required, add 4 g of calcium chloride (or 11 g of calcium gluconate) to 1000 mL of N/S. Run the infusion at 50 mL per h.
6 Correct concurrent hypomagnesaemia. *See Magnesium*. Aim for a serum magnesium concentration > 0.75 mmol/L.

⬤ Calcium channel blockers

Introduction

Calcium channel blocker drugs are used to treat hypertension and certain cardiac arrhythmias. They act by blocking the inward movement of calcium into the L-type 'long-acting' voltage-gated calcium channels in the heart, vascular smooth muscle and the pancreas. There are two types: dihydropyridines and non-dihydropyridines.

Dihydropyridines

These are used to treat hypertension as they are more effective in reducing vascular resistance than non-dihydropyridines. Examples include amlodipine, clevidipine, felodipine, nifedipine and nicardipine. They are also used to treat migraine and vaso-spastic angina.

Non-dihydropyridines

Non-dihydropyridines are favoured to treat some types of supraventricular arrhythmias. They inhibit the SA and AV nodes, slowing cardiac conduction, reducing heart rate and contractility. They are less potent vasodilators than dihydropyridines. Examples include verapamil and diltiazem.

Problems

1 Non-dihydropyridine drugs may worsen heart failure and cause bradycardia. They are contraindicated in patients with heart failure and reduced ejection fraction. They are also contraindicated if there is second or third degree heart block or sick sinus syndrome. *See Heart block (HB)* and *Sick sinus syndrome (SSS)*.

2 Dihydropyridine drugs may cause headaches and peripheral oedema.

◐ Calcium chloride 10%

Calcium chloride 10% contains 1 g of $CaCl_2$ in 10 mL. This equals 6.8 mmol or 14 mEq or 270 mg of elemental Ca^{2+} in 10 mL.

It is used to treat:

1 hypocalcaemia

2 hyperkalaemia

3 hypermagnesaemia

4 citrate toxicity due to massive transfusion.

◐ Calcium gluconate 10%

Calcium gluconate 10% contains 1 g of $C_{12}H_{22}CaO_{14}$ in 10 mL. This equals 2.2 mmol or 4.65 mEq or 93 mg of elemental calcium in 10 mL. Indications are the same as for calcium chloride.

◐ Cangrelor

Description

An intravenous $P2Y_{12}$ receptor antagonist antiplatelet drug. ($P2Y_{12}$ receptor antagonists are also called platelet adenosine diphosphate receptor antagonists.) It begins working within 2 min of administration and is fully effective in 30 min. It wears off after 60 min. It is used during percutaneous coronary artery revascularisation procedures, and as bridging therapy in high-risk patients with coronary artery stents undergoing non-cardiac surgery. Surgery can be performed 2 h after cessation of the infusion.

Dose

Adult

Start at 0.6 mcg/kg/min. Adjust infusion rate to maintain platelet reactivity levels between 80–180 units.

◐ Cannabis and cannabinoids

Definition

Cannabinoid drugs are either derived from the plant cannabis or are synthetic. The psychoactive properties (getting 'high') effects of cannabis are due to tetrahydrocannabinol (THC). Cannabidiol has little psychoactive effect. Both derivatives are used medically. Cannabis can be smoked, vaporised or ingested orally. Patients taking THC for medical purposes are not allowed to drive.

Use of medically prescribed cannabinoids

Cannabis-derived drugs may be useful for:

1 reducing opioid dependence

2 alleviating anxiety, depression and/or insomnia

3 treating nausea and pain

4 stimulating appetite.

Specific drugs

1 *Nabiximols*—used for multiple sclerosis-induced spasms, neuropathic pain and overactive bladder. It is sold as a mouth spray.
2 *Nabilone*—used to treat nausea and vomiting associated with cancer chemotherapy.
3 *Dronabinol*—used to treat refractory epilepsy in children.
4 *Non TGA-approved cannabinoids*—various uses.

Cannabis-derived drugs and anaesthesia

1 Drugs containing < 0.2% THC can be continued.
2 Drugs containing > 0.2% THC should be weaned prior to elective surgery if possible and clonidine used to treat withdrawal effects.

Cannabis use and anaesthesia

Acute use can be associated with:
1 tachycardia, serious arrhythmias (AF, VF, Brugada pattern)
2 coronary artery spasm if CAD present
3 airway hyperreactivity
4 pharyngeal and uvular oedema.

Chronic use can be associated with:
1 bradycardia/tachycardia/sinus arrest
2 postural/orthostatic hypotension
3 hyperreactive airway reflexes
4 intraoperative hypothermia
5 coronary artery spasm/infarction.

Synthetic cannabinoids used for drug abuse

There are novel psychoactive cannabinoids (designer drugs) created illegally, which have a greater potency than natural cannabis. They can have severe side effects such as psychosis, suicidal ideation, haemodynamic instability and respiratory difficulties.

⊙ Can't intubate, can't oxygenate (CICO)

*See **Difficult airway management**.*

⊙ Carbetocin (Duratocin)

Description

Long-acting uterotonic drug used post delivery in elective uncomplicated CS surgery performed under neuraxial anaesthesia. It causes uterine contraction.

Dose

100 mcg IV over 1 min. It is contraindicated in coronary artery disease. This drug can cause bronchoconstriction, pulmonary vasoconstriction and/or cardiac arrest. Do not use in patients with asthma or pulmonary hypertension.

⊙ Carbon monoxide poisoning

*See **Burns**.*

⊙ Carboprost (Prostin 15M)

Description

15-methyl-PGF2α prostaglandin analogue drug used to treat postpartum haemorrhage (PPH) due to uterine atony. ***See Postpartum haemorrhage (PPH)**.* Presented in ampoules of 1 mL containing 250 mcg of drug.

Dose

Mix 1–2 ampoules with 20 mL N/S. Give 250–500 mcg injected into the myometrium. Alternatively give 250 mcg IM.

▷ Carcinoid tumours and carcinoid syndrome

Carcinoid tumours

Carcinoid tumours are rare, malignant, neuroendocrine neoplasms, derived from enterochromaffin cells, also called Kulchitsky cells. These cells resemble chromaffin cells in the adrenal medulla. They occur most commonly in the gut (90%), especially the appendix and terminal ileum. They can also arise in the liver, pancreas, ovary, testicle, lung and bronchi. Around 8–20% of these tumours secrete substances such as serotonin, kallikrein, histamine, prostaglandins and other chemicals. These substances produce diverse effects, collectively known as 'the carcinoid syndrome'. The liver inactivates these substances. Therefore, gut carcinoid usually does not cause carcinoid syndrome unless there are liver metastases.

Carcinoid syndrome

Manifestations of carcinoid syndrome may sometimes be initiated by exercise, alcohol or ingestion of foods rich in tyramine such as blue cheese. Carcinoid syndrome effects include:

1 diarrhoea, abdominal pain, GIT bleeding
2 lacrimation
3 tachycardia, tachydysrhythmias, hypertension (due to serotonin), hypotension and bronchospasm (due to bradykinin)
4 mild hyperglycaemia
5 flushing
6 oedema.

Other effects of carcinoid tumours

1 Carcinoid tumours use tryptophan to make serotonin. This can deplete the body's tryptophan stores for the production of niacin (vitamin B3). This can result in niacin deficiency, causing pellagra (inflamed skin, diarrhoea, dementia and sores in the mouth).
2 Vitamin B12 and folate deficiency.
3 Clotting abnormalities due to malabsorption of fat-soluble vitamins.
4 Hypoproteinaemia.

Carcinoid heart disease

Typically affects the right side of the heart because the lung inactivates tumour secretions. Bronchogenic carcinoid can affect the left side of the heart, but this is very rare. Manifestations include:

1 Endocardial plaques of fibrous tissue that may involve the valve leaflets and sub-valvular apparatus. This can cause tricuspid and pulmonary valve stenosis, incompetence or both.
2 Fibrous thickening of the right pericardium.
3 Pulmonary stenosis can lead to high right-sided heart pressures, tricuspid incompetence and a pulsatile liver. Pulmonary valve surgery may be required before liver surgery, due to the risk of severe blood loss from the pulsatile liver.
4 Right heart failure may occur.

Carcinoid crisis

This can be precipitated by stress, GA, intraoperative tumour handling or radiological intervention. It is an extreme form of carcinoid syndrome. It is characterised by:

1 severe hypotension/hypertension
2 flushing
3 bronchospasm
4 hypercoagulability.

Diagnosis of carcinoid tumours

1 Measurement of the serotonin metabolite 5-hydroxyindoleacetic acid (HIAA) in a 24 h urine collection.
2 Serum chromogranin A is another useful test.
3 Endoscopy and biopsy may identify a carcinoid tumour.
4 CT, MRI, angiography.
5 I-123 metaiodobenzylguanidine (MIBG) scan or iridium-111 labelled octreotide scan can be used to localise metastatic disease.
6 Hyperglycaemia, hypoproteinaemia, elevated liver enzymes, electrolyte abnormalities.
7 Echocardiography to detect carcinoid heart disease.

Treatment

Treatment options include the following.

1 Octreotide (Sandostatin®) 200 mcg q 8 h subcut. It acts through somatostatin receptors to help relieve carcinoid symptoms. It inhibits the release of most carcinoid hormones and is the drug of choice for flushing and diarrhoea.
2 If octreotide is effective, lanreotide, which is a longer acting drug, can be trialled.
3 Chlorpromazine or antihistamines may help flushing.
4 Codeine, loperamide or diphenoxylate may relieve diarrhoea.
5 Steroids may be helpful to treat bronchospasm.
6 Surgical resection.
7 Chemoembolisation/radioembolisation of liver lesions. Chemoembolisation involves injecting chemotherapy drugs directly into the tumour. In radioembolisation, a thin flexible tube is used to inject radioactive beads into the liver.
8 Chemotherapy is usually ineffective.

Anaesthetic considerations

Anaesthesia requires involvement of, and planning with, the patient's endocrinologist. Other considerations include:

1 In addition to routine assessment, look for any evidence of heart disease, pellagra, electrolyte disturbance and dehydration from diarrhoea.
2 12 h before surgery, commence an octreotide infusion run at 100–200 mcg/h.[3]
3 Intraoperatively, continue the octreotide infusion at the same rate. Increase the rate, if necessary to control carcinoid effects, to a maximum of 500 mcg/h.
4 Use invasive arterial BP monitoring.
5 Do not use suxamethonium for intubation as it may increase intra-abdominal pressure and tumour secretion.
6 Avoid hypothermia, which may trigger a carcinoid crisis.
7 Bronchospasm is best treated with octreotide. Beta receptor agonists, such as salbutamol, may increase mediator release and worsen bronchospasm. Steroids may be helpful.

8 Beta receptor agonists such as adrenaline may stimulate the release of vasoactive substances from the tumour and cause hypotension.

9 Noradrenaline may increase bradykinin secretion, causing vasodilation and hypotension.

10 Avoid histamine-releasing drugs such as morphine and pethidine.

11 Treat hypotension due to carcinoid crisis (in addition to octreotide) IV fluid loading and phenylephrine. Vasopressin may be useful for vasoconstriction. *See **Vasopressin (Vasostrict, Pitressin)**.*

12 Treat hypertension with a beta blocker such as esmolol. *See **Esmolol (Brevibloc)**.* Ketanserin 10 mg IV over 3 min, followed by an infusion of 3 mg/h IV, may also be useful. *See **Ketanserin**.*

13 Continue octreotide infusion for 48 h post surgery, then wean slowly over the following week.

▶ Cardiac arrest, adult

Basic life support (BLS)

BLS is defined as the preservation or restoration of life by the establishment and/or maintenance of airway, breathing, circulation and related emergency care. The steps involved in doing this are summarised in the BLS chart below.

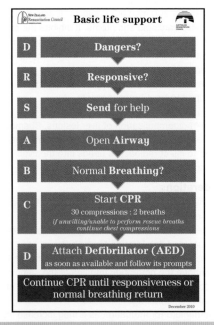

Figure C1 ARC BLS flow chart
Reproduced with permission from Australian Resuscitation Council.

D – **D**angers? Check the environment for danger to yourself, bystanders or the victim (e.g. electricity, fire, asphyxiating gases, water and/or sharps).

R – **R**esponsive? Establish whether the patient is responsive or non-responsive to verbal stimuli, touch and non-injurious vigorous physical stimulation ('talk, touch, torture').

S – **S**end for help. Notify nearby people/staff, activate the appropriate emergency response system (ERS) and send for available resuscitation equipment and a defibrillator.

A – Open **A**irway. Open the patient's airway with head tilt, jaw thrust; open the mouth.

B – Normal **B**reathing? Establish whether the patient is breathing or not breathing (or not breathing normally). A trained rescuer will also feel for a pulse.

C – Start **C**PR. Commence chest compressions, pressing on the lower half of the sternum at a rate of 100–120 compressions per minute. Depress the sternum ⅓ the anterior-posterior diameter of the chest. Provide two rescue breaths over two seconds after every 30 compressions, pausing the compressions while doing so. If an advanced airway is present (LMA or ET tube), provide continuous chest compressions and 6–10 ventilations per minute. Time the inspiratory phase with the chest recoil phase of the compressions.

D – Attach a **D**efibrillator, either a manual defibrillator or an automated external defibrillator (AED). Source a defibrillator as soon as possible and attach the pads to the patient. Shock a shockable rhythm (VF or pulseless VT) as soon as possible. If an AED is used, follow the prompts.

Advanced life support (ALS)

ALS is defined as BLS plus all other appropriate treatments, including drug therapy. Follow the ALS algorithm below.

Adult Advanced Life Support

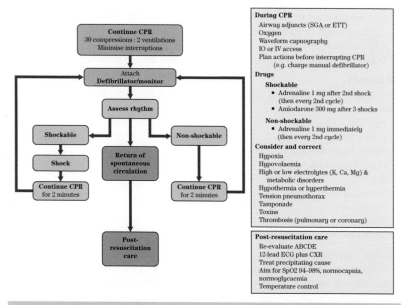

Figure C2 ARC ALS flow chart for adults
Reproduced with permission from Australian Resuscitation Council.

While BLS continues, attach the defibrillator pads and charge the defibrillator.

Shockable rhythm arrest

The shockable rhythms are VF and pulseless VT.

1 Give a 200 J shock, then recommence CPR immediately.
2 After nearly 2 min of CPR, charge the defibrillator.
3 Cease CPR and analyse the rhythm 2 min after the first shock.
4 If still in a shockable rhythm, give a second shock of 200 J or maximal energy, then immediately recommence CPR. Give adrenaline 1 mg IV. Repeat 1 mg of adrenaline after alternate shocks (about every 4 min).
5 After nearly 2 min of CPR, charge the defibrillator.
6 Cease CPR and analyse the rhythm 2 min after the second shock.
7 If still in a shockable rhythm, give a third shock and immediately recommence CPR. Give IV amiodarone 300 mg or 5 mg/kg.
8 Continue in this pattern. After the fifth shock, consider a second dose of amiodarone (150 mg or 2.5 mg/kg).
9 If amiodarone is unavailable or contraindicated, substitute lignocaine 1 mg/kg IV for the first dose and 0.5 mg/kg for the second dose.

Note: in certain circumstances, stacked shocks (three shocks in quick succession without CPR between shocks and checking the rhythm after each shock) can be considered. These circumstances are:

1 witnessed, monitored shockable rhythm arrest
2 cardiac ward post cardiac surgery
3 in the cardiac catheter lab

Non-shockable rhythm arrest

The non-shockable rhythms are asystole and pulseless electrical activity (PEA). If the defibrillator has been charged, dump the charge.

1 Give adrenaline 1 mg IV and repeat this every 3–5 min of arrest time.
2 Continue chest compressions.
3 Apply defibrillation pads.
4 Check rhythm every 2 min (charge the defibrillator prior to each rhythm check).

All arrests

Identify and treat the specific cause if possible. Always consider the 4Hs and 4Ts. These are:

1 Hypoxia
2 Hypovolaemia
3 Hyper/hypokalaemia
4 Hypo/hyperthermia
   and
1 Tension pneumothorax
2 Tamponade
3 Toxins
4 Thrombosis (pulmonary/coronary).

Consider other drugs such as:

1 magnesium—in cases of shock-resistant VF, pulseless VT, torsades de pointes
2 calcium—in cases of hyperkalaemia, calcium antagonist overdose, hypocalcaemia
3 potassium—in cases of hypokalaemia
4 sodium bicarbonate—in cases of prolonged arrest, acidosis prior to arrest, tricyclic antidepressant overdose

5 thrombolytic drug—if pulmonary embolism diagnosed or suspected
6 fluid therapy can be considered if hypovolaemia is known or suspected.

For prolonged resuscitation consider:
1 LUCAS device or other mechanical chest compressor
2 ECMO.

Cardiac arrest during neurosurgery

Cardiac arrest during neurosurgery produces special challenges, which include the following:
1 The patient may be positioned laterally or prone.
2 The head may be held in pins and clamped to the table (Mayfield clamp). CPR in this apparatus may result in skin laceration.
3 Excessive adrenaline may lead to severe cerebral bleeding and brain injury.

Modifications to standard adult BLS/ALS for neurosurgery arrest

1 Eliminate a surgical cause for asystole such as traction on cerebral structures. Pre-emptive use of atropine may reduce the risk of asystole from this cause.
2 Consider early release from the Mayfield clamp with the surgeon supporting the head while still in pins, before starting chest compression. The head may be lacerated by the pins if this is not done.
3 Chest compressions in the prone position may or may not be effective. If it is not, turn the patient supine.
4 If adrenaline is required, give it in increments of 50–100 mcg to a maximum dose of 1 mg. Subsequent doses of adrenaline should be 1 mg.
5 Minimise contamination of an open wound.

◐ Cardiac arrest, neonatal

See Neonatal resuscitation.

◐ Cardiac arrest, paediatric

Basic life support (BLS)

Asphyxia is a more common cause of cardiac arrest in children than it is in adults. However, a witnessed sudden cardiac arrest in a child (e.g. collapse while playing football) may be due to a cardiac cause. BLS is provided as described for the adult with the following caveats.
1 Give two ventilations prior to chest compressions.
2 Trained rescuers should use a compression to ventilation ratio of 15:2. Untrained rescuers should use a 30:2 ratio.
3 If the rescuer is alone, they should shout for help, then commence CPR for 1 min. If no help has arrived, the rescuer should go find help. If the child is small enough, the rescuer should carry the child with them.
4 If two rescuers are available, one should start CPR and the other should get help.
5 If the arrest is witnessed as a sudden collapse (potential cardiac cause) and the rescuer is alone, try to get help and a defibrillator first, then start CPR.
6 For children older than 8 years, standard AED pads can be used.
7 For children aged 1–8 years, an AED with paediatric pads and paediatric dose attenuation is preferred. If paediatric pads are unavailable, use adult pads, but ensure the pads are not in contact with each other when placed on the patient.

Follow the ALS algorithm below.

Advanced Life Support for Infants and Children

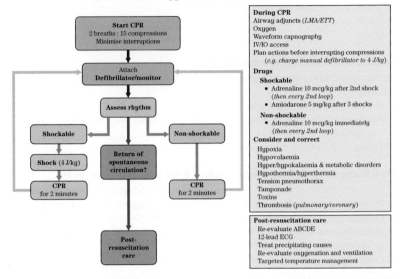

Figure C3 Advanced life support for infants and children
Reproduced with permission from Australian Resuscitation Council.

ALS in children is similar to that in adults, with the following caveats.

1 Use a defibrillation energy of 4 J/kg for all shocks.
2 If fluid therapy is required for hypovolaemia, give 10–20 mL/kg boluses of crystalloid.
3 Adrenaline dosage is 10 mcg/kg IV up to 1 mg.
4 Amiodarone dosage is 5 mg/kg IV up to 300 mg.
5 Calcium dosage is 0.15 mmol/kg IV.
6 Treat hypoglycaemia with 2mL/kg of 10% glucose IV.
7 Magnesium dosage is 0.1–0.2 mmol/kg IV. The infusion dose is 0.3 mmol/kg IV over 4 h.
8 Potassium dosage is potassium chloride 0.03–0.07 mmol/kg IV over several min.
9 Sodium bicarbonate dosage is 0.5–1 mmol/kg IV. It should only be used if there is a specific indication.

◑ Cardiac arrhythmias

This section is an overview of the enormous topic of cardiac arrhythmias. For more information on each specific type of arrhythmia, see their individual entry.

Tachyarrhythmias

Heart rate > 100 beats per minute. Sinus tachycardia may be physiological (e.g. exercise) or pathological (e.g. haemorrhage, fever). Other tachyarrhythmias are due to causes such as:

• heart conduction defects
• electrolyte abnormalities

- ischaemia
- drug effects e.g. cocaine.

Mechanisms of tachyarrhythmias due to electrical defects

Cardiac arrhythmias are due to three main mechanisms:
1 enhanced automaticity
2 triggered activity
3 re-entry.

Enhanced automaticity

This refers to acceleration of action potential formation by either normal cardiac tissue (e.g. the SA node leading to sinus tachycardia) or abnormal tissue (e.g. ectopic atrial tachycardia).

Triggered activity

This phenomenon results from depolarisation of myocardial cells due to mechanisms other than normal cardiac electrical conduction pathway activity. The electrical activity is triggered by an electrophysiological phenomenon called 'after-depolarisations'. For example, hypokalaemia or ischaemia may make ventricular cells hyperexcitable, leading to spontaneous depolarisations. These electrical effects can lead to an R-on-T type episode with precipitation of VF.

Re-entry

Re-entry means a continuous circuit is created so that, instead of a cardiac impulse dying out, it travels around the circuit and re-excites the heart after the refractory period has ended. Re-entrant tachycardias are also called re-entrant excitation, reciprocating tachycardias and reciprocal or echo beats. Onset and offset of the arrhythmia is usually abrupt. Re-entry tachycardias are divided into anatomical re-entry and functional re-entry. In anatomical re-entry there is an anatomically defined area of abnormality such as fibrosis. In functional re-entry, the location and size of the circuits vary. Examples include:
1 Wolff–Parkinson–White syndrome. **See Wolff–Parkinson–White (WPW) syndrome.**
2 atrial flutter/atrial fibrillation
3 AV nodal re-entry
4 atrioventricular re-entry using an accessory bypass tract
5 ventricular tachycardia and VF.

Tachyarrhythmias based on QRS duration

These can be divided into narrow complex and broad complex tachycardias.

Narrow complex tachycardias (NCTs)

If the QRS complexes are narrow (< 3 small squares or 120 ms), this suggests the arrhythmia originates above or within the His bundle. These are supraventricular tachycardias (SVTs). They can be regular or irregular.

Regular NCTs include:
1 sinus tachycardia
2 sinoatrial nodal re-entrant tachycardia (SANRT)
3 atrioventricular nodal re-entrant tachycardia (AVNRT)
4 atrial flutter.

Irregular NCTs include:
1 atrial fibrillation
2 atrial flutter with a variable block
3 multifocal atrial tachycardia (MAT).

Wide complex tachycardias (WCTs)

The QRS complexes are widened ($\geq$ 3 small squares or $\geq$ 120 ms). The arrhythmia originates below the His bundle in the Purkinje fibres or ventricles **or** there may be SVT with aberrant ventricular conduction e.g. LBBB. Most WCT are due to VT. It is safer to presume the diagnosis is VT and treat as such than treat VT as SVT with aberrant conduction.

Criteria which may help differentiate between SVT with aberrant conduction and VT are:

SVT with aberrant conduction
1 Young patients.
2 Structurally normal heart.
3 An irregular WCT usually suggests AF with aberrant conduction.

VT
1 Older patients.
2 Presence of heart disease.
3 Regular (with perhaps slight variation in the RR interval). Polymorphic VT will be irregular.
4 Very broad complexes > 160 ms.
5 An axis shift, extreme right axis deviation or bizarre axis.
6 Atrial rate slower than the ventricular rate (AV dissociation).
7 Capture and fusion beats. A capture beat is when the SA node sends an impulse at just the right time to cause normal conduction, resulting in a narrow QRS complex. A fusion beat is a hybrid complex of a supraventricular and a ventricular beat.
8 Concordance—all the QRS complexes in V1–V6 are monophasic, with the same polarity.

Regular WCTs are:
1 VT
2 regular SVT with aberrant conduction
3 sinus tachycardia with aberrant conduction
4 antidromic WPW.

Bradyarrhythmias
See Bradycardia.

◑ Cardiac failure

See Congestive cardiac failure (CCF)—chronic and Cardiogenic shock.

◑ Cardiac inherited channelopathies

1 Brugada syndrome—*see Brugada syndrome*.
2 Long QT syndrome (inherited form)—*see Long QT syndrome (LQTS)*.
3 Arrhythmogenic right ventricular dysplasia.
4 Catecholaminergic polymorphic ventricular tachycardia (CPVT).

◑ Cardiac investigations

See Cardiac risk for non-cardiac surgery.

◑ Cardiac output (CO), adult

This is defined as the volume of blood ejected from the left ventricle (LV) per minute (usually 5 L). It is equal to the stroke volume (SV) multiplied by the heart rate (HR), and is determined by preload, cardiac contractility and afterload.

Stroke volume—the amount of blood ejected from the left or right ventricle in a single contraction (usually 60–80 mL).

Preload—the end-diastolic ventricular wall tension (tension at the point of maximal filling). It is mainly determined by venous return and atrial contraction.

Afterload—the tension developed in the ventricular wall during systole (to eject blood). It is largely determined by systemic vascular resistance (SVR).

Systemic vascular resistance (SVR)—all the forces that oppose blood flow through the systemic circulation. It is primarily determined by the vasoconstriction of the arteriolar bed.

Contractility—a measure of the mechanical work the heart can do at a given preload and afterload.

Pulse pressure—SBP minus DBP.

Ejection fraction—the fraction of total blood in the left ventricle that is ejected per beat. This provides an index of contractility, and is normally 55–65%.

▶ Cardiac risk for non-cardiac surgery

About 4% of the population has major surgery each year, and 30% of these have cardiovascular comorbidities. Cardiac risk assessment is an evolving science with multiple approaches of varying complexity. This manual can only provide a general overview of this topic. For patients with cardiac stents, **see Coronary artery stents (CAS)**.

Surgery and 30-day risk of a major adverse cardiac event (MACE)

MACE includes myocardial infarction, stent thrombosis, cardiac failure and cardiac death.

Low risk < 1%
- Breast, superficial surgery, reconstructive surgery.
- Dental, eye, thyroid, minor gynaecological surgery.
- Minor orthopaedic surgery.
- Minor urological surgery including TURP.
- Asymptomatic carotid surgery (stenting or endarterectomy).

Intermediate risk 1–5%
- Intraperitoneal surgery e.g. cholecystectomy, splenectomy, hiatus hernia repair.
- Minor intrathoracic surgery.
- Symptomatic carotid surgery (stenting or endarterectomy).
- Peripheral arterial angioplasty.
- Endovascular aneurysm repair.
- Head and neck surgery.
- Neurological surgery.
- Major orthopaedic surgery.
- Major urological or gynaecological surgery.
- Renal transplant.

High risk > 5%
- Aortic and major vascular surgery.
- Open lower limb vascular surgery or amputation.

- Major upper gastrointestinal surgery/oesophagectomy.
- Perforated bowel repair.
- Adrenal resection.
- Total cystectomy.
- Pneumonectomy.
- Pulmonary or liver transplant.
- Emergency surgery.

Intermediate- and high-risk surgery may be referred to as 'elevated-risk surgery'.

Clinical risk factors

1 Coronary artery disease—elective surgery should be delayed for at least 60 days after acute myocardial infarction in the absence of coronary artery intervention.
2 Heart failure—patients with active heart failure are at a higher risk of perioperative death than patients with CAD. Risk is particularly high in patients with signs and/or symptoms of heart failure and/or an LVEF < 30%.
3 Cardiomyopathy—*see Cardiomyopathy*.
4 Valvular heart disease—*see Aortic stenosis*.

Very-high-risk patients

Patients who have:
1 experienced acute myocardial infarction within 60 days
2 acute coronary syndrome—*see Acute coronary syndrome*
3 decompensated heart failure
4 high-grade arrhythmias
5 haemodynamically significant valvular heart disease, especially aortic stenosis.

Functional capacity and blood tests

Functional capacity—the MET concept

MET stands for 'metabolic equivalent'.
- 1 MET—basal metabolic rate at rest.
- 4 METs—climb two flights of stairs, walk 100 m on level ground, run a short distance.
- > 10 METs—strenuous sport.

Poor functional capacity (< 4 METs) is associated with an increased incidence of postoperative cardiac events. When functional capacity is subjectively assessed as high, this may not accurately predict postoperative morbidity or mortality.[4]
See New York Heart Association (NYHA) functional classification of patients with heart failure.

Biomarkers of heart failure

These are B-type natriuretic peptide (BNP) and N-terminal-proBNP (NT-proBNP). They are produced by cardiac muscle cells in response to heart failure. *See B-type natriuretic peptide (BNP) and N-terminal-proBNP (NT-proBNP)*. BNP > 35 pg/mL or NT-proBNP > 125 pg/mL suggest heart failure.[5] These tests have good negative predictive value but a less reliable positive predictive value.

Biomarkers of myocardial ischaemia

These are the cardiac troponins. *See Acute coronary syndrome*.

Non-invasive testing

1 ECG—preoperative ECG is not recommended for patients who do not have risk factors and are having low-risk surgery. An ECG may be considered in patients having intermediate-risk surgery, who have no risk factors and are aged > 65 y. An ECG is recommended for patients with risk factors having intermediate- to high-risk surgery and should be considered if they are having low-risk surgery. ECG abnormalities are **not** predictive of MACE but a baseline ECG is important to help identify subsequent ECG changes.

2 Echocardiography—the simplest and easiest way to assess LV function and valve function. If the patient is asymptomatic, it can be *considered* if they are having high-risk surgery. A LVEF of ≤ 29% is associated with a significantly decreased survival after surgery compared with LVEF > 29%.[6] In patients with heart failure, the risk of death does not increase significantly until LVEF drops to < 40%. Systolic LV dysfunction carries a higher risk than diastolic LV dysfunction. *See Diastolic dysfunction grading*.

3 Exercise ECG—non-invasive test for ischaemic heart disease using ST segment analysis. It is not suitable for patients who are unable to exercise (see myocardial perfusion imaging tests below). Patients with a myocardial ischaemic response at low workloads are at significant risk of perioperative cardiac events. Patients with a myocardial ischaemic response at high workloads are at a slightly increased risk.

4 Myocardial perfusion imaging tests—such as the dipyridamole-thallium scan can assess the heart during stress and rest. This can give information about reversible defects and fixed defects (due to scar or non-viable heart tissue). Reversible defects in < 20% of the LV probably do not increase cardiac risk significantly. Reversible defects in > 20% of the LV increases risk. Reversible defects suggest a higher risk than fixed defects. A normal scan is highly suggestive of very low risk.

5 Stress echocardiography—in this test, echocardiography is combined with exercise- or drug-induced stress (e.g. by dipyridamole). These studies give information on LV function with rest and exercise, heart valve function, fixed function defects and reversible function defects. This test is very reassuring if normal but the positive predictive value is low for an abnormal result. Patients with resting wall motion abnormalities are at increased risk.

6 Cardiovascular MRI—can also detect myocardial ischaemia during stress and rest.

7 CT scanning to detect coronary artery calcium, and CT angiography to detect CAD can also be helpful.

Invasive testing—coronary artery angiography

Indications for coronary angiography are the same, regardless of whether or not the patient is having non-cardiac surgery. These are:

1 acute ST elevation myocardial infarction
2 non-ST elevation acute coronary syndrome
3 proven myocardial ischaemia and non-stabilised chest pain.

Preoperative treatment of myocardial ischaemia should be undertaken (medically or surgically) if surgery can be delayed. Coronary angiography should be *considered* in patients undergoing non-urgent carotid endarterectomy.

Risk calculators

These include NSQIP (*see NSQIP*) and Dr Lee Goldman's *Revised cardiac risk index for pre-operative risk* (updated January 2019). The latter predicts the 30-day risk of death, MI or cardiac arrest and consists of six variables:

1 elevated-risk surgery e.g. AAA repair
2 history of IHD—history of MI, positive exercise test, current myocardial chest pain, use of nitrate therapy, ECG with pathological Q waves
3 history of CCF—pulmonary oedema, bilateral rales or S3 gallop, paroxysmal nocturnal dyspnoea, CXR showing pulmonary vascular redistribution
4 history of cerebrovascular disease—TIA or stroke
5 preoperative treatment with insulin
6 preoperative creatinine > 176.8 µmol/L.

Other variables which may be helpful in predicting risk are:
1 poor functional capacity
2 atrial fibrillation
3 advancing age
4 obesity.

Peri-operative medical therapy

1 **Beta blockers**—patients on beta blockers should continue their therapy. It is debateable whether intermediate-risk patients benefit from perioperative beta blocker therapy. Atenolol or bisoprolol are preferred and should be carefully titrated to effect (to avoid excessive bradycardia/hypotension).
2 **Statins** provide coronary artery plaque stabilisation, which reduces the risk of plaque rupture. Patients on statins should continue these. If new statin therapy is to be commenced, it should be started at least two weeks before surgery.
3 **Angiotensin-converting enzyme inhibitors (ACE inhibitors) and angiotensin receptor blockers (ARBs).** These carry a risk of severe hypotension under anaesthesia, especially if patients are also on beta blockers. Stop ACE inhibitors and ARBs for 24 h prior to surgery.[7]

Collating the information

The American College of Cardiology/American Heart Association guidelines recommend at least 60 days between an acute coronary syndrome (*see Acute coronary syndrome*) and elective non-cardiac surgery. Prophylactic coronary revascularisation done exclusively to reduce peri-operative risk is currently not recommended, even for high-risk surgery.

Low- and intermediate-risk surgery

The majority of patients with stable heart disease can undergo low- and intermediate-risk surgery without further evaluation. Selected patients in this group may require more extensive evaluation due to:
1 complex heart disease e.g. congenital heart disease
2 low functional capacity
3 the potential for medical optimisation.

High-risk surgery

Patients with known cardiovascular disease, or who are at high risk for cardiovascular disease, should be considered for further investigation by a multidisciplinary team. Important considerations include:

1 Patients with moderate to severe valve stenosis or incompetence should have preoperative echocardiography unless this has been done in the previous 12 months and their condition has not deteriorated. If patients require repair or replacement of a cardiac valve, this should be considered before high-risk surgery.

2 Patients requiring urgent or emergency surgery who are high risk for MACE should, if possible, have urgent cardiologist review. There will probably be little time for additional investigation, but the cardiologist can provide invaluable advice on perioperative medical management and monitoring. They can also manage cardiac complications postoperatively.

3 There is no evidence that prophylactic revascularisation to prevent ischaemia at the time of surgery improves outcomes.

◗ Cardiac tamponade

Description

Cardiac tamponade is defined as mechanical compression of the heart by pericardial fluid, resulting in a decrease in cardiac output and shock. It is a life-threatening emergency and one of the causes of cardiac arrest. *See Cardiac arrest, adult.*

Causes

1 Blood is the most common cause of cardiac tamponade and may cause sudden, severe reduction or loss in cardiac output. Blood in the pericardial sac may be due to:
   a) penetrating or blunt trauma
   b) ventricular rupture after myocardial infarction
   c) aortic dissection
   d) post cardiac surgery
   e) complication of catheter-based procedures on the heart or pacemaker insertion.
2 Malignancy.
3 Mediastinal radiotherapy.
4 Infection of the pericardium (bacterial, viral such as HIV or TB).
5 Inflammation of the pericardium.
6 Chronic autoimmune diseases such as rheumatoid arthritis.
7 Heart failure.
8 Renal failure.
9 Hypothyroidism.

Pathophysiology

The fluid build-up causes compression of the chambers of the heart, preventing venous filling which, in turn, causes decreased cardiac output. Tachycardia is an early compensatory mechanism.

Clinical presentation

Beck's Triad consists of hypotension, elevated JVP and muffled heart sounds. Other manifestations include:

1 tachycardia
2 chest pain
3 dyspnoea/tachypnoea
4 pulsus paradoxus—a decrease in systolic blood pressure of more than 10 mmHg on inspiration
5 elevated JVP during inspiration (Kussmaul's sign)
6 agitation
7 syncope
8 altered mental status
9 cardiac arrest with pulseless electrical activity (PEA). *See Cardiac arrest, adult.*

Diagnosis

1 ECG—may show low-voltage complexes and electrical alternans (alternating height of consecutive QRS complexes).
2 CXR—enlarged heart shadow.
3 Echocardiography—will demonstrate the pericardial effusion and compression of the cardiac chambers. Diastolic collapse of the right atrium and right ventricle is diagnostic.

Treatment

1 Supportive measures—volume expansion with IV crystalloid, supplementary O_2, maintain a fast heart rate of 90–140 bpm.
2 Maintain SVR to support coronary artery perfusion.
3 Inotropic support may be required.
4 If cardiac arrest occurs, *see Cardiac arrest, adult.*
5 Emergency pericardiocentesis—see below.

Emergency pericardiocentesis

The following assumes that immediate cardiologist assistance is not available and the patient is in extremis or has arrested. If possible, this procedure should be performed under echocardiographic guidance. There is a risk of injury due to blind needle insertion. The next-best option to ultrasound guidance is ECG monitoring. This is achieved by attaching the chest lead of the ECG to the proximal shaft of the needle and the limb leads to the patient's limbs. Elevation of the ST segment or ectopics is an indication that the myocardium has been contacted. Elevation of the ST segment and/or ectopics suggest that the needle is in contact with the myocardium. Steps in the procedure are:

1 Position the conscious patient sitting in bed at 45°.
2 If available, use a Cook Medical pericardiocentesis kit. If the kit is unavailable, use a 10 cm 18 G spinal needle.
3 Sterilise the skin of the lower chest around the xiphoid process.
4 The insertion site is between the xiphisternum and left costal margin.
5 Use LA in the conscious patient.
6 Insert the spinal needle through the skin in the direction of the left shoulder with an entry angle of 40° to the skin. After puncturing the skin, remove the stylet and attach a three-way tap and 20 mL syringe.
7 Advance the needle towards the left shoulder while continuously attempting to aspirate fluid.
8 When the pericardium is punctured and fluid is aspirated, cease advancing.

9 Attach tubing to the three-way tap and drain as much fluid as possible. Removing 100–200 mL of fluid from an acute pericardial tamponade should produce dramatic improvement.

10 If utilising a kit, use a Seldinger technique to leave a pig-tail catheter in the pericardium. The steps are:

a) Identify the pericardial space as described above.

b) Pass the guide-wire through the needle, then remove the needle.

c) Nick the skin with a scalpel at the site of wire insertion, then dilate the skin and deeper structures with the 6Fr dilator.

d) Remove the dilator and pass the 6–8Fr pig-tail catheter over the wire into the pericardial sac. Then remove the wire.

e) Secure the catheter and use it to drain the pericardial fluid.

⊳ Cardiac transplant

*See **Heart transplant patient, non-cardiac surgery**.*

⊳ Cardiogenic shock

Description

Cardiogenic shock is a life-threatening emergency in which there is inadequate tissue perfusion, due to the heart being unable to pump sufficient blood. The reduced tissue perfusion results in decreased oxygen and nutrient supply to the tissues, which will lead to organ damage, multi-organ failure and death, if not rapidly reversed.

Causes

There are many causes of cardiogenic shock, and there can be combinations of causes. They include:

1 acute myocardial infarction—the most common cause

2 dysrhythmias such as VT

3 valvular heart disease. There can be sudden decompensation e.g. ruptured chordae of a degenerative mitral valve

4 thrombosed mechanical heart valve

5 end-stage cardiomyopathy

6 Takotsubo cardiomyopathy

7 hypertensive crisis

8 pulmonary embolus

9 aortic dissection.

Clinical effects

1 Altered mental status.

2 Dyspnoea.

3 Hypotension (SBP ≤ 90 mmHg).

4 Urine output ≤ 30 mL/h.

5 Cool, clammy skin.

6 Depressed cardiac index (< 2.2 L/min/m² body surface area).

7 Acute pulmonary oedema.

8 Abdominal tenderness due to liver distension.

9 Peripheral oedema.

10 Weak, rapid, thready pulse.

11 Elevated JVP.

12 Heart murmur(s).

Diagnosis

Diagnostic investigations should not delay treatment. Attempt to identify and treat the cause as soon as possible.

1 ECG.

2 CXR.

3 Blood screen—elevated lactate, renal and liver dysfunction.

4 ABG.

5 Cardiac echo.

Treatment

Seek urgent cardiologist/cardiac anaesthetist input. The following strategies are suggested:

1 Ensure adequate airway and breathing, supplementary oxygen; patient may require intubation.

2 Treat the cause of the cardiogenic shock if possible e.g. urgent coronary artery reperfusion for AMI, cardioversion for arrhythmia.

3 Establish invasive blood pressure monitoring and insert a central line.

4 Inotropic support is required, but the best inotrope/combination of inotropes is unknown. The main ones used are dobutamine, dopamine, noradrenaline and adrenaline.

   a) Dobutamine—a good starting point. It stimulates beta-1 receptors, increasing inotropy and lusitropy. It is a weak chronotrope, which is beneficial in a tachycardic patient. It does cause some vasodilation, which reduces afterload but may also reduce blood pressure. *See Dobutamine.*

   b) Dopamine—has effects similar to adrenaline but is less potent. It stimulates alpha and beta receptors. It will provide some increase in systemic vascular resistance (SVR), supporting blood pressure, but it will also increase afterload. *See Dopamine (Intropin).*

   c) Noradrenaline—a powerful vasoconstrictor (alpha-1) with some inotropic properties but little effect on heart rate. It is used for severe hypotension (SBP ≤ 70 mmHg), obviously a very critical situation. *See Noradrenaline (NA)/ norepinephrine.*

   d) Adrenaline—stimulates all adrenoreceptors and provides a mixture of beneficial and detrimental effects including increased inotropy and CO but also increased heart rate (HR) and myocardial oxygen consumption. Adrenaline is also arrhythmogenic. BP is increased but increased SVR results in increased afterload. *See Adrenaline/epinephrine.*

5 **Milrinone**—a phosphodiesterase III inhibitor. It increases myocardial contractility without increasing myocardial oxygen demand. It also improves lusitropy. Milrinone is beneficial in the situation of cardiogenic shock due to myocardial ischemia with persistent low blood pressure, despite an increase in SVR. It does cause some vasodilation, decreasing LV filling pressures. Milrinone is especially preferred in patients with severe pulmonary hypertension. *See Milrinone.*

6 **Levosimendan**—a cardiotonic drug that increases inotropy by enhancing the heart muscle's sensitivity to calcium. There is no increase in myocardial oxygen demand or rhythm effects. It also has vasodilator effects.

7 Preload optimisation—this is another difficult balancing act. Reducing preload decreases myocardial wall stress, myocardial oxygen consumption and physiological mitral and tricuspid regurgitation, improving forward flow. However, too much preload reduction will reduce CO and blood pressure. Give frusemide 40–120 mg IV. *See Frusemide*.

8 Afterload optimisation—if SVR is high it leads to increased myocardial workload and oxygen consumption, whereas SVR that is too low results in hypotension and decreased coronary artery perfusion. Vasodilators such as GTN are not advisable when there is hypotension.

9 Positive pressure ventilation with PEEP may improve ventilation perfusion mismatching and reduce LV preload favourably.

10 Mechanical assist devices such as an intra-aortic balloon pump.

11 ECMO.

12 Implanted ventricular assist device.

13 Transplant.

○ Cardiomyopathy

Definition
Cardiomyopathy is a progressive myocardial disorder in which the heart muscle is abnormal and weak, leading to impaired function.

Classification
1 Ischaemic cardiomyopathy.
2 Dilated cardiomyopathy. *See Dilated cardiomyopathy (DCM)*.
3 Hypertrophic cardiomyopathy. *See Hypertrophic cardiomyopathy (HCM) and hypertrophic obstructive cardiomyopathy (HOCM)*.
4 Restrictive cardiomyopathy. *See Restrictive cardiomyopathy*.
5 Arrhythmogenic right ventricular cardiomyopathy and/or dysplasia.
6 Peripartum cardiomyopathy. *See Peripartum cardiomyopathy*.
7 Alcoholic cardiomyopathy.
8 Cardiac sarcoidosis/amyloidosis.
9 Genetic cardiomyopathy.
10 Takotsubo cardiomyopathy. *See Takotsubo cardiomyopathy/syndrome (broken heart syndrome)*.

○ Cardioversion, electrical

Description
Cardioversion is the use of low-energy biphasic electric shocks to convert a dysrhythmia to normal sinus rhythm.

Technique
1 For elective cardioversion, the patient should be fasted and have an IV cannula. They should receive a GA or sedation.
2 Pads are usually applied in the anterior posterior position. The anterior pad is placed over the heart on the left side of the chest. The posterior pad is placed behind the heart, in between the scapulae.
3 Use synchronisation so the shock is synchronised with the R wave. Shock in expiration to minimise impedance.

4 Do not have oxygen flowing over the patient's chest during cardioversion.

5 Use up to three shocks.

Suggested shock initial energies in adults

Atrial fibrillation (AF)	100 J
Atrial flutter	50 J
Supraventricular tachycardia	25–50 J
Ventricular tachycardia (with pulse)	100 J

Note:

1 Prior to cardioverting AF/atrial flutter, ensure atrial clot is not present (usually by transoesophageal echocardiography). *See Atrial fibrillation (AF) and Atrial flutter.*

2 Do not cardiovert over an implanted device.

3 In pregnant patients, cardioversion is not a risk to the fetus.

⊙ Carotid endarterectomy/stenting/trans-carotid arterial revascularisation (TCAR)

Introduction

The aim of carotid endarterectomy (or stenting) is to reduce the risk of thromboembolic stroke.

1 Compared with endarterectomy, stenting has a lower risk of peri-operative myocardial infarction (MI) and cranial nerve palsy. However, the 30-day risk of stroke or death is higher in the stenting group than in the endarterectomy group, especially in symptomatic and older patients.

2 There is little benefit in asymptomatic patients compared with medical therapy unless stenosis > 80% and life expectancy > 5 y.

3 Patients with TIA or CVA (< 3 months) and > 60% stenosis have the most to gain from revascularisation.

4 There is no evidence that the type of anaesthetic used (GA vs LA) alters outcomes. The respective skills of both the surgeon and the anaesthetist in utilising their chosen technique are the most important factors affecting outcome.

5 Most patients have GA for carotid endarterectomy.

6 Whatever technique is selected, the peri-operative stroke rate should be < 2%.

7 Carotid intervention should be performed within 48 h of a TIA or minor stroke and, less ideally, within one week.

8 Carefully document the patient's pre-procedure neurological baseline.

Preoperative assessment and preparation

1 There are frequently co-morbidities that may require investigation and optimisation prior to surgery, such as IHD, hypertension, diabetes and lung disease.

2 Statins and beta blockers should be continued in patients already receiving these therapies, with the possible exception of metoprolol. *See Metoprolol.* All patients should be on aspirin. If the patient is on a second antiplatelet drug (DAPT), continuation needs to be discussed with the surgeon.

3 Hypertension should be controlled within reasonable limits. Aim to reduce SBP < 180 mmHg unless there is severe bilateral disease or frequent neurological events. Consider stopping ACE inhibitors and angiotensin II receptor blockers. *See Angiotensin converting enzyme (ACE) inhibitors and Angiotensin II receptor blocker (ARB) drugs.*

Anaesthetic aims

1 Provide haemodynamic stability intraoperatively, avoiding hypotension and hypertension. Towards this aim, use invasive arterial blood pressure monitoring. Maintain SBP < 170 mmHg, and (ideally) within 20% of the patient's preoperative BP.
2 Monitor the patient for myocardial ischaemia, and treat this promptly if it occurs.
3 Anticoagulate the patient with 5000 units of heparin at the time of carotid artery cross-clamping.
4 Ensure tight blood glucose control in diabetic patients, avoiding hypo- and hyperglycaemia.
5 The surgeon may or may not use a shunt from the common carotid artery to the internal carotid artery.
6 Surgical manipulation of the carotid sinus may result in hypertension and tachycardia or hypotension and bradycardia. Some surgeons will infiltrate LA into the carotid body or surrounding tissue.

General anaesthesia

1 The patient should be paralysed, intubated and ventilated with O_2, air and sevoflurane. Alternatively, GA can be maintained with TCI propofol.
2 A remifentanil infusion is also a reasonable option to help with haemodynamic stability.
3 Avoid hyper- and hypocapnia.
4 Shunting is a matter of surgeon preference. Some routinely shunt; others base their decision on some indicator of ipsilateral cerebral perfusion. One technique is measuring the internal carotid stump pressure after test clamping the internal carotid. A stump mean arterial pressure > 50–60 mmHg is considered as indicative of adequate perfusion. Other surrogate measures of brain perfusion include transcranial doppler, EEG, somatosensory evoked potentials and near infrared spectroscopy.
5 It is particularly important to avoid hypotension during the time of clamping. Consider increasing the patient's BP to 20% above baseline during cross-clamping.
6 Provide anti-nausea medication to reduce the risk of vomiting post procedure, which may increase the risk of bleeding.
7 Coughing on emergence is also undesirable.

Awake surgery (under LA or cervical plexus block)

1 In the awake patient, the need for shunting is indicated by the development of slurred speech, agitation or other evidence of inadequate brain perfusion.
2 Consider dexmedetomidine for sedation (LD 1 mcg/kg IV then infusion 0.3 mcg/kg/h IV).

Postoperative management

Most postoperative events occur within 8 h of surgery. The most dangerous are CVA and MI. Other possible issues include the following:
1 Hypertension—this may cause cerebral hyperperfusion syndrome (ipsilateral headache, focal neurological deficits, cerebral oedema, brain haemorrhage and death). Cerebral hyperperfusion syndrome can occur up to seven days post surgery. Treatment is to control the BP, aiming for an SBP of 100–150 mmHg.
2 Hypotension may occur due to exposure of the carotid sinus after plaque removal. Maintain SBP at 100–150 mmHg.
3 Hypoglossal and recurrent laryngeal nerve injury may occur.
4 Neck haematoma with airway compromise may occur. *See Neck haematoma management.*

Percutaneous carotid artery stenting

1 This procedure is usually performed under LA injected at the arterial puncture site.
2 Sedation can be provided with IV dexmedetomidine as described above.
3 GA is sometimes used. Spontaneous breathing with a LMA is appropriate in suitable patients.
4 Patients are usually stabilised on antiplatelet therapy (aspirin + clopidogrel) prior to the procedure, and this is continued postoperatively.
5 Patients are heparinised during the procedure.
6 Severe bradycardia/asystole may occur due to carotid body stimulation.
7 Potential complications include TIA, CVA, brain swelling, carotid artery perforation, arterial dissection or spasm.
8 There is a higher stroke rate with stenting compared with endarterectomy, but a lower MI rate. Death rate is about the same.

Trans-carotid arterial revascularisation (TCAR)

In this new technique:
1 This procedure can be performed under LA or GA.
2 A small incision is made low in the neck above the collarbone.
3 A sheath is placed into the carotid artery and connected to a neuroprotection system (NPS), which reverses blood flow away from the brain. High-rate reversed blood flow protects the brain from plaque-related stroke. The common carotid artery below the sheath is clamped.
4 The carotid artery blood flows under arterial pressure through a filtering system and is returned to the body via the femoral vein.
5 A wire is passed into the internal carotid artery and pre-dilation of the lesion is performed.
6 A stent is then passed into the internal carotid artery and the sheath removed. The carotid artery is then sutured closed.
This procedure can be done as a day case and may be safer than stenting.

◑ Carvedilol

An alpha and beta receptor blocker that is used to treat hypertension, angina and heart failure.

◑ Catecholaminergic polymorphic ventricular tachycardia (CPVT)

Description

In this syndrome, arrhythmias occur during exercise or times of severe emotional stress. It is due to an inherited disorder most commonly involving the ryanodine receptor, the same receptor involved in malignant hyperthermia. *See Malignant hyperthermia*. This receptor is involved in the release of calcium from the cardiac myocytes' sarcoplasmic reticulum, leading to contraction. It can cause sudden cardiac death. The heart is structurally normal and the resting ECG is normal.

Clinical effects

Symptoms manifest during exercise or emotional stress, including:
1 palpitations
2 dizziness, syncope, convulsions
3 sudden cardiac arrest.

Diagnosis

1 Genetic testing.
2 Exercise or emotion-induced bidirectional or polymorphic VT.

Treatment

1 Nadolol or propranolol.
2 Left cardiac sympathetic denervation.
3 Implantable defibrillator.

◑ Caudal anaesthesia

Introduction

Caudal (low epidural) anaesthesia is mainly used for postoperative analgesia in paediatric surgery below the umbilicus, and for adult chronic lower back pain relief. Paediatric operations appropriate for caudal anaesthesia include inguinal hernia repair, hypospadias repair, circumcision and peri-anal surgery.

Anatomy

In young children, the dural sac terminates at S3–4, and at S1–2 in adults. The dural sac can be entered via the sacral hiatus, which is triangular. The triangle is formed by the unfused lamina of S5 at the caudad base of the triangle and the medial sacral crest at the apex. It is roofed by the sacrococcygeal ligament, which corresponds to the ligamentum flavum.

Contraindications

1 Patient/guardian refusal.
2 Coagulopathy.
3 Infection at the site of insertion.
4 Sacral anomalies.
5 Spinal dysraphism such as tethered cord.

Technique

1 Establish IV access.
2 Position the patient laterally with the legs drawn up to the chest.
3 Palpate the medial sacral crest from cranial to caudal, until a gap is felt.
4 Using aseptic technique, puncture the skin, then the sacrococcygeal ligament with a 22 G short-bevelled needle angled at 45° to the skin in a cranial direction.
5 Once the ligament is punctured (often with a popping sensation), flatten the needle and insert it 2–3 mm into the sacral canal.
6 Aspirate for CSF or blood.
7 The 'whoosh test' helps confirm correct position. Place a stethoscope over the upper sacrum and inject air through the block needle, listening for a whooshing sound.

Dose

Use 0.125–0.25% bupivacaine or 0.1–0.375% ropivacaine 0.5 mL/kg for sacral dermatomes, or 1 mL/kg for lumbar dermatomes.

Complications

1 Periosteal injection causing pain that can last for weeks.
2 Dural puncture with total spinal anaesthesia.
3 Urinary retention.
4 Infection.
5 Neurological injury.

6 IV injection with LA toxicity.

7 Sacral osteomyelitis.

8 Rectal puncture.

◉ Celecoxib

Description

COX-2 inhibitor NSAID useful for treating post-surgical and inflammatory pain. **See *Non-steroidal anti-inflammatory drugs (NSAIDs)*.** It is contraindicated in patients with a history of sulfonamide allergy.

Dose—adult

For postoperative pain, 400 mg PO on day 1, then 100–200 mg PO bd (day 2–5).

◉ Cell salvage/cell saver

See *Blood salvage, intraoperative*.

◉ Cement implantation syndrome

See *Fat embolism syndrome (FES) and bone cement implantation syndrome (BCIS)*.

◉ Central anticholinergic syndrome

Description

Caused by a decrease in the inhibitory effects of acetylcholine in the brain. It can be due to inadequate acetylcholine or a muscarinic receptor blocker that crosses the blood–brain barrier such as atropine, hyoscine and scopolamine. There may be somnolence, confusion, agitation, hallucinations and many other effects.

Treatment

Physostigmine 0.03–0.04 mg/kg IV. **See *Physostigmine*.**

◉ Central cord syndrome

This condition is usually due to neck trauma or cervical spine disease and results in weakness that is worse in the arms than the legs. It is due to damage to the corticospinal tracts. There is variable sensory loss and bladder dysfunction.

◉ Central venous access

See *Internal jugular vein (IJV) central line* and *Subclavian vein central venous access*.

◉ Cerebral aneurysm and subarachnoid haemorrhage (SAH)

This is a vast topic that is controversial, complex and evolving. Each hospital will have its own protocols. Only a brief outline is offered in this manual.

Description

Cerebral aneurysms are arterial bulges in the subarachnoid space. They typically develop at bifurcations, are usually in the anterior circulation and are prone to rupture when larger than 7 mm. Most cerebral aneurysms are asymptomatic until they rupture, causing subarachnoid haemorrhage (SAH). Cerebral aneurysm rupture (CAR) causes 75% of cases of SAH. Other causes of SAH include bleeding from an arteriovenous malformation (AVM), extension of an intracerebral bleed into the subarachnoid space and head trauma. SAH is fatal in > 25% of cases, and > 50% of survivors will have persistent neurological deficits. Currently, endovascular repair is favoured. This involves inserting platinum coils into the sac of the aneurysm. More recently, polyalcohol-coated platinum coils and bioactive coils are being used. Flow-diverting stents may also be used.

Clinical presentation of unruptured cerebral aneurysms

These are usually clinically silent and discovered incidentally. However, patients may present with:

1 cranial nerve palsies
2 visual disturbance
3 facial pain
4 headache
5 seizures
6 ischaemic events due to emboli.

Clinical presentation of SAH

With rupture of the aneurysm, arterial blood flows into the cerebrospinal fluid of the subarachnoid space and intracranial pressure (ICP) rises to equal arterial pressure. This causes a sudden, severe headache. There may also be:

1 collapse, loss of consciousness
2 seizures
3 neck stiffness and pain
4 photophobia
5 nausea and vomiting
6 focal neurological deficits
7 cranial nerve palsies.

Hunt and Hess modified clinical grades[8]

Grade 0—unruptured

Grade I—asymptomatic or minimal headache, slight nuchal rigidity

Grade II—moderate to severe headache, nuchal rigidity, no neurological deficit except a cranial nerve palsy

Grade III—drowsiness, confusion, mild focal deficit

Grade IV—stupor, moderate to severe hemiparesis, possibly early decerebrate rigidity

Grade V—deep coma, decerebrate rigidity, moribund.

The original World Federation of Neurological Surgeons (WFNS) Scale included references to the presence or absence of focal deficit as well as the Glasgow Coma Score (GCS). The modified WFNS refers only to the GCS. The gradings of both versions are shown in Table C1.

Table C1 Gradings of original and modified WFNS Scales

Grade	Original WFNS Scale[9]	Modified WFNS Scale[10]
Grade I	GCS 15 without focal deficit	GCS 15
Grade II	GCS 13–14 without focal deficit	GCS 14
Grade III	GCS 13–14 with focal deficit	GCS 13
Grade IV	GCS 7–12	GCS 7–12
Grade V	GCS 3–6	GCS 3–6

Source: Sano H, Inamasu J, Kato Y, Satoh A, Murayama Y, Murayama Y. Modified World Federation of Neurosurgical Societies Subarachnoid Hemorrhage Grading System. Surg Neurol Int. 2016;7(Suppl 18):S502-3.

Investigations

1 Non-contrast CT scan within 3 days of SAH. If after 3 days since SAH, MRI is more sensitive than CT and therefore preferable.
2 Lumbar puncture looking for xanthochromia if CT scan inconclusive. Xanthochromia is the presence of bilirubin in CSF (it looks yellow). It may be the only sign of an acute SAH. It is typically present within 6–12 h of a SAH.
3 Four-vessel digital subtraction cerebral angiography to identify the site of the aneurysm. CT and MRI angiography are useful but less reliable for small aneurysms.

Complications of SAH

These can be neurological and non-neurological.
Neurological complications include:

1 hydrocephalus. *See Intracranial pressure (ICP) and treatment of raised ICP.*
2 seizures
3 rebleed—especially within the first 12 h
4 vasospasm—peaks at between 7–10 days after aneurysm rupture.[11] This can cause cerebral ischaemia. Hypovolaemia and raised ICP increase the risk of vasospasm.

Non-neurological complications include:

1 hyponatraemia—due to syndrome of inappropriate antidiuretic hormone secretion (SIADH). There may also be hypocalcaemia and hypokalaemia
2 neurogenic pulmonary oedema
3 dysrhythmias, troponin rise, neurogenic stress cardiomyopathy, regional wall motion abnormality on echo.

Preoperative management of ruptured cerebral aneurysms

1 Optimise electrolytes and blood pressure control. Aim for a SBP < 160 mmHg. Nimodipine, nicardipine, labetalol and esmolol may all be useful for blood pressure control.
2 Maintain normovolaemia.
3 Vasospasm prophylaxis with nimodipine. Give 60 mg PO q 4 h for 3 weeks post SAH. If oral therapy is not appropriate, use IV nimodipine 1 mg/h via a central line for 2 h. Increase to 2 mg/h if the patient's blood pressure is not significantly compromised. Nimodipine should be co-infused with N/S (20 mL/h per mg nimodipine/h), using a three-way tap to prevent nimodipine crystals forming.
4 Early surgery/endovascular therapy is usually preferred (24–72 h). Surgery involves clipping of the neck of the aneurysm and endovascular therapy involves obliterating the aneurysm with devices such as platinum coils. Both techniques involve risks such as intraoperative bleeding, vasospasm and thromboembolism.
5 If vasospasm with cerebral ischaemia occurs, consider elevating blood pressure with a vasopressor such as phenylephrine or noradrenaline. Other treatments include cerebral angioplasty and selective intra-arterial vasodilator therapy.
6 Aim for a haemoglobin of 80–100 g/L.
7 If a colloid is needed, use albumin.[11]

Anaesthesia for endovascular therapy

This can be done under sedation, but GA is usually preferred for reasons such as avoidance of patient movement. Surges in blood pressure must be avoided.

1 Establish invasive arterial blood pressure monitoring.
2 Induce anaesthesia with a technique that prevents the hypertensive response to intubation. **See** *Intubation—minimising hypertensive response.*
3 Catheterise the bladder.
4 Maintain anaesthesia with propofol, remifentanil, oxygen and air.
5 Maintain normal haemodynamics. Low blood pressure may decrease cerebral perfusion; high blood pressure may cause aneurysm rupture/bleeding.
6 Aim for normocapnia or mild hypercapnia.
7 Heparin therapy will be required as guided by the interventional neuroradiologist.

Rupture of cerebral aneurysm during endovascular repair

This is a crisis situation. Ensure the neurosurgeon is notified and be aware that immediate transfer to the operating theatre may be required. In addition:
1 Increase FiO_2.
2 Position the patient reverse Trendelenburg (head up).
3 Hyperventilate the patient.
4 Discuss with the interventional neuroradiologist the reversal of heparin with protamine. **See** *Protamine*. Administer protamine slowly after a test dose. It can cause hypotension.
5 Mannitol 0.25–1 g/kg IV infused over 15 min.
6 Nicardipine infusion 2.5–15 mg/h IV.
7 Maintain blood pressure in the normotensive range until bleeding is controlled (in the interventional radiological suite or the operating theatre).
8 Maintain euglycaemia and normothermia, and control seizures.

Intracranial aneurysm surgery

1 Monitor blood pressure invasively and aim for haemodynamic stability.
2 Use TCI with propofol, remifentanil, oxygen and air. Use fentanyl as needed.
3 Take extra precautions to avoid the hypertensive response to intubation. **See** *Intubation—minimising hypertensive response.*
4 Maintain adequate CPP—at least 70 mmHg. **See** *Cerebral perfusion pressure (CPP).*
5 Give antibiotic prophylaxis (e.g. cefazolin 2 g IV).
6 Give 10 mg IV dexamethasone and 1 g/kg mannitol IV on skin incision.
7 Use moderate hyperventilation to a $PaCO_2$ of 30 mmHg.
8 Ensure patient is fully paralysed with rocuronium throughout the procedure unless there is monitoring of motor evoked potentials (MEPs).
9 If EEG is monitored, use boluses of propofol for burst suppression in communication with neurophysiologist.
10 Use a phenylephrine infusion to maintain blood pressure.

Intraoperative aneurysm rupture

This is a crisis situation.
1 Resuscitate the patient with volume support, including blood if needed, and vasopressor therapy.
2 Increase FiO_2.
3 If rupture occurs before opening of the dura, treat abrupt increases in ICP with modest hyperventilation and mannitol 0.25–1 g/kg IV.
4 If rupture occurs after opening of the dura, reduce MAP to 50–59 mmHg to decrease bleeding.

5 Consider transient flow arrest with adenosine 0.3–0.6 mg/kg IV to enable surgeon to gain control of the bleeding site. This will produce flow arrest for 12–15 s. *See Adenosine.*

◑ Cerebral arteriovenous malformation (AVM)

Description

These lesions consist of a tangle of arterial vessels joined to venous vessels without a capillary network in between. The most common genetic cause is hereditary haemorrhagic telangiectasia (HHT). AVMs may form after birth. They may be an incidental finding or may be discovered due to complications such as:

1 intracranial haemorrhage
2 epilepsy
3 headaches
4 focal neurological defect.

Therapy aims at obliterating as many feeding arteries and fistulae as possible using:

1 radiological techniques—glues such as N-butyl cyanoacrylate (NBCA) or obstructive agents like Onyx® may be used to obliterate the feeder vessels
2 stereotactic radiosurgery
3 a neurosurgical approach.

Interventional radiological obliteration

1 GA is the best option for patient comfort and avoids patient movement.
2 Avoid hypertension—*see Cerebral aneurysm and subarachnoid haemorrhage (SAH)*. A TCI propofol/remifentanil anaesthetic is recommended.
3 Induced hypotension and/or transient asystole (with adenosine) are sometimes employed during placement of embolic material. This may lead to rebound hypertension. Consider a pre-emptive clevidipine infusion.
4 Aim for a smooth emergence with minimal coughing/bucking.

Complications

1 Intracranial haemorrhage.
2 Cerebral oedema.
3 Microcatheter retention.
4 Embolisation of non-target vessels.
5 Pulmonary oedema due to excretion of the solvent dimethyl sulfoxide by the lungs.

Neurosurgical approach to AVM

This is very similar to cerebral aneurysm surgery. *See Cerebral aneurysm and subarachnoid haemorrhage (SAH)*.

◑ Cerebral hyperperfusion syndrome

See Carotid endarterectomy/stenting/trans-carotid arterial revascularisation (TCAR).

◑ Cerebral oedema

See Intracranial pressure (ICP) and treatment of raised ICP.

◑ Cerebral perfusion pressure (CPP)

CPP is the difference between the mean arterial pressure (MAP) and jugular venous pressure (JVP) **or** intracranial pressure (whichever is the higher). *See Mean arterial* *pressure (MAP)* and *Intracranial pressure (ICP) and treatment of raised ICP.* Normal CPP is 60–80 mmHg. ICP is determined by intracranial volume (as the skull is a rigid box) and intracranial compliance. The intracranial contents are the brain, CSF and arterial and venous blood. Increased blood in the brain (SAH), increased CSF (hydrocephalus) or increased brain volume (cerebral oedema) increase ICP and decrease CPP. Adaptions to this include:

1 moving CSF to the spinal subarachnoid space
2 increasing MAP
3 cerebral vasoconstriction.

Autoregulation in the brain maintains CPP in the normal range between a MAP of 50–150 mmHg.

◗ Cerebral vasospasm angioplasty

This procedure is usually required urgently due to patient decompensation after SAH and before or after cerebral aneurysm clipping/obliteration. A balloon catheter is guided under fluoroscopy into the artery in spasm. The balloon is inflated and pharmacological agents, such as papaverine, verapamil or nicardipine, are injected. In general, maintain MAP 20–33 mmHg above baseline (unless the aneurysm is unclipped). *See Cerebral aneurysm and subarachnoid haemorrhage (SAH).*

◗ Cerebral venous sinus thrombosis (CVST)

Description

In this condition there is clot formation in the venous sinuses of the brain. This causes backpressure in the veins, which can result in blood leaking into the brain tissue and causing haemorrhagic cerebral infarcts. Elevated venous pressure can also cause vasogenic oedema, raised intracranial pressure and brain infarction. Risk factors include:

1 OCP
2 pregnancy and the postpartum period
3 thrombophilia e.g. antiphospholipid syndrome, protein C and S deficiency
4 cancer
5 collagen vascular diseases such as Wegener's granulomatosis
6 obesity
7 dural puncture resulting in decreased intracranial pressure.[12]

Clinical presentation

1 Headache, dizziness, blurred vision.
2 Nausea and vomiting.
3 Lethargy.
4 Seizures.
5 Hemiparesis.
6 Coma.
7 Death.

Differentiation between post dural puncture headache and CVST

1 History of previous thromboembolic disease favours CVST.
2 Presence of mental state changes, focal deficits and seizures favours CVST.
3 Little headache relief after blood patching favours CVST.

Diagnosis

MRI + venography is the standard test. CT scanning may only pick up about 30% of cases.

Treatment

1 Supportive measures.
2 Anticoagulation.
3 Endovascular treatments (thrombolysis, thrombectomy).
4 Neurosurgery such as decompressive craniotomy.

◉ Cervical plexus (CP) block

This block is used for anaesthesia/analgesia for carotid endarterectomy, superficial neck surgery and fractured clavicle. Only the technique for the superficial CP block will be described.

Anatomy

The cervical plexus originates from the anterior rami of C1–C4 and has both deep and superficial branches (Figure C4). The deep branches are:
1 phrenic nerve (C3–C5), which innervates the diaphragm
2 nerves to the geniohyoid and thyrohyoid muscles of the airway, and muscles for swallowing and speech.

The superficial branches are:
1 lesser and greater occipital nerves
2 transverse cervical nerve (anterior cutaneous nerve of neck)
3 supraclavicular nerves.

The superficial nerves emerge from the prevertebral fascia, between the longus capitis and the middle scalene muscle. The nerves run under the sternocleidomastoid (SCM) muscle, eventually emerging from behind the posterior border of the SCM at about where this border is crossed by the external jugular vein (EJV).

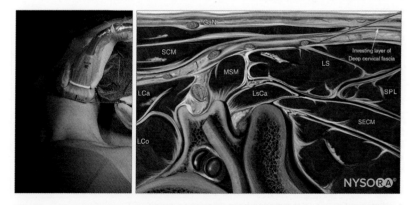

Figure C4 Probe position and anatomy for cervical plexus block. SCM = sternocleidomastoid muscle, MSM = middle scalene muscle, LsCa = longus capitus muscle
Image courtesy of NYSORA

Technique for the superficial CP block

Use 10 mL of ropivacaine 1%. The depth of the plexus is about 1–2 cm. See Figures C4 and C5 for the anatomy relating to the CP block.

1 Position the patient in the semi-reclined position, with the head turned away from the block side. Mark the posterior border of the SCM with a skin marker.
2 Take all usual precautions (IV cannula, sterility maintained throughout procedure).
3 Identify the SCM posterior border midway between the mastoid process and clavicle.
4 Place the transducer in a transverse orientation over the position described in point 3.
5 Identify the posterior edge of the SCM. The brachial plexus may be seen. **See Brachial plexus block (BPB)**. The muscles under the posterior border of the SCM are the anterior and middle scalene muscles.

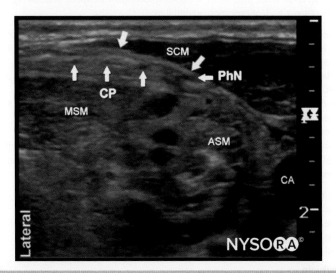

Figure C5 Sonoanatomy of the cervical plexus (CP). SCM = sternocleidomastoid muscle, MSM = middle scalene muscle
Image courtesy of NYSORA

6 Sliding the transducer caudally and cranially will identify individual nerves as small hypoechoic nodules located under the posterior border of the SCM.
7 Insert the needle in plane so the tip lies under the posterior border of SCM but superficial to the scalene muscles.
8 Inject a test dose of 1–2 mL of LA then 8 mL of LA.
9 The injection should result in a layer of spread between the SCM and scalene muscles.

⊙ CHA$_2$DS$_2$-VASc score

See Warfarin.

◐ Chemotherapy drugs and anaesthesia

Only two drugs will be discussed, bleomycin and doxorubicin.

Bleomycin (BLM)

This drug is a glycopeptide antibiotic-type anti-cancer drug. It is often used in the treatment of germ cell tumours (e.g. testicular cancer) and Hodgkin's lymphoma. It can cause pulmonary toxicity with subacute pulmonary damage that can progress to severe pulmonary fibrosis. This occurs in up to 10% of patients. Chronic lung damage may be indicated by:

1 dry cough, dyspnoea, pleuritic chest pain
2 hypoxaemia
3 crackles on chest auscultation.
4 CXR may show linear interstitial shadowing, confluent air-space shadowing, pneumothorax and/or pneumomediastinum.

Exposure to high concentrations of oxygen can cause rapidly progressive pulmonary toxicity, and the risk is life-long. Precautions to take with GA include the following:

1 Use air for ventilation when possible.
2 If patient is/becomes hypoxic, add sufficient oxygen to keep O_2 saturation at 88–92%.
3 High oxygen concentrations should only be used in an emergency to maintain an oxygen saturation of 88–92%.
4 Intraoperative PEEP should be used judiciously.

Postoperatively, oxygen therapy should be avoided, or used very carefully, to maintain an O_2 saturation between 88–92%. Physiotherapy and optimum fluid balance are also important.

Patients particularly at risk are:

1 those with evidence of pre-existing BLM toxicity
2 those who have had exposure to BLM in the last 1–2 months
3 those whose BLM dose > 450 mg
4 those whose creatinine clearance < 35 mL/min.

Doxorubicin

Doxorubicin is an anthracycline antibiotic cytotoxic. It causes cumulative dose-dependent cardiac toxicity, which can lead to cardiomyopathy, CCF and cardiogenic shock. It can also cause pulmonary toxicity.

◐ Chest drain/tube

Indication

A chest drain is required to drain a pneumothorax, haemothorax, pleural effusion or empyema (air, blood or other fluid in the pleural space). Positive pressure in the pleural space leads to lung collapse and impaired gas exchange. If the pneumothorax or pleural blood/fluid is small and not causing respiratory compromise, it may be appropriate to observe the patient for any deterioration. A tension pneumothorax is a life-threatening emergency and must be treated immediately.
See Pneumothorax.

Mechanics

A chest tube requires a system where air, fluid or blood can drain out of the pleural space but air cannot enter the pleural space through the tube. For a pneumothorax this can be achieved by inserting the proximal end of the chest tube into a bottle of sterile water with the end submerged 2 cm (a water seal). The bottle can vent air out. To drain blood or fluid, the chest tube needs to drain into a collection bottle. A second tube from the collection bottle then goes to the same system as for a pneumothorax, utilising a second bottle.

Up to this point, the system is passive. To make the process faster, suction can be applied but it must be very carefully controlled. This involves adding a third bottle. This has a higher level of water than the underwater seal. Air drains into the third bottle, which has suction applied to it. In the bottle there is a venting tube submerged in the water and open to air. The depth to which the venting tube is submerged (typically 20 cm) precisely controls the suction; too much suction can cause trauma.

Modern systems combine all three bottles into one multi-compartment unit such as the Atrium Ocean Chest Drainage System.

Insertion technique

For an adult, a size 26–28 Fr is appropriate for a pneumothorax and a size 36–40 Fr for a pleural effusion or haemothorax.

1 Insert an IV cannula and sit the patient up 30°. The site of insertion is the fourth or fifth intercostal space in the anterior axillary line. In the male, the fourth or fifth intercostal space is in line with the nipple.
2 Provide appropriate IV sedation/analgesia.
3 Surgically prep the site of insertion (chlorhexidine/drapes). Use a fully aseptic technique (gown, hat, gloves and mask).
4 Anaesthetise the skin and deeper tissues at the insertion point with LA.
5 Make an incision so the tube will pass over the rib, not underneath it. The incision should be big enough for the operator's index finger.
6 Blunt dissect with heavy forceps until the pleura is reached.
7 Break through the pleura with a finger, make sure you can feel inside the pleural cavity then introduce the tube held in the blunt forceps with the trocar pulled back. Clamp the tube unless air is escaping from the pleural space—in which case clamp the tube when the egress of air stops.
8 Direct the tube posteriorly and basally for fluid and apically for air. Insert the tube to a depth of about 12 cm.
9 Suture the wound with 3.0 silk so that it is closed snugly around the tube and the suture is tied to the chest tube. Place a separate suture so that the wound can be closed quickly when the tube is removed. Apply a suitable dressing.
10 Connect the tube to the drainage unit as described in the section on mechanics above.

○ Cholestasis of pregnancy

See *Intrahepatic cholestasis of pregnancy (ICP)*.

○ Cholinergic receptors

See *Acetylcholine receptors (cholinergic receptors)*.

○ Chronic hypertension and pregnancy

Description

Chronic hypertension (SBP > 140 mmHg ± DBP > 90 mmHg) is diagnosed when hypertension is detected before pregnancy, or before 20 weeks' gestation or when hypertension fails to resolve postpartum. There is an increased risk of preeclampsia, placental abruption, fetal growth restriction and other perinatal complications.

Antihypertensive drugs and pregnancy

1 Angiotensin converting enzyme (ACE) inhibitors and angiotensin receptor blocker drugs are contraindicated in pregnancy (teratogenic, renal dysfunction, skull hypoplasia).
2 Diuretics should be avoided because of the potential for fetal electrolyte disturbances.
3 Beta blockers should be avoided because they cause fetal bradycardia. However, labetalol and oxprenolol can be used.
4 Calcium channel blockers should be avoided because they can cause maternal hypotension and fetal hypoxia. However, nifedipine can be used.
5 Methyldopa, hydralazine and prazosin are all safe to use in pregnancy.

Doses of oral antihypertensive drugs in pregnancy

1 Labetalol—100–200 mg q 12 h, max 400 mg q 8 h.
2 Oxprenolol—40–80 mg q 12 h, max 80–160 mg q 12 h.
3 Nifedipine—10 mg q 12 h or 30 mg controlled release daily. Max 20–40 mg q 12 h or 120 mg controlled release daily.
4 Methyldopa—250 mg q 12 h. Max 500 mg q 6 h.
5 Hydralazine—25 mg q 12 h. Max daily dose 200 mg.
6 Prazosin—0.5 mg q 12 h. Max 3 mg total daily dose.

Safe antihypertensive drugs and breast feeding

1 Beta blockers—propranolol, metoprolol and labetalol are considered safe.
2 Nifedipine.
3 Captopril and enalapril.
4 Methyldopa.
5 Hydralazine.

▶ Cisatracurium

Description
Non-depolarising neuromuscular blocking drug. It is a benzylisoquinolinium.

Advantages
1 Broken down almost entirely by Hofmann elimination (it is not metabolised in the liver or kidney). Therefore, it can be used in patients with kidney or liver failure without accumulation.
2 Does not cause histamine release.
3 Dose requirements are not affected by anticonvulsants.

Disadvantages
1 Has a slow onset of action, which makes it unsuitable for a rapid sequence induction.
2 Requires refrigeration.
3 Laudanosine may accumulate with extended use in patients with liver and renal disease, resulting in seizures.

Dose
0.15 mg/kg IV. For a 70 kg patient use 10 mg, which lasts about 45 min. Repeat bolus doses 0.03 mg/kg (about 2 mg for a 70 kg patient). This will be effective for about 20 min.

Infusion

1.4 mcg/kg/min, 0.084 mg/kg/h. In a 70 kg patient, this equals 5–6 mg/h.

◘ Citrate toxicity

See Blood loss—assessment, management and anaesthetic approach.

◘ Clevidipine (Cleviprex)

Description

Dihydropyridine calcium channel blocker drug given IV by infusion. It decreases SVR by causing arterial vasodilatation, and is used to treat severe high blood pressure or control blood pressure during procedures such as cerebral aneurysm coiling. *See Hypertension.* It has a fast onset (2–4 min) and fast offset. It is metabolised by plasma esterases and has a half-life of about 1–3 min. It is formulated in an emulsion with soya oil and egg lecithin with a concentration of 0.5 mg/mL active drug.

Dose

Adults

The drug is given undiluted IV. Start at 1–2 mg/h and double the dose every 90 s until the desired MAP is achieved, to a maximum of 32 mg/h. Due to the lipid load, no more than 1000 mL of clevidipine should be given in a 24 h period.

Advantages

1 Clevidipine has little or no effect on myocardial contractility or cardiac conduction.
2 It has no effect on venous return to the heart.
3 Its elimination is not affected by kidney or liver function.

Disadvantages

1 It should not be used in patients in whom a reduction in SVR may be harmful e.g. severe aortic stenosis.
2 Due to its lipid content, the drug should not be used in patients with defects in lipid metabolism e.g. acute pancreatitis.
3 Its formulation can support microbial growth.
4 Reflex tachycardia may occur as MAP is lowered.
5 The drug is photosensitive and needs to be stored in cartons.
6 Clevidipine can cause extreme hypoxaemia by inducing pulmonary shunting and should be discontinued if no other cause for the hypoxaemia is found.[13]
7 There is a risk of rebound hypertension for up to 8 h after the infusion is ceased.
8 It is contraindicated in patients allergic to egg or soy products.

◘ Clonidine (Catapres)

Description

Antihypertensive alpha-2 adrenergic receptor partial agonist. Clonidine decreases noradrenaline release from sympathetic nerve endings and decreases sympathetic outflow by a central action. *See Adrenergic receptors.* It is also used for attention deficit hyperactivity disorder, drug withdrawal (e.g. alcohol), menopausal flushing, diarrhoea and certain pain conditions. It can also be used to treat migraine and recurrent vascular headache. Routes of administration are IV, intrathecal, epidurally, PO and as skin patches.

Anaesthetic uses

1 Antihypertensive.
2 Reduces anaesthetic agent and postoperative opioid requirement.
3 Reduces postoperative shivering.
4 Sedation in the critical care setting without causing respiratory depression.
5 Enhances the effect of LA drugs used via the neuraxial route.
6 Helps prevent emergence delirium and agitation in children.

Dose for hypertension

Adult

75–300 mcg IV. The maximum IV dose is 750 mcg/24 h. PO 50–100 mcg 8–12 h. The maximum oral dose is 600 mcg/day.

Child

IV 1–5 mcg/kg.

Dose for neuraxial block to prolong LA action

SAB—adult

Up to 150 mcg.

Epidurally—adult

Up to 150 mcg.

Dose for sedation

Adult

An infusion of 4 mcg/kg/h (although dexmedetomidine is preferred—*see Dexmedetomidine*).

Dose for analgesia

Give a LD of 5 mcg/kg then an infusion of 0.3 mcg/kg/h. This provides long-lasting analgesia with reduced opioid requirements.

Advantages

1 Long duration of action—up to 8 h.
2 Sedating with minimal effects on respiration.
3 Analgesic.

Disadvantages

1 Contraindicated if there is severe bradyarrhythmia due to sick sinus syndrome, or second- or third-degree heart block.
2 Can cause dry mouth.
3 Abrupt withdrawal can result in severe rebound hypertension.
4 Can cause hypotension and bradycardia.
5 No effect on peripheral nerve blocks.

◖ Clopidogrel (Plavix, Iscover)

Potent thienopyridine antiplatelet drug that irreversibly inhibits platelet function. It is a platelet adenosine diphosphate (ADP) receptor antagonist. *See Anticoagulant and antiplatelet drugs and surgery/neuraxial anaesthesia*.

Surgery and neuraxial block

Cease for at least five days before surgery and seven days for neuraxial block.

Complications

1 Intracranial haemorrhage.
2 Thrombotic thrombocytopenic purpura (TTP) may occur. *See Thrombotic thrombocytopenic purpura (TTP).*

Treatment of bleeding

Platelet transfusion is effective if given 4 or more hours after clopidogrel dose.

◐ Clotting pathways

Knowledge of the clotting pathways enables an understanding of the mechanism of action of anti-clotting and pro-clotting drugs, and the rationale behind tests of clotting. As this topic is the subject of entire textbooks, only a brief analysis is presented here.

Primary haemostasis

1 Trauma leads to tissue injury, including disruption of the endothelial lining of blood vessels.
2 Platelets become exposed to the underlying collagen.
3 Platelets bind to the collagen through their glycoprotein and integrin receptors. This binding is strengthened by von Willebrand factor. *See Von Willebrand disease (VWD).*
4 The platelets become activated and release various substances, including ADP, platelet activating factor (PAF) and thromboxane A_2.
5 Platelet receptor glycoprotein IIb/IIIa becomes activated and cross-links with fibrinogen to create a platelet plug. This essential platelet clot forms quickly but is weak.

Secondary haemostasis

Occurs through the extrinsic and intrinsic clotting pathways. See Figure C6.

Extrinsic pathway

The steps are as follows:
1 Trauma leads to tissue injury, including damage to the endothelium lining blood vessels.
2 Factor VII (FVII) comes into contact with tissue factor (TF) from the subendothelium (from stromal fibroblasts and leukocytes).
3 The activated complex TF-FVIIa is formed, which activates FIX and FX, beginning the common pathway.

Intrinsic pathway (also known as the 'contact activation' pathway)

The steps are as follows:
1 Tissue injury leads to the exposure of plasma factors to collagen.
2 This leads to activation of factor XII. Factor XII deficiency causes deranged clotting studies without a clinically significant bleeding tendency. Interestingly, it can be associated with recurrent miscarriages.

3 FXIIa activates FXI, which then activates FIX. Factor XI deficiency (haemophilia C) results in a mild bleeding tendency. Factor IX deficiency causes haemophilia B, also known as 'Christmas disease'. *See Haemophilia*.

4 FIXa and FVIII then activate FX, thus beginning the common pathway.

Common pathway

1 FXa + FV + calcium ions form the prothrombin conversion activator complex.

2 This complex converts prothrombin to thrombin (also called FII). Thrombin converts fibrinogen (FI) to fibrin monomers.

3 Fibrin stabilising factor (FXIII) converts the monomers to polymers, creating a fibrin mesh.

4 This mesh attracts platelets and phospholipids to form a stable clot.

An easy way to remember the intrinsic and common clotting pathway is to imagine a cheap item at a variety store costing $12. It does not sell so the price is reduced to $11.98. It still does not sell so the cost is progressively reduced to $10, $5, $2 and $1. The extrinsic pathway is just TF and factor VII. See Figure C7.

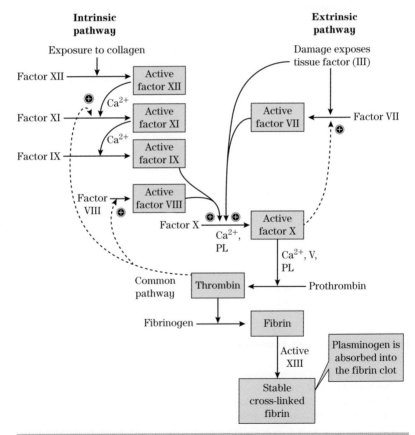

Figure C6 The clotting pathways (intrinsic, extrinsic and common).
Reproduced with permission from Kibble JD and Halsey CR: The Big Picture: Medical Physiology, New York, NY: McGraw-Hill, 2009.

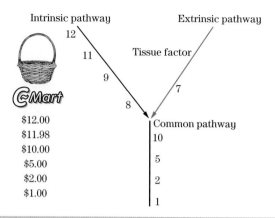

Figure C7 Clotting pathways in skeletonised form

Clotting studies

Activated partial thromboplastin time (APPT/aPPT)

Also known as partial thromboplastin time (PTT) or kaolin-cephalin clotting time (KCCT). It tests the intrinsic (or contact activation clotting pathway) and the common pathway, bypassing the extrinsic pathway. It measures factors XII, XI, IX, VIII, X, V, prothrombin and thrombin, and is carried out by:

- taking a sample of blood in a test tube containing citrate or oxalate—this binds calcium and prevents the blood from clotting
- centrifuging the sample and collecting the plasma
- mixing calcium with the plasma to reverse the effects of the citrate or oxalate
- activating the intrinsic pathway by an activator such as kaolin or silica.

NR 25–36 s. A prolonged APTT occurs with:

1 Heparin therapy—***see Heparin (unfractionated and low-molecular-weight heparins)***.
2 Decrease in the activity of clotting factors V, VIII, IX, X, XI, XII, prothrombin, thrombin and fibrinogen/fibrin. Haemophilia A is deficiency in FVIII and haemophilia B is deficiency in FIX.
3 Rivaroxaban/apixaban—these are activated factor X inhibitors.
4 Dabigatran—a direct thrombin inhibitor.

Prothrombin time (PT) and INR

These tests evaluate the extrinsic and common pathways of clotting. They measure the effectiveness of fibrinogen, prothrombin, FV, FVII and FX. Blood is drawn into a citrated tube (the citrate binds calcium, preventing clotting). A centrifuge is used to separate the plasma from the red cells. Calcium in a phospholipid suspension is added to the plasma and tissue factor. The time to clot is then measured.

NR is 12–13 seconds but is lab dependent. PT is prolonged with:

1 warfarin therapy—the main indication for the test
2 other anticoagulants—heparin, factor Xa inhibitors and direct thrombin inhibitors
3 FVII deficiency
4 vitamin K deficiency

5 increased factor consumption as in disseminated intravascular coagulation (DIC)
6 liver disease.

International normalised ratio (INR) enables standardisation of PT between different labs. The normal INR is ≤ 1.1.

Thrombin time (TT)

This test measures the final step in the clotting pathway, the conversion of fibrinogen to fibrin. It is performed by taking a blood sample in a citrated tube and separating the plasma. Thrombin is then added to the citrated plasma and time to clot formation is measured.

NR 14–19 s. A prolonged TT occurs with:

1 low fibrinogen
2 dysfunctional fibrinogen
3 fibrin degradation products
4 heparin (unfractionated)
5 dabigatran
6 high concentrations of serum proteins such as in multiple myeloma/amyloid.

❍ Coarctation of the aorta

Description

This condition is a congenital abnormality caused by narrowing of the aorta at the site of the ductus arteriosus, which becomes the ligamentum arteriosum after birth. 85% of patients with this condition have a bicuspid aortic valve with aortic stenosis or regurgitation. The patient may have an uncorrected condition or there may be aortic narrowing after correction. Coarctation can also be preductal or post ductal. It is more common in males and is frequently found in females with Turner syndrome (**see Turner syndrome**). Mortality of unrepaired coarctation of the aorta is about 90% by age 55.

Clinical features

1 Delayed femoral pulses with reduced blood pressure in the lower body.
2 Rib notching on CXR due to collateral vessels.
3 Hypertension with a BP differential between the right (higher BP) and left (lower BP) arm.
4 Systolic ejection murmur, left sternal edge.
5 Increased incidence of IHD and sudden death.
6 Increased risk of aortic rupture, dissection and aneurysm.
7 Heart failure.
8 Rupture of intracranial aneurysms.
9 Endocarditis.

Anaesthetic considerations for non-aortic surgery

There should be consultation and involvement of a cardiologist. Surgical correction or balloon dilatation may be required prior to other types of surgery. Surgery near dilated collaterals may result in severe bleeding.

❍ Cocaine abuse

Description

Cocaine is a common drug of abuse. Metabolised rapidly, it can cause euphoria, increased mental alertness and increased energy. It increases presynaptic release of catecholamines and blocks reuptake of norepinephrine, dopamine and serotonin. Cocaine reduces the production of nitric oxide.

It can be snorted, smoked or injected. Patients who are not cocaine toxic (no tachycardia or hypertension, no fever, no ECG changes) can be safely anaesthetised. Note that cocaine-using patients may self-medicate with the drug prior to their anaesthetic.

Patients who are cocaine toxic may show:

1 agitation, paranoia and aggression
2 ischaemic and haemorrhagic strokes
3 seizures
4 cardiac dysrhythmias, arrest
5 respiratory arrest
6 hypertension
7 tachycardia
8 hyperthermia
9 dilated pupils
10 tremors, muscle twitching
11 reduced platelet count
12 pulmonary hypertension
13 rhabdomyolysis
14 aortic dissection.

Chronic cocaine use effects

May include:
1 reactive airways (if it is smoked)
2 cardiomyopathy
3 atrophy of the brain
4 renal failure.

Chronic cocaine use and obstetrics

May cause:
1 intrauterine death
2 fetal growth abnormalities
3 neonatal withdrawal (crosses the placenta)
4 placental abnormalities, increased risk of abruption.
Cocaine abuse may mimic preeclampsia.

Treatment of acute cocaine intoxication and anaesthetic implications

1 Respiratory drive is usually maintained but if intubation is required, suxamethonium is contraindicated. This is because both drugs are metabolised by plasma cholinesterases so the effects of cocaine and suxamethonium may be prolonged. Use rocuronium.
2 Benzodiazepines are useful for agitation/aggression.
3 Hypertension can be treated with nitroglycerine or sodium nitroprusside.
   See Glyceryl trinitrate (GTN) and Sodium nitroprusside (SNP).
4 Treat hyperthermia as described in the section on malignant hyperthermia.
   See Malignant hyperthermia (MH).
5 Treat hypotension with phenylephrine.
6 Selective beta-1 antagonists such as esmolol can be used to treat tachycardia.

◑ Cocaine, medical uses

Amino-ester type LA and vasoconstrictor, used in nasal surgery. Presented as pastes and solutions in concentrations of 1–10%. Max topical dose is 3 mg/kg. Effects last 20–30 min. Medical use is disappearing.

◑ Codalgin forte

A trade name for a tablet containing a combination of codeine and paracetamol. **See Codeine.**

◑ Codeine

Description

Methylated morphine-derivative opioid drug suitable for mild-to-moderate pain. Acts primarily by conversion to morphine. Also used as a constipating and antitussive drug.

Dose

Adult

PO/IM 30–60 mg q 4–6 h.

Child

0.5–1 mg/kg q 4–6 h or subcut 1 mg/kg up to q 4 h. Maximum dose 3 mg/kg/day.

Advantages

Relatively low incidence of opioid side effects unless high dosages.

Disadvantages

1 Low analgesic potency and inter-patient variation in potency due to variation of conversion rate to morphine.
2 IV codeine not recommended as it may cause hypotension, possibly due to histamine release.
3 Codeine use in breast-feeding mothers has been implicated in neonatal death due to morphine toxicity. **See Breast feeding and maternal anaesthesia/postoperative care.**

◑ Combined spinal/epidural technique

See Subarachnoid block (SAB).

◑ Complement system

The complement system is part of the immune system. It 'complements' antibody-triggered responses, and its functions are:
1 identifying foreign materials and damaged cells by tagging them with complement protein C3
2 elimination of targets by lysis (membrane attack complex)
3 promotion of the inflammatory response.
There are the classical, lectin and alternative pathways, all of which activate C3, which then attaches to target material as C3b. This leads to the formation of the membrane attack complex (MAC), which attacks cell membranes and encourages phagocytosis by macrophages and neutrophils. Each pathway also promotes the inflammatory response. Inherited disorders of the complement system can predispose to bacterial infections or SLE.

▶ Compliance of the lung

The compliance of the lung is equal to the change in volume/change in pressure. In a compliant lung, a small change in pressure leads to large change in volume. In a non-compliant lung, a large change in pressure leads to a small change in volume.

▶ Compound sodium lactate

See Hartmann's solution/compound sodium lactate (CSL)/lactated Ringer's solution (LRS).

▶ Confusion, agitation, decreased level of consciousness post anaesthetic

See Delirium, postanaesthetic.

▶ Congenital heart disease (CHD) overview

Description

CHD is defined as an anatomical anomaly in the heart's structure that an individual is born with. About 0.9% of newborns have CHD. These cardiac defects can be mild, moderate or severe and can have clinical effects ranging from inconsequential to fatal. There can also be congenital defects that are outside the heart but affect the heart significantly, including coarctation of the aorta and patent ductus arteriosus. Anaesthetists will encounter patients who have either repaired, partially repaired or unrepaired CHD. Some of these patients will have cardiac decompensation as a result of their CHD.

Classification

CHD can be classified as acyanotic or cyanotic. Acyanotic heart disease may or may not be associated with a shunt. Cyanotic CHD is **always** associated with a shunt. There are two requirements for a shunt:

1 An abnormal anatomical connection between the systemic and pulmonary circulation.
2 A pressure difference between each side of the defect.

Acyanotic CHD can become cyanotic CHD if there is reversal of a left-to-right shunt called Eisenmenger syndrome. *See Eisenmenger syndrome/Eisenmenger complex.*

Acyanotic CHD

Specific defects include:

1 Ventricular septal defect (VSD).
2 Atrial septal defect (ASD).
3 Patent ductus arteriosus (PDA).
4 Atrioventricular septal defect (AVSD).
5 Aortopulmonary window (AP window).
6 Pulmonary stenosis (PS).
7 Aortic stenosis.
8 Coarctation of the aorta.

Note: VSD, ASD and PDA can become cyanotic if Eisenmenger syndrome develops. For more information on these defects, see the entries for each.

Cyanotic CHD

There is **always** a right-to-left shunt—meaning some venous blood bypasses the lungs and enters the systemic circulation. Lesions include:

1 Tetralogy of Fallot—*see Tetralogy of Fallot*.
2 Transposition of the great arteries.
3 Total anomalous pulmonary venous return (TAPVR).
4 Tricuspid atresia.
5 Truncus arteriosus.
   For more information on these conditions, see the individual section for each.

Effects of left-to-right shunt

A left-to-right shunt is not associated with cyanosis but still has progressively deleterious effects. More blood is flowing through the low-pressure pulmonary circulation than the high-pressure systemic circulation. Effects of this include:

1 Right ventricular overload, distension and hypertrophy. The RV must do more work than it was designed for, and may eventually fail.
2 There is excess pulmonary blood flow, which can lead to pulmonary congestion and pulmonary hypertension. Eventually, the pulmonary hypertension becomes irreversible.
3 Excess pressure in the pulmonary circulation can result in reversal of a left-to-right shunt (so it becomes a right-to-left-shunt).
4 Increased risk of lung infections.

Effects of right-to-left shunt

Think b**R**eath**L**essness. Effects include:

1 Cyanosis with polycythaemia and increased risk of thrombosis and CVA. May also have a low platelet count, impaired platelet function and coagulation factor deficiencies.
2 LV overload and eventual LV failure. LV distension can lead to mitral incompetence.
3 Increased risk of paradoxical embolus.

Types of circulation associated with CHD

1 Normal—the systemic and pulmonary circulations are in series and each circulation is supported by a ventricle. Even in corrected CHD with normal circulation, the surgeon may keep a small VSD or fenestrations as a pressure-relief mechanism.
2 Balanced—the pulmonary and systemic circulations are anatomically connected but mixing of the two is minimal, due to balance of the SVR and PVR. However, if the SVR and/or the PVR changes, the circulation will become unbalanced and shunting will occur.
3 Single ventricle physiology. Only one ventricle functions effectively, the other being rudimentary e.g. hypoplastic left heart syndrome. *See Single ventricle physiology and anaesthesia*.

CHD and anaesthesia

1 Haemodynamic stability is the main aim. Ideally there should be minimal effects on SVR, PVR, myocardial contractility, heart rate and blood pressure. The choice of agents should take this into account, but dosage and rate of administration are also extremely important considerations.
2 The main issues, as with any other type of heart disease, are the presence or absence of heart failure, arrhythmias, pacemaker/defibrillator and cardiac reserve.

3 Bacterial endocarditis risk must be considered, and gas embolus must be prevented in patients with right-to-left shunts. *See Bacterial endocarditis (BE) prophylaxis.*

4 Invasive arterial blood pressure monitoring is very helpful in the management of patients with significant lesions having significant surgery. Place the arterial line on the opposite side to a Blalock–Taussig shunt.[14]

5 Intraoperative transoesophageal echocardiography can also provide invaluable information.

6 A central line may be required for infusions of drugs such as dobutamine.

CHD and pregnancy

In general:[13]

1 More than 50% of women with cyanotic CHD deteriorate during pregnancy. Of women with acyanotic CHD, only 15% deteriorate during pregnancy.

2 If CCF is present, 30% of women will deteriorate during pregnancy compared with 5% in its absence.

3 The presence of pulmonary hypertension is associated with a 30% mortality.

4 There is a 50% risk of fetal death if the mother's oxygen saturation < 85% or haematocrit > 65%.

◖ Congestive cardiac failure (CCF)—chronic

See Cardiogenic shock.

Introduction

CCF occurs when the heart is unable to pump enough blood to meet the demands of the body. Disease impairs the ventricle's ability to fill and or expel blood. The three major risk factors for CCF are age, hypertension and coronary artery disease (CAD). Causes, which may overlap, include:

1 coronary artery disease/myocardioal ischaemia/acute myocardial infarction—the most common cause in developed countries

2 cardiac arrhythmias

3 cardiomyopathy

4 hypertension

5 valvular heart disease. This can cause heart failure, or be as a result of heart failure e.g. dilated cardiomyopathy causing mitral incompetence

6 congenital heart disease (CHD)

7 myocarditis

8 pericardial disease

9 pulmonary hypertension

10 thyrotoxicosis

11 infiltration of heart muscle with substances such as amyloid and sarcoid

12 toxins such as alcohol

13 severe obesity

14 diabetes mellitus

15 deficiency of vitamins such as thiamine.

Presentation

1 Palpitations/dysrhythmias.

2 Fatigue.

3 Chest pain.

4 Orthopnoea.

5 LV failure symptoms/signs—dyspnoea, orthopnoea, cough, paroxysmal nocturnal dyspnoea, pulmonary oedema, haemoptysis.

6 RV failure—leg oedema, elevated jugular venous pressure (JVP), liver distension/discomfort and ascites.

7 Gallop rhythm, third heart sound, regurgitant murmur(s).

8 Thromboembolism.

Pathophysiology

The heart becomes enlarged with hypertrophy of ventricular muscle and increased wall stiffness.

1 One or both ventricles may not empty properly—this is called systolic heart failure. The heart is weak and does not contract powerfully enough. The left ventricular ejection fraction (LVEF) < 50%.

2 One or both ventricles may not be able to relax properly—this is called diastolic heart failure. The heart is too stiff to relax, impairing diastolic filling. LVEF is preserved at least initially ($\geq$ 50%).

3 CCF with an ejection fraction of 40–50% are an intermediate group. LVEF < 40% is considered systolic failure and < 30% is severe disease.

4 There is dysfunction and/or death of cardiac myocytes, leading to decreased contractility and ventricular distension with decreased cardiac output (CO). This stimulates the renin-angiotensin system, leading to salt and water retention. This further increases ventricular distension.

5 Increased ventricular distension leads to increased CO (Frank–Starling Law) until overdistension occurs and CO falls again.

6 Over time, cardiac remodelling occurs, with myocardial hypertrophy and collagen deposition leading to stiffened ventricles with decreased compliance.

7 Ventricular filling is impaired by decreased ventricular compliance and hypertrophy.

8 The thickened ventricular walls have increased oxygen demands but with a less efficient oxygen supply, especially in the subendocardial regions.

9 A vicious cycle is established where cardiac energy expenditure becomes less and less efficient and myocardial oxygen requirements are increasingly compromised.

Grading heart failure (HF)

- Systolic HF (HF with reduced ejection fraction)—LVEF $\leq$ 40%.
- Diastolic HF (HF with preserved ejection fraction)—LVEF $\geq$ 50%.
- HF with mid-range ejection fraction—LVEF 41–49%.

Investigation

1 FBC (anaemia), UEC (electrolyte abnormalities/renal disease), TFTs.

2 CXR (cardiomegaly, pulmonary congestion, effusion).

3 ECG—arrhythmia, LVH, ST-T wave changes, conduction abnormalities.

4 Echocardiography—looking for changes such as dilated LV, reduced ejection fraction, increase in end-diastolic LV diameter, valvular dysfunction, mural thrombus.

5 Cardiac catheterisation—to elucidate coronary artery disease and investigate valvular heart disease.

6 Cardiac MRI.

7 Cardiac biomarkers such as B-type natriuretic peptide (BNP) and N-terminal pro-BNP (NT-proBNP) are produced by cardiac muscle cells in response to heart failure. *See B-type natriuretic peptide (BNP) and N-terminal-proBNP (NT-proBNP).*

Treatment

1 Treat the cause e.g. valve repair/replacement for valvular heart disease.
2 Dietary modification—salt and water restriction, reduction in excess weight.
3 Diuretics to decrease excess sodium and water in the body.
4 Angiotensin-converting enzyme (ACE) inhibitors e.g. enalapril to counteract the effects of the renin-angiotensin system. *See Renin-angiotensin system.* Angiotensin II receptor blocker (ARB) drugs can be used in patients who are intolerant of ACE inhibitors e.g. candesartan (Atacand). ACE inhibitors and ARBs should **not** be used together. *See Angiotensin-converting enzyme (ACE) inhibitors* and *Angiotensin II receptor blocker (ARB) drugs.*
5 Angiotensin receptor/neprilysin inhibitor drugs (ARNI). This is a combination of ARB and neprilysin inhibitor (e.g. sacubitril/valsartan).
6 Beta blocker therapy using selective beta 1 blockers. A popular drug is bisoprolol.
7 Hydralazine.
8 Nitrate therapy.
9 In diabetics—dapagliflozin, an SGLT2 inhibitor.
10 Mineralocorticoid receptor antagonist (MRA) e.g. eplerenone.
11 Cardiac glycosides—the most commonly used drug is digoxin and digitoxin.
12 Ivabradine—I_F ('funny' channel) blocker which acts on the SA node to slow heart rate. *See Ivabradine.*
13 Carvedilol is an alpha and beta blocker. *See Carvedilol.*
14 Soluble guanylate cyclase (sGC) stimulators e.g. vericiguat (Verquvo). These drugs, taken PO, reduce the risk of dying and repeat hospitalisations, for CCF. Their mechanism of action is complex. CCF is associated with decreased nitric oxide (NO) and decreased sGC activity, which is the receptor for NO. sGC catalyses the production of cyclic guanosine monophosphate (cGMP) which causes vascular smooth muscle relaxation and increased blood flow. cGMP also improves cardiac function and offsets damage caused by persistent activation of the renin-angiotensin-aldosterone system and the SNS.
15 Cardiac resynchronisation therapy (CRT).
16 Heart transplant (human or genetically engineered pig).
17 Ventricular assist device/mechanical heart e.g. the Carmat artificial heart.

Drugs which should be avoided in heart failure

1 NSAIDs—selective and non-selective.
2 Calcium channel blockers—amlodipine can be used if needed for angina or hypertension.
3 Metformin and thiazolidinediones.
4 Antiarrhythmic drugs, especially ibutilide and sotalol. Amiodarone is preferred in this situation.
5 Many other agents.

Anaesthetic risk and CCF

Patients with CCF are particularly at risk if:
1 there has been decompensation in the six months before surgery
2 the patient is unable to sustain four metabolic equivalents (METs) of exercise. *See Cardiac risk for non-cardiac surgery.*

Anaesthetic aims

1 Preserve preload. The ventricles are poorly compliant and need time to fill. Therefore, tachycardia is poorly tolerated. Also, atrial fibrillation reduces preload. Cardiac arrhythmias must be rapidly detected and treated. Hypovolaemia is poorly tolerated.
2 Maintain contractility—inotropic support with dobutamine or phosphodiesterase inhibitors may be required.
3 Increases in afterload will decrease CO and must be avoided.
4 The myocardial workload must be minimised—another reason why tachycardia/tachyarrhythmias are poorly tolerated. A carefully controlled reduction in afterload can increase CO and decrease myocardial workload.
5 Diastolic blood pressure must be maintained to ensure adequate coronary artery blood flow.

⊙ Coning/brain herniation syndrome/brain code

Description

Coning describes the catastrophic event of the cerebellar tonsils herniating through the foramen magnum with compression of the medulla oblongata. It is due to severe elevation of intracranial pressure. *See Intracranial pressure (ICP) and treatment of raised ICP.* This can be due to head injury, intracranial haemorrhage, brain tumour or encephalitis.

Clinical effects

1 Headache, decreased level of consciousness, coma.
2 Bradycardia, irregular breathing and hypertension (Cushing reflex).
3 Abnormal posturing—patient may be decorticate (arms flexed, legs extended) or decerebrate (arms and legs extended).
4 One or both pupils may be fixed and dilated.

Coning and lumbar puncture

A sudden release of CSF from a patient with raised intracranial pressure, such as a lumbar puncture, can cause coning. However, lumbar puncture is also a treatment for benign intracranial hypertension (BIH). Coning has been reported very rarely in the situation of BIH and lumbar puncture.[15] *See Benign intracranial hypertension (BIH).*

Treatment

This is a catastrophic and usually preterminal event.

1 Paralyse and intubate the patient, commence hyperventilation (to cause cerebral vasoconstriction and lower ICP).
2 Apply other measures to reduce ICP—*see Intracranial pressure (ICP) and measures to reduce elevated ICP.*
3 Control blood pressure.
4 Emergency craniectomy.

⊙ Conn's syndrome

Description

Conn's syndrome is due to excess aldosterone production by an adrenal gland adenoma, carcinoma or hyperplasia. Aldosterone is produced by the zona glomerulosa of the adrenal cortex, and is the main mineralocorticoid manufactured. It causes increased absorption of sodium in exchange for potassium and water from the renal tubules.

Clinical effects

1 Hypertension.
2 Low potassium.
3 Metabolic alkalosis.
4 Hypervolaemia.
5 Kidney damage.

Diagnosis

1 Measurement of aldosterone and renin levels.
2 Imaging of the adrenal glands.

Treatment

1 Antihypertensive medication. *See Hypertension*.
2 Potassium supplements.
3 Spironolactone to oppose the effects of aldosterone. *See Hypertension*.
4 Surgery to remove adenomas, carcinomas. Adrenal hyperplasia is usually treated medically.

Anaesthetic issues

Unilateral or bilateral adrenalectomy may be required.

1 The patient may be hypokalaemic. *See Potassium*. A potassium infusion may be indicated.
2 Adrenal handling may result in catecholamine secretion and hypertension.
3 Avoid hyperventilation, which may decrease serum potassium levels.
4 Hydrocortisone IV should be given intraoperatively if both adrenals are removed, followed by postop oral therapy.

◐ Cord prolapse

See Umbilical cord prolapse.

◐ Coronary artery balloon angioplasty

Balloon angioplasty may be used to dilate a coronary artery. Arterial recoil and acute thrombosis may occur in the first few hours or days after this procedure. Delay elective surgery for at least 4 weeks after coronary artery angioplasty.

◐ Coronary artery disease (CAD)

See Ischaemic heart disease (IHD).

◐ Coronary artery stents (CAS)

Description

Coronary artery stents may be bare metal or drug-eluting (DES). Up to 25–30% of bare metal stents undergo neointimal hyperplasia and in-stent restenosis. Drug-eluting stents (DES) were introduced to reduce this risk but can still be associated with stent thrombosis and restenosis. Stent thrombosis is usually due to platelet aggregation and antiplatelet drugs are used to mitigate this complication.

CAS and non-cardiac surgery (NCS)

About 12% of patients with stents will require NCS within 12 months of stent insertion. These patients may suffer a major adverse cardiovascular event (MACE), such as myocardial infarction, due to stent thrombosis. Stent thrombosis has a mortality of about 30% and is associated with interruption of dual antiplatelet therapy (DAPT) due to a rebound in levels of cyclooxygenase 1 (COX-1) and thromboxane A2 (TXA2). The risk of MACE is not increased if clopidogrel is ceased for < 7 days and aspirin continued, but cessation for longer than seven days increases the MACE risk. Bridging with heparin or LMWH is of little benefit because heparin does not inhibit platelet aggregation. Heparin can cause paradoxical platelet aggregation.

Bare metal stents (BMS)

These may be preferred when:

1 non-cardiac surgery (NCS) is required within four-to-six weeks of percutaneous coronary intervention (PCI)
2 patients have active bleeding at the time of PCI or are at very high risk of bleeding while taking dual antiplatelet therapy (DAPT)
3 patients are unlikely to comply with DAPT for more than four weeks.

Drug-eluting stents (DES)

These stents were developed to reduce the risk of restenosis and were introduced in about the year 2000. Examples of the drugs eluted include everolimus, zotarolimus and paclitaxel. Complications were reduced from about 30% with BMS to about 5–8%. Endothelisation of the stent occurs over about four months.

Dual antiplatelet therapy (DAPT)

For bare metal stents:

1 LD of 300–600 mg of clopidogrel is given before implantation.
2 Post-procedure aspirin 75–100 mg + clopidogrel 75 mg daily are continued for four-to-six weeks.
3 Aspirin is continued indefinitely.

For drug-eluting stents:

1 LD clopidogrel 300–600 mg before implantation.
2 post-implantation DAPT should continue for one year.

Guidelines for non-cardiac surgery (NCS)

Each patient must be individually assessed. Information required includes:

- when the stent was inserted
- type of stent
- patient co-morbidities
- patient exercise tolerance
- type of surgery
- urgency of surgery
- when DAPT can be restarted.

Discuss these issues with the cardiologist and surgeon. Significant surgery should be performed in a hospital with rapid access to an interventional cardiology suite.

1 Elective NCS should be delayed for four-to-six weeks after BMS insertion.
2 Delay elective NCS for at least six months after DES placement.
3 Cease clopidogrel for five days prior to the procedure if significant risk of bleeding but continue aspirin (if possible).
4 Restart clopidogrel as soon as safely possible.
5 In high-risk patients for MACE having high-risk surgery for bleeding e.g. brain surgery, consider the use of bridging therapy with IV cangrelor. *See Cangrelor.*

◑ Coronary perfusion pressure (CPP)

CPP equals aortic diastolic pressure minus left ventricular end-diastolic pressure. It is the pressure gradient that drives coronary artery flow. However, it is not the sole determinant of flow because there is variation in coronary artery resistance (vasodilation and constriction).

◐ Coronavirus

See COVID-19.

◐ Corticosteroids (corticoids)

Description

Corticoids are hormones produced in the adrenal cortex from cholesterol. They are divided into glucocorticoids and mineralocorticoids, and include:

1 cortisol—the main glucocorticoid
2 corticosterone
3 cortisone—an isomer of aldosterone
4 aldosterone—the main mineralocorticoid.

Glucocorticoids

These hormones bind to glucocorticoid receptors present on almost every cell of the body. Actions include:

1 anti-inflammatory
2 immunosuppressive
3 stimulating gluconeogenesis, especially in the liver
4 inhibiting glucose uptake in muscle and adipose tissue
5 stimulating fat breakdown to mobilise fatty acids
6 increasing protein breakdown and decreasing synthesis
7 increased sensitivity to endogenous pressor substances such as catecholamines and angiotensin II
8 reducing NO-mediated endothelial dilatation
9 increasing gastric acid secretion
10 decreasing thyroid hormone production.

Mineralocorticoids

Aldosterone acts mainly on the kidney, colon and salivary glands to retain sodium and excrete potassium and hydrogen ions in the urine. Water is retained with the sodium, helping to maintain normovolaemia. *See Renin-angiotensin system*.

◐ COVER ABCD A swift check

A comprehensive (although somewhat ungainly) algorithm for diagnosing the cause of an anaesthetic crisis situation. It works best if one rescuer reads and ticks off each item while other rescuers resuscitate the patient.

The letters relate to:
C – **C**olour, **C**irculation, **C**apnography
O – **O**xygen supply and **O**$_2$ reservoir, **O**xygen analyser
V – **V**entilation and **V**aporisers
E – **E**T tube and **E**liminate machine
R – **R**eview monitors and equipment

A – **A**irway (face mask, LMA, meticulous attention to ET)
B – **B**reathing (spontaneous ventilation, IPPV)
C – **C**irculation (pulse, blood pressure, ECG, blood loss)
D – **D**rugs (consider all given and not given, check all ampoules)
A – '**A**ir' (gas embolism), **A**wareness and **A**llergy

Swift check—make another assessment of the general situation of the patient, surgeon, effects of the surgery, drugs and infusions.

There are 24 specific sub-algorithms that are recommended by Runciman et al.[16] See the reference for more detail.

○ COVID-19

COVID-19 is the disease caused by SARS-CoV-2 virus (also referred to as 'coronavirus'), which emerged in Wuhan, China in December 2019. SARS stands for **s**evere **a**cute **r**espiratory **s**yndrome and CoV stands for coronavirus. SARS-CoV-1 resulted in the SARS epidemic in 2003. At the time of going to print, COVID-19 has caused a world-wide death toll of nearly 7 million. The delta strain has been the most aggressive form so far. The best preventative strategy is vaccination.

Symptoms

Symptoms begin two-to-four days after exposure. Infected persons are contagious for about two days before symptoms and for 10–20 days after symptoms start. The mortality rate is about 2.3% but is influenced by many factors such as the availability of effective treatments, vaccination status and the particular strain of COVID-19.

Infection results in a multisystem disorder, including:

1 cough, dyspnoea, runny nose, sore throat, loss of taste and or smell, chest pain
2 fever, muscle aches and pains, fatigue, headache
3 diarrhoea, nausea and vomiting
4 heart muscle damage, arrhythmias, pericarditis
5 respiratory failure
6 kidney failure
7 CNS manifestations, including strokes
8 long-term health problems, known as 'long covid'.

Diagnosis and investigation

Diagnosis is confirmed by:

1 Positive PCR test. PCR stands for 'polymerase chain reaction'. It tests for the presence of genetic material from the virus using a nasopharyngeal and pharyngeal swab.
2 Rapid antigen test (RAT)—this is a screening tool. It involves performing a nasal swab, after which the swab is placed in a chemical solution, with a result available in 10–15 min. The test identifies the presence of antigens on the surface of the virus. It is less accurate than a PCR test.
3 COVID-19 serology.

Severe illness

This is defined as a respiratory rate (RR) $\geq$ 30 breaths per minute, oxygen saturation $\leq$ 92% and a $PaO_2/FiO_2 \leq 300$.

Critical illness

Defined as:

1 Severe respiratory failure—$PaO_2/FiO_2 < 200$.
2 Acute respiratory distress syndrome (ARDS)
3 Patients who are deteriorating despite advanced forms of respiratory support i.e. non-invasive ventilation (NIV) or high-flow nasal oxygen (HFNO)
4 Hypotension, organ failure, altered mental state.

All patients require a COVID-19 serology baseline, FBC, UEC, LFTs, CRP, PCT, LDH, CK, troponin, ferritin, d-dimer, HbA1c, coagulation profile, ECG and CXR. Other illnesses (influenza, hepatitis, HIV, strongyloides, TB) should be excluded.

Management

About 19% of unvaccinated infected patients will become hypoxic, 14% will need oxygen therapy and 5% will need invasive ventilation. Of the ventilated patients, 60–70% develop ARDS and about 50% die. Patients should be managed in isolation, in a negative pressure room if possible. Full PPE precautions must be maintained to prevent spread of the infection. Patients may develop a viral pneumonia and/or ARDS.

Treatment can be divided into:

1 supportive measures
2 specific treatments.

Supportive measures

1 Oxygen therapy—can be nil, nasal prongs (1–4 L/min), high-flow nasal cannula (HFNC), non-invasive ventilation or invasive mechanical ventilation or ECMO. Aim to keep oxygen saturation > 93% but not higher than 96%. Non-invasive ventilation has a high failure rate and may be more of a risk to staff than HFNC. Patients should be referred to ICU if they are haemodynamically unstable, have rapidly worsening respiratory function or require ≥ 40% inspired concentration of O_2 to maintain an O_2 saturation ≥ 92%.
2 Anticoagulant therapy—Clexane 40 mg/day to prevent DVT/PE and microvascular thrombosis, especially in the lungs.
3 Ventilation strategies include low tidal volumes (TV), permissive hypercapnia and prone positioning for 12–16 h/day. *See Acute respiratory distress syndrome.* Consider recruitment manoeuvres. *See Recruitment manoeuvres.*
4 Neuromuscular blocker drugs should be considered if other parameters are optimised (driving pressure, PEEP) without hypoxaemia control, or if the patient is placed prone or there is persistent ventilator dyssynchrony or ongoing need for deep sedation.
5 Fluid therapy should be conservative as the incidence of heart failure is high.

Specific treatments

1 Dexamethasone—this drug should only be used in patients requiring any type of respiratory support/oxygen therapy. In adults administer 6 mg IV or PO daily for 10 days.
2 Remdesivir—broad-spectrum antiviral agent. It acts on coronavirus by inhibiting an RNA-dependent enzyme called RNA polymerase which enables the virus to reproduce itself. Dose, adult: 200 mg IV initially then 100 mg IV daily for five days. It is used in patients requiring oxygen therapy but not in patients on mechanical ventilation or ECMO, unless it was started before ventilation/ECMO. It is more effective in the early stages of the disease.
3 Baricitinib—a Janus kinase inhibitor normally used to treat moderate-to-severe rheumatoid arthritis by reducing inflammatory cascades. It is used in coronavirus patients requiring oxygen therapy **but not if they are mechanically ventilated or on ECMO**. Dose, adult: 4 mg PO daily for 14 days. It is not used in pregnancy; in pregnancy, tocilizumab (a monoclonal antibody treatment) is used as an alternative to baricitinib. Tocilizumab acts as an immunomodulator.
4 Sotrovimab—a monoclonal antibody treatment with a similar action to Ronapreve. It is used to prevent deterioration in patients not requiring oxygen therapy, who are at

a higher risk of death if COVID-19 progresses. These include patients with obesity, diabetes and renal impairment. The dose is 500 mg by IV infusion.

5 Ronapreve—monoclonal antibody treatment. Contains casirivimab and imdevimab. These antibodies prevent the virus from binding to human cells by attaching to the virus spike protein. Ronapreve is indicated to prevent COVID-19 infection before or after exposure, or to reduce the risk of severe disease in infected people. It is especially indicated in patients with compromised immune systems.

6 Convalescent plasma therapy—antibodies are removed from the plasma of people who have recovered from infection and given to newly infected people.

7 Specific antiviral drugs for COVID-19 are becoming increasingly available. These include molnupiravir and Paxlovid (nirmatrelvir + ritonavir). These drugs are taken orally and are intended to prevent COVID-19 infection from becoming life threatening.

Elective surgery after COVID-19 infection (advice based on *ANZCA Document PG68(A) Guideline on surgical patient safety for SARS-CoV-2 infection and vaccination 2023*, updated May 2023)

1 For most patients it is safe to proceed with elective surgery 2–3 weeks post COVID-19 infection, provided no ongoing symptoms are present.

2 Patients who are asymptomatic, have returned to baseline, are vaccinated, < 70 years of age and without co-morbidity can proceed with elective, minor surgery (day case) and endoscopy without delay beyond the infectious period.

3 Patients with ongoing symptoms, especially with non-return to baseline function and/or moderate or more severe COVID-19 infection should have elective surgery delayed for 7 weeks.

⏵ COX-1/COX-2 inhibitors

See Non-steroidal anti-inflammatory drugs (NSAIDs)

⏵ Creatine kinase (CK)/creatine phosphokinase (CPK)

CK (also known as CPK) is a protein enzyme found in skeletal and heart muscle and, to a lesser extent, in the brain. CK catalyses the addition of a phosphate group to creatine to create phosphocreatine (creatine phosphate), which is used by muscle for sudden bursts of energy. Muscle breakdown, as occurs in rhabdomyolysis, results in elevated CK levels. Intense exercise and muscle diseases can also increase CK levels. Normal CK levels are about 30–180 U/L for females and 60–220 U/L for males. *See Malignant hyperthermia.*

⏵ Creatinine clearance (CrCl)

See Renal function tests.

⏵ Cricoid pressure

This is the application of pressure to the cricoid cartilage with the index finger and thumb, with the aim of preventing regurgitation/aspiration. Pressure should be applied as the patient's eyes begin to close after induction of anaesthesia. The force should be about 30 N. Cricoid pressure should only be removed when the anaesthetist requests for this to happen. This is when intubation has been confirmed by detecting expired CO_2.

▶ Cricothyroid puncture/cricothyrotomy

See *Difficult airway management.*

▶ Critical arterial oxygen desaturation

This occurs at an oxygen saturation of 88–90%. This corresponds to the upper inflection point of the oxygen-haemoglobin dissociation curve. Oxygen saturation falls very steeply beyond this point.

▶ Cryoprecipitate

Cryoprecipitate is prepared from a single donated whole blood unit. Each bag has a volume of 30–40 mL and contains:
1 approximately 0.35 g of fibrinogen
2 factors VIII and XIII, von Willebrand factor and fibronectin.

A typical dose for a 70 kg adult is 8–10 bags (3–4 g of fibrinogen). Apheresis fibrinogen is prepared from FFP obtained from a plasmapheresis donor and contains about 0.8 g/bag of fibrinogen. A typical dose for a 70 kg adult patient is 4–5 bags of 60 mL each (3–4 g of fibrinogen). Cryoprecipitate should preferably be of the same blood group as the recipient. If this is not possible, use products that are ABO compatible with the patient's red cells. RhD status can be ignored. The order of preference of these products is shown in Table C2.

Table C2 Order of preference of plasma product ABO groups

Recipient's ABO group	Plasma product ABO group			
	First choice	Second choice	Third choice	Fourth choice
O	O	A	B	AB
A	A	AB	B	
B	B	AB	A	
AB	AB	A	B	
Unknown	AB	A		

▶ Cushing reflex

This describes the triad of responses to raised intracranial pressure—hypertension, bradycardia and irregular breathing. This level of raised ICP is usually preterminal and likely to be followed by coning. **See** *Coning* and *Intracranial pressure (ICP) and treatment of raised ICP.*

▶ Cyanide (CN) toxicity

Description
Cyanide is a potent cytochrome c oxidase inhibitor. It interferes with oxidative phosphorylation, which is needed for mitochondria to make ATP. Cells are therefore unable to utilise oxygen (a condition known as histotoxic hypoxia).

Cyanide poisoning causes headache, confusion, anxiety, nausea and vomiting, dyspnoea, chest pain, tachycardia, loss of consciousness, seizures and death. It can cause metabolic acidosis.

Causes

1 Sodium nitroprusside (SNP) infusion. *See Sodium nitroprusside (SNP)*.
2 Fumes from burning polymer products containing nitriles. *See Burns*.
3 Some insecticides.
4 Some foods such as flaxseed and cassava.

Treatment

1 Stop the source e.g. SNP infusion.
2 Administer 100% O_2.
3 Inhaled amyl nitrite—there is a lack of evidence of significant benefit.
4 IV sodium thiosulphate 150 mg/kg over 15 min, then an infusion of 30–60 mg/kg/h. This converts CN^- to thiocyanate.
5 Sodium nitrite—4–6 mg/kg slowly IV. This drug works by creating methaemoglobin, which binds to CN^-, removing it from mitochondria. Use with sodium thiosulphate.
6 Hydroxocobalamin IV—a dose of 100 mcg/kg is suggested. Binds to CN^-, forming cyanocobalamin.
7 Dicobalt edetate plus glucose. Cobalt chelates CN^- to cobalt cyanide. Glucose protects against cobalt toxicity.

❍ Cyclizine

Description

Piperazine-derivative antihistamine and anticholinergic drug used as an anti-emetic. Effects last about 4 h.

Dose

Adult

50 mg IV up to q 8 h to a maximum of 3 doses. Give 20 min before the end of surgery. The oral dose in adults is 50 mg.

Points to note

1 It is ineffective in patients given atropine.
2 Do not use in patients with severe heart failure, porphyria, glaucoma, urinary retention/prostatic hypertrophy.
3 Cyclizine, when combined with methadone, can cause strong psychoactive effects.
4 There is evidence of fetal damage in animal studies. Use during pregnancy and breast feeding is discouraged.

❍ Cyclo-oxygenase (COX)

See Non-steroidal anti-inflammatory drugs (NSAIDs).

Description

COX is also known as prostaglandin-endoperoxide synthase. It is an enzyme involved in the production of prostanoids such as thromboxane and prostaglandins such as prostacyclin. There are two isoenzymes of COX, COX-1 and COX-2.

COX-1

1 Stomach—protects gastric mucosa from acid.

2 Kidney—helps maintain normal renal function such as renin release and renal vasodilation and excretion.

3 Platelets—makes platelets more likely to adhere to each other and to other surfaces by increasing production of thromboxane A2 in platelets.

COX-2

COX-2 is found in macrophages, leukocytes and other immune cells. Its effects are pro-inflammatory.

○ Cystic fibrosis (CF)

Description

CF is an inherited autosomal recessive disease. It is the most common potentially lethal genetic disease in Caucasians and is due to a mutation of the CF transmembrane regulator (CFTR) gene on chromosome 7. There is disruption of the CFTR chloride channel on the apical border of epithelial cells lining most exocrine glands. This results in thick, sticky mucus instead of thin, watery mucus. Heterozygotes are unaffected. The carrier rate in the UK is about 1 in 25.

Clinical effects

1 Progressive lung disease with patchy atelectasis, airway inflammation and bacterial infection.

2 Bronchiectasis develops with chronic bacterial colonisation. Hypoxia and hypercapnia may occur.

3 Sinusitis.

4 Nasal polyps.

5 Pancreatic insufficiency with malabsorption of vitamins A, D, E and K and steatorrhea due to decreased fat absorption.

6 Pancreatic fibrosis and gland destruction leads to diabetes mellitus.

7 Liver cirrhosis and portal hypertension may occur.

8 Osteoporosis.

9 Subfertility/infertility—males and females.

10 Poor nutritional status.

11 Right ventricular hypertrophy/cor pulmonale/pulmonary hypertension. These are signs that suggest very advanced disease.

12 Distal intestinal obstruction syndrome (DIOS) may occur due to thick, tenacious stool.

13 Diminished or fluctuating functional status.

14 Clotting abnormalities (vitamin K deficiency, recurrent venous thrombosis related to central venous catheters).

15 Psychological issues—depression, anxiety.

Diagnosis

1 Elevated chloride levels in sweat test.

2 Lab evidence of abnormality of the CFTR gene.

Treatment

1 Physiotherapy and airway clearance techniques.

2 Inhaled bronchodilators and mucolytics. Dornase alfa (rhDNase) is a new drug which decreases the viscosity of secretions.

3 Inhaled hypertonic saline.

4 Mechanical devices such as high-frequency chest compression devices may help to clear mucus.

5 O_2 therapy/home non-invasive ventilation.

6 Anti-inflammatory drugs (steroids, NSAIDs). Inhaled steroids may be used.

7 Antibiotics (inhaled, oral, IV).

8 Diabetic medication.

9 Pancreatic enzyme replacement therapy e.g. Creon.

10 Nutritional support such as PEG feeding.

11 Gene therapy—in development.

12 Lung transplant (usually bilateral sequential single lung transplant—two lungs transplanted but the recipient retains their own heart). Transplanted patients will be on immunosuppressive drugs.

Anaesthetic management

These patients are obviously very complex, and anaesthesia is stressful for everyone involved. A multidisciplinary approach involving the patient's CF management team is essential. In general:

1 Optimise the patient for elective surgery (extra chest physio, medication review).

2 Understand the patient's baseline function—CXR, ABG, lung function tests. An obstructive pattern is usually seen. **See Lung function tests.** A decrease in FEV_1 to < 1 L, especially in hypoxic patients, is indicative of the potential need for postoperative ventilation.[17] An FEV_1 < 61% of predicted is also concerning.

3 Check usual preop blood tests and clotting studies.

4 Minimise the interruption to medical therapy and physiotherapy over the peri-operative period.

5 Minimise starvation time.

6 *Note:* an implanted IV access device may be present.

7 Transplanted patients must continue anti-rejection drugs.

8 Steroid cover if on significant steroid doses. **See Stress steroids.**

9 Consider preoperative proton pump inhibitor therapy due to the increased incidence of GORD in these patients.

10 Intraoperative nebulisation of patient's medication may be required—usually dornase alfa 2.5 mg. Hypertonic saline can be nebulised if dornase alfa is not available.

11 Creon should be continued every 4 h throughout the fasting period.

12 Avoid GA if possible (LA, nerve blocks, neuraxial).

13 Surgical site affects risk. The highest-risk operations are upper abdominal and thoracic surgery.

14 Nasogastric tube insertion is an independent risk factor for postoperative respiratory complications.[17] Avoid this if possible.

15 Appropriate diabetes mellitus management. **See Diabetes mellitus (DM).** Monitor patient's BSL.

16 A rapid sequence induction may be justified due to severe reflux.

17 Sevoflurane may provide some bronchodilation. TIVA is also acceptable.

18 Nasal intubation should be avoided due to the frequency of nasal polyps and infection risks.

19 Airway pressures should be kept low when IPPV is used to minimise the risk of pneumothorax. Use TV 6–8 mL/kg and PEEP 5–10 cm H_2O.[17]

20 Opioids should be used cautiously because of the risk of respiratory depression and DIOS.

21 Avoid long-acting drugs e.g. methadone. Reverse rocuronium with sugammadex.

22 Chest physiotherapy in recovery.

23 Resume patient's usual medications as soon as possible with early mobilisation if possible.

CF patients with failing RV[17]

1 Reduce afterload and preserve coronary artery perfusion.

2 Avoid acidosis, hypercarbia, hypoxia and hypothermia as these will all increase pulmonary vascular resistance.

3 Inotropes such as milrinone or enoximone will produce pulmonary vascular dilatation. However, SVR will also drop, so noradrenaline may be needed to maintain BP.

Patient with bilateral sequential single lung transplant[17]

1 The patient retains their own heart with full innervation.

2 The transplanted lungs have no cough reflex below the carina.

3 Expert advice is required for the management of immunosuppressive drugs.

4 FiO_2 should be minimised, as should ventilation times.

5 TV should be 6–8 mL/kg.

6 Keep inspiratory pressures < 30 cm H_2O.

7 Avoid hypervolaemia. The transplanted lungs have impaired lymphatics and are prone to low pressure pulmonary oedema.

8 Mucociliary clearance is poor and chest physio will be needed post surgery.

REFERENCES

1 Gao L, Zheng G, Han J et al. Effects of prophylactic ondansetron on spinal anaesthesia-induced hypotension: a meta-analysis. *Int J Obstet Anesth* 2015; 24: 335–343.

2 Lee AJ, Landau R, Mattingly JL et al. Left lateral table tilt for elective Cesarean delivery under spinal anesthesia has no effect on neonatal acid-base status: a randomised controlled trial. *Anesthesiology* 2017; 127: 241–249.

3 Powell B, Al-Mukhtar A, Mills GH. Carcinoid: the disease and its implications for anaesthesia. *Cont Educ in Anaesth Crit Care Pain* 2011; 11: 9–13.

4 Wijeysundera DN, Pearse RM, Shulma MA et al. Assessment of functional capacity before major non-cardiac surgery: an international, prospective cohort study. *Lancet* 2018; 391: 2631–2640.

5 Biccard BM, Devereaux PJ, Rodseth RN. Cardiac biomarkers in the prediction of risk in the non-cardiac surgery setting. *Anaesthesia* 2014; 69: 484–493.

6 Healy KO, Waksmonski CA, Altman RK et al. Perioperative outcome and long-term mortality for heart failure patients undergoing intermediate and high-risk noncardiac surgery: impact of left ventricular ejection fraction. *Congest Heart Fail* 2010; 16: 45–49.

7 Roshanov PS, Rochverg B, Patel A et al. Withholding versus continuing angiotensin-converting enzyme inhibitors or angiotensin II receptor blockers before noncardiac surgery: an analysis of vascular events in noncardiac surgery patients cohort evaluation prospective cohort. *Anesthesiol* 2017; 126: 16–27.

8 Hunt WE, Hess RM. Surgical risk as related to time of intervention the repair of intracranial aneurysms. *J Neurosurg* 1968; 28: 14–20.

9 Report of the World Federation of Neurological Surgeons Committee on a Universal Subarachnoid Haemorrhage Grading Scale. *J Neurosurg* 1988; 68: 985–986.

10 Sano H, Inamasu J, Kato Y et al. Modified World Federation of Neurosurgical Societies Subarachnoid Hemorrhage Grading System. *Surg Neurol Int.* 2016;7(Suppl 18): S502–503.

11 Abd-Elsayed AA, Wehby A, Farag E. Anesthetic management of patients with intracranial aneurysms. *Ochsner J* 2014; 14: 418–425.

12 Guner D, Tiftikcioglu BI, Uludag IF et al. Dural puncture: an overlooked cause of cerebral venous thrombosis. *Acta Neurol Belg* 2015; 115: 53–57.

13 Short JH, Fatemi P, Ruoss S, Angelotti T. Clevidipine-induced extreme hypoxaemia in a neurosurgical patient: a case report. *A A Pract* 2020; 14: 60–62.

14 Lovell A. Anaesthetic implications of grown-up congenital heart disease. *BJA* 2004; 93: 129–139.

15 Borire A, Lueck C, Hughes A. Tonsillar herniation after lumbar puncture in idiopathic intracranial hypertension. *J Neuroophthalmol* 2015; 35: 293–295.

16 Runciman WB, Kluger MT, Morris RW et al. Crisis management during anaesthesia: the development of an anaesthetic crisis management manual. *Qual Saf Health Care* 2005; 14: e1. Accessed online: https://pubmed.ncbi.nlm.nih.gov/15933282/PubMed (nih.gov), October 2022.

17 Dunstan C, Francis C, Simpson K. *Perioperative care for the cystic fibrosis patient.* CIG CYMRU NHS Wales Cardiff and Vale University Health Board, January 2020. Accessed online: https://www.cpoc.org.uk/sites/cpoc/files/documents/2021-03/Perioperative%20care%20for%20the%20cystic%20fibrosis%20patient.pdf, September 2022.

⭕ Dabigatran (Pradaxa)

Description

Dabigatran is a direct thrombin inhibitor (DTI) taken orally. It binds to thrombin thereby inhibiting the conversion of fibrinogen to fibrin. Dabigatran is effective after 2 h. It is contraindicated if the creatinine clearance (CrCl) < 30 mL/min.

Dose

Adult

1 VTE prevention (CrCl > 50 mL/min) 110 mg 1–4 h postop, then 220 mg/day. If CrCl 30–50 mL/min give 75 mg 1–4 h postop, then 150 mg/day. For hip surgery, give for 28–35 days. For knee surgery, give for 10 days.
2 Embolic stroke prevention—150 mg q 12 h. If elderly or creatinine clearance 30–50 mL/min, 110 mg q 12 h.
3 DVT/PE treatment—150 mg q 12 h after 5 days of heparin therapy. Use 110 mg q 12 h if patient is elderly, has high bleeding risk or creatinine clearance 30–50 mL/min.

When to cease dabigatran for surgery/neuraxial anaesthesia

Renal function can be assessed by creatinine clearance. If the calculated creatinine clearance is > 50 mL/min, then:
1 standard-risk procedures (e.g. cardiac catheterisation, colonoscopy without removal of large polyps, cholecystectomy)—cease dabigatran for 24 h
2 high-risk procedures and neuraxial anaesthesia, insertion of pacemakers, major surgery—cease dabigatran for 48 h.

If the calculated creatinine clearance is 30–50 mL/min, then:
1 standard-risk procedures—cease dabigatran for 48 h
2 high-risk procedures/neuraxial anaesthesia—cease dabigatran for 4 days.

When to restart dabigatran after surgery

This depends on the assessed post-surgical bleeding risk. Restarting in 1 day for low-risk surgery and in 2–3 days for high-risk surgery is usually considered reasonable. If an epidural catheter is removed, wait at least 2 h before initiating dabigatran.

Emergency reversal of dabigatran

The thrombin time is very sensitive to the presence of dabigatran. PT and INR are unaffected.
1 Idarucizumab (Praxbind) is a specific antidote for dabigatran. Give 5 g IV. Dabigatran can be resumed 24 h after idarucizumab. *See Idarucizumab (Praxbind).* If Praxbind is unavailable, consider FEIBA 50 U/kg and/or cryoprecipitate. *See FEIBA-NF (factor VIII inhibitor bypass activity).*
2 Tranexamic acid 1 g IV q 8 h.
3 Treatment as for any other major haemorrhage. *See Blood loss—assessment, management and anaesthetic approach.*

◉ Dalteparin (Fragmin)

A fractionated heparin. *See Heparin (unfractionated and low-molecular-weight heparins).*

◉ Danaparoid (Orgaran)

Description

Danaparoid is a low-molecular-weight heparinoid used in patients who require DVT/PE prophylaxis or treatment, but cannot have heparin/LMWH due to HIT type II. However, there is a risk of cross-reactivity with HIT antibodies. The drug acts mainly by inhibition of thrombin generation by:

1 indirect inactivation of FXa
2 inhibition of thrombin activation of FIX.

It is used IV and can also be used prophylactically subcut. Do not use if the creatinine clearance is < 30 mL/min. The duration of action is prolonged in patients with renal impairment.

Dose—adult

Prophylactic dose
750 units subcut 12 h.

Therapeutic dose
1 Patient < 55 kg IV bolus 1250 units.
2 Patient 55–90 kg IV bolus 2500 units.
3 Patient > 90 kg IV bolus 3750 units.

After the bolus, run an infusion of 400 units/h for 4 h, then 300 units/h for 4 h, then 150–200 units/h adjusted according to the Anti-Xa level. Aim for Anti-Xa levels of 0.5–0.8 units/mL.

Reversal and surgery/neuraxial anaesthesia

Danaparoid has a long half-life of 22 h. There is no antidote. It is unclear from the literature when it is safe to perform invasive procedures after ceasing danaparoid. 24 h is suggested.[1] No neuraxial block guidelines can be offered.

◉ Dantrolene (Dantrium)

Description

A hydantoin derivative (like phenytoin) which causes skeletal muscle relaxation. It acts directly on the muscle, probably by depressing excitation-contraction coupling by binding to the ryanodine receptor 1, thus decreasing intracellular calcium concentration.

Indications

1 Malignant hyperthermia. *See Malignant hyperthermia (MH).*
2 Neuroleptic malignant syndrome. *See Neuroleptic malignant syndrome (NMS).*
3 Chronic spasticity.

◉ D-dimer

D-dimer is a byproduct of intrinsic fibrin breakdown. Elevated levels suggest recent thrombus. *See Pulmonary embolism (PE).*

◐ Deep venous thrombosis (DVT) prophylaxis

Introduction

All inpatients should be assessed for their DVT risk. This risk depends on patient risk factors and the type of surgery being undertaken. DVTs are most likely to occur 2–10 days after surgery. The following recommendations are based on those of the Australian Commission on Safety, Quality and Health Care Venous Thromboembolism Clinical Care Standard 2018.

Patient risk factors

1 Malignancy.
2 Previous DVT/PE.
3 Thrombophilic disorder. *See Thrombophilia.*
4 Pregnancy.
5 Age > 60 y.
6 Immobile patients e.g. CVA patients or those with lower-limb weakness or amputations.
7 Obesity.
8 Smoking.
9 Varicose veins.
10 Dehydration.
11 Oral contraceptive pill or hormone replacement therapy.

Surgical risk factors

High risk (DVT risk 40–80%)

1 Major surgery in patients older than 60 y.
2 Major orthopaedic surgery (e.g. knee/hip replacement, hip fracture, pelvic fracture).
3 Multitrauma.
4 Abdominal or pelvic surgery for cancer.
5 Major surgery in patients aged 40–60 y with other risk factors.
6 Acute spinal cord injury with paresis.

Moderate risk (DVT risk 10–40%)

1 Major surgery in a patient aged 40–60 y.
2 Minor surgery in a patient aged 40–60 y with other risk factors.
3 Minor surgery in a patient aged over 60 y.

Low risk (DVT risk < 10%)

1 Minor surgery < 39 min in patients < 60 y.
2 Major surgery in patient < 40 y with no other risk factors.

Management of high-risk patients

1 Enoxaparin (Clexane) 40 mg daily, commenced 6–12 h post surgery (unless haemostasis not established). Delay for 24 h if high risk of postoperative bleeding. Alternatively, use dalteparin (Fragmin), 5000 units subcut daily.
2 Heparin 5000 units q 8 h or q 12 h can be used but low-molecular-weight heparin (LMWH) preferred for hip or knee replacement.
3 If patient < 50 kg or renal impairment, reduce above doses by 50%.
4 Intraoperative calf compressors.
5 Compression stockings on the ward.
6 Early mobilisation.

7 After hip replacement/fracture surgery, continue treatment for 28–35 days.

8 After total knee replacement, continue therapy for up to 14 days.

9 Continue fractionated heparin until the patient is mobile, or for 7–10 days.

10 After major general surgery, continue therapy for 1 week or until mobility returns to baseline.

11 Alternatively, rivaroxaban, dabigatran or apixaban can be used after hip or knee joint replacement.

Management of moderate-risk patients

1 Enoxaparin 20 mg/day or dalteparin 2500 units/day.

2 Calf compressors/compression stockings as described above.

3 Early mobilisation.

Management of low-risk patients

Consider intraoperative calf compressors plus early mobilisation.

Management of patients with heparin-induced thrombocytopenia (HIT) syndrome

Use fondaparinux 2.5 mg subcut daily (high- and moderate-risk patients).

Obstetric patients (labour and delivery)

These guidelines apply to patients with normal renal function. Wait longer if renal function is impaired.

1 For patients on, or commencing, prophylactic LMWH:
- No neuraxial anaesthesia for at least 12 h after last dose.
- No LMWH for at least 12 h after neuraxial anaesthesia (including if an epidural catheter has remained in situ).
- If the patient has had an epidural catheter in situ for more than 12 h, wait for at least 12 h after the last dose of LMWH before epidural catheter removal.
- Wait for at least 4 h after epidural catheter removal before the next dose of LMWH.

2 For patients on, or commencing, subcut unfractionated heparin:
- No neuraxial anaesthesia for at least 6 h after last dose.
- If an epidural is to remain in situ, wait at least 1 h before subcut heparin.
- No subcut heparin within 6 h of epidural catheter removal.
- Wait at least 1 h after epidural catheter removal before the next dose of subcut heparin.

Obstetric DVT prophylaxis postpartum

High-risk patients should have enoxaparin 40 mg subcut daily until discharge. High-risk patients are:

1 All Caesarean sections

2 All patients with BMI > 40

3 All vaginal deliveries with 4 or more risk factors. These are:
- **a)** age > 35 **or** booking BMI > 30 **or** parity ≥ 4 **or** major intercurrent illness
- **b)** preeclampsia/eclampsia
- **c)** major blood loss **or** instrumental delivery or labour > 12 h
- **d)** VTE in first degree relative
- **e)** heterozygous for factor V Leiden or prothrombin gene mutation
- **f)** immobility ≤ 4 days or gross varicose veins.

Very high-risk obstetric patients should have enoxaparin 40 mg daily for 8 weeks postpartum. This group includes patients with:

1 previous unprovoked spontaneous VTE

2 previous provoked VTE with thrombophilia. **See *Thrombophilia***

3 lupus anticoagulant or anticardiolipin antibody in high titre
4 deficiency of antithrombin III, protein C or protein S
5 factor V Leiden or prothrombin gene mutant homozygote or double heterozygote
6 paraplegia
7 homozygous sickle cell disease. ***See Sickle cell disease (SCD).***

Calf compressors are not recommended for CS intraoperatively, unless the patient is considered very high risk for DVT. Selective use of compression stockings on the ward is recommended for patients for whom postoperative enoxaparin is indicated.

Defibrillation

See Cardiac arrest and ***Cardioversion, electrical***.

Delirium, postanaesthetic

Introduction

Patients should be alert and cooperative after a maximum of 60 minutes post anaesthetic (unless there is a factor unrelated to GA, such as head injury). 'Delirium' is a catch-all term for all abnormal mental states after a general anaesthetic (GA), including agitation, aggression, confusion, repetitive purposeless movements and somnolence. There are three types of delirium:

1 hyperactive delirium—restlessness, irritability, combative behaviour, agitation, confusion and paranoia
2 hypoactive delirium—somnolence, lethargy and unawareness
3 mixed—features of the above two categories.

Some patients may have a prolonged recovery from delirium, and a small percentage never recover.

Perioperative risk factors

1 Elderly patient.
2 Clinical or subclinical dementia.
3 Opioids, especially pethidine.
4 Benzodiazepines.
5 Steroids.
6 Atropine, especially in the elderly.
7 Impaired hearing and/or vision.
8 Drug/alcohol withdrawal.
9 Decreased cognitive reserve/low educational achievement.
10 History of delirium associated with GA.

Prevention

1 Avoidance of GA.
2 Avoidance of full bladder, hypothermia and dehydration.
3 Good pain control.
4 Caution with the use of drugs associated with delirium.
5 Maintenance of sensory input (glasses, hearing aids).

Identification of common causes and initial management

1 Check all vital signs to detect/treat hypoxia, hypotension, hypertension, tachycardia and bradycardia. A slow respiratory rate suggests hypercapnia as a cause. Check pulse oximetry for hypoxia and arterial blood gases for hypercarbia.
2 Catheterise the patient if the bladder is full.

3 Consider drug effects or drug/alcohol withdrawal. Review all medications and consider an accidental overdose e.g. hydromorphone instead of morphine. Methadone can cause very prolonged somnolence. Ketamine may also cause neurological disturbance.
4 Consider prolonged effects of neuromuscular blockade.
5 Provide adequate pain control.
6 Always consider hypoglycaemia and electrolyte disturbances. Check BSL and electrolytes, looking for abnormalities such as low serum sodium, hypokalaemia and hypomagnesaemia.
7 Detect/treat acute coronary syndrome. Check ECG and cardiac troponins.
8 Administer carefully titrated doses of opioids if pain is a (suspected) cause of the delirium.
9 Give cautiously titrated doses of midazolam if alcohol/benzodiazepine or other drug withdrawal is suspected.
10 Treat (possible) atropine intoxication with physostigmine. **See *Anticholinergic syndrome*.**
11 Consider naloxone 100 mcg boluses for actual or suspected opioid intoxication. Check the dose of neuraxial opioid and consider accidental overdose as a cause of delirium.
13 Administer flumazenil if benzodiazepine sensitivity/overdose is a possible/likely cause.
14 Exclude/treat significant blood loss (check FBC, drains, look for abdominal distension). Consider concealed blood loss such as a retroperitoneal haematoma.
15 Consider local anaesthetic (LA) effects, including overdose, unintentional intravascular infusion, brainstem anaesthesia, high/total spinal anaesthesia and excessive epidural LA.

General treatments for delirium

1 Consider haloperidol for severe agitation—0.5–10 mg IM (preferred) or slow IV injection (maximum 20 mg/day). For strong/aggressive patients consider droperidol 4–8 mg IV.
2 Frequent orientation and reassurance of the patient.
3 Physical restraints as a last resort.

Rarer causes of delirium to consider

These include:
1 Liver failure with elevated serum ammonia levels.
2 Kidney failure with uraemia.
3 Check the anaesthetic record for any episodes of prolonged hypotension/hypertension/hypoxia. Consider the possibility of brain haemorrhage, ischaemic stroke, hypoxic brain injury or elevated intracranial pressure. Perform a neurological exam looking for any signs of brain injury such as unilateral or bilateral fixed dilated pupils. An urgent cranial CT should be considered.
4 Serotonin syndrome. **See *Serotonin syndrome*.**
5 An endocrine emergency e.g. severe hypothyroidism, thyrotoxicosis.
6 Status epilepticus. Consider emergency EEG.
7 Encephalitis.
8 Sepsis.
9 Poisons such as carbon monoxide.
10 Fat embolism or amniotic fluid embolism.
11 Methaemoglobinaemia.
12 Malignant hyperthermia/neuroleptic malignant syndrome.
13 Acute psychiatric illness or exacerbation of chronic illness.

⊙ DENPAX

This is a trade name for transdermal fentanyl patches providing doses ranging from 12–100 mcg/h.

▶ Depodur

This is an extended-release form of morphine for epidural use.

▶ Depth of anaesthesia monitoring

See *Awareness monitoring.*

▶ Dermatomes

Table D1 Key dermatome landmarks

Dermatome	Anatomical site	Dermatome	Anatomical site
C5–T1	Upper limb	T12–L1	Inguinal ligament
C7	Middle finger	L3	Front of knee
T3	Apex of axilla	L4	Medial side of calf
T4	Nipple	L5	Outer calf
T7	Tip of xiphoid	S1	Outer border of foot
T10	Umbilicus	S2	Back of knee

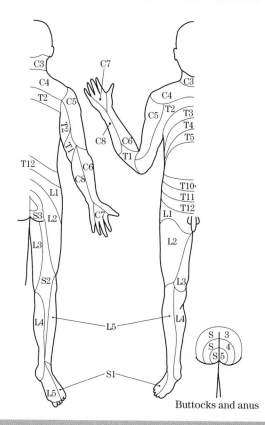

Figure D1 Dermatomes

◖ Desflurane

Description

Methyl ethyl ether inhalational anaesthetic agent, very similar in structure to isoflurane.

Dose

1 The MAC of desflurane is 6 but this varies with the age of the patient. For elderly patients, 5.2% inhalational concentration is suggested.

2 Following IV induction of anaesthesia, a reasonable initial vaporiser setting is 4–6%, with a fresh gas flow (FGF) of 3–5 L/min.

3 Gradually increase the delivered desflurane concentration by increments of 1% every few breaths, with a FGF of 4–6 L/min until the desired anaesthetic depth is reached.

4 FGF rates can then be turned down to a minimal flow rate.

Advantages

1 Rapid emergence—faster than sevoflurane. The clinical significance of this is dubious.

2 Metabolised to a very small extent (0.02%).

Disadvantages

In comparison with sevoflurane and propofol IV anaesthesia, the disadvantages of desflurane are substantial. Some authors have recommended that its use should be discontinued.[2] Significant issues include:

1 Requires a unique and complex vaporiser that is electrically heated to 39° and thermostatically controlled, with an internal pressure of 2 atmospheres.

2 Low potency.

3 Severely pungent, making it unsuitable for gaseous induction and asthmatics.

4 Can stimulate the sympathetic nervous system at higher doses, causing tachycardia and hypertension.

5 Impairs cerebral autoregulation at concentrations greater than 0.5 MAC, hence its use in neurosurgery is not ideal. It can cause cerebral vasodilation and increased ICP.

6 Interaction between desflurane and dehydrated CO_2 absorbers can result in significant carbon monoxide formation.

7 Desflurane can cause malignant hyperthermia.

8 Desflurane has very occasionally been associated with liver injury through trifluoroacetate formation.

9 Atmospheric pollutant. One tonne of desflurane is equivalent to 3714 tonnes of CO_2.[3] This is about 5–20 times more than sevoflurane, which is also considered environmentally hostile. Desflurane remains in the atmosphere for 14 years, whereas sevoflurane remains for 1.1 years. The environmental unsuitability of desflurane will see it disappear from anaesthetic practice.[4]

◖ Desmopressin (DDAVP)

Description

A synthetic analogue of vasopressin that is useful for:

1 treating von Willebrand disease (VWD) by increasing levels of von Willebrand factor (VWF). **See Von Willebrand disease (VWD)**

2 treating diabetes insipidus

3 increasing FVIII levels in mild haemophilia A, by increasing levels of VWF, which acts as a transport protein for FVIII. Unbound FVIII is broken down much faster than bound FVIII

4 improving platelet function in illnesses associated with platelet impairment such as renal failure
5 reducing the effect of antiplatelet drugs if bleeding is occurring
6 treating nocturnal enuresis.

Dose for improving platelet/clotting function

1 0.3 mcg/kg/12 h IV (maximum 20 mcg). Give diluted in 50 mL N/S over 30 min. This drug may cause vasodilation and hypotension.
2 DDAVP can also be given intranasally. Each spray is 150 mcg. The usual adult dose is 2 sprays q 12 h.

◐ DETECT

Description

This is an acronym used in detecting, and responding to, a deteriorating patient. The letters stand for:

D – **D**etect deterioration—use the ABCDEFG tool. *See ABCDEFG (A–G) assessment*.

E – **E**valuate your findings—look for early and late warning signs of deterioration; look for trends and consider the diagnosis and co-morbidities.

T – **T**reatment—provide initial treatment e.g. increase IV fluids, provide supplementary O_2, change patient's position. Use existing clinical pathways e.g. sepsis pathway.

E – **E**scalate your concerns (e.g. clinical review or rapid response). **Get help**.

C – **C**ommunicate—use ISBAR. *See ISBAR*. Use team strategies—utilise the team's knowledge and experience. Document your findings and formulate a treatment and review plan. Document expected outcomes and what to do if outcomes are not met.

T – **T**eams—provide leadership for the team. Ensure the team functions effectively. Assign roles for each team member and ensure effective team communication. Identify and communicate with other teams or individuals that are, or should be, involved.

◐ Dexamethasone

Description

Dexamethasone is a corticosteroid drug with many uses. These include:
1 preventing postoperative nausea and vomiting
2 acting as anti-inflammatory medication for many conditions such as arthritis and myocarditis
3 treating certain skin conditions
4 treating some cancers such as leukaemia, multiple myeloma and lymphoma
5 treating or preventing allergic reactions
6 treating some eye conditions (as eye drops)
7 treating some autoimmune disorders
8 reducing oedema associated with brain or spine tumours
9 treating raised intracranial pressure—*see Intracranial pressure (ICP) and treatment of raised ICP*
10 treating nausea and vomiting associated with chemotherapy
11 reducing swelling after dental/facial surgery
12 treating adrenal insufficiency
13 acting as an appetite stimulant in cancer patients

14 treating asthma

15 treating COVID-19 for patients requiring oxygen therapy of any type, including invasive ventilation. It reduces mortality in this group by one-third. *See COVID-19.*

16 dexamethasone (or betamethasone) can be used to accelerate fetal lung maturity when premature delivery is likely or necessary e.g. severe preeclampsia.

Dose for the prevention of PONV

Adult

4–8 mg IV.

Child

0.1–0.25 mg/kg maximum 8 mg.

It should be given at the beginning of surgery. There is no evidence of significant adverse effects such as hyperglycaemia in diabetics or delayed wound healing at these doses. Do not give dexamethasone IV to an awake patient. It can cause an unpleasant burning sensation in the lower pelvis through an unknown mechanism.

◯ Dexmedetomidine

Description

Dexmedetomidine is a highly selective alpha-2 adrenoreceptor agonist. It has 1600 × more affinity for the alpha-2 receptor compared to the alpha-1 receptor. It is useful for providing sedation and analgesia. It acts by decreasing noradrenaline (NA) release centrally and peripherally. This results in decreased sympathetic outflow from the CNS and decreases plasma NA levels.

Clinical use

Dexmedetomidine can be used for providing sedation in a wide range of clinical settings including:

1 the agitated patient in ICU

2 awake intubation, awake carotid endarterectomy and other procedures where patient cooperation is required.

It is also useful for minimising opioid analgesia requirements during GA and treating withdrawal syndromes such as from alcohol, benzodiazepines and opioids.

Dose for sedation/opioid sparing

Add 200 mcg (in 2 mL) to 48 mL of N/S (4 mcg/mL). Give an LD of 1 mcg/kg over 10 min, then an infusion of 0.2–0.7 mcg/kg/h. In a 70 kg patient, this equals a 17.5 mL LD and an infusion of 3.5–12 mL/h.

Advantages

1 Dexmedetomidine causes profound sedation without significant respiratory depression.

2 Despite deep sedation, patients are often able to cooperate.

3 It has anxiolytic, analgesic, amnesic and sympatholytic effects.

4 Dexmedetomidine 1 mcg/kg before skin incision may reduce PONV and pain in the first 24 h after laparoscopic surgery.

5 It potentiates all anaesthetic agents.

6 It decreases the haemodynamic stress response to intubation.

Disadvantages

1 Dexmedetomidine causes a dry mouth. This is unpleasant for the patient but may help with awake intubation.
2 It may cause hypertension (especially if given rapidly), followed by hypotension and bradycardia. This is why the drug **cannot be bolused**—it must be given by infusion.
3 The long infusion time is undesirable in time-pressured situations.
4 The infusion should not exceed 24 h. Longer-term use can result in a withdrawal syndrome of anxiety, agitation, headaches and hypertension.
5 Dose reductions may be required for patients with renal impairment.

◑ Dextropropoxyphene

Description

Dextropropoxyphene is a weak oral opioid analgesic drug, used to treat:
1 mild to moderate pain
2 restless legs syndrome
3 opioid withdrawal symptoms
4 cough (acts as a cough suppressant).
   Dextropropoxyphene has been removed from sale in the US and Europe due to concerns over addiction, fatal overdoses and heart arrhythmias. Di-Gesic is a combination of dextropropoxyphene 32.5 mg and paracetamol 325 mg.

Di-Gesic dose

Adult

Two tablets up to every 4 h; max 12 tablets per day. The maximum daily dose must not be exceeded as even a small overdose may be fatal.

Contraindications

1 Long QT syndrome. Dextropropoxyphene increases the QT interval.
2 May cause sudden death if combined with alcohol or other CNS depressants.
3 Must not be used in patients with depression or suicidal ideation.
4 Renal impairment/failure.
5 Elderly patient.

◑ Diabetes mellitus (DM)

Introduction

Diabetes mellitus is a chronic metabolic illness that is frequently encountered by anaesthetists. It is characterised by elevated blood glucose levels (NR: 3.9–6.2 mmol/L). In type 2 DM, the body becomes resistant to insulin and/or does not make enough insulin. In type 1 DM, the pancreas produces little or no insulin due to the destruction of islet cells. DM can cause severe damage to blood vessels, nerves and organ systems, resulting in many potential complications, including:
1 blindness
2 kidney failure
3 coronary artery disease/acute coronary syndrome
4 cerebrovascular disease/CVA
5 peripheral vascular disease/amputation

QUICK FLICK

D

6 peripheral neuropathy

7 autonomic neuropathy.

Type 2 DM drugs

About 95% of diabetics are type 2. The condition is strongly associated with obesity and decreased physical activity. The many types of drugs that are used to treat type 2 diabetes include the following:

1 **Biguanides**—metformin (Glucophage) is the only drug in this group. Its mechanism of action is not well understood. It is often used as a first-line drug in people who are overweight, as it causes weight loss.

2 **Dipeptidyl peptidase-4 (DPP-4) inhibitors**—these are the gliptin drugs, including alogliptin, linagliptin and saxagliptin.

3 **Glucagon-like peptide-1 (GLP-1) receptor agonists**—these drugs mimic the action of incretin hormone GLP-1 (increase insulin secretion for pancreatic beta cells, decrease glucagon secretion from pancreatic alpha cells and decrease gastric emptying and appetite). Examples include exenatide (Byetta), liraglutide (Victoza), dulaglutide (Trulicity) and semaglutide (Ozempic). These drugs are injected subcutaneously, varying from twice daily for exenatide to weekly for dulaglutide and semaglutide.

4 **Peroxisome proliferator-activated receptor (PPAR) gamma receptor agonists**— these drugs act by decreasing blood glucose levels in patients with insulin resistance and they also decrease hyperlipidaemia. An example is pioglitazone which is a thiazolidinedione. These drugs increase insulin sensitivity in the tissues, thus reducing insulin resistance.

5 **Sodium-glucose co-transporter-2 (SGLT2) inhibitors**—these are 'flozin' drugs and include:

a) canagliflozin

b) dapagliflozin (Forxiga)

c) empagliflozin (Jardiance)

d) ertugliflozin (Steglatro).

They may be combined with other oral hypoglycaemic drugs such as metformin. These combinations include:

• Jardiamet (empagliflozin and metformin)

• Glyxambi (empagliflozin and linagliptin)

• Xigduo (dapagliflozin and metformin)

• Qtern (dapagliflozin and saxagliptin)

• Segluromet (ertugliflozin and metformin).

These drugs help patients to lose weight and reduce cardiovascular risk factors.

6 **Sulfonylureas**—stimulate insulin release from the beta cells in the pancreas. They act by blocking ATP-sensitive potassium channels, reducing potassium permeability. This causes depolarisation of the beta cells and increases calcium entry, thus increasing insulin release. Examples include gliclazide, glimepiride, glipizide and tolbutamide.

7 **Insulin**—30% or more type 2 DM patients will eventually require insulin.

Type 2 DM and anaesthesia

1 All oral drugs should be omitted on the day of surgery.

2 Omit all drugs on the day before surgery if on clear fluids and bowel preparation for colonoscopy.

3 If renal impairment and intra-arterial contrast will be used, withhold metformin 24 h before surgery and for 48 h after surgery, due to the risk of lactic acidosis. In some countries, metformin is withheld for 24–48 h before all surgery.

4 Omit GLP-1 agonists if due on the day of surgery.

5 Patients on SGLT2 inhibitors should cease these drugs for 2 days before non-day case surgery or if bowel preparation is required for colonoscopy. See below for more details.

6 If a patient with type 2 DM is on insulin and is a morning case, omit the morning insulin dose and consider an insulin/glucose infusion, depending on blood glucose measurements on arrival at the hospital.

7 If a patient with type 2 DM is on insulin and is an afternoon case, they should have their usual nocte dose of insulin and an early light breakfast. On the morning of surgery:
- If on mane rapid- or short-acting insulin—50% of their usual dose.
- If on mane long- or intermediate-acting insulin—75% of their usual dose.
- If on premixed insulin—50% of their usual dose.

For a description of the types of insulin see below.

Glucagon-like peptide-1 (GLP-1) receptor agonists and anaesthesia

Elective surgery guidelines

1 For elective surgery patients on daily dosing, withhold these drugs on the day of surgery.

2 For patients on weekly dosing, withhold these drugs for 1 week before surgery.

3 For patients who have not ceased these drugs and who do not have GIT symptoms (nausea, vomiting, abdominal bloating or abdominal pain), proceed with 'full stomach' precautions. A gastric ultrasound may help to confirm whether or not the stomach is empty.

4 For patients who have not ceased these drugs and who have GIT symptoms, consider rescheduling surgery to a later date with cessation of the drug.

Emergency surgery guidelines

Treat the patient as a 'full stomach' risk.[5]

SGLT2 inhibitor euglycaemic ketoacidosis

In this condition, diabetic ketoacidosis can develop despite BSL not being particularly elevated (8–15 mmol/L). This condition can be fatal. It may develop several days after surgery. Causes include:

1 fasting

2 sepsis

3 any major intercurrent illness

4 stress

5 major surgery.

Prevention

Exact guidelines vary between hospitals and are thus not uniform. A basic guide to this issue is:

1 For day procedures not requiring bowel preparation, cease the SGLT2 inhibitor drug **on the day of surgery only.**[6]

2 For surgery requiring 1 or more days in hospital **or** bowel preparation for colonoscopy, cease SGLT2 inhibitor drug for the 2 days before surgery and the day of surgery. Monitor ketones pre- and postoperatively.

3 For patients having combination therapy (SGLT2 inhibitor and metformin or DPP-4 drug) **and** surgery requiring more than 1 day in hospital **or** bowel preparation, continue metformin or DPP-4 drug until the day of surgery. For example, if the patient is on Glyxambi, continue linagliptin for the 2 days prior to surgery.

4 If surgery is prolonged (> 2 h), commence an insulin/glucose infusion preoperatively.

5 For bariatric surgery, consider stopping SGLT2 therapy for longer than 3 days due to the higher risk of ketoacidosis.

6 Check blood ketones on **all** patients who have been on SGLT2 inhibitors. If the patient is clinically well and blood ketones < 1.0 mmol/L, proceed with surgery. Consider hourly BSL and blood ketones during the procedure and 2 h after the procedure until patient is eating and drinking.

7 If patient has been on SGLT2 inhibitor drug **and** is unwell **and** blood ketones > 1.0 mmol/L, measure base excess (BE). If BE < –5 mmol/L, presume diabetic ketoacidosis (DKA). If BSL < 14 mmol/L, presume euglycaemic diabetic ketoacidosis. Cancel elective surgery and seek urgent endocrinologist review.

Patient who has not ceased SGLT2 inhibitor drug (elective surgery)

1 If the patient is well, blood ketones < 1 mmol/L and BE > –5 mmol/L, proceed with day surgery. If more extensive surgery is required (requiring overnight stay or longer), discuss the issue with the endocrinology team **and consider** cancelling surgery. A perioperative insulin glucose infusion may decrease the risk of DKA. If Hb A1c > 9% and blood ketones > 0.6 mmol/L, the patient may be at a higher risk of DKA.[6]

2 If patient is well, blood ketones > 1 mmol/L and BE > –5 mmol/L, there is ketosis without acidosis. This may reflect starvation. Consider proceeding with surgery and perioperative insulin glucose infusion, to decrease the risk of DKA.

3 If the patient is well, blood ketones > 1 mmol/L and BE < –5 mmol/L, carefully consider cancelling non-urgent surgery. Consult with the endocrinology team.

4 Indications of an **unwell** patient are:
a) drowsiness
b) abdominal pain
c) nausea/vomiting
d) fatigue
e) unexplained deterioration.

When to restart SGLT2 inhibitor drug
Restart the drug when the patient is eating and drinking normally.

Insulin types used to treat Type 1 DM
Type 1 DM is treated with insulin. In general, rapid- or short-acting insulins are used 3 × per day with meals. Intermediate-acting insulins are used 2 × per day, and long-acting insulins once per day.

There are many different types of insulin. These can be categorised as:

1 **Rapid-acting insulin**—starts working after 2.5 min, peaks at 1–3 h and lasts about 5 h. Examples include insulin aspart (Fiasp, Novorapid), insulin lispro (Humalog) and insulin glulisine (Apidra).

2 **Short-acting insulin**—starts working after 30 min, peak effect in 2–5 h and lasts 6–8 h. Examples include neutral insulin (Actrapid) and Humulin R.

3 **Intermediate-acting insulin**—these insulins are cloudy and need to be mixed well. They include human isophane insulins (insulin mixed with protamine to slow absorption) e.g. Protaphane. Effects start after 60–90 min, peak at 4–12 h and last 16–24 h.

4 **Long-acting insulin**—Lantus, Toujeo (both glargine insulin). Injected once per day, lasts for 24 h. Levemir, another example, lasts for about 18 h and is injected once or twice daily.

5 **Mixed insulin**—these formulations combine either a rapid-acting or a short-acting insulin with an intermediate- or long-acting insulin. Available products are:
   a) Rapid-acting and intermediate-acting insulins—NovoMix 30, Humalog Mix 75/25 and Humalog Mix 50/50 (the numbers indicate the percentage of rapid-acting and intermediate-acting insulin in the mixture).
   b) Rapid-acting and long-acting—Ryzodeg.
   c) Short-acting and intermediate-acting—Mixtard 30/70, Mixtard 50/50 and Humulin 30/70.

Type 1 DM on morning list
1 Usual nocte insulin on the night before surgery.
2 No insulin on morning of surgery.
3 Commence an insulin glucose infusion preoperatively.

Type 1 DM on afternoon list
1 Usual nocte insulin on the night before surgery.
2 If on rapid- or short-acting insulin, have 50% of the usual dose mane.
3 If on intermediate- or long-acting insulin, have 75% of the usual dose mane.
4 If on premixed insulin, have 50% of the usual dose mane.
5 If on Levemir nocte, the patient must present to the hospital before 1100 hrs.
6 Start an insulin glucose infusion on arrival at the hospital.

Diabetes and Caesarean section (CS)

Type 2 DM/gestational DM
1 Omit metformin on the day of the procedure.
2 If on < 30 units insulin/day, omit insulin on the morning of CS.
3 If on insulin > 30 units/day, omit subcut insulin on the morning of CS and commence an insulin glucose infusion at 0600 hrs. Aim to keep BSL between 4–7 mmol/L.
4 Post CS, cease the insulin glucose infusion and assess the patient's blood sugar control.

Type 1 DM
1 If on an insulin pump, discontinue the pump and start an insulin glucose infusion at 0600 hrs. Post CS, recommence insulin pump at a basal rate.
2 For patients not on an insulin pump, omit the usual morning dose of subcut insulin and commence an insulin glucose infusion. Keep BSL between 4–7 mmol/L.
3 Post CS, recommence diet and usual insulin regime.

Insulin pumps
These are set to a basal rate and a meal-time bolus using short-acting insulin. Some pumps have an in-built interstitial glucose measuring system. If the pump stops working, there is a risk of developing hyperglycaemia and ketoacidosis over the next 4 h.
1 For emergency surgery, cease the insulin pump and commence an insulin glucose infusion.
2 Involvement of the endocrine team is invaluable in advising whether to cease or continue the insulin pump.
3 For short day-only procedures, the pump can probably continue.
4 For major surgery, the pump should be ceased and the patient converted to an insulin glucose infusion.

Blood glucose target

Maintain BSL at 6–10 mmol/L.

Insulin glucose infusion

1 Mix 50 units of Actrapid with 50 mL of N/S.
2 Prepare a 1000 mL bag of glucose 5%. Use 500 mL of glucose 10% if concerns about hypervolaemia e.g. renal failure.
3 Run the infusion as per local protocols for a sliding scale. These are usually very complex and will not be reproduced here.

◑ Diabetic ketoacidosis (DKA)

Description

This is a metabolic emergency. It usually occurs in patients with type 1 diabetes but can (although rarely) occur in type 2 diabetics. Due to lack of insulin, glucose is unable to enter cells. In response, the liver breaks down fat to form ketones for fuel. Ketones are acidic and result in a metabolic acidosis. Patients are typically young and slim. Expert urgent endocrinologist involvement is essential.

Pathophysiology

1 Insulin deficiency results in glucose being unable to enter cells for their metabolic needs.
2 This leads to an increased secretion of glucagon, catecholamines and cortisol.
3 These hormones mobilise fat stores which the liver uses to manufacture ketones.
4 These ketones can be used for fuel by cells but also cause metabolic acidosis. Blood ketone levels can be classified as:
   a) < 0.6 mmol/L—normal
   b) 0.6–1.5 mmol/L—increased risk of DKA
   c) 1.5–3 mmol/L—mild ketosis
   d) > 3 mmol/L—moderate/severe ketosis.
5 The hyperglycaemia and ketosis cause osmotic diuresis, leading to dehydration and electrolyte disturbances.
6 pH and bicarbonate levels indicate the severity of the ketoacidosis:
   a) Mild—pH 7.25–7.3, bicarb 15–18 mmol/L
   b) Moderate—pH 7.0–7.24, bicarb 10–14.9 mmol/L
   c) Severe—pH < 7.0, bicarb < 10 mmol/L.

Clinical effects

1 Severe thirst.
2 Diuresis due to renal excretion of glucose and ketones.
3 Dyspnoea.
4 Hyperventilation due to metabolic acidosis.
5 Headache, confusion.
6 Abdominal pain.
7 Nausea and vomiting.
8 Fatigue.
9 Ketone odour on breath.
10 Muscle stiffness and aches.

Causes

1 New-onset type 1 DM.
2 Inadequate insulin treatment.

3 Intercurrent illness e.g. acute coronary syndrome, CVA.
4 Trauma.
5 Alcohol/drug use.

Diagnosis

1 BSL elevated to at least 14 mmol/L.
2 Elevated anion gap metabolic acidosis—pH 7.3 or less, bicarbonate < 15 mmol/L.
3 Hypocapnia.
4 Elevated urinary and blood ketones.
5 Plasma sodium may be normal or decreased.
6 Serum potassium is usually normal despite profound losses of potassium. Patients will also be deficient in phosphate, magnesium and calcium. As treatment is provided, serum K^+ will fall due to K^+ entering the cells as acidosis is corrected.

Treatment

The priorities are to:
1 expand extracellular volume and stabilise the patient's haemodynamic state
2 correct K^+ deficiency and other electrolyte abnormalities
3 correct hyperglycaemia with insulin therapy.

Steps in the treatment of DKA include:
1 Rehydrate the patient. **This is the priority.** Total fluid deficit may be > 7 L.[6] Administer 0.9% saline 15–20 mL/kg (≥ 1 L) per h. If the patient is hypernatraemic, administer 0.45% saline for subsequent fluids.[7] Otherwise, continue with 0.9% saline.
2 Replace K^+ once urine output is established.
   a) If serum K^+ < 3.3 mmol/L, **withhold insulin**. This is because insulin will cause K^+ levels to fall by driving it into cells, which may result in arrhythmias. Give K^+ 20–40 mmol/h until K^+ > 3.3 mmol/L.
   b) Give 20–30 mmoL K^+ per L of 0.9% saline to keep K^+ between 4–5 mmol/L.
   c) If serum K^+ ≥ 5 mmol/L, do not add K^+ to 0.9% saline until K^+ < 5 mmol/L. Check serum K^+ levels every 2 h.
3 Commence insulin infusion (Actrapid). Start at 0.1 U/kg/h. Aim for a fall in BSL by 3–4 mmol/L/h. Keep doubling the insulin rate until this is achieved.
4 When BSL ≤ 14 mmol/L, start 5% glucose 80 mL/h. Follow local protocols.
5 Treat acidosis if pH < 7.0 after 1 h of rehydration. Administer bicarbonate 50 mL 8.4% in 50 mL sterile H_2O, infused over 1–2 h. Repeat dose until pH > 7.0. The use of bicarbonate is controversial and without consensus.[8]
6 Replace other electrolytes as guided by serial measurements.
7 Continue insulin glucose infusion until:
   a) ketonuria has resolved
   b) patient able to eat and drink
   c) pH > 7.3
   d) bicarbonate ≥ 18 mmol/L
   e) BSL < 11 mmol/L.
8 Commence/recommence subcut insulin therapy.
9 Treat the cause of DKA if known e.g. infection.

▶ Diacetylmorphine/diamorphine/heroin

Description

This is a synthetic diacetylated derivative of morphine. It is 1.5–2 × more potent than morphine. Heroin is a prodrug which acts through its metabolites 6 mono acetyl morphine (6MAM).

Dose

Adult

Analgesia—5–7.5 mg IM, IV boluses 2.5 mg titrated to effect up to 10 mg.

Epidural—2.5 mg.

Intrathecal—there is little consensus regarding optimal dose. 500–600 mcg is recommended by anaesthetists that use diamorphine in the UK.[q]

Advantages

1 Faster onset of action than morphine due to its higher lipid solubility.
2 Possibly less nausea and vomiting than morphine.

Disadvantages

1 Produces marked euphoria—highly addictive.
2 Banned in the USA due to the addiction potential, but used widely in the UK.

▶ Diastolic dysfunction grading

Left ventricular (LV) diastolic function is assessed by echocardiography. Diastolic dysfunction of the LV is due to impaired LV relaxation with increased LV stiffness and elevated filling pressures. It can occur when patients have a reduced ejection fraction or structural heart disease.

Grade I—decreased suction effect of the LV. Normal LV relaxation creates a suction effect. Grade I diastolic dysfunction is commonly seen in older adults.

Grade II—increased stiffness of the LV with elevated left atrial pressure (LAP). There may be LA enlargement.

Grade III—high LAP, non-compliant LV. May be reversible with reduction in preload (e.g. Valsalva manoeuvre). Also known as reversible restrictive diastolic dysfunction.

Grade IV—irreversible restricted LV filling. This leads to reduced LVEF. Also known as a 'fixed restrictive pattern'. It is only present in advanced heart failure and frequently associated with restrictive cardiomyopathies such as infiltrative cardiac amyloidosis.

▶ Diazepam

Description

Long-acting benzodiazepine drug used for:
1 sedation
2 anxiolysis
3 amnesia
4 muscle relaxation
5 status epilepticus. **See *Status epilepticus (SE)***
6 alcohol withdrawal.

Dose

1 Status epilepticus—*Adult:* 5–10 mg IV, may require up to 20–30 mg. *Child:* give 0.2 mg/kg/dose IV or 0.5 mg PR.

2 Sedation/anxiety—*Adult:* 2–60 mg/day in divided doses PO. *Child:* 0.2–0.5 mg/kg/dose PO q 8–12 h.

◗ Diazoxide (Proglycem, Balila)

Description

Non-diuretic benzothiadiazine antihypertensive drug that is useful for treating hypertensive emergencies. Diazoxide acts directly on arteriolar smooth muscle, causing relaxation. It can also be used to treat intractable hypoglycaemia by decreasing insulin secretion and inhibiting the peripheral utilisation of glucose.

Dose for hypertensive emergencies

Adult

Give bolus doses of 75–150 mg every 5–10 min up to 300 mg in 1 hour. Alternatively, give as an IV infusion of 15 mg/min to a maximum dose of 5 mg/kg.[10]

◗ Diclofenac (Voltaren)

Description

NSAID drug used to treat postoperative and arthritic pain. Non-selective COX inhibitor. *See **Non-steroidal anti-inflammatory drugs (NSAIDs)**.*

Dose

Adult

25–50 mg PO q 8 h with food.

Child

1 mg/kg (max 50 mg) PO q 8 h with food.

Note: Diclofenac has been associated with liver toxicity and, rarely, acute haemolytic anaemia.

◗ Difficult airway management

Introduction

This is a vast topic that is fundamental to anaesthetic practice, and it is challenging to encapsulate in a small manual. The difficult airway can be defined as the clinical situation where a trained anaesthetist has difficulty with mask ventilation or tracheal intubation or both. The worst type of difficult airway leads to the 'can't intubate, can't oxygenate' (CICO) crisis scenario. The difficult airway may be anticipated or unanticipated.

Anticipated difficult airway

Factors that may help predict a difficult airway in the adult include the following:

1 Previous anaesthetic history of a difficult airway and/or clues such as dental damage from intubation.

2 Mouth-opening ability. Less than 3 cm is particularly concerning.

3 Prominent teeth.

4 Mallampati score (modified). ***See Mallampati score (modified).***

5 Small, receding jaw.

6 Thyromental distance (distance between the thyroid notch and the lower border of the chin with the head extended). Less than 6.5 cm is concerning.

7 Inability to extend the head on the neck.

8 Obesity/history of OSA.

9 Short, fat neck.

10 Poor prognathic ability.

11 Numerous diseases affecting the neck such as ankylosing spondylitis.

12 Airway pathology e.g. dental abscess.

13 Pre-procedure nasal endoscopy suggesting difficult intubation.

14 Results of radiological/MRI assessment of the airway.

Management of the anticipated difficult airway

1 Consider alternatives to intubation e.g. neuraxial block, regional anaesthesia, sedation.

2 Assess the ease or otherwise of front of neck access (FONA).

3 Have a plan and discuss it with anaesthetic staff. Have back-up plans and prepare for failure. Ensure correct equipment is present (such as bougies, CICO kit).

4 Consider having a second anaesthetist present.

5 Optimise patient positioning—semi-recumbent, neck flexed and head extended (sniffing position).

6 Effective pre-oxygenation. *See Rapid sequence induction (RSI)*. Aim for end tidal expired $O_2 >$ 90%.

7 Consider awake video-endoscopic intubation. *See Awake intubation.*

8 Use a videolaryngoscope (McGrath, C-MAC, King Vision or other). A pre-curved steerable intubating guide (STIG) is an ideal bougie to use with the C-MAC. It has a steerable tip.

9 Awake tracheostomy may be the best option in certain circumstances.

10 If intubation is unsuccessful and the patient can be oxygenated, consider abandoning the procedure and waking the patient up.

11 See the Vortex implementation tool in Figure D2.

Management of the unanticipated difficult airway

This situation can occur electively or in a time-pressured emergency situation. The best approach (in the author's opinion) is to use the Vortex implementation tool, developed by Dr Nicholas Chrimes and Dr Peter Fritz. This is a simple three-dimensional implementation tool—only four things need to be remembered:

1 Have your best two or three attempts at intubation, preferably including the use of a videolaryngoscope.

2 Have your best two or three attempts at bag-mask ventilation—Guedel airway, nasal airway, two-person bag-mask ventilation.

3 Have your two or three best attempts at inserting a supraglottic airway (e.g. classic LMA, Ambu-type airway, i-gel).

4 If all these techniques fail to oxygenate the patient (CICO), move on to a surgical airway (FONA).

The Vortex implementation tool stresses the importance of not becoming fixated on any one technique. The operator must move on to the next technique after 2–3 attempts of the previous technique. Each technique can be thought of as a 'lifeline', and after three have been used, move on to FONA.

The Vortex implementation tool is a visual and three-dimensional (Figure D2). It is shaped like a funnel, with the green zone at the top representing oxygenation and the blue zone representing deoxygenation. The blue zone spirals down towards an emergency surgical airway.

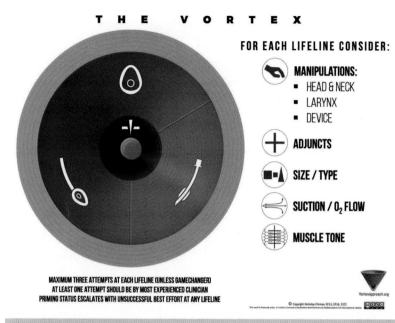

Figure D2 The Vortex Approach
Source: Copyright Nicholas Chrimes. Used with permission.

Emergency surgical airway

Figure D3 shows an algorithm for an emergency surgical airway.

Cannula cricothyrotomy/tracheotomy

The initial strategy is cannula cricothyrotomy. The steps are:

1. Obtain a 14 G Insyte cannula, 5 mL syringe, 2 mL of N/S, a Rapid-O₂™ insufflation device and a source of oxygen (cylinder or piped).
2. Extend the patient's head and neck.
3. Quickly wipe the skin with antiseptic solution if immediately available.
4. Attach the syringe containing 2 mL of N/S to the cannula hub.
5. Fix the larynx with the non-dominant hand and stab the 14 G cannula in a caudad direction through the cricothyroid membrane or trachea.
6. Aspirate air then insert cannula to the hub.
7. Again, make sure air can be aspirated from the cannula. Do not let go of the cannula.
8. Attach the Rapid-O₂™ insufflation device to the cannula hub and the O_2 source.
9. Turn the O_2 supply flowmeter to 15 L.
10. Occlude the Rapid-O₂™ insufflation device large yellow orifice with your thumb for 4 s—this will supply the patient with 1000 mL of O_2.
11. Allow time for the patient's O_2 saturation to rise to a satisfactory level (> 90%).
12. When the O_2 saturation falls by 5%, give a 2 s 'burst' (500 mL) of O_2. Repeat as needed.
13. If successful, consider your next step—this could be to wake the patient up or the conversion of the cannula to a definitive airway (see next page).
14. If this manoeuvre fails after three attempts or after 1 min and airway anatomy is palpable, go to the 'scalpel bougie' technique (see next page).

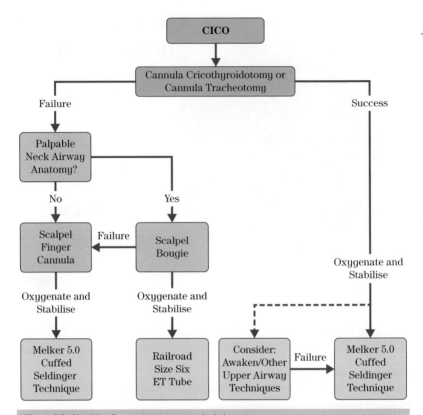

Figure D3 Algorithm for an emergency surgical airway.
Reproduced with permission from Heard AM, Green RJ, Eakins P. The formulation and introduction of a 'can't intubate, can't ventilate' algorithm into clinical practice. Anaesthesia. 2009;64(6):601-608.

Scalpel bougie technique

1 Obtain a Frova bougie, a size 6.0 ET tube and a size 10 scalpel blade and handle.
2 Stabilise the larynx with the non-dominant hand and stab the scalpel (blade edge towards yourself) through the cricothyroid membrane.
3 Twist the scalpel blade through 90° so the blade edge faces the patient's feet. Hold the scalpel handle vertically and pull it towards yourself, making a triangular-shaped incision.
4 Insert the tip of the Frova bougie into the trachea through the incision, with its distal end pointing away from you.
5 Pass the Frova bougie into the trachea while rotating the distal end towards the patient's head. Railroad the lubricated ET tube over the Frova using a rotational/ twisting action.
6 If this fails or airway anatomy is not palpable, go to the 'scalpel finger cannula' technique (see below).

Scalpel finger cannula technique

1 Using a scalpel, make a midline incision of 8–10 cm over the presumed position of the airway to the depth of the strap muscles.
2 Using fingers, separate the tissues until the airway is located.

3 Use the same technique as described for the cannula cricothyrotomy/tracheotomy technique above to oxygenate the patient.

4 If the cannula is unsuccessful, use a scalpel bougie technique.

5 If the cannula is successful, use the cannula to insert a Melker airway, using the technique described below.

Melker airway insertion

1 Insert a cannula into the airway as described above.

2 Pass the guidewire from the Melker kit through the cannula into the airway and remove the cannula. Make sure the guidewire moves freely in and out of the airway.

3 Use the scalpel blade tip to make a stab incision into the airway that includes the guidewire. Make sure the guidewire moves freely in the stab incision. Not including the wire in the incision is a common error.

4 Pass the cuffed size 5.0 mm tracheostomy tube pre-mounted on the dilator over the wire and insert both into the airway with a bidirectional rotational movement. Hold the dilator and tracheostomy tube assembly tightly so that they do not separate during insertion.

5 Remove the dilator and wire, inflate the cuff and ventilate the patient.

◗ Di-Gesic

This drug is a combination of dextropropoxyphene and paracetamol. *See Dextropropoxyphene.*

◗ Digibind

See Digoxin.

◗ Digital nerve block

Digital nerve block is useful for anaesthesia/analgesia for finger or toe surgery.

The digits are supplied by 4 digital nerves, 2 palmar/planter and 2 dorsal. The aim is to block the digital nerves on both sides of the base of the proximal phalanx.

Technique

1 Using a sterile technique, insert a 25G needle through the skin, from dorsal to palmer/planter, as close to the bone of the proximal phalanx as possible, almost transfixing the digit.

2 As the needle is withdrawn inject 2 mL of 2% lignocaine.

3 Repeat these steps on each side of the bone.

DO NOT USE ADRENALINE CONTAINING SOLUTIONS.

◗ Digoxin

Description

Digoxin binds to, and inhibits, the Na^+/K^+ ATP-ase enzyme, thus impeding the function of the Na^+/K^+ exchange pumps of the cardiac myocytes. This leads to a build-up of Na^+ in the myocytes, which is greater than can be compensated for by the Na^+/Ca^{2+} exchange pumps. Therefore, Ca^{2+} levels rise in the myocytes with a positive inotropic effect. Digoxin also decreases intracellular K^+ in the heart cells, causing a slowing of atrioventricular conduction and depolarisation of pacemaker cells. In addition, digoxin increases vagal activity.

Dose—adult

1 For atrial fibrillation and atrial flutter, **see Atrial fibrillation (AF)** and **Atrial flutter**.
2 Heart failure—250 mcg PO daily up to 250 mcg q 12 h. Measure the trough level 8 h after last dose (therapeutic range 0.5–0.9 ng/mL).

Digoxin toxicity

Digoxin has a narrow therapeutic index, and digoxin toxicity can easily occur. This can result in visual disturbances, nausea and vomiting and cardiac arrhythmias, which can be fatal. Hyperkalaemia is frequently seen with toxicity. Toxicity can also develop when the digoxin is in the therapeutic range due to:

1 hypokalaemia, hypomagnesaemia, hypercalcaemia
2 myocardial ischaemia
3 hypoxia
4 acid-base disturbances.

Treatment

1 Cease digoxin.
2 Administer IV Digibind. This contains digoxin-specific antibody Fab fragments. This drug binds to digoxin and stops it from binding to Na^+/K^+ ATP-ase enzyme. It also creates a concentration gradient so that digoxin is drawn out of the intracellular space. Dosing is very complicated and depends on how life-threatening the situation is. Each vial contains 38 mg of Digibind. Recommended doses for adults are:
   a) acute overdose—20 vials over 30 min, faster if cardiac arrest imminent or has occurred
   b) toxicity during chronic therapy—6 vials.

◖ Dilated cardiomyopathy (DCM)

Description

DCM is a major cause of heart failure and dysrhythmias in young adults, and may require heart transplant. There is mainly systolic dysfunction, with progressive enlargement of the ventricles. This leads to inefficient contraction, increased wall stress and myocardial oxygen demand and further systolic dysfunction in a vicious circle. There may be dilation of the atrioventricular rings with valvular regurgitation. The heart is 'weak and floppy'.

Causes

1 Idiopathic.
2 Post viral.
3 Part of another disorder e.g. IHD, alcoholism, neuromuscular disorder, hypothyroidism or pregnancy.
4 Inherited—familial dilated cardiomyopathy.
5 Exposure to certain drugs such as chemotherapy.

Clinical effects

As with heart failure from any cause, the following may be seen:

1 tachycardia, dysrhythmias
2 SOB, orthopnoea
3 decreased exercise tolerance, fatigue
4 pulmonary oedema, ascites, peripheral oedema, raised JVP
5 mitral regurgitation murmur
6 embolic events
7 sudden death.

Diagnosis

1 Clinical history.
2 CXR.
3 Echocardiography.

Treatment

Drugs commonly used to treat DCM are:
1 ACE inhibitors or angiotensin II receptor inhibitors
2 beta blockers
3 aldosterone inhibitors e.g. spironolactone
4 anticoagulants.

Surgical options are ventricular synchronisation therapy and transplant. DCM is a leading indication for heart transplant in young adults.[11]

Pre-anaesthetic preparation

These patients are at high risk of perioperative death or significant morbidity. A LVEF < 20% is predictive of a poor outcome.[11] LV hypokinesis and non-sustained VT are also highly concerning.

1 Co-ordinate patient preparation with their cardiologist to optimise medical management.
2 Ensure electrolytes are normalised and anaemia corrected.
3 If an AICD is present, *see Pacemakers.*

Induction and maintenance

Important aspects of management include:
1 Avoid myocardial depression and sudden hypotension.
2 Maintain adequate preload/normovolaemia.
3 Prevent increases in afterload, which will decrease CO and increase cardiac workload.
4 Avoid tachycardia.
5 Establish invasive arterial BP monitoring and a central line.
6 Induce anaesthesia carefully with low doses of propofol and a reasonable dose of fentanyl. Consider co-induction with sevoflurane. Avoid ketamine, which increases SVR.
7 Rocuronium is an appropriate muscle relaxant.
8 Sevoflurane is acceptable, but avoid high concentrations.
9 Transoesophageal echocardiography (TOE) provides a dynamic assessment of cardiac function intraoperatively.
10 Inotropic support may be required with agents such as phosphodiesterase inhibitors and dopamine.

See Congestive cardiac failure (CCF)—chronic and Cardiogenic shock.

❯ Dilaudid

Trade name for hydromorphone. *See Hydromorphone (Dilaudid, Jurnista).*

❯ Diltiazem

Description

A calcium channel blocker drug of the non-dihydropyridine type, like verapamil. *See Calcium channel blocker drugs.*

Indications

It is useful for treating:

1 arrhythmias such as paroxysmal supraventricular tachycardias
2 angina
3 hypertension.

Contraindications

1 Sick sinus syndrome. *See Sick sinus syndrome (SSS).*
2 Second or third degree heart block. *See Heart block (HB).*
3 Hypotension.
4 Severe heart failure.
5 Patients who have received dantrolene for malignant hyperthermia. Diltiazem or verapamil in this situation can worsen hyperkalaemia, myocardial depression and hypotension. *See Malignant hyperthermia (MH).*

Dose

30 mg PO q 8 h, increased gradually to a maximum of 360 mg/day. Optimum dose usually 180–240 mg/day.

◉ Diphenhydramine

Description

This antihistamine drug has many uses, including the treatment of motion sickness and allergy-related issues such as sneezing, itching and watery eyes. It is effective for treating acute dystonic reactions to dopamine-blocking drugs such as metoclopramide or prochlorperazine.

Dose

For dystonic reaction, give IV 1–2 mg/kg up to 100 mg. *See Dystonic reaction, acute.*

Note: Diphenhydramine reduces the tremor in Parkinson's disease, which is useful for awake surgery such as cataract operations.

◉ Direct laryngoscopy view grading

Grading of the view of the larynx by direct laryngoscopy provides information to subsequent anaesthetists regarding the ease or difficulty of intubation. In 1984, Cormack and Lehane originally suggested four grades, a system that has been progressively modified by Yentis and Lee[12] and Cook.[13]

Table D2 Modified Cormack and Lehane classification of the view obtained at laryngoscopy

Grade	View obtained
1	Most of vocal cords visible
2a	Posterior part of vocal cords visible
2b	Only arytenoids visible
3a	Epiglottis visible and liftable
3b	Epiglottis visible and adherent to pharynx
4	No laryngeal structures visible

◑ Disseminated intravascular coagulation (DIC)

Description

DIC is a maladaptive reaction caused by a disease process or injury manifesting with abnormalities of coagulation. It is due to procoagulants entering the blood stream and causing widespread clotting in small- and medium-sized blood vessels. This can cause organ ischaemia and damage, especially to the kidneys, lungs, brain and liver. As coagulation factors and platelets are consumed inappropriately, bleeding can occur. These procoagulants may be substances such as tissue factor, tissue thromboplastins or lipopolysaccharides from bacteria. As the clots break down, fibrin degradation products (FDPs) form. FDPs inhibit platelet aggregation and clot formation, making bleeding more likely.

DIC can develop acutely over hours to days or be more chronic (weeks to months). In acute DIC, clotting and haemorrhage predominate, whereas in chronic DIC, inappropriate clotting is the main issue.

Causes of acute DIC

1 Sepsis including severe COVID-19, malaria.
2 Complications of pregnancy e.g. preeclampsia, placental abruption, amniotic fluid embolus.
3 Fetal death in utero—**see Intrauterine fetal death**.
4 Major surgery.
5 Incompatible blood transfusion.
6 Massive blood loss.
7 Severe head injury.
8 Tissue damage due to burns, frostbite or major trauma.
9 Envenomation.
10 Anaphylaxis.
11 Pancreatitis.
12 Hypothermia.

Causes of chronic DIC

1 Certain types of cancer e.g. adenocarcinoma, acute promyelocytic leukaemia.
2 Aortic aneurysm.
3 Cavernous haemangiomas.

Clinical effects

The presence of DIC may be obscured by the causative disorder e.g. major trauma. DIC can have catastrophic effects on multiple organs. These include:

1 brain—confusion, decreased level of consciousness or loss of consciousness, seizures
2 lung—dyspnoea, hypoxia
3 fever
4 hypotension
5 bleeding, bruising, haematuria
6 jaundice.

Diagnosis

1 FBC—thrombocytopenia. In 50% of cases, platelet count < 50,000/mm³.
2 Deranged clotting studies—APPT, PT, INR.
3 Abnormal thromboelastographic studies. **See Thromboelastography/ thromboelastometry**.
4 Decreased fibrinogen levels (NR 1–3 g/L).

5 Elevated FDPs—NR < 10 mcg/mL. In DIC, levels may be > 40 mcg/mL.
6 Elevated D-dimer. D-dimer is a fibrin degradation product. Its normal level is < 0.5 mcg/mL.

Treatment

Treatment is complicated and difficult, and there are very few randomised trials to guide it. Seek expert haematologist advice. Suggested treatment strategies are:[14]

1 Treat/reverse the underlying disorder if possible e.g. antibiotics for infection.
2 Organ support e.g. ventilation to treat hypoxia, supporting blood pressure with inotropes.
3 Blood transfusion if Hb < 70 g/L.
4 If the patient is **not** bleeding, accept/maintain a platelet count > 10000/mm³.
5 If the patient is bleeding, treat coagulopathy and thrombocytopenia—platelet transfusions, FFP, cryoprecipitate (fibrinogen). Aim for platelets > 50000/mm³.
6 Pro-clotting drugs (tranexamic acid, prothrombin complex concentrates) may increase the risk of thrombotic complications.
7 If bleeding is not present and blood clotting is the most significant manifestation, consider heparin therapy.

◔ Dobutamine

Description

This drug is a sympathomimetic amine used as an inotropic agent to treat congestive heart failure. **See Congestive cardiac failure (CCF)—chronic** and **Cardiogenic shock**. Dobutamine stimulates beta-1 and -2 receptors, and also alpha-1 receptors (**see Adrenergic receptors**). It augments stroke volume and decreases peripheral vascular resistance. It is a potent inotrope and a weaker chronotrope.

Dose

Dobutamine is given by IV infusion. Mix 250 mg with 100 mL 5% glucose. Initial dose is 0.5–1 mcg/kg/min. In a 70 kg patient, this equals 0.8–1.6 mL/hr. Maintenance 2–20 mcg/kg/min (70 kg patient, 3.2–32 mL/h). The maximum dose is 40 mcg/kg/min. It can be given peripherally through a large-bore cannula. Titrate to heart rate and blood pressure.

Adverse effects

1 Increased risk of rapid ventricular response in patients with AF.
2 Hypotension may occur.
3 Can cause hypokalaemia.
4 Contraindicated in acute coronary syndrome, sulfite allergy, myocarditis, pericarditis and hypertrophic obstructive cardiomyopathy.

◔ Dolasetron (Anzemet)

Description

Long-acting single daily dose anti-emetic that acts through selective 5-HT₃ (serotonin) receptor antagonism.

Dose

Adult

Prevention of nausea/vomiting 12.5 mg IV over 30 s or 50 mg PO. Treatment of established nausea/vomiting 12.5 mg IV over 30 s.

Note: Dolasetron prolongs the QT interval and can increase the risk of developing torsades de pointes. **See *Torsades de pointes***. The FDA has issued a warning that IV dolasetron must not be used in adults or children to treat chemotherapy-induced nausea and vomiting.

Doloxene

This a trade name for dextropropoxyphene. **See *Dextropropoxyphene*.**

Domperidone (Motilium)

Description

Domperidone is a dopamine D2 receptor antagonist used to treat nausea and vomiting. It is also a prokinetic agent that is useful for treating delayed gastric emptying. Domperidone can also be used to initiate and promote breast milk production.

Dose

Adult

10 mg PO q 8 h as needed.

Advantages

1. Domperidone is useful for treating nausea and vomiting in patients with Parkinson's disease because minimal amounts cross the blood–brain barrier.
2. Can be used rectally.

Disadvantages

Contraindicated in patients taking drugs that prolong the QT interval such as amiodarone.

Dopamine (Intropin)

Description

Sympathomimetic catecholamine drug used to treat low cardiac output states, hypotension and shock. Dopamine acts on dopamine receptors (**see *Dopamine receptors***). It also acts on alpha and beta adrenergic receptors.

Dose

Mix 200 mg dopamine with 100 mL 5% glucose. Administer **only** via a central line.

Low-dose infusion: 0.5–3 mcg/kg/min—vasodilation in coronary, renal, mesenteric and cerebral vascular beds. Increases urine output.

Intermediate-dose infusion: 3–10 mcg/kg/min. Acts on beta-1 receptors, causing noradrenaline (NA) release and inhibition of reuptake. This leads to increased SVR. Increased myocardial contractility and increased electrical conductivity occurs, increasing heart rate.

High-dose infusion: 10–20 mcg/kg/min. Alpha-1 effects predominate—marked vasoconstriction and inotropic effects.

Precautions

Dopamine may cause:

1. tachycardia and tachydysrhythmias
2. depressed respiratory drive
3. increased intrapulmonary shunt.

◑ Dopamine receptors

Dopamine is a neurotransmitter and precursor to noradrenaline. Dopamine receptors are found in the CNS and many other parts of the body. Subtypes D1 and D5 are members of the D1-like family and D2, D3 and D4 are members of the D2-like family. All types are found in the brain. Additional sites are:

1 D1—smooth muscle in the proximal renal tubule and cortical collecting duct. Stimulation causes increased urine output. D1 receptors are also found in the pulmonary artery. Stimulation of these causes relaxation of pulmonary artery smooth muscle.
2 D2—pre-synaptic on renal nerves and within glomeruli and the adrenal cortex. Also found in the brain.
3 D3—possibly only found in the brain.
4 D4—the atria, pulmonary artery.
5 D5—pulmonary artery.

◑ Double inlet left ventricle (DILV)

In this form of congenital heart disease, both atria are connected to the left ventricle (LV), usually with a hypoplastic right ventricle (RV). The vestigial RV may be on the opposite side of the heart to normal. There is usually transposition of the great vessels, with the aorta connected to the vestigial RV and the pulmonary artery to the LV. The LV and RV must be connected by a ventricular septal defect, and this is a single-ventricle circulation. There are often other defects such as pulmonary atresia.

Treatment

1 Bidirectional Glenn shunt or hemi-Fontan procedure.
2 Fontan procedure.

◑ Double lumen tube

See *One-lung ventilation (OLV).*

◑ Double outlet right ventricle (DORV)

In this congenital condition, both the aorta and pulmonary artery arise from the right ventricle (RV). No arteries are connected to the left ventricle (LV). There is always a ventricular septal defect. Systemic venous blood enters the LV and passes to the RV, from where it enters both the pulmonary and systemic arterial system. This exposes the pulmonary circulation to high pressures.

Types of DORV

There are many different types of DORV with associated abnormalities. The most common types are:

1 DORV with subaortic VSD—similar to tetralogy of Fallot (ToF) but without pulmonary outflow obstruction. Repair involves placing a patch in the RV to direct LV flow towards the aorta.
2 Taussig–Bing anomaly—the VSD is sub-pulmonary. Blood from the LV is directed towards the pulmonary artery and RV blood is directed towards the aorta. This is a similar situation to transposition of the great vessels. Treatment can include an arterial switch operation with a patch in the RV. This directs flow to the artery adjacent to the VSD.

3 Doubly committed VSD—RV and LV blood flow is equally directed to the aorta and pulmonary artery.

4 Non-committed VSD—blood from RV and LV simply mixes and may go anywhere between the aorta and pulmonary artery. A Fontan procedure may be undertaken to palliate this abnormality.

◗ Down syndrome

Description

This condition is due to an extra copy of chromosome 21 (Down syndrome is also referred to as 'Trisomy 21'). 40–60% of Down syndrome individuals are born with cardiac abnormalities such as atrial and ventricular septal defects and tetralogy of Fallot. *See Tetralogy of Fallot (ToF)*. It is the most common chromosomal-related illness. Other types of Down syndrome are:

- Translocation Down syndrome—an extra chromosome 21 is present (or part of it is present) but is attached to a different chromosome (about 3% of Down syndrome cases).
- Mosaic Down syndrome—some cells have three chromosome 21 copies and some have two. The manifestation of Down syndrome type depends on the percentage of cells affected.

Clinical features

1 Flattened face, flattened nasal bridge and small ears.

2 Flattened occiput, microcephaly.

3 Almond-shaped eyes that slant upwards with prominent epicanthic folds.

4 Brushfield spots (light-coloured spots) near the periphery of the iris.

5 Short neck.

6 Large tongue.

7 Atlantoaxial instability (about 15–20%). Spinal cord compression may occur.[15,16]

8 A single line across the palm of the hand (Simian crease).

9 Poor muscle tone.

10 Loose joints.

11 Short stature.

12 Duodenal atresia.

13 IQ in the mild to moderately low range.

14 Hearing loss.

15 OSA.

16 Between 5% and 10% of people with Down syndrome have epilepsy.[15]

17 About 50% of patients are hypothyroid.

18 Increased incidence of respiratory tract infections.

19 Increased risk of gastro-oesophageal reflux.

20 Down syndrome is associated with acute lymphoblastic leukaemia.

Cause

The cause of Down syndrome is unknown but it is more common in pregnancy after age 35 years. Pregnancy at age 45 is associated with a 1:40 risk of Down syndrome.

Prenatal screening

1 Fetal ultrasound indicating the amount of fluid at the back of the fetal neck (nuchal translucency).
2 Chorionic villus sampling, amniocentesis and percutaneous umbilical blood sampling for genetic testing.
3 NIPT involves identifying and genetically testing fetal cells in the maternal bloodstream.

Anaesthesia

Pre-anaesthetic phase

1 Assess the patient carefully for any congenital heart disease such as atrial septal defect or patent ductus arteriosus. Unrepaired lesions may be associated with Eisenmenger syndrome. *See Eisenmenger syndrome/Eisenmenger complex.* Obtain an ECG and echocardiography if there are any concerns. Pulmonary vascular disease may be present.
2 There may be atlantoaxial subluxation as suggested by neurological symptoms or signs or limited head movement or neck pain. If this is suspected, consider a lateral cervical spine X-ray with flexion and extension views.

Anaesthetic phase

1 Airway management may be difficult due to a large tongue, subglottic stenosis and enlarged tonsils and adenoids. Use gentle head positioning in case atlantoaxial joint instability is present.
2 Intubation may be difficult and a smaller than expected ET tube may be required due to subglottic stenosis. Avoid extreme neck flexion/head extension. Use a videolaryngoscope.
3 There is an increased risk of infection in Down syndrome patients. Use strict asepsis and appropriate antibiotic prophylaxis. Also consider antibiotics for prevention of bacterial endocarditis in patients with structural heart disease.

Post-anaesthetic phase

Observe the patient closely for airway obstruction post GA due to OSA and hypotonia. Drugs that depress respiration, such as opioids, should be used cautiously.

⊙ Driving pressure

This is defined as plateau airway pressure minus peak end expiratory pressure (PEEP). *See Plateau pressure.* It is also the ratio of tidal volume to respiratory system compliance.

⊙ Droperidol

Droperidol is a butyrophenone-derivative drug that blocks dopamine 2 receptors. It also has post-synaptic GABA receptor and alpha adrenoreceptor blocker effects. It is useful for:

1 PONV prevention
2 treatment of emergence agitation in adults.

There is a risk of sudden cardiac death if used in doses of greater than 25 mg.

Dose

Adult

1 PONV prevention—0.625–1.25 mg IV given at the end of surgery.
2 Emergence agitation—4–8 mg IV.

Child
PONV prevention—10–20 mcg/kg IV.

Points to note
1 Causes prolongation of the QTc interval. At anti-emetic doses, this is similar to the effects of ondansetron. Do not use droperidol if the QTc interval is prolonged. **See Long QT syndrome (LQTS).**
2 Can cause a dystonic reaction as can occur with metoclopramide.
3 Causes dose-dependent sedation.
4 Can cause neuroleptic malignant syndrome.

◑ Durogesic

A trade name for transdermal fentanyl patches providing 12–100 mcg/h of fentanyl. **See Fentanyl.**

◑ Durotram-XR

A trade name for tramadol. **See Tramadol (Tramal).**

◑ Dutran

A trade name for fentanyl patches providing transdermal fentanyl. Available in 2 strengths—75 mcg/h and 100 mcg/h. **See Fentanyl.**

◑ Dynastat

See Parecoxib (Dynastat).

◑ Dysfibrinoginaemia

This is an inherited or acquired disorder that is characterised by having abnormal fibrinogen. This can lead to an increased or decreased ability to form clots. About 50% of people with the inherited disorder have an increased tendency to bleed, and 10% have a pro-thrombotic disorder or a combined bleeding and pro-thrombotic disorder. The acquired disorder is more common and is associated with liver disease such as cirrhosis and liver tumours.

◑ Dystonic reaction, acute

Description
This syndrome is due to an idiosyncratic reaction to drugs that block central dopamine 2 receptors in the basal ganglia. It is characterised by involuntary contractions of the muscles of the face, neck (torticollis), eyes (oculogyric crisis), extremities, larynx and other areas. Laryngeal dystonia can cause laryngospasm and pharyngeal muscle spasm with the potential for airway obstruction. Macroglossia may occur where the tongue protrudes and feels swollen but does not actually swell. There may also be trismus and blepharospasm.

Causative agents
- **Anti-emetics**—metoclopramide, prochlorperazine.
- **Antipsychotics**—haloperidol, droperidol, fluphenazine, clozapine, olanzapine.
- **Antidepressants**—SSRIs e.g. fluoxetine.
- **Antibiotics**—erythromycin.
- **Recreational**—cocaine.

Treatment

Adult

1 Benztropine 0.02 mg/kg IV to a maximum of 1 mg, followed by the same dose orally q 12 h for 2 days.
2 Diphenhydramine 1 mg/kg IV to a maximum of 50 mg.
3 Benzodiazepines in the doses described above.
4 Benzodiazepines (second-line therapy)—lorazepam 0.05–0.1 mg/kg IV or IM or diazepam 0.1 mg IV.

Child

Benztropine 0.02 mg/kg max 1 mg. Can be repeated once. Give the same dose orally bd for 2 days.

REFERENCES

1 South Eastern Sydney Local Health District. *SESLHDPR/600 Protocol for the Safe Use of Danaparoid.* Version 2, October 2021. Accessed online: https://www.seslhd.health.nsw.gov.au/sites/default/files/documents/SESLHDPR600.pdf, November 2023.
2 Shelton CL, Sutton R, White SM. Desflurane in modern anaesthetic practice: walking on thin ice(caps)? *Br J Anaesth* 2020; 125: 852–856.
3 Ryan SM, Claus J. Global warming potential of inhaled anaesthetics: application to clinical use. *Anaesth Analg* 2010; Jul; 111(1): 92–98. doi: 10.1213/ANE.0b013e3181e058d7. Accessed online: https://pubmed.ncbi.nlm.nih.gov/20519425/, August 2022.
4 Naggs T. Pick your poison. *Australian Anaesthetist* September 2022; 10–12.
5 Joshi GP, Abdelmalak BB, Weigel WA et al. American Society of Anesthesiologists consensus-based guidance on preoperative management of patients (adult and children) on glucagon-like peptide-1 (GLP-1) receptor agonists. *American Society of Anesthesiologists News.* Published 29 June 2023. Accessed online: https://www.asahq.org/about-asa/newsroom/news-releases/2023/06/american-society-of-anesthesiologists-consensus-based-guidance-on-preoperative, November 2023.
6 Australian Diabetes Society/New Zealand Society for the Study of Diabetes, ALERT UPDATE January 2020. *Periprocedural Diabetic Ketoacidosis (DKA) with SGLT2 Inhibitor Use.* Accessed online: https://www.diabetessociety.com.au/documents/ADS_DKA_SGLT2i_Alert_update_2020.pdf, February 2023.
7 Chiasson JL, Aris-Jilwan N, Bélanger R et al. Diagnosis and treatment of diabetic ketoacidosis and the hyperglycaemic hyperosmolar state. *CMAJ* 2003; 168: 859–866.
8 Chua HR, Schneider A, Bellomo R. Bicarbonate in diabetic ketoacidosis - a systemic review. *Ann Intensive Care* 2011; 1: 23. Accessed online: https://pubmed.ncbi.nlm.nih.gov/21906367/, December 2022.
9 Alderman J, Sharma A, Patel J et al. Intrathecal diamorphine for perioperative analgesia during colorectal surgery: a cross-sectional survey of current UK practice. *BMJ Open* 2022; 12: e057407. Accessed online: https://bmjopen.bmj.com/content/bmjopen/12/8/e057407.full.pdf, December 2022.
10 Thien T, Koene RA, Schijf C et al. Infusion of diazoxide in severe hypertension during pregnancy. *Eur J Obstet Gynecol Reprod Biol.* 1980; 10: 367–374.
11 Ibrahim RI, Sharma V. Cardiomyopathy and anaesthesia. *BJA Educ* 2017; 11: 363–369.

12 Yentis SM, Lee DHJ. Evaluation of an improved scoring system for the grading of direct laryngoscopy. *Anaesthesia* 1998; 53: 1041–1044.

13 Cook TM. A new practical classification of laryngeal view. *Anaesthesia* 2000; 55: 274–279.

14 Leung L. Evaluation and management of disseminated intravascular coagulation (DIC) in adults. *UpToDate*. Accessed online: www.uptodate.com/contents/evaluation-and-management-of-disseminated-intravascular-coagulation-dic-in-adults, September 2022. Topic last updated 16 December 2021.

15 Melarkode K. *Anaesthesia for children with Down's syndrome*. WFSA Tutorial 139 June 2009. Accessed online: https://resources.wfsahq.org/atotw/anaesthesia-for-children-with-downs-syndrome-anaesthesia-tutorial-of-the-week-139/, January 2023.

16 Meitzner MC, Skurnowicz JA. Anesthetic considerations for patients with Down syndrome. *AANA J* 2005; 73: 103–107.

◖ Ebstein's anomaly

Description

A rare congenital cardiac abnormality that has the following characteristics:

1 Malformed tricuspid valve leaflets displaced downwards with adherence of the septal and posterior leaflets to the myocardium. The valve is usually regurgitant but may be stenotic (this is rare). The anterior leaflet may be redundant and may be fenestrated.
2 Downward displacement of the tricuspid valve annulus.
3 The part of the right ventricle (RV) adjacent to the valve is atrialised, thus reducing RV function.
4 In 50% of cases, there is a patent foramen ovale (PFO) or atrial septal defect (ASD) through which right-to-left shunting may occur, causing cyanosis.

Pathophysiology

1 The RV contracts poorly and may dilate, contributing to tricuspid valve incompetence.
2 PFO or ASD may result in right-to-left shunt and increased risk of paradoxical embolus. This is even more likely if pulmonary stenosis is present. **See Pulmonary stenosis (PS)**.
3 Varying degrees of tricuspid regurgitation.
4 Right atrial (RA) dilatation may cause arrhythmias.
5 As the demarcation of the RA and RV is disrupted, WPW occurs in about 20% of cases.[1] **See Wolff–Parkinson–White (WPW) syndrome**.
6 There may be left heart involvement with impaired left ventricular (LV) systolic/diastolic dysfunction. This may be due to the dilated RV displacing the ventricular septum and compressing the LV and impairing filling.
7 CO tends to be 'fixed'.
8 There may be pooling and recirculation of blood in the right atrium.
9 Pulmonary hypertension may be present.

Clinical features

The patient's condition may range from asymptomatic to critically ill.

1 Fatigue.
2 Heart murmur—pansystolic.
3 Cyanosis.
4 Paradoxical embolus.
5 Heart failure.
6 Arrhythmia.

Diagnosis

1 Echocardiography.
2 Cardiac MRI.
3 ECG—tall, wide P waves, first degree AV block.

Anaesthesia

This condition is rare and varies in severity. Advice is difficult to give as there are relatively few case reports. Patients require review by a cardiologist and appropriate preoperative investigation. Surgery under LA or regional block is preferred. Involvement of a cardiac anaesthetist is advisable. Also, consider the following.

1 Antibiotic prophylaxis for relevant defects/surgery. **See Bacterial endocarditis (BE) prophylaxis**.

2 Etomidate may be considered for anaesthetic induction due to its negligible effects on heart function. **See Etomidate**. Etomidate is not currently available in Australia.

3 Aim for haemodynamic stability, avoiding hypotension and hypertension, and bradycardia and tachycardia. Hypovolaemia and new-onset arrhythmia may be poorly tolerated. Maintain preload and afterload.

4 Avoid any measures that would increase pulmonary vascular resistance in patients with right-to-left shunt (N_2O, hypoxia, hypercarbia, acidosis, high intrathoracic pressures).

5 Avoid introducing any IV air, which may result in paradoxical embolus.

6 Consider invasive monitoring (arterial line, CVP).

7 Postoperative DVT prophylaxis is extremely important.

Obstetrics

Women with Ebstein's anomaly who are not cyanosed and not in heart failure may tolerate pregnancy well. In sicker patients, its clinical effects may worsen during pregnancy due to increased blood volume and other physiological changes. **See Physiology of term pregnancy**. There may be increased tricuspid incompetence and increased right-to-left shunting and cyanosis. Involvement of a cardiologist with an obstetric interest is essential.

Labour

1 An epidural anaesthetic for labour should be titrated cautiously, with a vasopressor infusion available. Invasive arterial blood pressure monitoring is required.

2 Do not use solutions that contain adrenaline.

Caesarean section

1 Topping up an epidural placed in labour or a carefully titrated epidural as described above would be appropriate. Also, a CSE with a low-dose spinal component can be considered. For the epidural component use ropivacaine 0.75% + fentanyl 5 mcg/mL to avoid solutions containing adrenaline.

2 SAB alone would be inappropriate due to the sudden decrease in SVR, which would worsen the right-to-left shunt.

3 GA may be safest in very unstable patients, but must be conducted thoughtfully and carefully with arterial line monitoring.

4 Syntocinon should be administered cautiously to avoid vasodilatation. Ergometrine should be avoided due to its vasoconstrictive effects on the pulmonary vasculature.

◗ Edoxaban (SAVAYSA, Lixiana)

Description

Direct-acting Xa inhibitor. Used orally to decrease the incidence of thromboembolism after hip or knee joint replacement, prevention of stroke in non-valvular AF and treatment of DVT and PE (after 5–10 days of fractionated/unfractionated heparin).

Dose

60 mg PO daily.

Antidote

Andexanet alfa. *See Andexanet alfa (Andexxa®).*

⬥ Ehlers–Danlos syndrome (EDS)

Description

EDS describes a group of inherited connective tissue disorders characterised by defective collagen with joint hypermobility and instability. There is also fragility of blood vessels and soft tissues. Patients with EDS may have smooth, velvety skin and 'glassy' eyes. It is a spectrum of disorders from subclinical to severe. The patient may be prone to joint injury and dislocation. Blood vessels or organs may rupture. There may be severe skin fragility with defective wound healing and kyphoscoliosis. The gastrointestinal tract, gravid uterus, lungs and spleen may be prone to rupture.

Anaesthesia[2]

1 Attempt to elucidate the specific manifestations of the patient's EDS. For example, vasculature fragility may suggest that an arterial line may cause radial arterial wall dissection.
2 Position the patient carefully to avoid skin shear stresses and external pressure forces.
3 Be very cautious with the eyes, which may be prone to retinal detachment, globe rupture or corneal injury.
4 Tapes may cause skin damage (especially highly adhesive tapes).
5 Be careful not to cause jaw dislocation due to temporomandibular joint laxity.
6 There may be atlanto-occipital joint instability.

⬥ Eisenmenger syndrome/Eisenmenger complex

Description

This occurs when a left-to-right shunt due to an uncorrected atrial septal defect (ASD), ventricular septal defect (VSD) or patent ductus arteriosus (PDA) becomes a right-to-left shunt or bidirectional shunt due to the development of irreversible pulmonary hypertension. Pulmonary vascular resistance (PVR) exceeds systemic vascular resistance (SVR). It is due to excessive pulmonary blood flow permanently damaging the pulmonary vasculature. The Eisenmenger complex consists of a large VSD with an overriding aorta and hypertrophy of the right ventricle (RV).

Clinical picture

1 Heart murmur.
2 Hypoxaemia, cyanosis.
3 Coagulation disorders—due to such effects as polycythaemia and hyper-viscosity. Consider phlebotomy or autologous donation if haematocrit > 55–60%.
4 Fatigue.
5 Haemoptysis.
6 RV hypertrophy/failure.
7 Increased bleeding tendency due to such causes as thrombocytopenia and platelet dysfunction.
8 Clubbing.
9 Peripheral oedema.

Treatment

1 Heart/lung transplant.
2 Medications to reduce PVR such as bosentan and sildenafil. Inhaled nitric oxide or prostacyclin may also be of benefit.
3 Heart failure medication. *See Congestive cardiac failure (CCF)—chronic.*

Anaesthetic approach

Anaesthetising a patient with Eisenmenger syndrome involves significant risk. There should be involvement of a multidisciplinary team, in particular a cardiologist. The overriding aim during GA is to maintain haemodynamic stability by keeping the PVR and SVR balanced—a very challenging task. The main anaesthetic strategies are:

1 Every precaution must be taken to avoid/treat increases in PVR which can be precipitated by:
   a) hypoxia
   b) acidosis
   c) hypercarbia
   d) hypothermia
   e) high lung inflation pressures/PEEP
   f) elevated catecholamine levels
   g) use of N_2O.
2 Avoid factors that decrease SVR. These include:
   a) hypovolaemia
   b) decreased sympathetic tone e.g. spinal anaesthesia
   c) vasodilating drugs such as propofol.
3 An increase in SVR can lead to acute RV failure and must also be avoided.
4 Following from points 1–3, maintain the pre-anaesthetic PVR:SVR ratio.
5 Use invasive monitoring (arterial line, central line) unless surgery is minor e.g. cataract surgery.
6 Use a vasoconstrictor IV infusion e.g. metaraminol or phenylephrine, to maintain SVR. Vasopressin is also useful as it increases SVR without increasing PVR. Experience with vasopressin in obstetric surgery is limited.[3]
7 Induce anaesthesia slowly and carefully to minimise myocardial depression and a fall in SVR. Agents such as propofol, fentanyl and rocuronium are appropriate.
8 Maintain anaesthesia with a propofol infusion or sevoflurane or both. Use O_2 and air.
9 Use IPPV with low inflation pressures and minimal PEEP. Aim for a low/normal $ETCO_2$.
10 Bacterial endocarditis prophylaxis will be required for procedures involving at-risk patients. *See Bacterial endocarditis (BE) prophylaxis.*
11 Patients **must** be protected from paradoxical embolus. Meticulous care must be taken to avoid the introduction of any IV gas bubbles.
12 Maintain euvolaemia. Keep patients well hydrated. Treat haemorrhage promptly.
13 Minimise myocardial depression. Avoid bradycardia and tachycardia.
14 Start thromboembolism prophylaxis when it is surgically safe to do so.
15 Avoid excess opioids postoperatively due to the risk of respiratory depression.

Laparoscopic surgery

This may be hazardous in patients with Eisenmenger syndrome due to:

1 decreased venous return
2 elevated airway pressures due to elevated intra-abdominal pressure, which can increase PVR
3 hypercarbia associated with CO_2 insufflation, in turn causing elevated PVR.

If laparoscopic surgery is performed:

1 intra-abdominal pressure should be kept < 15 mmHg
2 avoid Trendelenburg positioning.

Obstetric considerations

Maternal mortality in late pregnancy is high (30–50%).[4] Pregnancy should be discouraged, and early termination considered. Pregnancy is associated with a decrease in SVR, which can lead to patient decompensation.

Epidural anaesthesia for labour

1 Insert an arterial line.
2 Ensure that the patient is well hydrated.
3 Titrate the epidural slowly and carefully. Do not use solutions containing adrenaline.

Caesarean section under neuraxial anaesthesia

1 Insert an arterial line.
2 Make sure the patient is well hydrated.
3 Use a carefully titrated epidural anaesthetic or CSE with a low-dose spinal component e.g. 1.2 mL heavy bupivacaine 0.5% 1.2 mL. Do not use adrenaline containing solutions for the epidural component.
4 SAB as the sole anaesthetic is inappropriate due to the effect on SVR.
5 Do not give an oxytocin bolus as this may decrease SVR. Use an infusion of oxytocin instead.
6 Carboprost should be avoided as it may cause a significant PVR increase.

Caesarean section under GA

GA may be used in situations where neuraxial anaesthesia is not appropriate such as severe dyspnoea when lying flat or thrombocytopenia. Follow the guidelines suggested above.

◗ Elbow blocks

See Arm blocks in the elbow region.

◗ Electrocardiography (ECG)—a brief guide

Normal values

ECG graph paper is divided into small squares of 1 mm and large squares of 5 mm. Standard recording speed is 25 mm/s, 1 cm on the horizontal axis = 0.4 s and 1 mm = 0.04 s. 1 cm on the vertical axis (two large squares) = 1 mV.

PR interval—NR 3–5 small squares = 0.12–0.2 s.
QRS—NR < 3 small squares = 0.12 s.
QT interval—needs to be corrected for HR to calculate QTc (corrected). Abnormal QTc intervals are > 0.450 s for males and > 0.470 s for females.
Normal axis— −30° to +120°.
J point—the end of the QRS complex.

Some important diagnostic ECG patterns

Axis abnormalities

Look at leads I, II and III. A positive QRS in I and a negative QRS in II and III indicates left axis deviation. A negative QRS in I and II and a positive QRS in III indicates right axis deviation.

Abnormal extra ECG waves

1 U wave occurs after the T wave. An inverted U wave in leads I, II and V5 may be seen in ischaemic heart disease and hypertension. They can also occur with hypokalaemia.
2 Delta wave is a slurred upstroke on the R wave. This is classically seen in Wolff–Parkinson–White syndrome. *See Wolff–Parkinson–White (WPW) syndrome.*
3 J wave is a rounded hump on the down stroke of the R wave. It is also called an Osborn wave. It is seen in hypothermia.

P wave

1 P mitrale is a bifid P wave associated with left atrial hypertrophy, as can occur with mitral stenosis.
2 P pulmonale is a tall, peaked P wave associated with right atrial enlargement, as can occur with pulmonary hypertension.
3 P wave flattening occurs in hyperkalaemia.

R wave

Tall R waves occur in ventricular hypertrophy.

PR interval

1 PR interval is prolonged in hyper/hypokalaemia/hyper/hypomagneseamia. The PR interval is also prolonged in first degree heart block (by definition).
2 The PR interval is shortened in Wolff-Parkinson-White syndrome.

Strain pattern

Depression of the ST segment and T wave inversion. This pattern may be seen with myocardial ischaemia.

QRS

Widened QRS (> 0.12 s) can occur with hyperkalaemia, hypermagnesaemia, hypercalcaemia, LBBB.

QT interval abnormalities

1 Prolonged QTc interval is seen in long QT syndrome. *See Long QT syndrome.* It is also prolonged by hypomagnesaemia, hypocalcaemia, hypokalaemia, slow heart rate, drugs such as sotalol.
2 Shortened QTc is seen with digoxin therapy, hyperthermia, hyperkalaemia, hypercalcaemia, acidosis.

T wave abnormalities

1 Tall, peaked T waves occur with hyperkalaemia.
2 Diminished or inverted T wave can occur with hypokalaemia.
3 Flattened, widened T wave may be seen with hypercalcaemia.
4 T wave inversion may occur with myocardial ischaemia, hypocalcaemia.

S wave abnormalities

Deep S wave can occur with hyperkalaemia.

Electrolyte disturbances

1 Hyperkalaemia—prolonged PR interval, widened QRS, flattening of the P wave, tall, peaked T wave, deep S wave. Ultimately get a sine wave ECG which proceeds to asystole.
2 Hypokalaemia—prolonged PR interval, T wave amplitude diminishes then becomes inverted. U wave may develop.

3 Hypermagnesaemia—increased PR interval, widened QRS due to non-specific intraventricular conduction system delay. Sinoatrial (SA) and atrioventricular (AV) nodal block may occur. *See Preeclampsia/eclampsia*.

4 Hypomagnesaemia—increased PR and QT intervals and myocardial irritability.

5 Hypercalcaemia—increased PR interval and widened QRS and a shortened QT interval. T wave flattening and widening. AV nodal block progressing to complete heart block may occur.

6 Hypocalcaemia—prolonged QT interval, T wave inversion, heart block, VF.

7 Hyponatraemia—Na < 115 mmol/L: widened QRS, ST segment elevation. Na < 100 mmol/L: may see VF or VT.

Bundle branch conduction defects

1 Right bundle branch block (RBBB)—rSR pattern in V1, broad and slurred S wave in V5, V6. With incomplete RBBB, the QRS complex duration is between 0.10 and 0.12 s. With complete RBBB, the QRS duration is > 0.12 s.

2 Left bundle branch block (LBBB)—QRS > 0.12 s, wide-notched M-shaped QRS in V5, V6. There may be left axis deviation.

3 Left anterior hemiblock—left axis deviation, tall R wave in aVL, deep S wave in II, III and aVF. QRS is widened but < 0.12 s.

4 Left posterior hemiblock—right axis deviation and prominent S wave in I and aVL. Tall R waves in II, III and aVF (but especially III).

5 Bifascicular block—a combination of RBBB and left anterior or left posterior hemiblock. RBBB and left anterior hemiblock causes a RBBB pattern with left axis deviation. RBBB and left posterior hemiblock causes a RBBB pattern, right axis deviation, prominent S wave in I and aVL, tall R waves in II, III and aVF.

6 Trifascicular block—true trifascicular block is third degree heart block with a ventricular escape rhythm. Some authors describe trifascicular block as first or second degree heart block + RBBB + left anterior or posterior hemiblock.

Heart block (HB)

1 First degree HB—PR interval longer than 5 small squares (> 0.2 s).

2 Second degree HB. There are 2 types of second degree heart block:

   a) Wenckebach or Mobitz Type 1—PR interval gets progressively longer and longer until a dropped beat occurs, then the cycle repeats. The electrical defect is in the AV node.

   b) Mobitz Type 2—there are intermittent non-conducted P waves without a lengthening of the PR interval. The PR interval may be short or long but its length is constant. This type of block is much more serious than a Mobitz Type 1 block. The defect is in the His–Purkinje system. Atropine may make this block worse, and those afflicted need a pacemaker.

   The block may be of a fixed ratio in Mobitz Type 1 or 2 block (ratio of P waves to QRS complexes e.g. three P waves for every QRS complex).

3 Third degree HB/complete HB—no relationship between P waves and QRS complexes. *See Heart block (HB)*.

Ventricular hypertrophy

1 Right ventricular hypertrophy—suggested by right axis deviation, large R waves in V1 and V2 with an initial slur. May also see inverted T waves in V2, V3 and strain pattern in V1–V4, with prominent S waves in I, II and III.

2 Left ventricular hypertrophy—left axis deviation. Tall R wave in V5, V6. Deep S wave in V1, V2. S wave in V1 + R wave in V5 or V6 > 35 mm.

Myocardial ischaemia

Horizontal or down-sloping ST depression (1 mm or more) with an upright or inverted T wave. LBBB may occur with left axis deviation. Sharply pointed symmetrical T waves may be seen.

Myocardial infarction (MI)

1 ST segment elevation—occurs in minutes.
2 Tall and widened T waves—occurs in minutes.
3 Inversion of T waves.
4 Appearance of pathological q waves over hours or days. These are q waves which are > 0.04 s wide and > 0.2 mV (2 mm vertical).
5 Localising the site of MI:
   a) inferior—II, III, aVF
   b) posterior—ST depression, tall R waves and tall, wide asymmetrical T waves in leads V1–V3; these are reciprocal changes
   c) antero-septal—V1–V4
   d) antero-apical—V3–V4
   e) extensive anterior/anterolateral—I, aVL, V1–5.

Pulmonary embolus

May cause acute right ventricular strain with RBBB, right axis deviation, prominent S wave in I, Q wave in III and inverted T wave in III. May also see non-specific ST changes and T inversion in anterior leads, P pulmonale and atrial dysrhythmias.

Pulmonary hypertension

May see right axis deviation, right ventricular hypertrophy, P pulmonale and RBBB.

◐ Eliquis

See Apixaban (Eliquis).

◐ Endone

This is a brand name for oral oxycodone. *See Oxycodone.*

◐ Endotracheal tube (ET) size based on age

Table E1 Appropriate size (mm internal diameter) non-cuffed endotracheal (ET) tube based on age

Age	Non-cuffed ET tube size (mm internal diameter)
Term newborn (2–3 kg)	3.0
Term newborn > 3 kg	3.0–3.5
Infant up to 6 months	3.5
Infant 7–12 months	4.0
Child > 1 y	Age (y)/4 + 4

◐ Endovascular stroke therapy

See Acute stroke.

Table E2 Appropriate size (internal diameter in mm) cuffed endotracheal (ET) tube based on age

Age	Cuffed ET tube size (mm)
Term newborn > 3 kg	3.0
Infants up to 1 year	3.5
Child 1–2 yrs	4.0
Child > 2 yrs	Age (yrs)/4 + 4
Adult male	8.0
Adult female	7.0

◗ End-tidal expired carbon dioxide (ETCO₂) levels

This is defined as the partial pressure of CO_2 in expired gas at the end of expiration. The NR of end tidal CO_2 is 35–45 mmHg. It is slightly lower than blood partial pressure of CO_2 under normal circumstances.

Causes of elevated ETCO₂

Causes may be respiratory or non-respiratory.

Respiratory causes
1 Hypoventilation—either inadequate tidal volume (TV) or respiratory rate or both. However, if TV is very low, only the anatomical dead space is being ventilated and $ETCO_2$ will be much reduced.
2 Lung disease.
3 Rebreathing CO_2 e.g. exhausted CO_2 absorber.

Non-respiratory causes
1 Increased CO_2 production e.g. thyrotoxicosis, malignant hyperthermia. *See Malignant hyperthermia (MH)*.
2 Sodium bicarbonate therapy.

Causes of reduced ETCO₂

Causes can be respiratory or non-respiratory.

Respiratory causes
1 Hyperventilation.
2 Small TV with mainly/only dead space ventilation.
3 Lung embolism—gas, fat, amniotic fluid, clot.
4 Ventilation perfusion mismatch e.g. pneumonia.
5 Hyper-expanded alveoli (air trapping).

Non-respiratory causes
1 Reduced cardiac output resulting in decreased lung perfusion.
2 Sampling line leak.
3 Breathing circuit leak.
4 Decreased metabolism e.g. hypothermia.

◗ Enoxaparin (Clexane)

A low-molecular-weight heparin. *See Heparin (unfractionated and low-molecular-weight heparins)*.

◗ Enoximone (Perfan)

Description

Enoximone is a PDE-III inhibitor. Its main effects are positive inotropy and vasodilatation. **See *Phosphodiesterase-III (PDE-III) inhibitors*.** Enoximone is useful for the treatment of:

1 acute or chronic heart failure
2 weaning from bypass/post cardiac surgery
3 as bridging therapy to heart transplant.

Dose by infusion

Administer a LD of 500 mcg/kg no faster than 12.5 mg/min followed by an infusion of 5–20 mcg/kg/min. The total dose over 24 h should not exceed 24 mg/kg.

Oral dose

25–50 mg q 8 h.

◗ Entropy

See Awareness monitoring.

◗ Ephedrine

Description

Sympathomimetic drug derived from the ma huang plant. Stimulates alpha and beta receptors directly and also causes endogenous release of noradrenaline (NA). It is useful for the treatment of hypotension.

Dose

Adult

3–9 mg IV boluses titrated to desired effect. Lasts for about 1 h. Can also give ephedrine sulphate 15 mg IM when a sustained effect on BP is needed. **Ephedrine hydrochloride is not recommended for IM use.**

Child

0.25 mg/kg IV.

◗ Epidural abscess, spinal

Description

An abscess in the epidural space. It can be intracranial or spinal. In the spine, an epidural abscess can compress the spinal cord.

Causes

The causative organism is usually *Staphylococcus aureus*. Streptococci, gram negative rods and fungi may also be causative organisms. Mechanism of entry for a spinal epidural abscess can be:

1 epidural anaesthesia, SAB
2 back surgery
3 vertebral osteomyelitis
4 infection in another part of the body e.g. UTI

5 illicit IV drug use

6 immunosuppressive state e.g. alcoholism, HIV

7 diabetes mellitus is a common risk factor.

Clinical effects

1 Back pain.

2 Fever.

3 Neurological deficit.

4 Pain on straight leg raising.

5 Urinary retention/incontinence.

6 Bowel incontinence.

7 Motor weakness or paralysis.

8 Sensation changes.

Diagnosis

1 MRI with gadolinium contrast.

2 Myelography followed by CT scan is also highly sensitive for diagnosis.

3 C-reactive protein and WBC are usually raised.

4 Positive blood cultures are only obtained in about 25% of cases.

5 Send any pus obtained from an epidural puncture site for culture.

6 If an epidural catheter is still in situ, remove and send the tip for culture.

7 Lumbar puncture must not be done.

Treatment

1 Urgent neurosurgical consultation. Emergency spinal surgery with drainage of pus and spinal decompression is usually needed if neurological signs are present.

2 IV antibiotic therapy. While gram stain and sensitivities are being processed, treat the adult patient with vancomycin 15–20 mg/kg q 8–12 h + ceftriaxone 2 g q 12 h.[5] An infectious diseases specialist should be consulted to guide antibiotic selection.

3 IV antibiotics are usually required for 6–8 weeks.

4 In special circumstances, IV antibiotics without surgical intervention is recommended. These circumstances include when patients do not have neurological signs or refuse surgery.

◉ Epidural anaesthesia/analgesia

See also Ultrasound-assisted neuraxial anaesthesia.

Anatomy

The spinal epidural space is a potential space containing nerve roots, fat, lymphatics, blood vessels and areolar tissue (a form of loose connective tissue). It extends from the foramen magnum to the sacral hiatus and surrounds the dura (Figure E1). In adults the dural sac terminates at S1–2, and in children it terminates at S3–4.

It is bounded anteriorly by the posterior longitudinal ligaments of the spinal column and laterally by the intervertebral foramina and pedicles. Posteriorly it is bounded by the ligamentum flavum. The structures encountered when inserting the epidural Tuohy needle are:

1 skin, subcutaneous tissue

2 supraspinous ligament, interspinous ligament

3 ligamentum flavum.

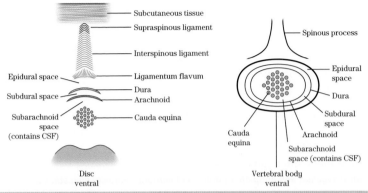

A **Dorsal (between spinous processes)**

- Subcutaneous tissue
- Supraspinous ligament
- Interspinous ligament
- Ligamentum flavum

Epidural space
Subdural space
- Dura
- Arachnoid

Subarachnoid space (contains CSF)
- Cauda equina

Disc
ventral

B **Dorsal (through spinous process)**

- Spinous process
- Epidural space
- Dura
- Subdural space
- Arachnoid

Cauda equina
Subarachnoid space (contains CSF)

Vertebral body
ventral

Figure E1 Anatomy of the epidural space. **A** indicates the structures that will be penetrated by the Tuohy needle to reach the epidural space.

Epidural analgesia/anaesthesia can be used for:
1 relieving labour contraction pain
2 anaesthesia for surgery such as caesarean section (CS)
3 postoperative analgesia.

Contraindications
Absolute:
1 infection at the site of insertion
2 coagulopathy (pathological or drug induced)
3 patient refusal (as for any other procedure).
Relative:
1 anatomical abnormalities e.g. tethered cord as can occur with dwarfism, spina bifida
2 previous spinal surgery in region of epidural insertion site
3 hypovolaemia
4 systemic sepsis not treated with antibiotics.

Risks
Major risks:
1 nerve damage (lasting < 6 months 1:1000, lasting > 6 months 1:13 000)
2 severe nerve injury/paralysis 1:250 000
3 epidural haematoma with spinal cord compression (1:170 000)
4 epidural abscess (1:50 000)
5 meningitis (1:100 000)
6 total spinal anaesthesia due to misplaced catheter.
Minor risks:
1 postdural puncture headache
2 hypotension
3 nausea
4 shivering/shaking.

Thrombocytopenia

1 If the platelets are functioning normally, a count $> 75\,000/mm^3$ is considered safe.
2 If the count is between $50\,000$ and $75\,000/mm^3$, a carefully performed epidural can be considered if the benefits outweigh the risks.
3 A platelet count $< 50\,000/mm^3$ is an absolute contraindication to epidural placement.
4 In patients with preeclampsia, platelet function may not be normal. An epidural can be considered if coagulation studies are normal and the platelet count $> 75\,000/mm^3$.
5 If there is severe preeclampsia/eclampsia, do not perform an epidural unless the platelet count $> 100\,000/mm^3$ and the coagulation studies are normal.
  See Preeclampsia/eclampsia.

Anticoagulant and antiplatelet drugs

See Anticoagulant and antiplatelet drugs and surgery/neuraxial anaesthesia.

Lumbar epidural

Technique

1 Fully inform the patient about what the procedure entails and the risks involved, and obtain consent. Identify any contraindications.
2 Insert an IV cannula (18 G or larger).
3 Commence IV Hartmann's solution, aiming for about 500 mL to be given during the procedure.
4 Position the patient (sitting or lateral in the fetal position). Educate the patient on how to maximally flex the spine.
5 For an obstetric epidural, the target space is L3–4. Tuffier's line is a line between the highest points of the iliac crests. It should pass through L4 or the L4–5 interspace. The spinal cord ends at about the L1–2 interspace in the adult, continuing as the cauda equina. The L4–5 interspace is also suitable and safe. Spaces above L3–4 can be used recognising the increased risk of spinal cord injury.
6 A 2% chlorhexidine + 70% alcohol applicator is very useful for prepping the skin. Allow this to fully dry. Use a fully aseptic technique—sterile gown, gloves, drapes, mask and theatre cap.
7 Use 1% lignocaine to anaesthetise the skin at the site of insertion.
8 Use a loss of resistance (LOR) to saline technique. Insert the Tuohy needle 1–2 cm, remove the trocar and attach a LOR syringe filled with 5 mL saline and push the needle slowly and incrementally towards the epidural space.
9 Resistance to the advancing needle will increase just before the epidural space— this is the ligamentum flavum being penetrated.
10 Advance the needle using mainly hydraulic pressure on the syringe plunger. There will be a sudden LOR and some saline will fill the epidural space. In 80% of cases, the depth of the epidural space from the skin is 4–6.5 cm.[6]
11 Remove the syringe and examine the hub of the epidural needle for a CSF leak. It is normal for a few drops of saline to dribble out, but a continuous flow of CSF indicates dural puncture. Management of recognised dural puncture is described below.
12 Insert the epidural catheter so that 3–5 cm lies in the epidural space. The catheter should pass easily. Some discomfort on insertion may occur but should be transitory. If discomfort/pain persists, remove the epidural needle and catheter.

13 Remove the epidural needle and attach the connector to the catheter. Use a syringe to test aspirate for blood/CSF. If blood is aspirated, withdraw the catheter so that there is still sufficient in the epidural space, flush the catheter with saline then re-aspirate. If there is no aspirated blood, use the catheter carefully, being vigilant for evidence of intravascular injection (see below). If there is still blood being aspirated, remove the catheter and re-site. The risk of epidural catheter insertion into an epidural vein can be reduced by injecting 5 mL of N/S through the Tuohy needle and keeping the plunger depressed for 20 s, prior to insertion of the catheter.[7]

14 If negative aspiration, attach the filter to the connector and give a 5 mL test dose of LA.

15 Apply a sterile dressing and tape the catheter to the patient's back so that the connector and filter are accessible at the patient's shoulder.

Important points

1 Do not advance the Tuohy needle during a contraction as this increases the risks of a dural puncture and/or puncturing an epidural blood vessel.

2 Do not pull the epidural catheter out through the Tuohy needle as this might shear off the catheter. Remove the needle and catheter together.

LA drugs and dosages

For a patient in labour the following drugs and dosages are recommended.

1 5 mL test dose of bupivacaine 0.125% + fentanyl 5 mcg/mL.

2 Establish the block with a further 15 mL of the above solution.

3 An alternative is to use ropivacaine 0.2% + fentanyl 5 mcg/mL in the same volumes as above.

4 To maintain the block, use a combination of programmed intermittent epidural bolus (PIEB) plus patient controlled epidural analgesia (PCEA). Use ropivacaine 0.1% + 2 mcg/mL fentanyl. The initial settings are:

a) PIEB 8 mL

b) PIEB dose range 0–15 mL

c) PIEB lockout interval 60 min

d) PCEA dose 5 mL

e) PCEA lockout interval 10 min

f) Hourly limit 25 mL

g) Delay time to first PIEB 30 min.

5 Alternatively, give an infusion of bupivacaine 0.125% + fentanyl 2.5–5 mcg/mL run at 8–14 mL/h. Give a bolus of 10 mL for breakthrough pain.

6 Alternatively, use midwife-initiated boluses of bupivacaine 0.125% + fentanyl 5 mcg/mL 2–4 h as needed for pain.

Combined spinal epidural (CSE) used for labour

In patients who are extremely distressed in labour, this technique can be quite useful to get faster pain relief. For performance of the technique, *see Subarachnoid block (SAB)*. Inject 2 mL of the standard premixed solution (bupivacaine 0.125% + fentanyl 5 mcg/mL) through the spinal needle then remove it. Insert the epidural catheter then commence the PIEB catheter protocol once the pain reoccurs. An alternative would be to do a subarachnoid block with 2 mL of the premix solution, then perform the epidural when pain is controlled.

Epidural used for CS

Top up the epidural with lignocaine 2% + adrenaline 1:200000 + fentanyl 5 mcg/mL. Between 15 and 25 mL (given incrementally) will be required. *See Caesarean section*. If only 2% lignocaine is available, add 1 mL of 1:10000 adrenaline (1 mg adrenaline in 10 mL ampoule) to 19.5 mL of 2% lignocaine. This will give an adrenaline concentration of 1:200 000 (5 mcg/mL). Another option is using ropivacaine 0.75% with fentanyl 5 mcg/mL. 1 mL ropivacaine 0.75% is equivalent to 1 mL 2% lignocaine with adrenaline.

Accidental epidural catheter misplacement

The catheter can be misplaced into three sites: the subdural space, intrathecally or intravascularly.

Subdural block

In this situation, the tip of the catheter has penetrated the dura but is not intrathecal (it has not penetrated the arachnoid layer). This results in a 'funny block' typified by:
1 unexpectedly high sensory block
2 asymmetrical patchy block without adequate pain relief and sacral sparing
3 sparing of autonomic and motor function and moderate (rather than severe) hypotension
4 Horner's syndrome, trigeminal nerve palsy, nasal stuffiness, decreased level of consciousness, respiratory incoordination/apnoea may occur.

There may be neural damage due to compression of nerve roots or compression of the arteries supplying nerve roots.

Treatment

1 Recognise what is happening.
2 Attend to ABC—support airway, breathing, circulation.
3 Remove the catheter.
4 Re-site the catheter at a different level.
5 If an urgent CS is required, consider a CSE with a low-dose spinal component or GA. Do not use the subdural catheter.

Total spinal due to intrathecal injection of LA

In this situation there is a progressive symmetrical ascent of decreased sensation and motor block. Typical signs are:
1 restlessness, inability to speak
2 ascending weakness including arms
3 profound hypotension
4 dyspnoea, loss of consciousness, apnoea.

Management of total spinal

This is a crisis situation. **Recognise what is happening and activate the emergency response system.**
Notify the obstetrician and resuscitate the patient using:
1 A – **A**irway: support the airway, provide supplementary O_2; intubation may be required using conservative doses of propofol, midazolam + muscle relaxant.
2 B – **B**reathing: support ventilation.
3 C – **C**irculatory support: IV fluids, vasopressors, atropine for bradycardia, left lateral positioning to reduce aortocaval compression. CPR may be required.
4 Emergency LSCS may be required.

5 Attempt to aspirate CSF/LA from the catheter. Aspirate 20–30 mL then inject 20 mL of N/S.
6 Death from total spinal anaesthesia should be completely preventable.

Intravascular injection of epidural solution

Typically there is evidence of IV LA such as ringing in the ears and tingling of the lips or tongue. *See Local anaesthetic (LA) toxicity*, which describes more severe LA reactions. There will also be little or no block.

Treatment

1 Treat LA toxicity if required.
2 Reassure the patient.
3 Re-site the epidural.

Recognised dural puncture

In this situation, CSF is seen to be leaking from the epidural needle hub or is aspirated through the epidural catheter when doing the aspiration test. CSF can be differentiated from N/S in the following ways:

1 CSF is warm, N/S is cool.
2 Using a urinary dipstick—CSF contains protein, a trace of glucose and pH $\geq$ 7.5. N/S has a pH of 7.5 and contains no protein or glucose.

Fully disclose this complication to the patient. The following strategy is suggested.

1 Ensure about 4 cm of catheter is in the subarachnoid space and remove the epidural needle. Make sure the catheter is labelled 'subarachnoid catheter'.
2 The anaesthetist must take sole responsibility for establishing the block and providing 'top-ups'.
3 Administer 2 mL bupivacaine 0.125% + fentanyl 5 mcg/mL every 1–3 h.
4 If CS is required, give 100 mcg morphine, 20–25 mcg fentanyl and 0.5 mL boluses of bupivacaine 0.5% heavy solution until a satisfactory level of block is established.
5 Remove the catheter after delivery and follow the patient up. A postdural puncture headache may occur.

Another option is to simply re-site the epidural and top it up carefully as there may be some intrathecal spread of LA through the dural tear.

Thoracic epidural

Thoracic epidurals are useful for the management of post-operative pain (thoracic and abdominal) and chest pain due to causes such as fractured ribs. The site of insertion is determined by the mid-dermatomal level of the site of pain. Suggested levels are:

1 upper abdominal surgery T6–T8
2 lower abdominal surgery T9–T10
3 fractured ribs e.g. fractured ribs 3–7, insert epidural at T5.

The vertebral prominence at the base of the neck corresponds to C7. The inferior angle of the scapula corresponds to T7. The width of the epidural space is only 0.5–3 mm at T6, compared with 5–6 mm at L3.

Technique

This procedure has a risk of spinal cord damage and must be performed with utmost care.

1 Place an IV cannula and position the patient sitting. Use full aseptic technique.
2 Sterilise and drape the back. Ask the patient to arch their back.
3 Anaesthetise the skin and deeper structures.

4 Insert the epidural needle using a midline approach and a loss of resistance technique. Note that the thoracic spines are angulated, which may make finding the epidural space difficult.

5 If unable to locate the space in the midline, consider a paramedian approach. Insert the epidural needle 1.5 cm lateral to the spinous process and identify the lamina. Attempt to walk the tip of the epidural needle off the lamina in a slightly angled inwards and cephalad direction until bone is no longer encountered. Then advance the Tuohy needle with extreme care until LOR is achieved.

6 Insert the epidural catheter ensuring 3–4 cm is in the epidural space.

7 Attach the connector and aspirate for blood or CSF. If no blood or CSF is aspirated, attach the filter and give a test dose of 3 mL of 2% lignocaine. Assess for any evidence of spinal block. Secure the catheter with a sterile dressing.

Dose

1 Intraoperatively establish the block with 0.25% bupivacaine with adrenaline 1:200 000 + fentanyl 5 mcg/mL. Give 5 mL boluses to a maximum of 15 mL, depending on the patient's physiological response.

2 Commence an infusion of bupivacaine 0.125% + fentanyl 2.5 mcg/mL at 4–12 mL/h.

3 Alternatively, establish the block with 5 mL boluses of ropivacaine 0.75% + fentanyl 5 mcg/mL up to a total of 15 mL.

4 Then commence an infusion of ropivacaine 0.2% + fentanyl 2.5 mcg/mL at 4–12 mL/h.

Short-term thoracic epidural technique

In this technique:

1 A thoracic epidural is sited pre-operatively.

2 The block is established with incremental 5 mL boluses of bupivacaine 0.25% with adrenaline 1:200 000 + fentanyl 5 mcg/mL to a total of 15 mL.

3 Near the end of surgery 3 mg of epidural morphine is administered.

4 Another 5 mL of the bupivacaine/fentanyl solution may be injected at the discretion of the anaesthetist just before emergence.

5 In recovery, the patient is assessed for pain and, if present, 5 mL boluses of ropivacaine 0.2% are given until the patient is pain free.

6 The epidural is then removed and a low-dose PCA is provided (e.g. fentanyl 10 mcg boluses and a 10 min lockout).

Thoracic epidural for rib fractures

1 Insert the thoracic epidural at the midpoint of the fractures e.g. fractured ribs 4–10, insert the epidural at T6 or T7.

2 Establish the block with 8–10 mL of ropivacaine 0.2% + fentanyl 5 mcg/mL.

3 Run an infusion of ropivacaine 0.2% + fentanyl 2 mcg/mL at 6–12 mL/h.

◗ Epidural haematoma, spinal

Description

An epidural haematoma can be intracranial or spinal. A spinal epidural haematoma may occur as a complication of epidural or spinal anaesthesia. The incidence of epidural haematoma after epidural anaesthesia is about 1:150 000, and about 50% of cases are associated with catheter removal.[8] Risk factors include:

1 anticoagulant therapy

2 haemostatic abnormalities such as thrombocytopenia

3 difficult epidural catheter insertion
4 blood in the epidural catheter
5 elderly patients.
See Anticoagulant and antiplatelet drugs and surgery/neuraxial anaesthesia for guidelines on anticoagulant drugs and neuraxial anaesthesia.

Clinical effects

Symptoms and signs typically occur 0–2 days after epidural catheter insertion or removal or spinal anaesthesia. Effects include:

1 Back pain or radicular pain (pain that radiates into one or both arms, or one or both legs). Pain may not be present in most cases associated with epidural anaesthesia.[8]
2 Motor and/or sensory deficits. Motor block may be a more sensitive indicator than sensory block.[8]
3 Bowel/bladder dysfunction such as urinary retention.

Diagnosis

Urgent MRI. If MRI is not available, CT myelography is the next best option.

Treatment

An epidural haematoma is a neurosurgical emergency. It must be treated promptly to avoid the risk of permanent neurological injury. The patient requires emergency decompressive laminectomy/surgical drainage. A good outcome is likely if surgery is performed within 8 h of the onset of symptoms. Full recovery after a delay of 72 h is rare. Very occasionally conservative management is undertaken e.g. mild, resolving neurological deficit. A neurosurgeon must be consulted and must be in agreement with this approach.

◗ Epiglottitis

Description

Epiglottitis is an infection in which there is swelling and inflammation of the epiglottis. This can cause fatal airway obstruction. Before immunisation of children with *Haemophilus influenzae* vaccine, epiglottitis was commonly seen in young children (ages 2–6 y). It is now more commonly seen in adults. In the past, the most common causative organism was *Haemophilus influenzae* type b (Hib). Now the most common causative bacteria are group A *Beta-haemolytic streptococci.*[9]

Presentation—child

1 Child usually previously well.
2 Stridor (usually inspiratory), difficulty breathing.
3 Drooling, sitting up, tongue protruding.
4 Absence of coughing.
5 Fever, tachycardia.
6 Muffled voice.
7 Severe sore throat.
8 Complete airway closure can occur at any time.

Presentation—adult

1 May have underlying medical condition such as diabetes mellitus.
2 Inflammation may be more supraglottic (uvula, pharynx, base of tongue) than in children.
3 Dysphagia.
4 Voice changes.

5 Very sore throat.

6 Complete airway obstruction less likely in adults.

Diagnosis—child

1 Clinical presentation.

2 Swollen 'cherry red' epiglottis at laryngoscopy. **Never** attempt to examine a child's throat while awake as complete airway obstruction may occur.

3 Oedematous epiglottic folds.

4 Throat swab to identify infecting organism.

Diagnosis—adult

1 Clinical presentation.

2 Soft-tissue lateral neck X-ray.

3 Nasoendoscopy.

Treatment—child

1 Transfer to the operating theatre and have a surgeon skilled at tracheostomy present.

2 Do **not** attempt IV access.

3 Gaseous induction with O_2/sevoflurane with child sitting on parent's lap.

4 Perform laryngoscopy when the child is deeply anaesthetised.

5 Secure the airway with an oral ET tube.

6 Secure IV access.

7 Administer cefotaxime IV 50 mg/kg q 12 h.

8 When the situation is completely controlled, change the oral tube to a nasal tube.

9 Transfer to paediatric ICU.

Treatment—adult

Only about 15% will require urgent airway intervention.

1 Urgent ENT review with nasoendoscopy.

2 Nebulised adrenaline may be helpful (4 mg in 4 mL).

3 Monitor in a high-dependency setting.

4 Stridor, respiratory distress and rapid progression suggest a threatened airway. To secure the airway, transfer the patient to the operating theatre and have an ENT surgeon present. Perform awake endoscopic nasal intubation with sedation. **See Difficult airway management.** Gaseous induction would be the next best option.

5 Antibiotic therapy with cefotaxime and metronidazole.

◗ Epilepsy, status

See Status epilepticus (SE).

◗ Eptacog alpha (activated)

See Recombinant activated factor VII (rFVIIa).

◗ Erector spinae plane (ESP) block

Indications

This block is useful for:

1 analgesia for rib fractures

2 thoracoscopy

3 breast surgery

4 spine surgery.

It is also called a paraspinal fascial plane block. It acts like a paravertebral block, but the ESP block is safer and has less risk of a pneumothorax. It can be done with the patient sitting, lateral or prone.

Anatomy

The erector spinae muscles stabilise the spine and run from the skull to the sacrum. They are divided into three parts. These are, moving from medial to lateral, the spinalis part, the longissimus part and the iliocostalis part. These muscles lie superficial to the vertebrae. The spinal nerves are formed from a sensory nerve root from the dorsal part of the spinal cord and a motor nerve from the ventral part of the spinal cord. The nerves emerge from the intervertebral foramina and lie deep to the erector spinae muscles and superficial to the transverse processes. The nerves then divide into the dorsal primary ramus and the ventral primary ramus. The dorsal primary ramus supplies the posterior chest and abdomen (motor and sensory). The ventral primary ramus supplies the anterior chest and abdomen (motor and sensory). How the ESP block actually works is not clear, but it is presumed the block spreads to the paravertebral space.

Ultrasound anatomy

1 Position the patient sitting up.
2 With the probe orientated in the sagittal plane, the spinous processes are easily identified centrally as a series of bumps in the midline.
3 Move the probe in a parasagittal direction to be about 2 cm from the midline to identify the tip of the transverse process. See Figure E2.
4 Above T5 the layers seen are trapezius (stabilising the neck and thoracic spine), rhomboid (stabilising the thoracic spine) and the erector spinae. Below T5 only two layers are seen, trapezius and erector spinae. If the probe is too lateral, ribs are seen; if too medial, the laminae are seen.

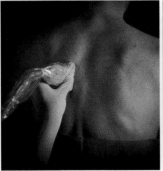
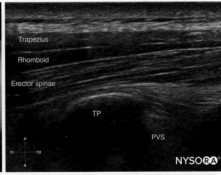

Figure E2 Probe position and sonoanatomy for erector spinae plane block. TP = transverse process
Image courtesy of NYSORA

Performing the block

Orientate the ultrasound probe as described in the previous section and in figure E2. A linear probe can be used for the upper spine. A curvilinear probe can be considered for the lower spine because the structures are deeper. As a rough guide: T5 is an appropriate level for chest surgery, T10 is an appropriate level for abdominal surgery and L2 or L3 is an appropriate level for lumbar spine surgery.

1 Use chlorhexidine antiseptic at the injection site, a sterile probe cover, sterile gloves and mask.
2 Insert the block needle in-plane either cranio-caudally or vice versa.
3 The tip should lie in contact with the transverse process.
4 Inject 2–3 mL of LA to visualise spread deep to the erector spinae muscle layer. The muscle should be seen to be lifting off the transverse process.
5 Complete the block with 20–30 mL LA e.g. ropivacaine 0.5%.
6 For surgery crossing the midline, use 30 mL of ropivacaine 0.2% each side.
7 If a catheter is used, run an infusion of ropivacaine 0.2% at 8–10 mL/h.
8 About 4 dermatomal levels above and below the site of injection will be covered in the thoracic region (8 in total). In the lumbar region about 4 dermatomal levels in total will be covered.

◗ Ergometrine

See Syntometrine.

◗ Esmolol (Brevibloc)

Relatively selective beta-1 adrenoreceptor blocker. It is short acting and only used IV. Esmolol is metabolised by hydrolysis via plasma esterases with an elimination half-life of 10 min. It is used for:

1 hypertension and control of the hypertensive response to intubation
2 acute supraventricular tachydysrhythmias such as supraventricular tachycardia (SVT), atrial fibrillation and atrial flutter
3 angina.

Dose

Esmolol is presented in ampoules of 10 mL containing 100 mg (10 mg/mL). Time to onset of effect is 5–10 min. Effects cease after about 20 min.

1 The LD is 500 mcg/kg over 1 minute (70 kg patient = 3.5 mL).
2 Infuse esmolol at 50 mcg/kg/min for 4 min. If adequate response, continue at this rate (70 kg patient = 21 mL/h).
3 If inadequate response, give the same LD (optional) then infusion at 100 mcg/kg/min for 4 min. If adequate response, continue at this rate (70 kg patient = 42 mL/h).
4 If inadequate response, give the same LD (optional) then infusion at 150 mcg/kg/min for 4 min. If adequate response, continue at this rate.
5 If inadequate response, increase infusion rate to a max of 200 mcg/kg/min (70 kg patient = 84 mL/h).

Bolus dose

For a rapid effect prior to intubation, give 1 mg/kg over 30 s.

Contraindications/cautions

See Beta-adrenergic receptor blocker drugs.

⏵ Etomidate

Description

Carboxylated imidazole short-acting IV anaesthetic agent unrelated to other anaesthetic drugs. Can be used to induce anaesthesia or for procedural sedation e.g. relocation of dislocated joint.

Dose for anaesthesia

0.2–0.6 mg/kg.

Advantages

1 Excellent haemodynamic stability with minimal histamine release. Etomidate is useful in haemodynamically compromised patients e.g. hypovolaemic shock, heart disease.
2 Reduces intracranial pressure (ICP) and intraocular pressure (IOP).
3 Ventilation is not significantly affected.

Disadvantages

1 Pain on injection. May be reduced by adding lignocaine.
2 No analgesic properties.
3 Etomidate anaesthesia can be associated with involuntary patient.
4 Causes adreno-cortical suppression and is not suitable for prolonged use by IV infusion because of this effect. It should be avoided in patients with sepsis.
5 Contraindicated in porphyria. *See Porphyria*.
6 Causes more nausea and vomiting than thiopentone. *See Thiopentone*.
7 Dissolved in propylene glycol, which causes a high incidence of thrombophlebitis.
8 Not available in Australia.

⏵ EXIT procedure

See Ex utero intrapartum treatment (EXIT) procedure.

⏵ Extracorporeal membrane oxygenation (ECMO)

Description

More than a brief description of this highly complex therapy is beyond the scope of this manual. ECMO is an invasive technique used for respiratory support or cardiorespiratory support in highly compromised patients in the ICU. It is a last resort strategy used in patients with reversible or potentially treatable respiratory or cardiac failure. There are two types of ECMO: veno-venous ECMO (VVECMO) for respiratory failure and veno-arterial ECMO (VAECMO) for heart failure.

Contraindications

These are many and include:
1 disseminated malignancy
2 severe brain injury
3 peripheral vascular disease
4 prolonged CPR without adequate tissue perfusion.

VVECMO

Indications are also many and include COVID-19-related ARDS, severe intractable asthma, paraquat poisoning and bridge to lung transplant.

1 The patient is anticoagulated.
2 Large cannulas are inserted into major veins e.g. common femoral vein for drainage and the internal jugular for infusion.
3 Alternatively, a single double-lumen cannula can be inserted into the right atrium.
4 Blood is passed through a heat exchanger and oxygenator where O_2 is added and CO_2 is removed
5 Blood is then returned to the patient
6 The patient's heart provides the pumping force
7 Pulmonary blood flow is maintained.

VAECMO

The multitude of indications include cardiogenic shock, refractory cardiac arrhythmias and myocarditis. The steps are as follows:

1 Large cannulas are inserted into a major vein and artery e.g. the common femoral vein and the femoral artery, or the SVC or right atrium and carotid artery.
2 The patient is anticoagulated.
3 The heart and lungs are bypassed.
4 Blood is removed from the venous system, oxygenated and then pumped into the arterial system.

Complications

There are many potential complications of this highly invasive therapy including:

1 haemorrhage due to anticoagulation and loss of platelets
2 thromboembolism
3 cerebral infarction
4 infection
5 limb ischaemia/major tissue loss/amputation.

◖ Ex utero intrapartum treatment (EXIT) procedure

Description

The EXIT procedure involves performing a caesarean section in such a way that uteroplacental circulation is maintained until the fetal airway is secured. The most common indications are masses of the head and neck such as cystic hygroma or mandibular hypoplasia. Lung or mediastinal masses may require EXIT to ECMO. *See Extracorporeal membrane oxygenation (ECMO).*

Medical staff and extra equipment required

1 Obstetric anaesthetist.
2 Paediatric anaesthetist.
3 Obstetric surgeon.
4 Paediatric airway surgeon (if tracheostomy required).
5 Neonatologist.
6 Ventilator for the neonate.
7 Cell salvage machine. *See Blood salvage, intraoperative.*

Anaesthetic approach

1 Prepare for massive blood loss—have two large-bore IV cannulas, arterial line, group and hold available.
2 Prepare a glyceryl trinitrate infusion. *See Glyceryl trinitrate (GTN).*
3 Induce GA as described in *Caesarean section.*

4 It is very important to keep the mother warm with strategies such as a forced-air warming blanket.

5 Place patient in lithotomy position so that the neonatal team can work between the mother's legs.

6 Provide uterine relaxation with high-dose inspired sevoflurane (2.8–4.5%) for 20 min prior to skin incision. In addition, give 50 mcg boluses of GTN 5 min before skin incision + an infusion run at 6 mL/h (50 mg GTN in 100 mL 5% glucose).

7 Use a remifentanil infusion for maternal analgesia and to reduce the respiratory drive of the fetus. Use a dose of around 0.15 mcg/kg/min.

8 Support blood pressure with a metaraminol or phenylephrine infusion and IV fluids.

9 Ensure the mother is fully relaxed with rocuronium.

10 The uterus will be incised and the fetal head and one arm delivered.

11 The neonatal team will cannulate the fetus and provide additional fetal anaesthesia/muscle relaxation with fentanyl and rocuronium. It is very important that the fetus does not attempt to breathe.

12 The obstetrician will maintain uterine amniotic fluid volume with infused warm Hartmann's solution or N/S.

13 Blood loss from the uterine incision can be reduced by uterine sutures or staples.

14 Once the neonatal airway is secured and the baby is delivered, cease GTN infusion and reduce the inhaled volatile concentration to a level sufficient for anaesthesia.

15 Give oxytocin 5 units and start an oxytocin infusion (40 IU in 1000 mL Hartmann's solution over 4 h).

16 Give appropriate maternal analgesia as described in *Caesarean section*.

17 Treat postpartum haemorrhage as described in *Postpartum haemorrhage*. There may be persistent uterine atony.

Eye blocks

Eye blocks are performed for surgery such as cataract extraction and insertion of an intraocular lens.

Innervation of the eye

1 Sensation of the cornea and conjunctiva is provided by the ophthalmic division of the trigeminal nerve.

2 VI cranial nerve (abducens) supplies the lateral rectus.

3 IV cranial nerve (trochlear) supplies the superior oblique muscle.

4 The rest of the muscles are supplied by cranial nerve III (oculomotor).

Types of eye block

Two types of eye block will be described—peribulbar and sub-Tenon's. Establish IV access before performing the eye block and use a careful aseptic technique.

Peribulbar eye block

There are many variations of the peribulbar block.

1 Draw up 10 mL lignocaine 2% + 30 units/mL hyalase (hyaluronidase).

2 Use a 25 G 33 mm orbital block needle.

3 Anaesthetise the conjunctiva with topical amethocaine 1%.

4 Prep the skin around the eye with 5% povidone iodine.

5 With the patient supine, ask them to fix their gaze on an object on the ceiling (eye in the neutral position).

6 Identify the junction of the medial two-thirds and lateral one-third of the lower rim of the orbit. This is the insertion point.

7 Elevate the globe by pushing on the skin below the eye with the non-dominant hand.

8 Insert the needle with the bevel facing towards the globe.

9 Insert the needle very close to the floor of the orbit until past the equator of the eye (orbital floor bone may be encountered), then direct the needle slightly upward and medially.

10 Make sure the eye can move freely.

11 Aspirate for blood.

12 Inject 4–8 mL of LA slowly. Ptosis and mild protrusion of the eyeball should occur.

13 Massage the eye with the eyelid closed using fingers and gauze.

14 If the block is inadequate, a second injection can be performed 2 mm inferior and 2 mm medial to the supraorbital notch.

15 Insert the needle about 15 mm in a direction 90° to the orbit.

16 Inject 2–3 mL of LA and repeat eye massage.

Risks of peribulbar eye block

1 Globe perforation.

2 Damage to other eye structures e.g. optic nerve.

3 Periorbital haemorrhage.

4 Retrobulbar haemorrhage.

5 Brainstem anaesthesia. *See Brainstem anaesthesia*.

Sub-Tenon's eye block

Tenon's capsule is a dense layer of white connective tissue surrounding the globe and the extraocular muscles at the front of the orbit. It lies directly under the conjunctiva and overlies the sclera. Sub-Tenon's space is a potential space between the sclera and the Tenon's capsule. The capsule is avascular, mucoid, mobile and may be poorly defined. The sclera is white, dense, avascular and fibrous. Use a 50:50 mix of lignocaine 2% and ropivacaine 1% plus hyalase 30 units/mL. Do not perform the block if there is a large pterygium, a retinal band or a scleral buckle.

Technique

1 Anaesthetise the eye with amethocaine 1%.

2 Sterilise the conjunctiva with 5% povidone-iodine.

3 Clean the upper and lower eyelids by wiping them with 5% povidone iodine and sterile gauze.

4 Position the eyelid speculum to keep the eye open. The patient should look upwards and outwards.

5 Use the Moorfield non-toothed forceps to pick up the conjunctiva and capsule at the inferonasal point at least 7 mm from the edge of the iris. This is the entry point.

6 Use a pair of Westcott scissors to make a 1–2 mm cut through the conjunctiva and capsule, avoiding conjunctival blood vessels while holding the tissue elevated with the forceps.

7 The closed scissors are gently advanced through the cut, opened slightly, withdrawn, closed and advanced again. This is repeated until the tips of the scissors are around the globe and nearly vertical.

8 Still holding the conjunctiva and Tenon's capsule opening with the forceps, insert the lacrimal cannula (Southampton needle). Follow the curve of the globe towards

the back of the eye between the attachments of the medial and inferior rectus. Hydro-dissection, used gently, may assist the passage of the cannula by breaking adhesions between the sclera and Tenon's capsule.

9 Insert the cannula fully.

10 Inject 3–4 mL of LA + hyalase over 15–30 s. Use the forceps to pinch around the cannula gently. Consider changing the cannula tip position slightly after each mL. Conjunctival distension may indicate the injection is subconjunctival rather than sub-Tenon's.

11 After the injection, remove the cannula and eye speculum. Massage the closed eye with gloved fingers and gauze.

Complications

1 Conjunctival haemorrhage.

2 Chemosis.

◐ Eye injury, penetrating

Description

A penetrating eye injury with perforation of the globe can result in expulsion of intraocular contents if intraocular pressure (IOP) increases. The normal value for IOP is 16 ± 5 mmHg. Increases in IOP > 24 mmHg are pathological. IOP can be increased by:

1 Drugs such as suxamethonium or ketamine. Suxamethonium increases IOP by 6–12 mmHg. However, see comments below regarding its use in a GA with a full stomach scenario.

2 Coughing, straining, vomiting. These actions can increase IOP up to 30–40 mmHg.[10]

3 Laryngoscopy, intubation.

4 Hypoxia, hypercarbia.

5 Head-down position.

6 Hypertension.

Eye injury and the full stomach

The factors to consider are as follows.

1 Can surgery wait until the stomach is empty?

2 Is the eye salvageable?

3 Can the injury be repaired with topical anaesthesia or an eye block?

General anaesthesia with full stomach

1 Consider measures to decrease the risk/effects of aspiration—metoclopramide 10 mg IV, sodium citrate 0.3 M 30 mL PO.

2 Midazolam 2–3 mg IV in the adult.

3 Position the patient sitting up at 15–20°.

4 Pre-oxygenate without pressure on the injured eye.

5 Give lignocaine 1.5 mg/kg IV and fentanyl 2–3 mcg/kg IV two minutes before induction.

6 Perform a modified rapid sequence induction with an appropriate dose of propofol and rocuronium 1.2 mg/kg. If rocuronium cannot be used the next best safest option is suxamethonium 1.5 mg/kg IV. Even though this drug increases IOP, vitreous extrusion with suxamethonium in this situation is extremely rare.[11]

7 Ensure full paralysis has occurred before laryngoscopy (using a nerve stimulator).

8 Administer ondansetron 4 mg and dexamethasone 4–8 mg to reduce the risk of postoperative nausea and vomiting.

9 Give lignocaine 1.5 mg/kg IV before extubation to reduce the risk of coughing.

10 After the completion of surgery, extubate the patient on their left side when they are able to protect their own airway.

REFERENCES

1 Gite JV, Gangakhedkar GR, Nadkarni M. Anaesthetic management of caesarean section in a patient with Ebstein's anomaly. *Indian J Anaesth* 2018; 62: 915–916.

2 Wiesmann T, Castori M, Malfait F, Wulf H. Recommendations for anaesthesia and perioperative management in patients with Ehlers-Danlos syndrome(s). *Orphanet J Rare Diseases* 2014; 9: 109.

3 Arendt KW. Anesthesia for labor and delivery in high-risk heart disease: specific lesions. *UpToDate* July 2022. Accessed online: www.uptodate.com/contents/anesthesia-for-labor-and-delivery-in-high-risk-heart-disease-specific-lesions#!, December 2022.

4 Fang G, Tian YK, Mei W. Anaesthesia management of caesarean section in two patients with Eisenmenger's syndrome. *Anesthesiol Res Pract* 2011; 972671. Accessed online: https://europepmc.org/article/MED/21961000, December 2022.

5 Sexton DJ, Sampson JH. Spinal epidural abscess. *UpToDate* May 2022. Accessed online: www.uptodate.com/contents/spinal-epidural-abscess, December 2022.

6 Brown DL, Wedel DJ. Spinal, epidural and caudal anaesthesia. In: Miller RD (ed). *Anaesthesia,* 3rd edn. Churchill Livingstone, New York, 1990: 1397.

7 Evron S, Gladkov V, Sessler D et al. Predistension of the epidural space before catheter insertion reduces the incidence of intravascular epidural catheter insertion. *Anesth Analg* 2007; 105: 460–464.

8 Vandermeulen EP, Van Aken H, Vermelyn J. Anticoagulants and spinal-epidural analgesia. *Anesth Analg* 1994; 79: 1165–1177.

9 Lichtor L, Rodriguez MR, Aaronson N et al. Epiglottitis: it hasn't gone away. *Anesthesiol* 2016; 124: 1404–1407.

10 Kelly DJ, Farrell SM. Physiology and role of intraocular pressure in contemporary anesthesia. *Anesth Analg.* 2018; 126: 1551–62. https://doi.org/10.12.1213/ANE:0000000000002544.

11 Redelinghuys C. Anaesthesia for open eye injuries. *Southern African J Anaesth Anag.* 2021;27:210–213. https://doi.org/10.36303/SAJAA.2021.27.6.S1.2718.

○ Factor V Leiden mutation

FV acts as a cofactor for FXa. Protein C degrades FV. The factor V Leiden mutation inhibits this degradation process, leading to thrombogenic disease.

○ Factor VIII concentrate

Description

FVIII may be derived from plasma or be a recombinant product. It is used to treat haemophilia A. *See Haemophilia*. There are standard life products (half-life 8–12 h) and extended life products.

Dose

1 unit/kg will increase FVIII levels by 2%. 50 units/kg will increase FVIII levels by 100%. Round dose up to nearest vial. For patients with severe bleeding or surgery, give as an IV bolus LD then an infusion of 3 units/kg/h.

○ Factor IX concentrate

Description

FIX may be derived from plasma or created by recombinant technology. Used to treat haemophilia B. *See Haemophilia*. 1 unit/kg increases FIX levels by 0.7–1%. 50 units/kg would increase levels by 30–50%.

Dose

For patients with severe bleeding or surgery, give a bolus dose 100 units/kg then infusion of 3 units/kg/h.

○ Fascia iliaca block

Indications and rationale

This block is used for analgesia for hip injury such as fractured neck of femur and hip surgery such as joint replacement. It can also be used for femoral shaft fractures.
The aim of the block is to anaesthetise the femoral, lateral femoral cutaneous and the obturator nerves. These nerves are sandwiched between the fascia iliaca and the iliopsoas muscle.
Use 20 mL of ropivacaine 1% mixed with 40 mL N/S (total volume 60 mL) and an 80 mm short-bevelled block needle.

Anatomy

The medial surface of the ilium is lined by the iliacus muscle. The psoas muscle attaches proximally to the vertebral bodies of T12 to L4. These muscles fuse to form the iliopsoas muscle, which passes under the inguinal ligament to insert into the lesser trochanter. Overlying these muscles are the fascia lata and, more deeply, the fascia iliaca. The femoral artery and vein lie under the fascia lata but are superficial to the fascia iliaca, whereas the femoral nerve is deep to both fasciae.

Contraindications

1 Infection at the site of insertion.
2 Anticoagulation.
3 Inguinal hernia or repaired inguinal hernia.
4 Femoral artery surgery.
5 Patient refusal (as for any other procedure).

Technique

1 Position the patient supine and insert an IV cannula.
2 Using aseptic technique, place the ultrasound (U/S) probe on the anterior superior iliac spine (ASIS). This bony prominence is obvious on U/S.
3 Orientate the probe so the marker end is pointing halfway between the xiphisternum and the umbilicus.
4 Move the probe 2.5 cm laterally and slightly caudally.
5 The target image is the 'hour glass' or 'bow tie' shape. The marker end of the probe will show the internal oblique muscle and the other end will show the sartorius muscle (two sides of the 'bow tie'). Deep to the 'bow tie' is the fascia iliaca and, beneath that, the iliopsoas muscle. Use colour doppler to identify blood vessels in the needle path.
6 Insert the needle in-plane in a caudal-to-cranial direction through the sartorius muscle to pierce the centre of the 'bow tie' and perform the injection, after negative aspiration and a 2 mL test dose (Figures F1 and F2).

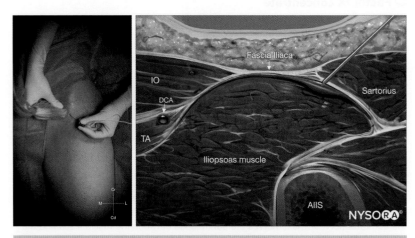

Figure F1 Correct probe and needle position for fascia iliaca block. IO = internal oblique muscle, TA = transversus abdominus muscle, AIIS = anterior inferior iliac spine
Image courtesy of NYSORA

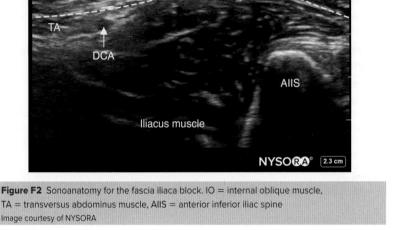

Figure F2 Sonoanatomy for the fascia iliaca block. IO = internal oblique muscle, TA = transversus abdominus muscle, AIIS = anterior inferior iliac spine
Image courtesy of NYSORA

An alternative approach is:

1 With a probe parallel and just caudal to the inguinal ligament, identify the femoral artery, vein and nerve. See Figure F3 in *Femoral nerve block*.
2 Insert the block needle in-plane from lateral to medial to pierce the fascia lata and fascia iliaca (two pops) lateral to the femoral nerve.
3 Inject the LA at this site.

◗ FAST

This is a screening tool for stroke. The letters of this acronym stand for:

F – **F**acial asymmetry—ask the patient to smile.
A – **A**rms—ask the patient to raise their arms.
S – **S**peech—is the patient's speech slurred?
T – **T**ime—time is of the essence.

◗ Fasting prior to anaesthesia

These fasting guidelines are based on ANZCA guideline PG07(A) Appendix 1, July 2021 *Guideline on pre-anaesthesia consultation and patient preparation*. They apply to patients undergoing GA, major regional anaesthesia and sedation.

Adult

1 Limited solid food can be consumed up to 6 h prior to anaesthesia.
2 Clear fluids (water, clear juices, glucose-based drinks, cordials, black tea and black coffee) up to 400 mL can be consumed up to 2 h before anaesthesia. Clear fluids must be transparent with no solids in the fluid. Jelly is not included.
3 Although not in the current ANZCA guidelines, sips of water are probably acceptable anytime.[1]

Child

1 Children over 6 months of age can have limited solid food or formula up to 6 h before anaesthesia. Breast milk can be given up to 4 h before anaesthesia and clear fluids (up to 3 mL/kg) up to 1 h before anaesthesia.
2 Children under 6 months can have formula up to 4 h before anaesthesia and breast milk up to 3 h before anaesthesia. Clear fluids (up to 3 mL/kg) can be given up to 1 h before anaesthesia.

◐ Fat embolism syndrome (FES) and bone cement implantation syndrome (BCIS)

Fat embolism

Description

Fat embolism is a condition in which fat globules and bone marrow elements embolise and can cause life-threatening brain and lung effects. How fat causes FES is unknown. There may be an element of mechanical obstruction of blood vessels and/or a reaction to the fat, resulting in the production of substances which damage cells.

Causes

1 Long bone fractures (especially femur and tibia) and pelvic fractures.
2 Surgery on the long bones e.g. intramedullary nailing.
3 Bone marrow transplant.
4 Liposuction.

Clinical effects

1 Respiratory distress, hypoxia, pulmonary oedema.
2 Confusion, restlessness, coma.
3 Petechial rash, especially in the upper half of the body, conjunctiva and mucous membranes of the mouth.
4 Fever.
5 Retinal exudates and haemorrhages. Fat droplets may be seen traversing retinal blood vessels.
6 Coagulopathy/thrombocytopenia.

Diagnosis

There is no specific diagnostic test.
1 CXR may show diffuse pulmonary infiltrates.
2 ECG may show right ventricular strain pattern—RBBB, right axis deviation, prominent S wave in I, Q wave in III and inverted T wave in III.
3 ABG may show hypoxia, large A-a gradient (*see A-a gradient*).
4 Fat globules may be visible in urine or sputum.
5 A fall in end tidal CO_2 during anaesthesia may indicate a fat embolus is occurring.
6 MRI may be diagnostic of fat embolism to the brain.

Treatment

Supportive measures mainly concerning oxygenation and haemodynamic support. Treatment may include:
1 O_2 therapy
2 non-invasive ventilation
3 IPPV + PEEP
4 ECMO—*see Extra corporeal membrane oxygenation (ECMO)*
5 IV fluids, vasopressors, inotropes.

Bone cement implantation syndrome (BCIS)

Description

BCIS can occur with cemented total hip replacement surgery during the peri-cementation period. Material that embolises may include:

1 fat
2 bone powder
3 bone marrow elements
4 bone cement (unlikely).

Clinical effects

Effects vary from mild and unnoticed to fatal. Presentation may include:

1 sudden loss of consciousness if having surgery awake under neuraxial anaesthesia
2 hypotension
3 hypoxaemia
4 pulmonary hypertension
5 cardiac arrhythmias
6 cardiac arrest
7 sudden fall in end tidal CO_2.

Diagnosis

Diagnosed on clinical grounds.

Treatment

Supportive, including:

1 supporting blood pressure with IV fluids, vasopressors
2 inotropes if needed
3 maintaining oxygenation as for FES.

◗ Fatty liver of pregnancy

See Acute fatty liver of pregnancy (AFLP).

◗ FEIBA-NF (factor VIII inhibitor bypassing activity)

Description

This drug is used to control or prevent bleeding episodes in patients with haemophilia A or B with inhibitors (antibodies) to FVIII or FIX. *See Haemophilia*. It can also be considered for the treatment of bleeding associated with oral factor Xa inhibitors (rivaroxaban, apixaban). It contains factors II, VII, IX and X plus activated factor VII. It may be helpful in treating bleeding patients on fondaparinux.

Dose

50–100 IU/kg IV every 12 h for bleeding episodes.

◗ Femoral nerve block

Anatomy

The femoral nerve is derived from L2, 3, 4 of the lumbar plexus. It is sensory to the anterior thigh, and through the saphenous nerve branch, supplies sensation to the medial lower leg, ankle and foot. *See Adductor canal block*. The femoral nerve supplies the quadriceps muscle and other muscles of the anterior thigh. It enters the thigh beneath the inguinal ligament lateral to the femoral artery. Note that the femoral nerve is below the fascia lata and enveloped by the fascia iliaca. The femoral artery is **between** the fascia lata and iliaca. *See Fascia iliaca block (FIB)*.

Femoral nerve block is useful for analgesia following:
1 knee surgery
2 surgery on the anterior thigh e.g. quadriceps tendon repair
3 surgery on the medial lower leg
4 femoral shaft and neck fractures.

Technique using ultrasound

Secure IV access and sterilise the target area—the mid-inguinal ligament and anterior upper thigh.
1 Identify the femoral artery in transverse view (probe parallel and below the inguinal ligament) in the femoral crease.
2 The femoral nerve is triangular and lateral to the artery (like a hat on the head of a reclining clown).
3 Anaesthetise the skin, then insert a short-bevelled block needle in-plane from lateral to medial.
4 Penetrate the fascia lata and the fascia iliaca near the apex of the triangular nerve. Two 'pops' should be felt.
5 Aspirate to check for blood.
6 After a 2 mL test dose, inject 10 mL of ropivacaine 1%, which should push the nerve downwards.
7 Reposition the needle towards the lower part of the nerve, aspirate and then inject a further 10 mL of ropivacaine 1%.

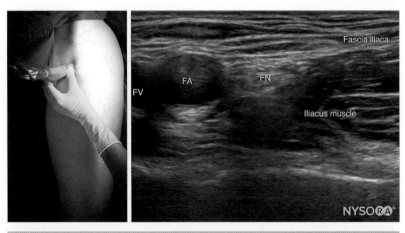

Figure F3 Probe position and sonoanatomy of the femoral nerve. FN = femoral nerve, FA = femoral artery, FV = femoral vein. The femoral nerve sits like a clown's hat on the femoral artery
Image courtesy of NYSORA

▶ Fenoldopam

Description

Fenoldopam is used to treat severe hypertension. It is a synthetic benzazepine derivative which acts on selective D_1 receptors as a partial agonist. The D_1 receptor is a dopamine receptor found in the CNS and cardiovascular system (CVS). **See *Dopamine receptors*.** Activation of D_1 receptors in the CVS causes a reduction in systemic vascular resistance (SVR). It does this by activating adenyl cyclase, increasing intracellular cyclic AMP, which causes vasodilation in most arterial beds. It decreases afterload and promotes renal perfusion and sodium excretion by the kidney. It also increases diuresis. It has no beta effects but may have some alpha-1 and alpha-2 agonist effects.

Dose

Adult

1. Initiate treatment with an IV infusion run at 0.1–0.3 mcg/kg/min.
2. Increase by 0.05–0.1 mcg/kg/min at 15 min intervals until desired BP is reached or a maximum of 1.6 mcg/kg/min is reached.

Advantages

1. It is the only antihypertensive agent that improves renal perfusion. It may be of benefit in severely hypertensive patients with chronic kidney disease.
2. Can be used in liver and kidney disease.

Disadvantages

1. A reflex tachycardia may occur—this may cause/exacerbate angina.
2. The drug increases intraocular pressure so may be unsuitable in patients with glaucoma.

Fenpatch

This a trade name for transdermal fentanyl patches that provide fentanyl at 12–100 mcg/h.

Fentanyl

Description

Synthetic opioid drug with a similar structure to pethidine. It is the most popular opioid used in anaesthetics by anaesthestists due to its advantages as described below. It has a short duration of action at doses < 10 mcg/kg but it becomes long acting at higher doses (50–100 mcg/kg).

Dose

Adult

Depending on the type and duration of surgery, doses of 100–500 mcg are commonly used. 50–100 mcg will last 30–60 min. In cardiac surgery, very large doses may be used e.g. 1–1.5 mg. The effects of very large doses last about 6 h.

1. *Epidural*—50–100 mcg.
2. *SAB*—20–25 mcg.
3. *IV infusion*—50 mcg/kg in 50 mL N/S run at 1–4 mL/h (1–4 mcg/kg/h).
4. *PCA*—20–30 mcg boluses with a 5 min lockout.
5. *Fentanyl patches*—available in five different strengths: 12, 25, 50, 75 and 100 mcg/h. The patches are applied for 72 h. They should be continued post-surgery if the patient has been on them long term. Fentanyl 50 mcg/h is equivalent to 135–244 mg/day oral morphine.
6. *Fentanyl intranasal spray*—nasal fentanyl is about 70% as effective as IV fentanyl. It is available in strengths of 50, 100 and 200 mcg.

7 *Fentanyl buccal tablets*—these are rapidly effective and provide analgesia in 10–15 min.

8 *Fentanyl lollipop*—used to treat patients who are unable to take oral medications, severe cancer pain, and novel situations such as soldiers injured in combat.

Child

Depends on the type and duration of surgery—1–2 mcg/kg is a reasonable starting point.

Advantages

1 Very high margin of safety with little myocardial depression. It may cause bradycardia.

2 Rapid onset when used IV (< 1 min), with peak effects in 2–5 min.

3 Very potent (100 × more potent than morphine, 50 × more potent than heroin).

4 Safe to use in renal failure. It is metabolised renally with no active metabolites.

5 Does not cause histamine release.

Disadvantages

1 Shorter-acting (1–2 h) than morphine (about 4 h).

2 More addictive than morphine. Fentanyl and its analogues account for more deaths than any other opioid in the USA.[2] Opioids are involved in more than 70 000 overdose deaths per year in the USA.[2]

3 Has serotonergic properties and is a medium-risk drug for inducing serotonin syndrome. **See *Serotonin syndrome*.**

4 Muscle rigidity can occur with high doses. Wooden chest syndrome can occur— sudden rigidity of abdominal and chest muscles and diaphragm, leading to respiratory failure.[3]

◖ Fentanyl Sandoz

This is a trade name for fentanyl patches providing transdermal fentanyl at a rate of 12–100 mcg/h.

◖ Fetal death in utero

*See **Intrauterine fetal death**.*

◖ Fetal resuscitation in utero

*See **Intrauterine fetal resuscitation**.*

◖ Fetal scalp blood sampling

This can be used as an indicator of fetal welfare. pH and lactate can be measured to help determine the optimal delivery time.

Table F1 Fetal scalp blood pH and lactate and its significance

Fetal scalp pH	Lactate mmol/L	Comment
7.25–7.35	< 4.2	Normal
7.2–7.24	4.2–4.8	Non-reassuring—repeat in 30 min
< 7.2	4.9–5.7	Consider immediate delivery
	> 5.7	Immediate delivery

● Fibrinogen

Fibrinogen is a glycoprotein complex clotting factor that is manufactured in the liver. The NR is 2–4 g/L. Thrombin converts fibrinogen to fibrin monomers in the common clotting pathway. **See *Clotting pathways*.** It is available clinically as:

1 Fresh frozen plasma (FFP). **See *Fresh frozen plasma (FFP)*.** 1 g of fibrinogen is present in 4 units of FFP.
2 Cryoprecipitate (**see *Cryoprecipitate*).**
3 Fibrinogen concentrate (**see *Fibrinogen concentrate).***

When used therapeutically in severe haemorrhage, fibrinogen improves clot firmness, decreases blood loss and increases survival rates.

Fibrinogen level and bleeding

Aim for a plasma fibrinogen level > 1.5 g/L in non-obstetric haemorrhage and > 2 g/L in obstetric haemorrhage.

● Fibrinogen concentrate

There is 1 g of fibrinogen in 50 mL of fibrinogen concentrate. For hypofibrinogenaemia give 25–50 mg/kg.

● Fluid replacement therapy (maintenance)

Adult

Use the formula 40 mL + 1 mL/kg = mL/h. A heathy 70 kg patient requires about 110 mL/h maintenance fluid.

Child (hourly rate maintenance fluid)

4 mL/kg first 10 kg + 2 mL/kg next 10 kg then 1 mL/kg rest of weight—therefore a 32 kg child requires 72 mL/h. Standard fluid in child < 1 year: N/4 saline + 5–10% glucose. Older child: N/4 saline + 3.75% glucose. Potassium requirements are 3 mmol/kg/day. Ensure urine output is established before giving potassium.

● Flumazenil

Description

An imidazobenzodiazepine drug which is a competitive antagonist of benzodiazepine drugs such as midazolam. It acts by binding to the benzodiazepine receptor site on the GABA/benzodiazepine receptor complex.

Dose

Adult

Give 200 mcg IV over 15 s, then 100 mcg at 60 s intervals up to 1 mg (up to 2 mg in ICU). Effects last 15–140 min and re-sedation may occur. The IV infusion dose range is 100–400 mcg/h.

Child

1 5–10 mcg/kg (max 200 mcg) IV bolus. Repeat dose at 60 s intervals to a max dose of 50 mcg/kg or 1 mg, whichever is less.
2 IV infusion dose 2–10 mcg/kg/h.

❖ Focal atrial tachycardia (FAT)

Description

This supraventricular tachycardia (SVT) arises from a single focus in either the right or left atrium. Rate > 100 bpm. Attacks are usually paroxysmal and self-limiting. It may be associated with chronic heart disease or occur in normal hearts. Incessant FAT can result in cardiomyopathy.

Treatment

1 Reverse associated pathology.
2 Vagal manoeuvres.
3 Adenosine.
4 Metoprolol or diltiazem.
5 Amiodarone.
6 Cardioversion.
7 Ablation therapy.

❖ Fondaparinux

Description

This pentasaccharide drug is a selective inhibitor of factor Xa and is used as an anticoagulant. It can be used in patients who cannot have heparin due to HIT. *See Heparin-induced thrombocytopenia (HIT).*

Dose

Adult

* Prophylactic dose—2.5 mg/day subcut. Reduce to 1.5 mg/day if renal insufficiency.
* Therapeutic dose—5–10 mg/day. Effects can be monitored by measuring anti-FXa activity.

Points to note:

1 Renally excreted—not suitable for patients with severe renal impairment/failure.
2 Experience with neuraxial anaesthesia and fondaparinux is limited. Do not perform SAB within 3–4 days of the last dose. Do not use epidural catheters. *See Anticoagulant and antiplatelet drugs and surgery/neuraxial anaesthesia.*
3 Recombinant activated FVII may be effective in a bleeding emergency associated with fondaparinux. Give 90 mcg/kg IV. Factor VIII inhibitor bypassing activity (FEIBA) contains variable amounts of activated clotting factors and may be helpful in a patient that is bleeding while on fondaparinux. Give 50 U/kg IV. *See FEIBA-NF (factor VIII inhibitor bypassing activity).*

❖ Fontan procedure/Fontan circulation

Description

This procedure is used to palliate congenital heart disease (CHD) when there is only one functioning ventricle. It endeavours to divert systemic venous blood from the inferior and superior vena cava (IVC and SVC) towards the pulmonary artery (PA), bypassing the right ventricle (RV). Conditions in which it is used include:

1 hypoplastic left heart syndrome or hypoplastic right heart syndrome
2 tricuspid, pulmonary or mitral valve atresia

3 double inlet left ventricle
4 double outlet right ventricle
5 complete atrioventricular septal defects
6 other complex types of CHD where definitive repair is impossible or ill advised.

Blood is not 'pumped' through the lungs—it flows through the lungs under venous pressure. Therefore, central venous pressure (CVP) and pulmonary vascular resistance (PVR) are critical. If PVR rises or CVP falls, lung blood flow is reduced.

Stages of the repair

1 Blalock–Taussig shunt procedure—a graft is placed between the right subclavian artery and the right pulmonary vein.
2 Bidirectional Glenn procedure (hemi-Fontan)—the SVC is disconnected from the right atrium and attached to the right pulmonary artery.
3 Fontan–Kreutzer completion—the IVC is disconnected from the heart and attached to a pulmonary artery. This may be done using graft material.

There are many variations of this highly oversimplified description. One variation is to place a baffle in the right atrium to partition systemic and pulmonary venous blood. Systemic venous blood goes to the lungs and pulmonary venous blood goes to the functional ventricle to be pumped around the body. Small holes can be made in the baffle so if PVR rises, blood can be directed away from the pulmonary arteries (acting as a 'pop-off' valve).

Pathophysiology of Fontan circulation[4]

1 The dominant limiting factor in ventricular function is preload.
2 Blood flow from the systemic circulation into the lungs is entirely passive.
3 Arrhythmias can occur.
4 Shunts. Due to such effects as baffle fenestrations and drainage of coronary sinus blood into the systemic circulation, right-to-left shunting and desaturation may occur. Left-to-right shunting may occur through aorto-pulmonary collaterals.
5 Volume overload of the functioning ventricle with dilation, hypertrophy and reduced contractility.
6 Increased pulmonary vascular resistance (PVR) due to high pulmonary blood flow.
7 Protein-losing enteropathy—there is a loss of protein from the plasma into the gut. This may be due to high SVC pressure impeding drainage of the thoracic duct. There may also be mesenteric inflammation. This can cause:
a) oedema
b) immunodeficiency
c) ascites
d) malabsorption of fat
e) hypocalcaemia/hypomagnesaemia.
8 Chronic hepatic congestion with cirrhosis/fibrosis with an increased tendency to thromboembolic disease.

Anaesthesia and Fontan circulation

Many patients with a Fontan repair will undergo a gradual decline in exercise capacity and have a shortened lifespan. Patients may be taking diuretics, steroids and octreotide for protein-losing enteropathy. All patients are prone to thromboembolism and will be on warfarin or antiplatelet drugs. Some patients may be on antiarrhythmic drugs.

The principles of anaesthetic management are as follows:

1 Defend CVP—avoid hypovolaemia and decreased SVR. Maintain sinus rhythm (SR).

2 Avoid drugs with negative inotropic effects such as beta blockers and excess volatile anaesthetic.

3 Avoid drugs and other factors that increase pulmonary vascular resistance. *See Pulmonary hypertension.*

4 Invasive arterial monitoring should be used except for very minor procedures.

5 Transoesophageal echocardiography (TOE) can help intraoperatively to assess ventricular filling and function.

6 Maintain O_2 saturation $> 95\%$. Increased O_2 requirement is indicative of increased right-to-left shunt through a fenestration or intrapulmonary shunts. Exclude/treat:
   a) decreased ventricular function
   b) increased PVR
   c) increased mean intrathoracic pressure.

7 For patients that are paralysed and ventilated, use low respiratory rates, short inspiratory times, low PEEP values and tidal volumes of 5–6 mL/kg.

8 Consider the need for bacterial endocarditis prophylaxis. *See Bacterial endocarditis (BE) prophylaxis.*

9 Postoperative management should be in ICU/HDU following significant surgery.

Obstetrics and Fontan circulation

The physiological changes of pregnancy may stress the Fontan circulation in the following ways.

1 Increased blood volume may lead to atrial distension and arrhythmias.

2 Increased risk of thromboembolic complications.

Labour

Epidural block in labour should be titrated cautiously with adequate fluid loading. Epidural anaesthesia is helpful in avoiding excessive straining in the second stage of labour, which can reduce pulmonary blood flow by increasing intrathoracic pressure. Forceps-assisted delivery may further reduce straining.

Caesarean section

1 Use epidural anaesthesia or CSE with a low-dose spinal component.

2 Consider invasive arterial monitoring.

3 Avoid vasopressors with alpha agonist properties as these may increase PVR.

4 Avoid ergometrine, which may cause coronary artery spasm and increased PVR.

5 Avoid prostaglandin F2 alpha, which may cause bronchospasm, intrapulmonary shunting and severe hypoxaemia.

Laparoscopic surgery

Laparoscopic surgery can result in adverse effects in Fontan circulation. The following should be considered.

1 Use low intra-abdominal inflation pressures. Abdominal pressure < 10 mmHg will increase venous return and CO, but pressures > 15 mmHg will compress the IVC and have the opposite effect.

2 CO_2 distension of the abdomen may increase blood CO_2 levels, leading to increased PVR. Avoid/treat hypercarbia.

3 Fenestrations in the baffle may increase the risk of CO_2 embolism entering the systemic arterial circulation.

◗ Forehead block

This block is useful for surgery on the forehead and anterior scalp to the vertex.

Anatomy

The supraorbital nerve supplies the upper eyelid medially, and the forehead and scalp to the vertex. The supratrochlear nerve supplies the conjunctiva and the skin of the medial upper eyelid, the skin of the medial orbit and the root of the nose.

Technique

About 8 mL of 2% lignocaine is required. Using a sterile technique:

1 Identify the supraorbital notch (in the same sagittal plane as the pupil in the neutral position).
2 Insert the needle just below the eyebrow in the same plane as the eyebrow, aiming towards the midline. Inject 1 mL of LA just above the notch to block the supraorbital nerve.
3 Advance the needle 1 cm further medially and inject 1 mL of LA to block the supratrochlear nerve.

◗ Fresh frozen plasma (FFP)

FFP is plasma separated from a whole blood donation. It contains all the coagulation factors, albumin and other plasma proteins. The volume of 1 bag is 250–334 mL. A typical dose for a 70 kg adult is 10–15 mL/kg (3–4 bags). Thawed FFP can be accepted back into inventory if it has been out of controlled storage (2–6° C) for 30 min or less on one occasion only. FFP can be stored for 12 months at minus 25° C or below. Thawed FFP kept at 2–6° C can be used for up to 24 h. It is preferable to give FFP that is of a compatible blood group for the recipient. AB FFP can be given to any recipient. Matching Rh status is not necessary. Group O FFP can **only** be given to a blood group O recipient.

Table F2 Compatibility of transfused FFP based on recipient's blood group

Recipient blood group	FFP donor blood group
O	O, A, B, AB
A	A, AB
B	B, AB
AB	AB

◗ Frusemide/Furosemide

Description

Frusemide is a loop diuretic that inhibits the sodium-potassium chloride co-transporter in the thick ascending limb of the loop of Henle. It does this by binding to the chloride transport channel. This causes increased excretion of sodium, chloride, potassium and water. Frusemide is a sulphonamide derivative.

Indications

Frusemide is used to treat oedema associated with:

1 Congestive cardiac failure. *See Congestive cardiac failure (CCF)—chronic.*
2 Liver cirrhosis.
3 Kidney disease.
4 Hypertension. *See Hypertension.*
5 Raised ICP. *See Intracranial pressure (ICP) and treatment of raised ICP.*

Dose

Adult

PO initial dose 20–80 mg. IV dose 40–80 mg. Frusemide can be given by infusion, commencing at 5–10 mg/h.

Points to note

1 Frusemide is contraindicated in patients who are allergic to sulfonamides.
2 Bolus IV therapy should be given slowly due to the risk of ototoxicity.

REFERENCES

1. Friedrich S, Meybohm P, Kranke P. Nulla per os (NPO) guidelines: time to revisit? *Curr Opin Anaesthesiol* 2020; 33: 740–745.
2. National Institute of Drug Abuse website. *Drug overdose death rates.* 9 February 2023. Accessed online: https://nida.nih.gov>research-topics>trends-statistic, February 2023.
3. Rosal NR, Thelmo FL, Tzarnas S et al. Wooden chest syndrome: a case report of fentanyl induced chest rigidity. *J Investig Med High Impact Case Rep* 2021; 9: 23247096211034036. Accessed online: https://www.ncbi.nlm.nih.gov/pmc/articles/PMC8312149, February 2023.
4. Nayak S, Booker PD. The Fontan circulation. *Cont Educ in Anaesth Crit Care* 2008; 1: 26–30.

▷ Gabapentin (Neurontin) and pregabalin (Lypralin, Lyrica)

Description

Gabapentin and pregabalin are termed gabapentinoids and are used orally. They are useful for treating epilepsy, neuropathic pain (such as postherpetic neuralgia), alcohol withdrawal and for reducing postoperative pain when given preoperatively. These drugs act by affecting pre-synaptic voltage-gated calcium channels. They also increase the synthesis of GABBA. There is a limitation on gabapentin's oral bioavailability due to saturation of absorption pathways. Pregabalin oral absorption is not limited.

Dose

Adult

Neuropathic pain—gabapentin 300 mg PO q 8 h to a maximum of 3600 mg/day. Pregabalin 75 mg q 12 h, increase to 150 mg q 12 h after 3—7 days, to a maximum of 300 mg q 12 h.
Postoperative pain—preoperative gabapentin 600–1200 mg PO may significantly reduce postoperative pain and PCA use.[1]

Advantages

1 Gabapentin and morphine have synergistic analgesic effects.[2]
2 Eliminated unchanged in urine but is removed by haemodialysis.
3 Extremely safe without serious toxicity, even after massive overdose.

Disadvantages

1 May cause somnolence, dizziness, ataxia and fatigue.
2 Use with caution in patients with renal impairment.
3 May cause acute reversible kidney transplant dysfunction.[3]
4 Can cause convulsions (although rarely).
5 Not recommended for use while breast feeding as it is excreted in breast milk and the effects on the neonate are unknown.
6 Gabapentinoids my cause depression, aggressive behaviour and suicidal ideation.

▷ Gas embolism

Description

The term 'gas embolism' describes gas entering a vein or artery or gas forming in the blood stream. This can cause many adverse effects and/or death.

Causes of venous gas embolism

1 Exposure of cut veins or venous sinuses to air when a pressure gradient favours the entry of air into the vein. This is particularly likely with neurosurgery and liver surgery.
2 Gas entry into the vein through IV access devices—cannula, central line (including removal of a central line).
3 Operations and procedures involving gas insufflation e.g. laparoscopy, colonoscopy.
4 Trauma.
5 Pulmonary barotrauma.

6 Decompression sickness.
7 Exposure to vacuum.

Causes of arterial gas embolism

1 Paradoxical embolism—venous gas enters the arterial system via the lungs, patent foramen ovale or a heart defect such as ventricular septal defect (VSD).
2 Decompression sickness.
3 Trauma.
4 Pulmonary barotrauma.
5 Accidental injection of air into an artery during procedures such as a cervical plexus block.
6 Exposure to vacuum.

Pathophysiology of venous and arterial gas embolism

1 Arterial gas embolism causes obstruction of small vessels, causing ischaemia of the tissue beyond the bubble(s).
2 Venous air embolus causes obstruction of flow from the heart and through the pulmonary vasculature.
3 Venous air also causes an endothelial inflammatory response, which can lead to pulmonary oedema and bronchospasm.

Clinical effects of venous gas embolism

1 Small bubbles of gas are usually benign unless they enter the arterial circulation.
2 A large volume of gas (100–300 mL), entering the venous system quickly, can cause obstruction of right ventricle (RV) outflow at the pulmonary outflow tract (air lock), causing cardiac arrest.
3 Gas entering more slowly may be trapped in pulmonary arterioles, causing pulmonary arterial hypertension and acute RV failure.
4 The type of gas is important—CO_2 is better tolerated than air due to its solubility.
5 Dyspnoea, tachypnoea.
6 Tachycardia, hypotension.
7 Altered mental state.

Clinical effects of arterial gas embolism

1 Small bubbles of gas can cause severe effects by blocking blood supply to parts of organs, most importantly the brain (stroke) and heart (ischaemia, infarction, arrhythmias).
2 The kidneys (haematuria/proteinuria) or spinal cord (paralysis) may be damaged.
3 It is a leading cause of death in scuba divers.

Diagnosis of venous gas embolus

If the patient is awake there may be dyspnoea, gasping, wheezing, chest pain, acute distress and a feeling of impending doom. There may be headache and confusion. If the patient is anaesthetised, signs include:

1 an abrupt decrease in end tidal CO_2 levels
2 hypoxia
3 ECG changes—ST depression, right-heart strain pattern (RBBB, RAD, prominent S wave in I), peaked P waves, dysrhythmias
4 hypotension, haemodynamic collapse
5 elevation of jugular venous pressure (and central venous pressure if a central line is present)
6 'mill-wheel' murmur (splashing sound) on heart auscultation

7 visible gas in the right atrium (RA), RV on cardiac echocardiography

8 sound change on precordial Doppler (irregular roaring noise).

Treatment of venous gas embolus

1 Notify the surgeon and stop more gas entering the venous system.

2 If air is entering the venous system via the surgical field, ask the surgeon to flood the surgical field with saline. The anaesthetist should lower the surgical field to a position below the heart if possible.

3 Ventilate the patient with 100% O_2.

4 IV fluid loading to increase venous pressure.

5 Support blood pressure with vasopressors, inotropes.

6 A Valsalva manoeuvre and/or neck compression (for brain surgery) may decrease air entry. It may also reveal the site of air entry to the surgeon by causing bubbles in the flooded field.

7 If cardiac arrest occurs, the performance of chest compressions may break up the air bubble.

8 If a central line is present, attempt to aspirate air from it. Consider attempting to site a central line, with the tip at the junction of the SVC and RA. The Bunegin–Albin multi-orifice central venous catheter can be used for this purpose, if available.

9 Positioning the patient left lateral and head down (Durant's manoeuvre) may move the air lock away from the RV outflow tract.

10 Surgical removal of air by thoracotomy.

Diagnosis of arterial gas embolus

1 Stroke-like effects including confusion, focal neurological deficit such as partial paralysis, sensation changes, seizures.

2 Spinal cord ischaemia.

3 Acute coronary syndrome, dysrhythmias, hypotension, cardiac arrest.

4 Purple/blue skin blotching, pale tongue.

5 Blood and/or protein in urine.

6 Severe pain anywhere in the body (but especially joints).

Treatment of arterial gas embolus

1 Stop gas from entering the arterial system.

2 Supportive measures.

3 Hyperbaric 100% oxygen is the most effective treatment.

4 Recompression, if the embolism is due to nitrogen bubbles.

◐ Gelofusine

Description

Synthetic colloid solution containing 4% succinylated bovine gelatin in saline. It is manufactured from the hydrolysis of beef collagen and has an average MW of 30 000 Daltons.

Constituents

1 Sodium 154 mmol/L.

2 Chloride 120 mmol/L.

3 pH 7.4 +/− 0.3.

4 Beef gelatin.

Uses

Hypovolaemia—plasma elimination half-life 4–5 h.

Problems

1 Risk of anaphylaxis.
2 In patients taking ACE inhibitors that are hypotensive under GA, gelofusine may worsen the hypotension.
3 Bovine spongiform encephalitis ('mad cow disease') may be transmissible in gelofusine.

◐ Gestational hypertension

This is the commonest form of hypertension seen during pregnancy. It can occur after 20 weeks' gestation but, more usually, after 37 weeks. There are no other manifestations of preeclampsia and the condition normally resolves by 12 weeks postpartum. It is associated with an increased risk of adverse outcomes e.g. placental abruption.

◐ Gestational thrombocytopenia (GT)

Up to 12% of obstetric patients develop thrombocytopenia (platelet count < 150 000 per mm³) in pregnancy. The platelet count is < 100 000 per mm³ in < 1% of pregnant patients.[4] Apart from GT, thrombocytopenia in pregnancy may be due to immune thrombocytopenia or thrombocytopenia due to preeclampsia/eclampsia. Typically, the platelet count is > 75 000 per mm³ and the patient is asymptomatic. The cause is unknown. If the platelet count is < 50 000 per mm³, then the cause is not GT.

◐ Glasgow coma scale (GCS)

The GCS was originally developed to grade the severity of head injury and predict its outcome.[5] If the left and right motor responses are different, use the highest-scoring side. There are three parts to the GCS, summarised by the letters EMV:

1 Eyes open
2 Best motor response
3 Best verbal response.

Table G1 Glasgow coma scale

Eyes open	Score
Spontaneously	4
To speech	3
To pain	2
Nil	1
Best motor response	
Obeys commands	6
Localises pain	5
Withdraws to pain	4
Abnormal flexion	3
Extensor response	2
Nil	1
Best verbal response	
Orientated	5
Confused	4
Inappropriate words	3
Sounds other than words	2
Nil	1

Source: Courtesy of University of Glasgow. https://www.thelancet.com/article/S0140-6736(74)91639-0/fulltext

◐ Glenn shunt

A Glenn shunt procedure involves the anastomosis of the superior vena cava to the right pulmonary artery to increase pulmonary blood flow. **See Bidirectional Glenn shunt.**

◐ Glucagon (GlucaGen)

Description

Peptide hormone produced by alpha cells in the pancreas. It is released in response to hypoglycaemia. Glucagon causes the liver to increase glycogenolysis (converting glycogen to glucose). The glucose is released into the blood stream to increase blood glucose levels.

Drug uses of glucagon

1 Treatment of hypoglycaemia.
2 Gastrointestinal motility inhibitor for procedures such as endoscopy, ERCP.
3 As a treatment of beta blocker overdose.
4 Treating anaphylaxis resistant to adrenaline, in patients taking beta blockers. **See Anaphylaxis.**

Dose

Adult

Hypoglycaemia—1 mg IV. Can be given IM or subcut if no IV access.
Gastrointestinal motility inhibitor—1 mg IV.
Beta blocker overdose—50 mcg/kg IV LD then continuous infusion of 1–15 mg/h titrated to response. Glucagon increases heart rate, contractility and AV conduction.
Anaphylaxis—**see Anaphylaxis.**

Contraindications

1 Phaeochromocytoma.
2 Insulinoma.
3 Glucagonoma.

◐ Glucose-6-phosphate dehydrogenase (G6PD) deficiency

Description

G6PD is an enzyme in red blood cells (RBC) which, through a biochemical pathway, prevents oxidative damage to the erythrocyte by substances such as hydrogen peroxide. G6PD deficiency is an X-linked inherited disorder, in which exposure to a triggering event or substance, results in haemolytic anaemia. This results in jaundice and dark urine. Splenomegaly may occur. There are multiple classes of G6PD deficiency. Class I is the most severe, with haemolysis even in the absence of triggering agents. Classes II and III G6PD deficiency may offer some protection against malaria. G6PD deficiency can cause neonatal jaundice.

Triggering events for haemolytic anaemia episodes

Haemolytic anaemia and jaundice may occur between 24–72 h after exposure to a trigger. Triggers include the following:
1 Bacterial and viral infections.
2 Eating fava beans (favism is a severe acute haemolytic anaemia).

3 Many drugs are considered possible triggers. Drugs that are **definite** triggers are dapsone, methylene blue, nitrofurantoin, phenazopyridine, primaquine, rasburicase and toluidine blue.

4 Acidosis such as diabetic ketoacidosis.[6]

Diagnosis

1 The fluorescent spot test is a screening test.

2 Demonstration of low G6PD levels in RBCs.

3 Genetic testing.

Treatment

1 Cease the trigger agent or treat the triggering infection.

2 Supportive measures (O_2 therapy, IV fluids).

3 Blood transfusion if the haemolytic reaction is severe.

Anaesthesia and G6PD deficiency

1 Avoid the use of triggering drugs.

2 Sevoflurane may or may not be safe.[7]

3 These patients are at increased risk of developing methaemoglobinaemia (MetHb). This is because G6PD deficiency results in reduced NADPH supply. Avoid drugs which can cause MetHb, such as glyceryl trinitrate. Although methaemoglobinaemia can be treated with methylene blue, **this drug cannot be used** in patients with G6PD deficiency. *See Methaemoglobin (MetHb).*

⬤ Glyceryl trinitrate (GTN)

Description

GTN acts by its conversion to nitric oxide (NO), which causes vasodilation of veins, coronary arteries and small arterioles. It produces arterial dilation at higher doses. It is useful for the treatment of acute angina (sprays and tablets), chronic angina (patches) and hypertension. GTN is also useful for producing uterine relaxation to treat conditions such as uterine inversion. Another indication is for the treatment of acute LV failure associated with acute myocardial infarction. GTN is also indicated for the management of autonomic dysreflexia associated hypertension and hypertension due to Irukandji syndrome. *See Spinal cord injury (pre-existing) and anaesthesia.*

   The use of nitrates is contraindicated in patients that have recently taken PDE V inhibitor drugs such as sildenafil or tadalafil, as severe hypotension may occur. *See Nitrate drugs.*

Acute angina

Sublingual tablets are either 300 mcg or 600 mcg. Take 1 tablet and repeat after 5 min if needed. If using spray use 1–2 sprays (400–800 mcg). Repeat after 5 min if needed.

Chronic angina

Transdermal patch 0.2–0.8 mg/h, one patch (25 mg or 50 mg) per day (remove at night for 12 h).

IV infusion for acute coronary syndrome or hypertensive emergency (adult)

1 Add 50 mg of GTN to 500 mL of N/S in a glass bottle (remove 10 mL N/S prior to adding GTN). This gives a concentration of 100 mcg/mL.
2 Administer via an approved giving set to reduce absorption into plastics.
3 Increase the infusion rate until the desired effect is achieved.
4 Start at 5 mcg/min = 3 mL/h. Increase infusion rate by 5 mcg/min every 3–5 min up to 20 mcg/min.
5 Once 20 mcg/min is reached, increase dose by 10–20 mcg/min every 3–5 min.
6 Max dose is 200 mcg/min = 120 mL/h. GTN has a wide therapeutic range.
7 Adverse effects include tachycardia, headache, nausea, vomiting, apprehension.
8 Boluses of 50–100 mcg can be used for immediate effect.

GTN for uterine relaxation

1 Remove 1 mL from an ampoule of GTN 50 mg in 10 mL (5 mg).
2 Dilute this in 9 mL of N/S.
3 Remove 1 mL of this solution (0.5 mg)
4 Mix with 9 mL of N/S, giving a final concentration of 50 mcg/mL.
5 Give 1 mL boluses. 100–200 mcg is usually effective.
6 Alternatively, sublingual GTN spray can be used. Give 400 mcg (1 spray) which can be repeated after 1 min to a maximum of 3 sprays.

◑ Glycopyrronium/glycopyrrolate

Description
A quaternary ammonium anticholinergic drug with similar actions to atropine but, unlike atropine, does not cross the blood–brain barrier. It has no central actions and causes less tachycardia than atropine.

Uses
1 Antisialagogue for procedures such as awake endoscopic intubation.
2 Treatment of bradycardia.
3 Mitigation of side effects of neostigmine used to reverse the effects of non-depolarising neuromuscular blocking drugs (NDNMBDs).

Dose
1 When used with neostigmine to reverse NDMBDs, use 400 mcg glycopyrronium with 2.5 mg neostigmine.
2 200 mcg is an effective antisialagogue in adults.

◑ Granisetron

First-generation 5-HT$_3$ receptor antagonist used to prevent/treat postoperative nausea and vomiting. *See Postoperative nausea and vomiting (PONV).*

Dose

Adult
1–3 mg IV.

◯ Greek alphabet

The Greek alphabet is often used in physiology to describe different types of similar things e.g. receptors or strains of COVID. Usually, the lower case is used. The Greek letters and their names are:

α – alpha	ν – nu
β – beta	xi – ξ
γ – gamma	o – omicron
δ – delta	π – pi
ε – epsilon	ρ – rho
ζ – zeta	σ/ς – sigma
η – eta	τ – tau
θ – theta	υ – upsilon
ι – iota	φ – phi
κ – kappa	χ – chi
λ – lamda	ψ – psi
μ – mu	ω – omega

REFERENCES

1 Srivastava U, Kumar A, Saxena S et al. Effect of preoperative gabapentin on postoperative pain and tramadol consumption after mini-lap open cholecystectomy: a randomised double-blind, placebo-controlled trial. *Eur J Anaesthesiol* 2010; 27: 331–335.

2 Ekhardt K, Ammon S, Hofmann U et al. Gabapentin enhances the analgesic effects of morphine in healthy volunteers. *Anesth Analg* 2000; 91: 185–191.

3 Gallay BJ, De Mattos AM, Norman DJ. Reversible acute renal allograft dysfunction due to gabapentin. *Transplantation* 2000; 70: 208–209.

4 Bauer ME, Arendt K, Beilin Y et al. The Society for Obstetric Anesthesia and Perinatology Interdisciplinary Consensus Statement on neuraxial procedures in obstetric patients with thrombocytopenia. *Anesth Analg* 2021; 132: 1531–1544.

5 Teasdale G, Jennett B. Assessment of coma and impaired consciousness. A practical scale. *Lancet* 1974; 13: 81–84.

6 Goi T, Shionoya Y, Sunada K et al. General anaesthesia in a glucose-6-phosphate dehydrogenase deficiency child: a case report. *Anesth Prog* 2011; 66: 94–96.

7 Cho H, Lee SY, Kim GH et al. Anaesthetic management of a patient with glucose-6-phosphate dehydrogenase deficiency undergoing robot-assisted laparoscopic surgery—a case report. *Anesth Pain Med* 2017; 12: 243–246.

▷ Haemaccel

Description

Plasma volume expander. Made from polygeline, manufactured from urea-linked bovine gelatin. Also contains:

1 sodium 145 mmol/L
2 potassium 5.1 mmol/L
3 calcium 6.25 mmol/L
4 chloride 145 mmol/L
5 pH 7.4 +/− 0.3
6 osmolarity 301 mOsm/L.

Uses

Colloid plasma volume expander. Plasma half-life about 4 h.

Potential problems

1 Transfused blood should not be mixed with Haemaccel because it contains calcium. This may result in clotting. Flush Haemaccel out of the IV line before transfusion.
2 Can cause anaphylaxis.
3 Can cause increased bradykinin production, leading to hypotension especially in patients taking ACE inhibitors.
4 There is concern about bovine illnesses being transferred to humans.
  See Gelofusine.

▷ Haematocrit (Hct)

Haematocrit is the ratio of the total volume of the red blood cells (RBC) to the total volume of the blood (RBC + plasma) in a blood sample. Normal Hct values are:

1 males 0.47–0.50
2 females 0.36–0.48.

The Hct as a percentage can be estimated as 3 × the haemoglobin (Hb) level in g/100 ml. If the Hb is 12, the Hct is 36% or 0.36.

▷ Haemochromatosis

Description

Primary haemochromatosis is an inherited disorder in which too much iron is absorbed from the diet. The iron cannot be excreted and is stored in the liver, heart, pancreas and other parts of the body such as joints. Secondary haemochromatosis is due to a large number of blood transfusions or excess iron in the diet. **See Iron overload.**

Defect in primary haemochromatosis

A fault in the HFE gene causes primary (or hereditary) haemochromatosis. Normal total body iron in men is 3.5 g and 2.5 g in women. Symptoms may not occur until > 10–20 g has accumulated.

Clinical effects

1 Systemic symptoms—weakness, lethargy, weight loss.
2 Skin hyperpigmentation—bronze or grey skin colour.
3 Liver cirrhosis, hepatocellular carcinoma.
4 Heart damage/cardiomyopathy.
5 Pancreatic damage with resulting diabetes mellitus.
6 Arthritis.
7 Abdominal pain.

Diagnosis

1 Elevated serum ferritin, fasting serum iron and transferrin saturation.
2 Liver biopsy.
3 Genetic testing for HFE gene mutations.

Treatment

1 Phlebotomy once or twice per week (500 mL per session). Each session removes 0.25 mg of iron so removal of 10 g of iron requires 40 phlebotomy sessions.
2 Iron chelation therapy if phlebotomy not an option e.g. anaemia and iron overload. Desferrioxamine is an example of a chelating agent. It acts by binding with iron and enabling its excretion in urine.
3 Dietary modification—avoid substances which increase iron absorption such as excess alcohol and vitamin C.
4 Treatment of organ damage such as diabetes mellitus.
5 Regular screening for hepatocellular carcinoma.

Anaesthesia and haemochromatosis

1 Assess the patient carefully for cardiac involvement/cardiomyopathy with investigations such as echocardiography.
2 Assess for liver impairment—check liver function tests and clotting studies.

⊙ Haemodynamic instability defined

Haemodynamic instability is defined as the presence of one or more of the following:
1 hypotension (SBP < 90 mmHg or MAP < 65 mmHg)
2 altered mental state
3 chest pain
4 dyspnoea
5 heart failure.
Treatment of the patient with haemodynamic instability is an emergency.

⊙ Haemoglobin A1c

This is also known as a glycated haemoglobin test or glycohaemoglobin. The test measures how much glucose is bound to haemoglobin. It gives an indication of the average blood sugar level over the past 2–3 months.

For adults with Type II diabetes that is diet controlled, ± single agent, aim for a HbA1c of ≤ 6.5%. A value of 7.5% or higher indicates the need for escalation of therapy.

Table H1 Interpretation of HbA1c results

HbA1c test result	Significance
4–5.6%	Normal
5.7–6.4%	Prediabetes
≥ 6.5%	Diabetes
≤ 6.5%	Good diabetic control
> 7%	Poor diabetic control

◐ Haemoglobin (Hb) and haemoglobinopathies

Normal adult haemoglobin (HbA)

Haemoglobin is a massive molecule contained in red blood cells. Normal adult haemoglobin (HbA) is made up of four subunit proteins (two alpha and two beta). Each subunit contains an embedded haem group, and the type of subunit affects how O_2 binds to the haem group. Each haem group contains one iron atom, making four altogether. Each iron atom can bind with one O_2 molecule, making a maximum of four O_2 molecules bound to each Hb molecule. Hb can bind 1.34 mL O_2 per gram, and there are 12–20 g Hb/100 mL blood. Hb is 70 × more efficient at transporting O_2 than plasma. It is found in all vertebrates except for the white-blooded fish, which relies on the solubility of O_2 in its plasma. Hb also carries about 20–25% of the body's respiratory CO_2 (carbaminohaemoglobin).

Hb outside the erythrocytes

Red cell haemolysis results in free Hb in the plasma—haemoglobinaemia. Hb is also found in many other cells such as macrophages. In these other cells, Hb acts as an antioxidant and helps in the regulation of iron metabolism.

Types of physiological Hb

1 HbA (adult)—(two alpha and two beta subunits)—the main type of Hb found in the adult (about 90%).
2 HbA2—(two alpha and two delta subunits)—a small percentage of this type is found in adult blood (about 5%).
3 HbF—(two alpha and two gamma subunits)—found in fetal red blood cells and young children. It has a higher affinity for O_2 than HbA. Adult levels of HbA are reached after about 1 year of age.
4 Hb Gower—(two zeta and two epsilon subunits)—this is the first form of Hb in the embryo. From about 7 weeks, Hb Gower is replaced by HbF.

Types of abnormal Hb (haemoglobinopathies)

1 HbS—sickle cell Hb. This disease is due to an abnormal beta subunit. *See Sickle cell disease (SCD)*.
2 HbC—a disease with abnormal beta subunits. Its main effects are anaemia, gall stones and splenomegaly. *See Haemoglobin C (HbC) disease*.
3 HbSC—a combination of sickle cell and haemoglobin C disease.
4 Thalassaemia. *See Thalassaemia*.

5 HbH—Hb made up of beta subunits only. It occurs in alpha thalassaemia minor. *See Thalassaemia.*

6 HbE—*see Haemoglobin E (HbE)* below.

Haemoglobin C (HbC) disease

Description

This inherited haemoglobinopathy is due to Hb with abnormal beta subunits (*see Haemoglobin (Hb) and haemoglobinopathies* above). It is a common structural Hb trait. Patients can be homozygotes (HbC) or heterozygotes termed HbAC or HbC trait. HbC trait patients are asymptomatic. In patients with HbC, the RBC are less deformable but, unlike sickle cell disease, vaso-occlusion does not occur. *See Sickle cell disease (SCD).* HbC does not polymerise at low O_2 tensions but crystals can form. RBC survival time is shortened. HbC may be protective against malaria (heterozygotes and homozygotes).

Clinical effects

1 Mild anaemia.

2 Splenomegaly.

3 Increased frequency of pigmented gall stones.

Treatment

Folic acid to replace depletion due to high RBC turnover.

Haemoglobin E (HbE)

This is an abnormal Hb formed when there is a specific beta subunit gene mutation. It is a form of thalassaemia. *See Thalassaemia.*

Haemoglobin H (HbH) disease

This is a form of alpha thalassaemia where three of four alleles for the alpha subunit of Hb are deleted. *See Thalassaemia.*

Haemophilia

Introduction

Haemophilia is an inherited disorder of blood clotting due to reduced or absent clotting factors. Haemophilia A (the most common) is due to FVIII deficiency and haemophilia B ('Christmas disease') is due to FIX deficiency. Both haemophilia A and B are X-linked and therefore almost never occur in females. However, women who are carriers may have reduced clotting factor levels. Haemophilia C is FXI deficiency. It is not sex linked and can occur in females. Haemophilia can be mild, moderate or severe, depending on the level of clotting factor present. The normal clotting factor range is 50–200%. In mild haemophilia, 6–50% of the factor is present. In moderate disease 1–5% is present, and in severe disease < 1% is present. APTT is the most useful clotting test. PT is usually normal. There may also be inhibitors present which attack the factors administered. These inhibitors are antibodies produced by the patient.

Haemophilia A (classical haemophilia)

The normal level of FVIII is 0.5–1.5 IU/mL.[1] Expert haematologist advice is required before surgery. Treatment includes the following:

1 Desmopressin may be useful for increasing FVIII levels in mild disease in patients having minor surgery.
2 FVIII replacement therapy. Each IU/kg will raise FVIII levels by 2%.
3 Emicizumab is a monoclonal antibody drug that acts in the same way as FVIII. It can be used in patients with or without FVIII inhibitors. It is not useful if a bleeding episode is occurring.
4 FEIBA (factor VIII inhibitor bypassing activity) can be used to control or prevent bleeding episodes in patients with haemophilia A or B **with inhibitors**. *See FEIBA-NF (factor VIII inhibitor bypassing activity).*

Haemophilia B
The normal level of FIX is 0.5–1.5 IU/mL.[1] Expert haematologist input is required before surgery. Treatment includes:
1 FIX replacement therapy. Each IU/kg given will increase levels by 1%.
2 Administering FEIBA if inhibitors are present.

Haemophilia and surgery
1 There should be a multidisciplinary approach involving haematologist, surgeon, anaesthetist and patient.
2 Surgery must be performed in an appropriate centre with access to factor concentrates in sufficient quantities.
3 Give factors in appropriate doses 30–60 min prior to surgery. Repeat as needed as per haematologist guidance. Correction to 80–100% is required for major surgery and needs to be maintained for 1–6 weeks.
4 Use FEIBA if inhibitors are present. Consider recombinant activated FVII.
5 Do not give drugs which may worsen bleeding such as aspirin/NSAIDs.

Haemophilia and haemorrhage
1 Use specific factors if available.
2 If factors are not available, use cryoprecipitate.
3 If cryoprecipitate is not available, use FFP.
4 Recombinant activated FVII. *See Recombinant activated factor VII/rFVIIa/Eptacog alfa-activated (NovoSeven RT).*
5 Prothrombin complex concentrate can be used as a source of FIX.
6 Tranexamic acid may be helpful. *See Tranexamic acid (TXA) (Cyklokapron).*

◗ Haemoptysis, life-threatening

Description
Bleeding in the airway is a crisis situation and can result in death from asphyxiation. Life-threatening haemoptysis can be defined as blood loss in the airway sufficient to be life threatening due to impairment of oxygenation, obstruction of the airway by blood clots or exsanguination. Patients are more likely to die from asphyxiation than exsanguination.

Causes
There are two potential sources of haemoptysis: the low-pressure pulmonary circulation and the arterial supply to the bronchi at systemic pressure. About 90% of haemoptysis is from the bronchial circulation. Causes of haemoptysis include:
1 infection—TB, aspergilloma, necrotising pneumonia, hydatid cyst
2 bronchiectasis

3 bronchogenic carcinoma

4 vascular disease—arteriovenous malformation, aortic aneurysm with erosion, pulmonary infarct or embolism

5 trauma e.g. penetrating chest injury

6 Wegener's granulomatosis, Goodpasture's syndrome, Behçet's disease, SLE

7 bleeding disorders

8 complication of surgery e.g. lung transplant

9 iatrogenic e.g. complication of airway instrumentation or pulmonary artery catheter.

Initial management

There is no 'one size fits all' management strategy for life-threatening haemoptysis. Obtain expert respiratory physician assistance as soon as possible.

1 If the patient is conscious, sit them up and tilt them forward to help them expel blood while assisting them with suctioning.

2 Exclude haematemesis or bleeding from the nose/throat (e.g. post tonsillectomy).

3 Wear appropriate PPE—there may be an infective cause or co-existing blood-borne disease.

4 If it is known whether the bleeding is from the left or right lung, consider putting the patient on their side, bleeding lung lowermost. Assist expulsion of the blood with suctioning.

5 Resuscitate the patient—two large-bore IV cannulas, IV fluids (crystalloid, colloid, blood).

6 Send blood for cross-match, coagulation studies, FBC, electrolytes, fibrinogen. Correct any coagulopathy.

7 Obtain a mobile CXR if time permits.

8 If the situation is critical, induce anaesthesia with appropriate doses of fentanyl/propofol, suxamethonium 1–1.5 mg/kg or rocuronium 1–1.2 mg/kg and intubate the patient using a rapid sequence induction. ***See Rapid sequence induction (RSI)***. Use the largest ET tube that will fit e.g. 8.5–9 mm tube for a male, 8–8.5 mm tube for a female. This is to enable inspection and instrumentation of the airway with a flexible bronchoscope.

9 Maintain anaesthesia with a propofol infusion.

10 Insert a large bronchoscope and identify which side is bleeding. If successful, insert a bronchial blocker into the bleeding bronchus to isolate the bleeding lung from the non-bleeding lung. Alternatively insert the ET tube into the non-bleeding lung main stem bronchus to seal it off from the bleeding lung.

11 If unable to tell which side is bleeding, or bleeding is from both sides, ventilate both lungs.

12 Use of a double lumen tube (DLT) is not currently recommended in this situation. The small lumens of the DLT can easily become blocked blood clot and only a very small diameter bronchoscope can be inserted. This makes interventional therapy difficult.

Subsequent management

1 Flexible bronchoscopy through the ET tube may identify the source of bleeding and allow treatment with iced saline lavage, topical adrenaline, topical vasopressin or insertion of balloon blockers. Insertion of a rigid bronchoscope may be required to facilitate therapy. More advanced techniques include endobronchial stent tamponade, balloon tamponade, topical cellulose mesh and application of a biocompatible glue.[2]

2 Bronchoscopic laser therapy, electrocautery and argon plasma coagulation may also be options in specialist centres.[3]

3 Angiographic bronchial artery embolisation. This may require pre-procedural chest CT and descending thoracic aortogram to identify the origins of the bronchial arteries from the aorta.
4 Emergency thoracic surgery for e.g. chest trauma or pulmonary artery haemorrhage due to a resectable lung tumour.
5 In terms of other treatments for immunologically diffuse alveolar haemorrhage, steroids, cytotoxic therapy and/or plasmapheresis may be of benefit.

Haemorrhage

See *Blood loss—assessment, management and anaesthetic approach*.

Haloperidol

Butyrophenone antipsychotic drug useful for the treatment of acute psychosis and severe behavioural disturbance. In adults give 2–10 mg IM (use 0.5–2 mg in the elderly). It also has anti-emetic effects.

Halothane

Description

Obsolescent halogenated hydrocarbon volatile inhalational general anaesthetic agent. Only used in developing countries. MAC 0.75 vol%.

Advantages

Sweet, non-irritating odour. Very well tolerated for inhalational induction.

Disadvantages

1 Requires thymol as a preservative, which can interfere with vaporiser function.
2 Can cause halothane hepatitis. Avoid repeated exposure. Do not use twice within a 6-month period. A history of unexplained jaundice or pyrexia after halothane is an absolute contraindication to a subsequent halothane anaesthetic.
3 Sensitises the heart to catecholamines. Use of adrenaline may result in tachydysrhythmias.
4 Prolongs QT interval. Increased risk of torsades de pointes. **See *Long QT syndrome (LQTS)*** and ***Torsades de pointes*.**
5 Causes vagal stimulation, which can lead to bradycardia.
6 Potent trigger of malignant hyperthermia. **See *Malignant hyperthermia (MH)*.**

Hartmann's solution/compound sodium lactate (CSL)/ lactated Ringer's solution (LRS)

Description

IV crystalloid solution intended to more closely resemble plasma than N/S. It contains:
1 sodium 131 mmol/L
2 potassium 5 mmol/L
3 calcium 2 mmol/L
4 chloride 111 mmol/L
5 lactate 29 mmol/L
6 osmolarity 274 mOsm/L
7 pH 5–7.

QUICK FLICK H

Comparison with other IV fluids

1 Contains potassium hence unsuitable for patients with hyperkalaemia.
2 Due to a lower chloride content than N/S, it does not cause hyperchloraemic metabolic acidosis.
3 Contains calcium, which may cause clotting if mixed with citrated blood during transfusion. N/S and Plasma-Lyte 148 do not contain calcium.
4 Lactate in Hartmann's solution is metabolised by both gluconeogenesis and oxidation (mainly in the liver) to bicarbonate and glucose. Hartmann's solution therefore maintains a more stable pH than N/S.
5 The metabolism of lactate to glucose may result in increased blood glucose levels if the insulin response is impaired. The significance of this in diabetic patients is unclear. However, Hartmann's solution should probably not be used in patients with brittle diabetes.
6 Lactate metabolism is impaired in liver disease and in severe shock.
7 Normal plasma osmolarity is 280–296 mOsm/L. Hartmann's solution is slightly hypotonic and therefore less suitable for patients with cerebral oedema.

◗ Heart block (HB)

Heart block occurs when P wave conduction to the AV node is delayed or ineffective. There are three types.

1 *First degree HB*—the PR interval is longer than five small squares (0.2 s). Each P wave is followed by a QRS complex. It does not require intervention but may be indicative of underlying heart disease.
2 *Second degree HB*—there are two types. One type is Wenckebach or Mobitz type 1 block; the PR interval gets progressively longer, then a non-conducted P wave occurs. It is not life threatening in itself, but is concerning in terms of underlying cardiac pathology. In Mobitz type 2, there are intermittent non-conducted P waves, without lengthening of the PR interval. The PR interval may be short or long but its length is constant. The block may be in a fixed ration of P waves to QRS complexes e.g. 2:1 block, 3:1 block.
3 *Third degree HB*—there is no relationship between P waves and the QRS complexes, which are widened.

Treatment

First degree and Mobitz type 1 HB usually do not require treatment because HR is usually well maintained. Mobitz type 2 may require treatment because of bradycardia. Third degree heart block requires pacing either emergently if haemodynamic instability is present or semi-urgently. *See Pacing.*

◗ Heart failure

See Congestive cardiac failure (CCF)—chronic.

◗ Heart transplant patient, non-cardiac surgery

Introduction

There are several unique aspects to providing anaesthesia for the heart transplant patient, including:

1 physiology of the transplanted heart
2 special pharmacological considerations

3 effects of immunotherapy
4 chronic co-morbidities due to pre-transplant heart failure or the disease necessitating transplant.

Physiology of the transplanted heart

1 The heart is denervated—it has no rapid response to the sympathetic and parasympathetic nervous systems. Carotid sinus stimulation and vagal manoeuvres have no effect on heart rate.
2 Despite attachment to the recipient's atrial remnant, electrical impulses do not cross the suture line. Two P waves may be present on the ECG.
3 The transplanted heart can increase or decrease its cardiac output slowly by the Frank–Starling mechanism—stroke volume increases as end-diastolic volume of the ventricle increases until the ventricle is overstretched. Therefore, preload is of utmost importance for cardiac output.
4 The transplanted heart tends to have a high resting heart rate, typically 90–110 bpm with less heart rate variability than the non-transplanted heart.
5 The ECG frequently indicates sinus rhythm, often with a first degree heart block. About 10–20% of patients will have a pacemaker.
6 Circulating catecholamines will increase heart rate and contractility.
7 The patient will not feel angina if the myocardium is ischaemic unless partial reinnervation occurs, which takes many years. Myocardial ischaemia may present as LV dysfunction or arrhythmia.
8 There is accelerated atherosclerosis in the transplanted heart. This tends to start in the smaller non-stentable coronary arteries and spread proximally to the larger vessels. Even if atherosclerosis is absent, the coronary arteries may narrow significantly.[4]
9 Mild to moderate mitral and tricuspid valve regurgitation may occur.
10 New-onset dysrhythmias may indicate acute rejection. Other effects of rejection include unexplained weight gain, fever, dyspnoea and peripheral oedema.

Special pharmacological considerations

1 Atropine and glycopyrrolate have no effect on heart rate.
2 Neostigmine will not cause bradycardia unless the heart has reinnervated, in which case it can cause cardiac arrest.
3 The transplanted heart is extremely sensitive to adenosine. Use this drug very cautiously at a reduced dose. The effects will be prolonged compared with the normal heart.
4 Isoprenaline and dobutamine have similar effects on the transplanted heart as they do on the non-transplanted heart. Adrenaline and isoprenaline are useful to treat bradycardia. Adrenaline will also treat hypotensive emergencies, but exercise caution with the dose.
5 Indirect-acting vasopressors such as ephedrine will have no effect on the heart.
6 The response to vasodilating agents such as propofol, glyceryl trinitrate and sodium nitroprusside may be profound hypotension due to the lack of a compensatory reflex tachycardia. Use vasodilatory drugs with **extreme** caution.
7 Beta blockers are usually avoided because they blunt the effects of increased circulating catecholamines during exercise.

Effects of immunotherapy

1 Azathioprine—withdrawal of this drug may precipitate bleeding in patients who take warfarin. The combination of azathioprine and allopurinol may cause severe bone marrow suppression, pancreatitis and liver toxicity.
2 Tacrolimus—associated with a high incidence of postoperative wound infection.[5]
3 Cyclosporine—may cause hypertension.
4 Steroid therapy—may cause diabetes mellitus, myopathy and leukopaenia.

Chronic co-morbidities

1 Patients with congenital heart disease requiring transplant may have damage to other organs or associated congenital/genetic abnormalities.
2 Renal impairment due to chronic hypoperfusion.
3 Prolonged liver congestion leading to fibrosis or cirrhosis.

Anaesthetic considerations

If possible, elective surgery should be delayed for the first 6–12 months after heart transplant.[6]

Preoperative phase

Consultation with the patient's cardiologist is of utmost importance.
Special pharmacological considerations are discussed above.

1 Assess the patient for any evidence of rejection including the review of the most recent investigations such as endomyocardial biopsy.
2 The patient's exercise capacity is helpful in estimating cardiopulmonary function.
3 Appropriately manage the patient's pacemaker if one is present. *See Pacemakers.*
4 Minimise interruption to the patient's immunotherapy treatment.
5 Arrange appropriate preoperative tests, including ECG, FBC, UEC, LFTs.
6 Maintain preoperative hydration to prevent hypovolaemia.
7 Give stress steroids if the patient is taking 10 mg or more of prednisone daily. *See Stress steroids.*

Intraoperative phase

1 Ensure appropriate prophylactic antibiotic therapy is administered. Heart transplant patients with abnormal heart valves are at increased risk of bacterial endocarditis. *See Bacterial endocarditis (BE) prophylaxis.*
2 If inserting a central line, avoid using the right internal jugular vein, which is used for endomyocardial biopsies.
3 Do not insert a nasal ET tube unless absolutely necessary due to the risk of infection from nasal microbes.
4 If blood transfusion is required, give CMV-negative blood.
5 Phenylephrine is an effective vasoconstrictor if hypotension occurs.
6 These patients are critically preload dependent—ensure venous return is maintained.
7 Vasodilation due to GA drugs can result in a severe drop in blood pressure. It is recommended to have a vasopressor infusion running e.g phenylephrine.
8 Neuraxial anaesthesia must be used with great caution. The resultant loss in sympathetic tone can result in greatly decreased systemic vascular resistance (SVR) without a compensatory increase in heart rate and contractility. This can result in severe hypotension. Preload patients with 500–1000 mL of IV crystalloid. Titrate epidural anaesthesia slowly and carefully with a phenylephrine infusion.

If CSE is used, a low-dose spinal component is advised. SAB with a surgical dose of LA may be quite hazardous.

9 Avoid hyperventilation due to reduced seizure thresholds associated with cyclosporine and tacrolimus.

Postoperative phase

1 Remove invasive monitoring (central line, arterial line) as soon as they are not needed to reduce the risk of infection.

2 Ensure immunotherapy is resumed as soon as this is practical. Consider IV therapy if the patient is unable to resume oral intake.

Obstetric anaesthesia and heart transplant

1 Preeclampsia occurs in about 20% of patients.[4]

2 There is an increased incidence of gestational diabetes.

3 If an epidural is required for labour or CS, it should be carefully titrated with IV fluid loading and a phenylephrine infusion available. If CSE is used for CS, use a low-dose spinal component. A SAB is not recommended.

⊙ HELLP syndrome

This acronym describes a pattern of complications that may occur with severe preeclampsia/eclampsia. HELLP stands for:

H – **h**aemolysis

E L – **e**levated **l**iver enzymes

LP – **l**ow **p**latelets.

*See **Preeclampsia/eclampsia**.*

⊙ Heparin (unfractionated and low-molecular-weight heparins)

Heparin (unfractionated)

Description

Heparin is a highly sulphated glycosaminoglycan that binds reversibly to antithrombin III and activates it. Antithrombin III inactivates thrombin, FXII, FXI, FX and FIX. It also inhibits platelet activation by fibrin. It is an anticoagulant drug that is used for:

1 prevention of venous thromboembolism (VTE)

2 treatment of deep venous thrombosis/pulmonary embolus (DVT/PE)

3 any situation requiring immediate anticoagulation such as unstable angina, cardiac bypass surgery

4 priming of machines to prevent extracorporeal clotting such as dialysis machines, cell-saver machines.

Dose

Adult

1 *Prophylactic (subcut)*—5000 U q 8–12 h. Do not perform neuraxial anaesthesia within 6 h of the last dose.

2 *Therapeutic (infusion)*—100 U/kg IV loading dose (usually 5000 U) then 1000 U/h. Adjust dose depending on APTT values aiming for APTT to be 1.5–2.5 × normal (60–85 s). The first APTT should be done after 4 h. Do not perform neuraxial anaesthesia within 6 h of the heparin infusion being ceased. Check APTT to ensure the heparin effect has worn off.

Reversal

Heparin can be reversed by protamine at a dose of 1 mg/100 U heparin. **See Protamine**. If protamine cannot be used, consider recombinant platelet factor IV, or heparinase-I, which cleaves heparin.

Heparin-induced thrombocytopenia (HIT)

See *Heparin-induced thrombocytopenia (HIT)*.

Heparin (fractionated)

Fractionated heparin is also referred to as low-molecular-weight heparin (LMWH). Examples include dalteparin (Fragmin) and enoxaparin (Clexane). LMWHs act by catalysing the inhibition of factors IX, X, XI and XII by antithrombin III.

Advantages of LMWH compared with heparin

1 Inhibits platelets less than heparin and may cause less intraoperative bleeding.
2 Longer duration of action than heparin.
3 Less risk of causing HIT.
4 Monitoring of the anticoagulant effect is not required due to greater predictability of effect.
5 Therapeutic treatment at home is a practical option.

Disadvantages of LMWH compared with heparin

1 More difficult to measure the anticoagulant effect. This is done by measuring anti-Xa activity. The TR for established DVT/PE is 0.3–0.8 anti-Xa units/mL at 3–5 h after dose.
2 In cases of bleeding, LMWH is more difficult to reverse than heparin. See below.
3 Patients susceptible to HIT type II cannot have LMWH due to 90% cross-reactivity.
4 The long duration of action of LMWH may be a disadvantage when the timing of surgery is uncertain.

Dose

Adult

Prophylactic—enoxaparin (Clexane) 40 mg subcut daily; dalteparin (Fragmin) 5000 IU subcut daily.
Therapeutic—Clexane 1 mg/kg q 12 h or 1.5 mg/kg subcut daily. Fragmin 200 IU/kg subcut daily up to 18 000 IU/day.

LMWH and neuraxial anaesthesia

Prophylactic doses—do not perform neuraxial anaesthesia within 12 h of the last dose. Do not give LMWH until 12 h after neuraxial anaesthesia. Do not give LMWH until 4 h after removal of an epidural catheter.

Therapeutic doses—do not perform neuraxial anaesthesia for 24 h after therapeutic dose (wait longer if renal impairment). Do not remove an epidural catheter within 24 h of last dose (longer if renal impairment). Do not give next dose of LMWH within 12 h after epidural catheter removal or SAB.

◖ Heparin-induced thrombocytopenia (HIT)

Types of HIT

There are two types of HIT.
1 HIT Type I is non-immunological, transient and associated with a mild drop in platelet count without thrombosis. It is a benign condition.

2 HIT Type II is an immunological reaction involving IgG antibodies which activate platelets. It occurs in 1–5% of patients treated with heparin. The antibodies persist after heparin is stopped.

HIT Type II

1 Usually occurs 5–10 days after commencing heparin.
2 An immune complex forms between heparin and platelet factor 4 (PF4).
3 The body produces IgG antibodies to the heparin-PF4 complexes.
4 When antibodies attack the heparin-PF4 complexes, the platelets are activated and destroyed.
5 This platelet activation leads to thrombus formation due to the release of platelet microparticles which activate thrombin.
6 There is a 50% drop in platelet count and an increased risk of venous and arterial thrombosis causing DVT/PE, myocardial infarction and skin necrosis.
7 Thrombosis is a much more significant risk than bleeding.

Diagnosis
1 C14 serotonin release assay.
2 Heparin induced platelet activation assay.
3 Falling platelet count.

Treatment of HIT
Cease heparin and start a non-heparin anticoagulant such as danaparoid, lepirudin or argatroban.

❍ Hepatic surgery

See Liver resection surgery.

❍ Hereditary angioedema (HAE)

See Angioedema.

❍ Hydralazine

Description

Hydrazinophthalazine derivate. Acts directly on vascular smooth muscle, causing arteriolar vasodilation by inhibiting intracellular accumulation of calcium in vascular smooth muscle. Used to treat moderate to severe hypertension in conditions such as preeclampsia and to treat severe heart failure. It is available in oral and IV forms.

Dose

Adult
5–10 mg IV boluses every 20 min to a max dose 20–40 mg. Lasts 2–6 h.

Points to note
1 Giving diazoxide to patients who have had hydralazine can result in severe hypotension.
2 Monoamine oxidase inhibitors (MAOIs) can increase the effects of hydralazine.
3 Hydralazine is contraindicated in porphyria.

● Hydromorphone (Dilaudid, Jurnista)

Description

Opioid analgesic drug that is five times more potent than morphine. It is a semi-synthetic modification of morphine. It is particularly useful in opioid-tolerant patients. Hydromorphone is mainly a mu agonist with lesser effects at delta and kappa receptors. *See Opioid receptors*. It is available as a sustained-release (SR) tablet, trade name Jurnista, and in immediate-release (IR) form, trade name Dilaudid (as tablets and syrup). It is also available in parenteral form.

Dose PRN

Adult

1 *PO*—1–8 mg q 4 h.
2 *IM/subcut*—1–2 mg q 4–6 h.
3 *IV*—0.5–1 mg q 4–6 h.
4 *PCA*—50 mg in 50 mL N/S, start with 0.2 mL bolus (200 mcg) with a 5 min lockout.

Child

1 *PO*—0.05–0.1 mg/kg q 4 h.
2 *IM/subcut*—0.02–0.05 mg/kg q 4–6 h.
3 *IV*—0.01–0.02 mg/kg q 4–6 h.
4 *Infusion*—add 0.1 mg/kg to N/S to a total volume of 50 mL. Infuse at 0–4 mL/h (0–8 mcg/kg/h). For painful procedures, give 1–2 mL of this solution.

Advantages

1 Hydromorphone may have a lower incidence of side effects than morphine (e.g. sedation, pruritis, nausea and vomiting).
2 It is a potent opioid.
3 It is a popular alternative to fentanyl PCA in renal failure patients. However, it should be considered a second-line drug, with minimisation of dosage and careful monitoring of the patient. This is because the metabolite hydromorphone-3-glucuronide can accumulate and cause dose-dependent neuro-excitatory effects.

Disadvantages

1 Overdose can occur due to a lack of understanding that this drug is 5 times more potent than morphine.
2 Like morphine, hydromorphone causes histamine release.
3 It cannot be used in patients on monoamine oxidase inhibitor drugs unless they have been stopped for 14 days.

● Hydrops fetalis/fetal hydrops

This disease is characterised by severe oedema in the fetus. It can be due to:
1 alpha thalassaemia major (Bart's disease)
2 infections
3 fetal cardiac malformations
4 fetal or placental tumours
5 twin-to-twin transfusion syndrome
6 rhesus isoimmunisation.

Hydrops fetalis can cause mirror syndrome in the mother. **See *Mirror syndrome*.** Fetal hydrops can be diagnosed by fetal ultrasound.

5-Hydroxytryptamine 3 (5-HT_3) receptors and antagonists

5-HT_3 receptors

These receptors are neurotransmitter-gated ion channels that respond to serotonin (hydroxytryptamine). Receptors are present in many sites, including the brain, with the highest levels in the brainstem. 5-HT_3 receptor blockers are thought to act directly on the area postrema and nucleus tractus solitarius, which are responsible for the vomiting reflex. Another important site of action is thought to be in the vagal afferent neurones. Nausea and vomiting are theorised to be triggered by the release of serotonin from enterochromaffin cells of the intestinal mucosa.

5-HT_3 antagonists

These are among the most effective anti-nausea drugs. They include ondansetron, tropisetron, granisetron, dolasetron and palonosetron. Other 5-HT_3 receptor blocker drugs are used to treat irritable bowel syndrome and include alosetron. **See *Postoperative nausea and vomiting (PONV)*.**

Hyper/hypocalcaemia

See *Calcium*.

Hyper/hypocapnia

Hypercapnia

Hypercapnia is defined as an increase in the partial pressure of CO_2 in the blood > 45 mmHg. It can be due to:

1. hypoventilation
2. increased CO_2 production as occurs with malignant hyperthermia. **See *Malignant hyperthermia (MH)*.**
3. rebreathing of CO_2 e.g. exhausted soda lime
4. sodium bicarbonate administration
5. iatrogenic source of CO_2 e.g. CO_2 used for laparoscopic surgery.

Hypocapnia/hypocarbia

This is defined as a decrease in blood CO_2 partial pressure < 35 mmHg. It is usually due to hyperventilation. Another cause is reduced metabolism, as occurs with hypothermia.

Hyper/hypokalaemia

See *Potassium*.

Hyperosmolar hyperglycaemic state (HHS)

Description

This is a diabetic endocrine emergency usually associated with severe intercurrent illness. **See *Diabetic ketoacidosis (DKA)*.** It tends to occur in older, obese patients with Type 2 diabetes. It has a mortality 10–20 times greater than DKA due to the seriousness of the associated illness. It was previously called hyperglycaemic hyperosmolar non-ketotic coma.

QUICK FLICK H

Causes

1 Ceasing oral medication—refusal, difficulty swallowing, nausea.
2 Acute infections.
3 Severe intercurrent illness.

Clinical effects

1 Polydipsia.
2 Thirst.
3 Nausea.
4 Dry skin.
5 Confusion, drowsiness, seizures, eventual coma. 22–50% of cases are comatose.
6 Severe dehydration. Fluid deficit can exceed 10 L.

Diagnosis

1 Severe hyperglycaemia (> 33 mmol/L).
2 There is an absence of severe ketosis due to patients having enough endogenous insulin to suppress ketogenesis. Acidosis, if present, is mild.
3 High plasma osmolality (> 320 mOsm/L).

Treatment[7]

1 IV N/S rehydration. Give 1000 mL in first hour then 250–500 mL/h, depending on clinical assessment. If hypernatraemia, give 0.45% saline. Hydration alone may decrease plasma glucose levels precipitously. Measured sodium levels should be adjusted for hyperglycaemia, which can cause dilutional hyponatraemia. Add 1.6 mmol/L to the measured sodium concentration for every 5.6 mmol/L of glucose above a glucose measurement of 5.6 mmol/L. For example, if BSL is 40 mmol/L, add 10 mmol to measured serum sodium.
2 Correction of hypokalaemia and potassium replacement therapy.
   a) Serum K^+ < 3.3 mmol/L—40 mmol/h.
   b) Serum K^+ 3.3–4.9 mmol/L—20–30 mmol/h.
   c) Serum K^+ > 5 mmol/L—withhold potassium.
3 IV insulin infusion (commence if/when serum K^+ > 3.3 mmol/L).
4 Commence IV glucose when BSL < 16 mmol/L.
5 Treat the precipitating illness.

❂ Hypertension

Introduction and definitions

Hypertension is a major risk factor for stroke, myocardial infarction, heart failure, vascular disease and chronic kidney disease. The following definitions are from the ACC/AHA guidelines.[8]

1 Normal BP: SBP < 120 mmHg and DBP < 80 mmHg.
2 Elevated BP: SBP 120–129 mmHg, DBP < 80 mmHg.
3 Stage 1 hypertension: SBP 130–139 mmHg or DBP 80–89 mmHg.
4 Stage 2 hypertension: SBP ≥ 140 mmHg, DBP ≥ 90 mmHg.

Causes of chronic hypertension

1 Idiopathic/essential.
2 Renal causes e.g. polycystic kidney disease, renal ischaemia.
3 Coarctation of the aorta.
4 Vasculitis.
5 Collagen vascular disease.

6 Endocrine disorders—primary aldosteronism, phaeochromocytoma, hyperthyroidism.

7 Oral contraceptive pill.

8 Pregnancy.

9 Neurogenic—brain tumour, intracranial hypertension.

10 Obesity/OSA.

11 Drugs—alcohol, cocaine.

Treatment of hypertension

Generally, aim for a BP < 130/80 mmHg. Treat the cause if possible.

1 Angiotensin-converting enzyme inhibitors (ACEIs) or angiotensin receptor blockers (ARBs)—especially if diabetes or chronic kidney disease. *See Angiotensin-converting enzyme (ACE) inhibitors* and *Angiotensin II receptor blocker (ARB) drugs.*

2 Calcium channel blockers. *See Calcium channel blocker drugs.*

3 Thiazide diuretics—these help other antihypertensive drugs work by limiting volume expansion.

4 Spironolactone—opposes the sodium and water retention effects of aldosterone. It is also a potassium sparing diuretic.

5 Beta blockers—especially if heart failure and/or following MI. *See Beta adrenergic receptor blocker drugs.*

6 Alpha-2 adrenoreceptor agonists e.g. clonidine. *See Clonidine.*

Intraoperative hypertension

Intraoperative hypertension is frequently encountered and usually responds to simple measures. These include the following:

1 Deepening anaesthesia with a bolus of propofol or increasing sevoflurane inhaled concentration.

2 Bolus of opioid if nociceptive stimulation is suspected as the cause.

3 Clonidine 75 mcg IV. *See Clonidine.*

4 Hydralazine 5–10 mg IV boluses. *See Hydralazine.*

5 Remifentanil infusion. *See Remifentanil.*

If simple measures are not effective, further management overlaps with the more aggressive treatment strategies described below.

Hypertensive urgency

This occurs when blood pressure spikes but does not cause damage to the body's organs. BP readings are up to about 180/110 mmHg. Blood pressure needs to be brought down over the next few hours with oral medication.

Hypertensive emergencies (malignant hypertension)

This is defined as BP that is high enough to cause organ damage, especially to the brain, heart and kidneys. Damage may result in encephalopathy, cerebral oedema, retinopathy, intracerebral haemorrhage, myocardial ischaemia, acute left ventricular failure with pulmonary oedema, acute aortic dissection and renal failure. Immediate reduction in blood pressure is required. Typical BP readings are 180/120 mmHg or higher.

Causes of hypertensive emergencies

1 Preeclampsia/eclampsia. *See Preeclampsia/eclampsia.*

2 Phaeochromocytoma. *See Phaeochromocytoma.*

3 Discontinuation of BP medication.

4 Drugs such as cocaine, amphetamines.
5 CNS trauma e.g. intracranial haemorrhage.
6 Aortic dissection.
7 Autonomic dysreflexia. *See Spinal cord injury (pre-existing) and anaesthesia.*

Treatment of hypertensive emergencies

Treatment aims at reducing blood pressure by 20–25% over 1 h, then to 160/100–110 mmHg over next 2–6 h, then cautiously to normal over 24–48 h. Always consider the possibility of phaeochromocytoma. **Patients with, or suspected of having, phaeochromocytoma must not receive beta blockers without alpha receptor blockade.**

Options for treatment of hypertensive emergencies include:

1 Clevidipine—*see Clevidipine*. This drug should be used cautiously in acute heart failure due to negative inotropic effects.
2 Glyceryl trinitrate infusion—*see Glyceryl trinitrate (GTN)*. This is a vasodilator that affects veins more than arteries. It is preferred for hypertension associated with acute coronary syndrome. *See Acute coronary syndrome*. It is also preferred when there is pulmonary oedema or a history of ischaemic heart disease.
3 Labetalol.
4 Fenoldopam. *See Fenoldopam*.
5 Sodium nitroprusside. *See Sodium nitroprusside (SNP)*.
6 Magnesium infusion for the treatment of hypertension associated with preeclampsia/eclampsia and phaeochromocytoma. *See Preeclampsia/eclampsia* and *Phaeochromocytoma*.

⊙ Hypertensive response to intubation

See Intubation—minimising hypertensive response.

⊙ Hypertrophic cardiomyopathy (HCM) and hypertrophic obstructive cardiomyopathy (HOCM)

Description

HCM is an inherited autosomal dominant disease in which there is thickening of the left ventricular (LV) wall without an identifiable cause such as hypertension. The right ventricle (RV) can also be involved. Normal LV wall thickness is 7–10 mm. With HCM, the LV wall thickness is at least 15 mm. In about 70% of HCM patients there is obstruction to the LV outflow tract (LVOT).[q] This is the obstructive form of HCM known as HOCM, also referred to as idiopathic hypertrophic subaortic stenosis (IHSS).

Pathophysiology

1 The LV becomes hypertrophied, which can be asymmetrical, concentric, diffuse or focal. It typically involves the anterior interventricular septum.
2 The ventricle becomes stiff (less compliant) and the LV cavity reduces in size.
3 There is excessive contractility in systole but decreased effectiveness of diastolic relaxation.
4 This results in a high diastolic filling pressure and the left atrium (LA) has to work harder to fill the LV.
5 If AF develops, it is poorly tolerated due to the loss of atrial 'kick' for LV filling.
6 The thickened ventricle with impaired diastolic relaxation is prone to ischaemia leading to chest pain, myocardial irritability and the development of dysrhythmias.

7 Hypertrophy of the interventricular septum can lead to LV outflow tract obstruction (LVOTO). Underfilling of the LV may make the obstruction worse. The whole situation is worsened if LV myocardial contractility increases e.g. activation of the sympathetic nervous system (SNS). Cavity size will be reduced, LV filling further impaired and there is increased obstruction to LV outflow.

8 A fall in SVR increases LV emptying but this will result in increased outflow obstruction because the LV is not being 'splinted open'.

9 This situation can be further worsened by the anterior mitral valve leaflet being pulled away from the posterior leaflet and towards the septum during systole (called systolic anterior motion of the mitral valve). This causes mitral valve incompetence and can completely obstruct the outflow tract.

10 LV fibrosis can lead to worsening systolic function and end-stage disease.

Clinical effects

HOCM effects range from asymptomatic to highly debilitating. Symptoms and signs may include:

1 chest pain, especially during exercise
2 fainting, especially during or just after exertion
3 heart murmur, typically a systolic ejection murmur (SEM)
4 a mitral regurgitant murmur may be present
5 palpitations—AF, SVT and ventricular arrhythmias
6 dyspnoea, particularly during exercise
7 hypotension
8 low-volume pulse
9 sudden death, especially in young athletes, due to VF or pulseless VT.
See Cardiac arrest.

Diagnosis

1 ECG may show high-voltage complexes, ST abnormalities, T wave inversion and P wave abnormalities. 90% of patients with HCM/HOCM will have ECG abnormalities.[9]
2 Cardiac echo shows LV wall thickening. Typically, the interventricular septum thickness is $> 1.3 \times$ the LV free wall thickness. It will also enable calculation of the LV outflow tract gradient. LVOT gradient > 30 mmHg is significant and > 50 mmHg is severe.[10]
3 Cardiac MRI if echocardiography inconclusive.
4 Cardiac catheterisation/angiography—to obtain direct measurements of filling pressures and LVOT gradient.

Treatment

1 Avoiding high-intensity exercise.
2 Beta blockers—to slow the heart rate (HR) and reduce the effect of exercise or excitement on the heart. Slowing the HR allows more time for ventricular filling.
3 Calcium channel blockers may improve diastolic relaxation, increase ventricular filling and increase exercise tolerance.
4 Sotalol—useful for its beta blocker and antiarrhythmic effects.
5 Amiodarone—for management of supraventricular and/or ventricular dysrhythmias.
6 Anticoagulant therapy such as warfarin—in patients with AF to reduce the risk of thromboembolism.
7 Automatic implantable cardioverter-defibrillator (AICD). *See Pacemakers.* Used to treat malignant dysrhythmias (VF, pulseless VT).

8 Dual-chamber pacemaker to induce apical pre-excitation to alter the timing of septal contraction and reduce outflow obstruction.

9 Catheter-based alcohol septal ablation.

10 Surgery—septal myotomy, myomectomy, cardiac transplant.

Anaesthesia and HCM/HOCM

Consult with the patient's cardiologist. Take appropriate pacemaker precautions if one is present. *See Pacemakers*.

The aims of anaesthetic management are as follows.

1 Maintain preload. Keep the LV well filled.

2 Prevent increases to myocardial contractility, which will paradoxically result in decreased cardiac output. Phenylephrine and vasopressin are preferred vasoconstrictors. Adrenaline and ephedrine should not be used as they will increase heart rate and contractility.

3 Prevent increases in HR to allow more time for LV filling. An HR of 60–80 bpm is optimal.[10]

4 Maintain SVR to reduce LV emptying and keep the LV 'splinted open'.

5 Treat arrhythmias such as new onset AF promptly as LV filling may be compromised.

Preoperative preparation

1 Maintain preload. The patient should be well hydrated but not over-hydrated.

2 Consider invasive blood pressure monitoring.

3 Have a defibrillator readily available.

Anaesthetic phase

1 Induce GA slowly and carefully with appropriate doses of midazolam, fentanyl and propofol. Ketamine is less suitable because it may increase HR. Use rocuronium for muscle relaxation. Ensure adequate opioid has been given to mitigate sympathetic stimulation due to intubation.

2 Maintain anaesthesia with propofol TCI or sevoflurane. Desflurane and N_2O should not be used.

3 Maintain afterload with a metaraminol or phenylephrine infusion. Do not use ephedrine, which will increase HR. Neuraxial anaesthesia, by decreasing SVR, may be particularly hazardous in these patients.

4 Treat hypotension with volume loading followed by boluses of metaraminol or phenylephrine. DBP should be > 70 mmHg to ensure adequate coronary artery perfusion of the hypertrophied LV.

5 Do not use drugs which increase contractility such as dobutamine.

6 Avoid high airway pressures, PEEP and Valsalva manoeuvres, which will increase intrathoracic pressure and decrease preload. Smaller tidal volumes and higher respiratory rates are preferable.

7 Treat hypertension with increased concentration of inhaled sevoflurane or boluses of propofol. If ineffective, use esmolol. *See Esmolol (Brevibloc)*. Do not use vasodilators such as GTN or SNP.

8 The use of transthoracic echocardiography (TOE) can help fluid management optimisation by assessing LV filling and assessment of the degree of LVOT obstruction.

9 Use sugammadex to reverse rocuronium to avoid tachycardia associated with atropine or glycopyrrolate.

HCM/HOCM and obstetrics

A team approach involving patient, obstetrician, cardiologist and anaesthetist should be utilised.

Preterm labour

Salbutamol is contraindicated if LV outflow tract obstruction is present. Consider magnesium therapy instead.

Epidural for labour

Early placement of an epidural in labour should be considered to avoid pain-induced tachycardia. The following is recommended:

1 Volume load the patient with IV crystalloid to maintain preload.
2 Use invasive BP monitoring if severe disease.
3 Maintain SVR with a phenylephrine infusion titrated to blood pressure.
4 Do not use adrenaline containing solutions.

Caesarean section

1 Use invasive arterial blood pressure monitoring if significant disease.
2 SAB is inappropriate for the reasons explained above.
3 An epidural can be used but must be slowly and carefully topped up using the precautions described above. A CSE with a low-dose spinal component can be considered.[10]
4 Have an infusion of phenylephrine running.
5 In severely compromised patients, CS should probably be managed with GA.
6 Give oxytocin by infusion post delivery rather than as a bolus which may cause vasodilation.

◖ Hypoglycaemia

Defined as a blood sugar level (BSL) of < 4 mmol/L (72 mg/dL).

Causes

1 Islet cell tumours—insulinoma.
2 Leucine-sensitive hypoglycaemia—hypoglycaemia provoked by the amino acid leucine or high-protein meals.
3 Drugs such as sulfonylurea toxicity or insulin overdose.
4 Missing a meal or excessive exercise after insulin therapy.
5 Liver failure
6 Congenital hyperinsulinism.

Clinical effects

1 Headache, hunger, mood change.
2 Dysphoria.
3 Dizziness.
4 Irregular or rapid heart rate.
5 Pale skin.
6 Sweating.
7 Numbness of lips, tongue and/or cheeks.
8 Confusion.
9 Decreased level of consciousness.
10 Seizures.

Patients that have asymptomatic hypoglycaemic episodes are at particular risk of losing consciousness.

Treatment

1 Oral glucose—**not if patient unconscious**.
2 IV glucose—50 mL of 50% glucose. If alcoholism is suspected, give IV thiamine 100 mg before glucose to avoid precipitating Wernicke's encephalopathy.
3 Glucagon 1 mg IV or IM if no IV access (e.g. out of hospital 'hypo').
4 Diazoxide. *See Diazoxide*.

◗ Hypotension

Definition

Systemic hypotension is defined as an SBP < 90 mmHg and a DBP < 60 mmHg. A MAP < 50 mmHg is particularly concerning. There are many causes of hypotension, and it is a frequently encountered problem in anaesthesia.

Causes

These can be divided into inadequate preload, cardiac causes and reduced systemic vascular resistance (SVR), also termed afterload. The following list is not exhaustive.

Inadequate preload

1 Venodilation due to depression of the sympathetic nervous system by anaesthetic drugs.
2 Hypovolaemia due to fasting, haemorrhage, dehydration, vomiting and/or diarrhoea.
3 Decreased venous return due to high intrathoracic pressures in ventilated patients.
4 Anaphylaxis with transudation of intravascular fluid into the tissues.
5 Supine hypotensive syndrome.

Cardiac causes

1 Cardiac depression by anaesthetic drugs.
2 Myocardial ischaemia due to coronary artery disease, hypotension, hypoxia.
3 Cardiac tamponade.
4 Tension pneumothorax.
5 Cardiac arrhythmias.
6 Other cardiac disease such as cardiomyopathy.

Reduced afterload

1 Neuraxial anaesthesia.
2 Hypotensive drugs causing arterial relaxation e.g. clonidine, hydralazine.
3 Sepsis.
4 Systemic inflammatory response syndrome.
5 Endocrine issues—adrenal suppression from long-term steroid therapy, adrenal haemorrhage.

Treatment

The urgency, aggressiveness and type of treatment depends on the severity of the hypotension and the presumed cause e.g. massive blood loss. A general approach is as follows:

1 Attempt to identify and treat the specific cause e.g. treat haemorrhage with IV crystalloid, colloid, blood.

2 Check all the other monitors—exclude hypoxia, check capnography, look for arrhythmia on ECG.
3 Start treatment with vasoconstrictors such as metaraminol, ephedrine or phenylephrine. An infusion of metaraminol or phenylephrine may be required.
4 Give IV crystalloid to improve preload.
5 Look at the patient. Is there any evidence of anaphylaxis, swelling, rash? Look at the neck veins for any evidence of distension suggesting tamponade. Listen to the heart for any evidence of failure or new murmurs. Listen to the lungs— bronchospasm, uneven chest movement. Feel for subcutaneous emphysema.
6 Check all drug infusions and dosages. Check what drugs have been given and if any drugs have been given accidently.
7 If vasoconstrictors are inadequate, insert an arterial line and central line. Commence catecholamine therapy with noradrenaline. If cardiac failure is thought to be the cause, **see Cardiogenic shock**. Summon skilled assistance. Intraoperative transoesophageal echocardiography can provide invaluable diagnostic information.
8 Consider other drugs such as adrenaline and vasopressin.

⊙ Hypoxia/hypoxaemia

Definitions
Hypoxia is defined as an inadequate supply of oxygen to the tissues. There are five types.
1 Hypoxic hypoxia—inadequate supply of oxygen e.g. altitude-related hypoxia.
2 Pulmonary hypoxia—lung disease causing inadequate oxygenation.
3 Hypoxaemic hypoxia—inadequate oxygen carried by the blood e.g. severe blood loss, anaemia, carbon monoxide poisoning, methaemoglobinaemia.
4 Stagnant hypoxia—inadequate blood flow to the tissues e.g. cardiac failure, use of a tourniquet.
5 Histotoxic hypoxia—cells are unable to utilise available oxygen e.g. cyanide poisoning, hydrogen sulphide poisoning.
   Hypoxaemia is a partial pressure of oxygen in arterial blood < 60 mmHg.
An oxygen saturation of < 90% on pulse oximetry is indicative of hypoxaemia.

Causes of hypoxaemia
There are many causes, and the anaesthetist must identify and treat the cause quickly to avoid brain damage, cardiac arrest and death.

Issues of equipment other than the ET tube or LMA
1 Contaminated O_2 supply e.g. N_2O being delivered instead of O_2.
2 Inadequate O_2 supply—fresh gas flow too low or hypoxic mixture due to user error, ventilator switched off.
3 Disconnection.
4 Blocked ventilator tubing.
5 Blocked filter.

Issues with the ET tube or supraglottic device
1 Blocked ET tube or supraglottic device—herniated cuff, foreign body (FB) in the lumen.
2 Kinked ET tube, device being bitten by patient.
3 Accidental extubation or dislodgement or malposition of supraglottic device.
4 Oesophageal intubation.
5 Endobronchial intubation.

QUICK FLICK **H**

Patient ventilation/airway issues

1 Laryngospasm.
2 Inadequate patient self-ventilation.
3 Foreign body in the airway.
4 Laryngeal swelling (anaphylaxis, angioedema).
5 Tracheal compression—mediastinal mass.
6 Bronchospasm.

Lung issues

1 Ventilation/perfusion (V/Q) mismatch.
2 Shunt.
3 Diffusion limitation—alveolar O_2 has difficulty entering the pulmonary capillaries e.g. pulmonary oedema.
4 Pneumothorax.
5 Pulmonary embolus—gas, fat, blood clot, amniotic fluid.
6 Smoke inhalation.

Hypoxaemia due to other causes

1 Anaemia.
2 Inadequate blood volume.
3 Inadequate cardiac output.
4 Hypermetabolic states—malignant hyperthermia.
5 Methaemoglobinaemia.
6 Carbon monoxide poisoning.
7 Other poisons e.g. cyanide.
8 Consider catastrophic causes such as amniotic fluid embolus, pulmonary embolus.

Hypoxia drill

1 Always check that the pulse oximeter is attached properly.
2 Maintain situational awareness, including surgical factors.
3 A quick scan of the anaesthetic machine, circuit and patient may quickly reveal the cause of the hypoxia.
4 Always check all other monitors, especially capnography, ECG and blood pressure. Patients who are hypoxic while receiving anaesthesia can be divided into two groups:

1 The awake or sedated patient (receiving e.g. neuraxial block or regional block such as brachial plexus block).
2 The patient receiving GA via supraglottic airway or ETT.

Awake or sedated patient

A – is the **a**irway patent? Open airway. Look for any evidence of airway compromise—vomitus, swelling suggesting anaphylaxis. Give supplementary oxygen. Is there laryngospasm?

B – is the patient **b**reathing, and breathing adequately—look and listen to the chest.

C – **c**irculation—check pulse, blood pressure, ECG.

D – always consider **d**rug effects e.g. phrenic nerve block with brachial plexus block, high spinal block, excess opioid medication, volatile being delivered to the patient unintentionally.

E – check **e**quipment—has supplementary oxygen become disconnected?

GA

A – check the monitors—is the oxygen flowmeter indicating O_2 flow? Does the oxygen analyser reflect the presence of O_2 and the correct inspired concentration? Look at the patient for any obvious issues. Change to bag ventilation with 100% O_2. This provides very useful information including:

- spontaneously breathing patient—is the bag moving? Is minute ventilation adequate? Is there laryngospasm? Is the patient biting the airway? Is the patient regurgitating/aspirating?
- intubated patient—does the compliance feel normal? Is there an obstruction? Is there a disconnection? Is the patient biting the tube? Is the tube kinked? Pass a Y-suction catheter down the tube to ensure it is patent. 'If in doubt, take it out' and reintubate.

B – could there be a circuit/filter problem? Change to ventilation with a self-inflating bag and cylinder oxygen with the filter removed. If no effect, return to machine ventilation. If a supraglottic airway is being used, intubate the patient. Listen to the lungs; check for breath sounds; is chest expansion equal, and is there any evidence of pneumothorax or bronchospasm?

C – check pulse, blood pressure, ECG. Any evidence of haemodynamic instability (blood loss, cardiac dysrhythmia)?

D – always consider anaphylaxis and drugs causing hypotension leading to hypoxia. Check IV lines for any entrainment of air (gas embolism).

E – check all equipment. This has basically been done when the anaesthetic machine was excluded. Check for other causes like carbon monoxide poisoning. Perform an ABG to confirm hypoxia. Obtain an urgent CXR and consider bronchoscopy.

REFERENCES

1   Shah U, Narayanan M, Smith J. Anaesthetic considerations in patients with inherited disorders of coagulation. *Cont Educ Anaesth Crit Care & Pain* 2015; 15: 26–31.

2   Peralta A, Chawla M, Lee RP. Novel bronchoscopic management of airway bleeding with absorbable gelatin and thrombin slurry. *J Bronchology Interv Pulmonol* 2018; 25: 204–211.

3   Kathuria H, Hollingsworth HM, Vilvendhan R, Reardon C. Management of life-threatening haemoptysis. *J Intens Care* 2020; 8. Accessed online: https://pubmed.ncbi.nlm.nih.gov/32280479, September 2022.

4   Qi X, Wang X, Huang X et al. Anaesthesia management for caesarean section 10 years after heart transplantation: a case report. *Springerplus* 2016; 5: 993.

5   Choudhury M. Post-cardiac transplant recipient: implications for anaesthesia. *Indian J Anaesth* 2017; 61: 768–774.

6   Conte AH, Lubin LN. Anaesthetic considerations after heart transplantation. *UpToDate* December 2021. Accessed online: www.uptodate.com/contents/anesthetic-considerations-after-heart-transplantation, September 2022.

7   Brutsaert EF. MSD Manual Professional Version. *Hyperosmolar Hyperglycaemic State (HHS)*. September 2022. Accessed online: www.msdmanuals.com/professional/endocrine-and-metabolic-disorders/diabetes-mellitus-and-disorders-of-carbohydrate-metabolism/hyperosmolar-hyperglycemic-state-hhs, December 2022.

8   Whelton PK, Carey RM, Aronow WS et al. 2017 ACC/AHA/AAPA/ABC/ACPM/AGS/APhA/ASH/NMA/PCNA Guideline for the prevention, detection, evaluation and management

of high blood pressure in adults: a report from the American College of Cardiology/ American Heart Association Task Force on Clinical Practice Guidelines. *Hypertension* 2018; 71: e13.

9 Ibrahim IR, Sharma V. Cardiomyopathy and anaesthesia. *BJA Education* 2017; 17: 363–369.

10 Mulaikal TA, Moitra VK. Anaesthesia for patients with hypertrophic cardiomyopathy undergoing noncardiac surgery. *UpToDate*, updated 18 May 2021. Accessed online: www.uptodate.com/contents/anesthesia-for-patients-with-hypertrophic-cardiomyopathy-undergoing-noncardiac-surgery, December 2022.

▶ Idarucizumab (Praxbind)

Description
Monoclonal antibody fragment that binds to dabigatran (Pradaxa), stopping its thrombin-blocking effect.

Dose
5 g IV given as two injections of 2.5 g over 5–10 min. A second 5 g dose can be given if needed. Praxbind is effective within 5 min of administration. Dabigatran can be restarted 24 h after Praxbind.

▶ Ideal body weight (IBW)

IBW is defined as the weight associated with the lowest mortality (as calculated from actuarial studies) and is calculated from the patient's height. IBW calculators are available online. Numerous equations can be used, including Broca or Robinson.

The Broca formula is:
Women: IBW (kg) = (height in cm − 100) + [(height in cm − 100) × 0.15]
Men: IBW (kg) = (height in cm − 100) + [(height in cm − 100) × 0.1]

The Robinson equation is:
Women: IBW (kg) = 49 kg + 1.7 kg × (height in inches − 60)
Men: IBW (kg) = 52 kg + 1.9 kg × (height in inches − 60)

▶ Ilioinguinal and iliohypogastric nerve blocks

Introduction
The iliohypogastric nerve supplies sensation to the skin above the inguinal ligament, the suprapubic region and the lateral thigh. The ilioinguinal nerve supplies sensation to the medial upper thigh, scrotum and pubic area. Blocking these nerves is useful for inguinal hernia and scrotal surgery.

Anatomy
These nerves are branches of the L1 spinal nerve from the lumbar plexus, with a branch from T12. The L1 primary ventral ramus enters the upper part of the psoas muscle, where it branches into the ilioinguinal and iliohypogastric nerves.

The two nerves emerge at the lateral border of the psoas muscle, and pass anterior to the quadratus lumborum muscle. They then run in a plane between the internal oblique and transversus abdominis muscles. The ventral rami of the nerves then pierce the internal oblique and lie between the internal and external oblique muscle layers.

Block using ultrasound in the adult
Use aseptic technique. Prepare a syringe with 15 mL of 1% ropivacaine and a short-bevelled block needle.
1   Place the ultrasound probe medial to the anterior superior iliac spine (ASIS), angled upwards on an imaginary line between the ASIS and the umbilicus.

2 The nerves are seen between the muscle layers very near to the ASIS, at a depth of about 3 cm. At this point the nerves are consistently between the internal oblique and rectus abdominis muscles.

3 Insert the needle in-plane from medial to lateral so the needle tip lies near the nerves between the muscle layers.

4 After a negative aspiration test, inject 10–15 mL of LA.

5 Note that this anatomical site is just above the iliacus muscle. An injection in the plane between the iliacus muscle and the rectus abdominis may result in a femoral nerve block.

◗ Iloprost

This drug is an analogue of prostacyclin. It is used by inhalation to treat primary or secondary pulmonary hypertension. *See Pulmonary hypertension*. It may also be helpful in the treatment of Raynaud's phenomenon and scleroderma. The dose is 2.5 mcg by nebuliser 6–9 times per day during waking hours as tolerated.

◗ Immune thrombocytopenic purpura (ITP)

Description

ITP is due to antiplatelet glycoprotein antibodies which result in increased platelet destruction in the spleen. It was formerly referred to as idiopathic thrombocytopenic purpura. There are two types of ITP:

1 Acute thrombocytopenic purpura—usually affects children after an acute viral infection and lasts < 6 months. Treatment is usually not needed.

2 Chronic thrombocytopenic purpura—usually affects adults, mainly females. Lasts longer than six months and may be lifelong.

Causes

ITP is due to some trigger causing antiplatelet antibodies to be made. This trigger can be drugs or infections such as hepatitis C. It is also associated with pregnancy and immune disorders such as rheumatoid arthritis. Low-grade lymphomas and leukaemias may result in antiplatelet antibodies.

Clinical effects

1 Bleeding.
2 Bruising.
3 Petechial rash.

Diagnosis

1 FBC showing low platelets.
2 Antiplatelet antibody test.

Treatment

1 Cease suspected drug cause.
2 Treat suspected infective cause e.g. hepatitis C.
3 Steroid therapy.
4 IV gamma globulin (IVGG).
5 Danazol and azathioprine.
6 Rh immune globulin.
7 Splenectomy.
8 Platelet transfusion.
9 Rituximab—slows antiplatelet antibody production.
10 Drugs that stimulate increased platelet production such as romiplostim.

Anaesthesia and ITP

1 Platelet count should be > 50000 per mm^3 for surgery and > 75000 per mm^3 for neuraxial anaesthesia and deep nerve blocks.
2 A platelet transfusion is required for significant surgery if the platelet count is $< 50000/mm^3$ but should **not** be carried out simply to provide neuraxial anaesthesia.

ITP and pregnancy

1 If the platelet count is less than $30\,000/mm^3$ before 36 weeks' gestation, administer oral prednisone 1–2 mg/kg/day or IV immunoglobulin (1 g/kg) once.
2 Splenectomy if severe refractory thrombocytopenia.
3 The neonate may also be affected.
4 Neuraxial anaesthesia can be considered if the platelet count is > 75000 per mm^3.

◗ Immunosuppressive drugs—side effects

General effects of immunosuppression

1 High-dose immunosuppression increases the risk of malignancies, including skin cancers and lymphoma.
2 Renal impairment.
3 Increased risk of infections.
4 Liver, pancreatic and/or bone marrow toxicity.
5 Hypertension.

Azathioprine

1 Withdrawal of this drug in patients taking warfarin may precipitate bleeding.
2 May cause severe bone marrow depression and/or pancreatitis.
3 Liver toxicity and biliary stasis may occur.
4 Infants born to mothers on azathioprine may have pancytopenia and severe immunosuppression.
5 Increased duration of effect of suxamethonium.
6 Inhibition of non-depolarising NMBDs.

Cyclosporin

May cause:
1 hypertension
2 gingival hyperplasia
3 decreased seizure threshold
4 renal toxicity
5 hepatic insufficiency
6 biliary stasis.

Mycophenolate

Pregnant patients may be at increased risk of miscarriage and oro-facial clefts in the fetus.

Tacrolimus

This drug is associated with:
1 increased incidence of postoperative infection
2 increased risk of diabetes mellitus
3 decreased seizure threshold
4 nephrotoxicity.
Tacrolimus and ketamine may interact, with resultant confusion.

◉ Infraorbital nerve block

Introduction

The infraorbital nerve is a branch of the maxillary division of the trigeminal nerve. A block of this nerve is useful for surgery on the lower eyelid, cheek, upper lip and side of nose. It also supplies the upper incisor, canine, premolar and root of the first molar tooth. It emerges from the infraorbital foramen.

Anatomy

The infraorbital nerve provides sensory innervation to the lower eyelid, cheek, upper lip and side of nose. It also supplies the upper incisor, canine, premolar and root of the first molar tooth. It emerges from the infraorbital foramen 1.5 cm below the inferior orbital rim. This foramen lies about 2 cm from the lateral border of the nose and is in line with the pupil when the eye is in the neutral position.

Technique

Use an aseptic technique. Sterilise the injection site.

1 Pass a 23 G needle 0.5 cm below the infraorbital foramen and inject 2 mL of 2% lignocaine at the foramen orifice.
2 Alternatively, insert the needle through the mucosa adjacent to the upper gum above the first premolar tooth, aiming the needle towards a finger of the opposite hand, held over the foramen. The bevel of the needle should be facing the bone.
3 Inject 2 mL of 2% lignocaine near the foramen.

◉ Inherited bleeding disorders

These include:

1 haemophilia. *See Haemophilia*
2 Von Willebrand disease—the most common inherited coagulopathy.
   See Von Willebrand disease (VWD)
3 rare bleeding disorders due to factor deficiencies in addition to those described in the *Haemophilia* section.
4 hereditary haemorrhagic telangiectasia—tangled blood vessels that can bleed.

◉ Intercostal nerve block

Introduction

Intercostal nerve blocks are useful for treating pain from the chest wall and upper abdomen e.g. pain associated with fractured ribs, breast surgery and post-herpetic neuralgia.

Anatomy

The intercostal nerves lie in the intercostal grooves at the lower edge of each rib. T2–T6 supply the chest and T7–T11 supply the abdomen (sensory and motor innervation). *See Dermatomes* to identify the correct ribs and associated intercostal nerves to block. For fractured ribs, block each fractured rib.

Technique

Use aseptic technique. Explain the procedure and the potential complications to the patient (see below). Position the patient prone with the arms in front of the head and the chest on a pillow. The best place to block the nerve is behind the midaxillary line.

1 Identify the target rib and pull the skin up slightly cephalad.
2 Insert a 23 G sharp-bevelled needle at 90° to the skin onto the middle of the rib after anaesthetising the skin.

3 Walk the needle towards the caudad edge of the rib.
4 Angle the needle cephalad and insert the needle about 2 mm so that the point is in the intercostal groove.
5 Perform test aspiration then inject 3–5 mL bupivacaine 0.5%.
6 If using ultrasound, place the probe over the lateral ribs in a cephalad caudad plane. The rib shadows, pleura and intercostal muscles are easily visualised.
7 Insert the block needle from caudad to cranial direction so the needle tip is in the intercostal groove.
8 Do not insert the needle through the bright white line (the pleura).

Complications
Pneumothorax is the main risk. Be careful not to inject the LA intravascularly.

◖ Internal jugular vein (IJV) central line

Anatomy
The IJV originates from the jugular foramen at the base of the skull and terminates between and behind the sternal and clavicular heads of the sternomastoid muscle. Here it joins the subclavian vein to form the brachiocephalic vein. At its origin the IJV is posterior to the internal carotid artery, but as it descends it becomes lateral to the common carotid artery (CCA) and anterior to it. Sometimes the IJV overlies the CCA and sometimes it is medial to it. See Figure I1.

Technique with ultrasound (adult patient)
This must be done as a fully sterile procedure with all precautions, including sterile gown, gloves and drapes.
1 Position the patient supine with 10–20° of Trendelenburg positioning.
2 Prep the neck with antiseptic solution on the side of insertion. The target area is about midway between the mastoid process and the clavicle, over the sternomastoid muscle.
3 Prepare the central line. Flush all lumens with N/S and attach three-way taps in the closed position to all lumens except the brown (distal) one.
4 Place sterile drapes over the neck with the head turned away slightly from the side of insertion.
5 Place a sterile sheath over the ultrasound probe and scan the neck. Identify the IJV (which should be 'squishy') and CCA (pulsatile and usually medial and deeper). Orientate the probe to give a transverse view of the vessels.
6 If the patient is awake, anaesthetise the entry point with 1% lignocaine.
7 Attach a 5 mL syringe to the Seldinger needle and, using an out-of-plane approach, penetrate the IJV while providing aspirating force constantly on the syringe. A tactile 'pop' may be felt.
8 If venous blood is not aspirated, put the probe down and aspirate while withdrawing the needle.
9 When venous blood is easily aspirated, remove the syringe and insert the J-tip of the guidewire through the needle.
10 Use the probe to confirm the wire is in the vein. Ectopics may be noted on the ECG display due to the wire irritating the endocardium. Withdraw the wire slightly if this occurs.
11 Using the scalpel, make a small cut through the skin at the entry point of the wire. This must be large enough to enable insertion of the dilator over the wire.

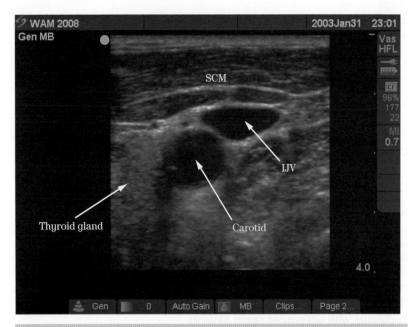

Figure I1 Ultrasound image of the internal jugular vein (IJV)
SCM = sternomastoid muscle
Image courtesy of Dr Alwin Chuan

12 Pass the dilator over the wire to dilate the puncture wound and deeper tissues, then remove the dilator.

13 Pass the central line over the wire. Make sure the proximal end of the guidewire is visible before insertion of the central line into the patient.

14 Insert the central line to a depth of about 12–15 cm for the right IJV and about 14–18 cm for the left IJV on average. The ideal position of the tip is the lower SVC just proximal to the right atrium.

15 Remove the wire and ensure blood can be aspirated from each lumen and then flush each lumen with N/S. Ensure each lumen is **not** open to air.

16 Place the white and blue clips over the central line where it enters the neck and suture the clips to the neck.

17 Curve the central line around gently so the lumens will not be brushing against the patient's face. Suture the proximal end of the central line to the skin.

18 Apply a sterile dressing.

19 Perform a post-procedure CXR to check the position of the tip of the central line.

Differences between the right IJV and left IJV

1 The left IJV provides a longer, less direct route to the SVC.

2 The left IJV tends to have a smaller calibre.

3 The dome of the lung is higher on the left.

4 The thoracic duct enters the circulation at the base of the IJV or subclavian vein.

Complications

1 Carotid artery puncture. Arterial blood will usually be seen spurting out from the needle hub. Remove the needle and apply pressure, then reattempt IJV puncture.

2 Dilation of the carotid artery. If this occurs, leave the dilator in place and capped. Contact a vascular surgeon urgently to explore the arterial injury.

3 Pneumothorax.

4 Infection.

5 Inability to thread the wire. This can be due to the needle slipping out of the vein or venous thrombus or stenosis of the vein may be present.

6 Placement of the tip in the RA. Under sterile conditions withdraw the central line sufficiently, so it is just proximal to the right atrium.

○ International normalised ratio (INR)

The INR was developed to improve comparability of measures of prothrombin time (PT) between different laboratories. *See Prothrombin time (PT)*. NR for INR 0.9–1.2. Surgery and neuraxial anaesthesia can be performed if INR < 1.5, assuming there are no other coagulation issues. *See Warfarin*.

○ Intra-arterial injection of drugs (unintentional)

This section is based on published case reports and the author's experience of accidental intra-arterial injection of drugs, presented in alphabetical order.

1 Atropine—no effects[1]

2 Buprenorphine—can produce peripheral limb ischaemia[2]

3 Dexmedetomidine—no ill effects

4 Diazepam—potentially ischaemia and tissue necrosis

5 Etomidate—no effect[3]

6 Fentanyl—no effect

7 Flucloxacillin/penicillin—severe effects with arterial vasospasm/gangrene[3]

8 Glycopyrrolate—no effect[1]

9 Ketamine—can cause ischaemia and necrosis

10 Midazolam—no effect[4]

11 Morphine—no effect

12 Neostigmine—no effect[1]

13 Pancuronium—no effect

14 Phenytoin—can cause vascular complications

15 Propofol—can cause pain, local blanching and transient decrease in blood flow to the distal limb. Full recovery is expected[5]

16 Mannitol—no effect (author experience)

17 Promethazine—very severe tissue damage/gangrene

18 Succinylcholine—no effect

19 Thiopentone—severe arterial spasm, intense pain, gangrene.

Treatment of harmful intra-arterial injection

1 Disconnect infusion tubing from the cannula, aspirate residual drug from the cannula and then flush the cannula with saline.

2 If there is any evidence of arterial spasm, consider:

  a) papaverine 40–80 mg in 20 mL N/S intra-arterially

  b) tolazoline 25–50 mg intra-arterially

  c) reserpine 1.25 mg IV

  d) phenoxybenzamine 0.5 mg IV

  e) anti-clotting/antiplatelet agents used systemically.

3 Iloprost, a thromboxane inhibitor, with dextran 40, given intra-arterially, may be helpful.[6] Dextran is an anti-sludging agent.

4 Urokinase, given intra-arterially, can be used to dissolve arterial blood clot.
5 A brachial plexus block can be used to treat severe upper limb pain and provide sympathetic blockade.

◗ Intracranial pressure (ICP) and treatment of raised ICP

Description

ICP is the pressure exerted by the cerebrospinal fluid (CSF) inside the skull and on brain tissue. ICP is defined as the pressure in the lateral ventricle or in the space over the convexity of the cerebral cortex.

1 Normal ICP is 13 cm H_2O (10 mmHg).
2 20–25 cm H_2O is equivocal.
3 > 25 cm H_2O (18.4 mmHg) is raised ICP.

Patients with a normal blood pressure remain alert up to an ICP of 54 cm H_2O. Above this level, there is decreased level of consciousness, with brain infarction and death above 67 cm H_2O (50 mmHg).

Symptoms/signs of raised ICP

1 Headache—worse on coughing, sneezing or bending over.
2 Vomiting.
3 Visual disturbance/papilloedema.
4 Back pain.
5 Decreased level of consciousness.
6 Ocular palsies—especially the abducens nerve (sixth cranial nerve—moves eye laterally).
7 Pupillary dilatation.
8 Cushing's triad—hypertension with an increased systolic blood pressure and widened pulse pressure, bradycardia and an irregular breathing pattern. The abnormal breathing is due to impaired brainstem function. This triad is also called the Cushing reflex.
9 Coning—the ICP is so high that the brain (specifically the cerebellar tonsils) herniates through the foramen magnum. **See Coning/brain herniation syndrome/ brain code.**

Causes of raised ICP

1 Brain tumour.
2 Brain injury.
3 Subarachnoid haemorrhage.
4 Epidural or subdural haematomas in the skull.
5 Cerebral oedema.
6 Cerebral infarction.
7 Encephalitis/meningitis/brain abscess.
8 Hydrocephalus.
9 Malignant hypertension with brain haemorrhage. **See Hypertension.**
10 Cerebral venous sinus thrombosis.
11 Overproduction of CSF e.g. due to choroid plexus tumour.
12 Decreased resorption of CSF e.g. meningeal granulomas.
13 Elevated central venous pressure e.g. due to SVC obstruction. **See Superior vena cava syndrome (SVCS).**
14 Benign intracranial hypertension.

Measurement of ICP

1 Lumbar puncture (LP) and measurement of the height of CSF in a plastic tube. However, performing a LP may result in coning if raised ICP is due to conditions such as cerebral oedema/space-occupying lesion. Exclude these pathologies with a cerebral CT prior to LP.

2 Intraventricular catheter inserted through a burr hole, penetrating the brain and entering the lateral ventricle. This is the most accurate method of measurement and allows CSF to be removed to decrease ICP.

3 Subdural screw bolt—a hollow screw is inserted through a burr hole and into the subdural space over the brain. CSF cannot be removed with this device.

4 Epidural sensor—a sensor is inserted through a burr hole and sits in the dural tissue. CSF cannot be removed with this device.

5 Trans-cranial doppler ultrasonography.

Treatment of raised ICP

1 Identify and treat the cause e.g. extradural haematoma.

2 Reverse Trendelenburg position 15–30°.

3 Ensure there is no venous obstruction (e.g. tight ETT tie around the neck) and that the head is in the neutral position.

4 Ensure muscle relaxation in the anaesthetised patient as increased thoracic/abdominal tone can increase ICP. Also coughing, bucking and straining will increase ICP.

5 If the patient is having a GA use propofol TCI. Do not use volatile/N_2O.

6 Ensure optimal ventilation to prevent hypoxia and hypercarbia. If necessary, hyperventilate the patient to an $ETCO_2$ concentration of 30 mmHg. Use minimal PEEP.

7 Mannitol 20% solution 0.25–1 g/kg (up to 2 g/kg) IV over 20 minutes. **See Mannitol.** Effects start in about 10 min and peak effects occur at 45 min. If ICP remains elevated, give mannitol 20% 0.25–0.5 g/kg IV q 6 h. The effects of mannitol are enhanced by giving frusemide 0.3 mg/kg. Frusemide can be given instead of mannitol at a dose of 1 mg/kg IV.

8 Hypertonic saline (1.6–7.5%) by continuous IV infusion run at 0.1–1 mL/kg/h.

9 Steroid drug for brain tumours/vasogenic oedema—dexamethasone 16 mg IV LD then 4 mg q 6 h.

10 CSF drainage.

11 Maintain glucose control (7.8–10 mmol/L).

12 Avoid hyperthermia > 38°C.

13 In rare circumstances barbiturate coma is used e.g. thiopentone 10 mg/kg IV over 30 min, then 5 mg/kg/h IV for 3 h, then 1 mg/kg/h.

14 Cold saline irrigation of the brain by the surgeon.

15 Decompressive craniotomy.

○ Intracranial venous thrombosis (IVT)

See Cerebral venous sinus thrombosis (CVST).

○ Intrahepatic cholestasis of pregnancy (ICP)

Description

This condition occurs in about 0.7% of pregnancies. There is impaired release of bile from liver cells into the biliary tree. This leads to subsequent impairment of liver function. There is a build-up of bile acids and other toxic substances in the blood. ICP is the most common liver disease specific to pregnancy. The condition usually presents in the third trimester of pregnancy with:

1 intense itch without rash
2 jaundice
3 loss of appetite/nausea
4 premature birth, meconium-stained amniotic fluid
5 sudden and unpredictable intrauterine death
6 deranged LFTs
7 coagulopathy (rarely).

Causes

The cause is usually unknown, but 15% of patients have an autosomal dominant inherited genetic mutation of ABCB11 and ABCB4 genes. There is a higher incidence of ICP in women with a history of liver disease and non-singleton pregnancies. It tends to reoccur with subsequent pregnancies. Full recovery after pregnancy is a feature of this illness.

Management

1 Relief of itching with ursodeoxycholic acid, which decreases serum bilirubin.
2 Rifampicin is used as a second-line drug.
3 If bile acid levels are > 100 μmoles/L, consider induction of labour/Caesarean section between 34 and 37 weeks.
4 If bile acid levels are < 100 μmoles/L, consider induction of labour/Caesarean section at 37–38 weeks.

Anaesthesia

Coagulopathy is rare in patients presenting for Caesarean section with ICP. While it is prudent to check coagulation status prior to neuraxial blockade, in an emergency Caesarean section neuraxial blockade should not be withheld purely because of the diagnosis of ICP.[6]

◗ Intralipid for the treatment of ropivacaine/bupivacaine toxicity

In the event of serious toxicity with possible or actual cardiac arrest:

1 Give intralipid 20% solution, 1.5 mL/kg IV bolus (70 kg patient = 100 mL).
2 Commence IV infusion of intralipid 20% at a rate of 15 mL/kg/h (70 kg patient = 1000 mL/h).
3 Double the rate of intralipid infusion (30 mL/kg/h) if haemodynamic stability is not restored or deterioration occurs.
4 Repeat intralipid bolus 1.5 mL/kg IV q 5 min × 2 if needed.
   The suggested maximum total dose of intralipid 20% is 12 mL/kg.

◗ Intraoperative blood salvage

Description

This strategy involves suctioning of blood from the operative site, adding heparin to the collected blood and filtering out impurities such as tissue and clots. Suction pressure should not exceed 150 mmHg. Do not suck up non-blood substances such as amniotic fluid, sterile water, hydrogen peroxide or iodine. The blood is transferred to a reservoir and then to a centrifuge, which separates the red blood cells (RBC) from all other substances. The RBC are then washed and suspended in N/S (haematocrit 40–60%) and reinfused into the patient through a blood filter. *See Blood filters.*

Indications

1 Any situation where significant blood loss may occur. In obstetric surgery, suction away all the amniotic fluid before salvage and use a leukocyte depletion filter for the reinfused blood. There is a risk of infusing fetal RBC.
2 Jehovah's Witnesses patient.
3 Patient with pre-existing anaemia.
4 Patient that is difficult to cross-match.

Contraindications

1 Infected material at the site of surgery.
2 Faecal contamination.
3 Sickle cell disease due to RBC sickling. ***See Sickle cell disease (SCD).***
4 Beta thalassaemia trait is a theoretical risk due to RBC fragility. ***See Thalassaemia.***
5 Phaeochromocytoma—due to the risk of adrenaline and noradrenaline being mixed with the salvaged blood. ***See Phaeochromocytoma.***
6 Malignancy? This is a highly controversial area, and some researchers feel that malignancy is an absolute contraindication unless the infusate is irradiated.[7] However, there is little evidence of harm. A leukocyte depletion filter should be used.[8]

Intraoperative myocardial ischaemia

Introduction

Intraoperative myocardial ischaemia is rare, but has a high morbidity and mortality. The following section concerns patients having general anaesthesia. Over 30% of perioperative deaths are due to cardiac complications.[9]

Pathophysiology

Intraoperative myocardial ischaemia occurs when the O_2 supply to the heart muscle does not meet the heart's demand. Factors determining O_2 supply include:

1 calibre of the coronary vessels
2 coronary artery perfusion pressure (aortic diastolic blood pressure minus LVEDP). Hypotension reduces coronary artery perfusion pressure. The ischaemic threshold is estimated to be a MAP < 55 mmHg in normal patients[10]
3 time spent in diastole which is determined by heart rate
4 O_2 saturation (+ small amount of O_2 dissolved in plasma)
5 haemoglobin level
6 cardiac output.

Factors determining O_2 demand include:

1 end diastolic left ventricular wall tension, which is determined by preload and cardiac compliance
2 myocardial contractility
3 heart rate
4 systemic vascular resistance (afterload)
5 sympathetic outflow to the heart.

Diagnosis of intraoperative myocardial ischaemia

1 ECG changes—usually ST segment depression, T wave inversion, new bundle branch blocks and arrhythmias. ***See Electrocardiography (ECG)—a brief guide.***
2 Regional wall changes on transoesophageal echocardiography (TOE).

3 Haemodynamic disturbance—hypotension, tachycardia, bradycardia.

4 Fall in O_2 saturation/hypoxaemia.

5 Rapid troponin test positive. **See *Acute coronary syndrome*.**

Management

Notify the surgeon and expedite surgery. Obtain urgent expert cardiologist advice and, if possible, the assistance of a cardiac anaesthetist. In addition:

1 Optimise O_2 supply—increase FiO_2 to 100% initially until the patient is stabilised and then reduce FiO_2 to a level that maintains reasonable oxygenation.

2 Reduce sympathetic outflow to the heart due to nociceptive stimulation with adequate opioid therapy. Exclude/treat awareness.

3 Ensure adequate Hb level (80–100 g/L) and adequate blood volume. Has there been acute blood loss?

4 Optimise blood pressure. Aim for SBP > 90 mmHg. Phenylephrine is a reasonable choice of vasoconstrictor.

5 Optimise preload. A TOE is very useful for assessing cardiac filling.

6 Treat arrhythmias.

7 Correct bradycardia/tachycardia. In patients with HR > 100 bpm with stable SBP, consider slowing HR with beta blocker therapy.

8 Insert an arterial line and send blood for ABG analysis.

9 Correct electrolyte abnormalities.

10 Commence a glyceryl trinitrate infusion to increase the calibre of coronary arteries and decrease preload, thus reducing ventricular wall stress. Sublingual GTN 0.4 mg q 5 min up to 3 doses can be given while the infusion is prepared. GTN is also a preferred treatment in the setting of myocardial ischaemia and hypertension. It may be necessary to combine GTN with phenylephrine to prevent/treat GTN-induced hypotension.

11 If there is no surgical contraindication, give aspirin 160–325 mg down a nasogastric tube.

12 If heart failure occurs, **see *Cardiogenic shock*.** If inotropes are required, this may result in tachycardia and increase myocardial O_2 demand. Noradrenaline may be a reasonable first choice. Also consider a combination of dobutamine and milrinone. Vasopressin should also be considered.

13 Mechanical circulatory support e.g. intra-aortic balloon pump may be required.

14 Obtain a 12 lead ECG as soon as practically possible. A STEMI suggests an acute thrombus is present in a coronary artery and is much less likely to be treated successfully with medical therapy alone.[10]

15 Post-procedure, a decision must be made by the cardiologist and surgeon as to which therapy poses the least risk to the patient, the choices being:

a) medical therapy—more likely to be chosen if NSTEMI, stable patient, high bleeding risk

b) double antiplatelet therapy, coronary revascularisation procedure—more likely to be chosen if STEMI, unstable patient, low bleeding risk.

⊙ Intraosseous (IO) access

Description

IO access can be used as an alternative to IV access when the latter is not possible (difficult veins, burns). This procedure has become feasible thanks to the development of the Arrow EZ-IO drill with specially designed needles.

Technique

1 Surgically prep the insertion site. The two favoured sites in the adult are:
   a) anteromedial surface of the tibia—2–3 cm below the tibial tuberosity.
   b) upper lateral humerus 1 cm above the surgical neck. The surgical neck is where the greater tuberosity joins the rest of the bone.

2 For the humeral approach—the patient flexes the elbow to 90° and the palm of the hand is placed onto the upper abdomen. For the left arm approach, the operator places the medial edge of his/her left hand along the axilla, and the edge of the right hand over the lateral humerus. Where the thumbs meet is in the area of the surgical neck (it feels like a golf ball on a tee). Go 1 cm above this point. The patient cannot adduct their arm after needle placement as the needle may be displaced by the coracoid process.

3 For the tibial approach, palpate the flat medial surface of the tibia 2–3 cm below the tibial tuberosity.

4 In the awake patient, anaesthetise the skin and periosteum at the entry point.

5 Poke the needle through the skin until bone is contacted. If this is not done, skin can become twisted in the rotating drill needle. Drill the needle into the bone until the hub is flush with the skin. A loss of resistance sensation should be felt with correct positioning.

6 Unscrew the needle cap and remove the trocar. Place the sterile IO stabiliser dressing over the hub then attach the IO needle connector (pre-primed with N/S or LA in the awake patient).

7 Aspirate bone marrow or blood. Inject 5 mL of 1% lignocaine slowly in the awake patient. If anaesthetised or unconscious patient inject 10 mL N/S (which is very painful if patient is awake).

8 Blood aspirated from the IO needle can be used for cross-match.

9 There are three sizes of needle—pink for paediatric, blue (25 mm) for most adults and yellow (45 mm) for the humeral site or if excess adipose tissue.

10 Any drug can be given through the IO needle.

11 To remove the needle, attach a Luer lock syringe. Rotate the needle clockwise and then pull the needle out.

Special points

1 Do not use the IO needle in a fractured bone or if there is infection at the site of insertion.

2 Do not leave the IO needle in the bone for more than 24 h.

3 If an IO needle has been inserted into a bone and then removed, do not insert a second IO needle into the same bone.

◑ Intrathecal anaesthesia

See Subarachnoid block (SAB).

◑ Intrauterine fetal death

Intrauterine fetal death can be associated with coagulopathy that can be severe. Disseminated intravascular coagulopathy may occur. *See Disseminated intravascular coagulopathy (DIC).* This is probably due to the release of fetal thromboplastin. DIC rarely occurs unless the fetus has been dead for days or weeks. Delivery soon after fetal death will usually prevent DIC from occurring. Perform coagulation studies before neuraxial anaesthesia. There is also an increased risk of sepsis.

⊙ Intrauterine fetal resuscitation (IUFR)

Description

IUFR is required when there is a non-reassuring fetal heart trace suggesting fetal hypoxia/acidosis. Fetal scalp blood monitoring can definitively identify fetal acidosis. *See Fetal scalp blood sampling.* IUFR aims at enhancing uterine and placental blood flow until urgent CS can be initiated. This may involve resuscitating the mother.

Causes

1 Increased uterine activity.
2 Poor maternal positioning with aortocaval compression.
3 Umbilical cord issues (prolapse, cord compression, cord around the neck, knotted cord).
4 Placental abruption.
5 Uterine rupture.
6 Maternal haemorrhage.

Strategies

1 Correct maternal hypotension (IV fluids, vasoconstrictors).
2 Positioning the mother left or right lateral to relieve aortocaval compression.
3 Reduce uterine contraction intensity/frequency by ceasing oxytocin infusion and/or using tocolytic drugs such as terbutaline or GTN. *See Terbutaline* and *Glyceryl trinitrate (GTN).*
4 Maternal oxygen supplementation to increase oxygen supply to the fetus.
5 Cord compression can be treated by manually elevating the presenting part, filling the bladder with saline or by Trendelenburg or knee-chest positioning.
6 Bolus of 1000 mL of Hartmann's solution. This has been shown to improve fetal condition even when there is no evidence of maternal hypotension.[11]

⊙ Intubation—minimising hypertensive response

This is required in specific clinical situations such as:
1 cerebral aneurysm surgery
2 phaeochromocytoma
3 preeclampsia/eclampsia.

Strategies

In addition to an appropriate dose of propofol:
1 fentanyl 5 mcg/kg IV
2 lignocaine 1.5 mg/kg 2–3 min before intubation
3 esmolol 0.5 mg/kg IV. *See Esmolol*
4 remifentanil 1 mcg/kg IV over 2 minutes during induction, then an IV infusion run at 0.05 mcg/kg/min
5 spray the vocal cords with 3 mL of topical lignocaine prior to intubation
6 use a nerve-stimulator to ensure the patient is fully paralysed before intubation.

⊙ Intubation without muscle relaxant

This can be achieved by:
1 awake intubation using LA to anaesthetise the airway. *See Awake intubation*
2 propofol 2 mg/kg IV + remifentanil 4–5 mcg/kg IV 2.5 min before intubation.[12]

◐ Iron overload

Description

Iron overload describes a condition in which there is excess storage of iron in the body. Normally, only 1–2 mg of iron is absorbed and excreted per day. There can be primary overload as occurs with haemochromatosis or secondary overload due to frequent blood transfusions. Iron can harm the body in two ways:

1 accumulation of iron in organs
2 circulation of unbound iron (iron not bound to transferrin) can damage tissues directly. Unbound iron is a powerful oxidising agent.

Causes

1 Haemochromatosis. **See Haemochromatosis.**
2 Frequent blood transfusion required for conditions such as severe thalassaemia. **See Thalassaemia.** One unit of RBC contains about 200–250 mg of iron. Individuals are at risk of iron overload after 20–40 units of blood.

Effects

1 Asymptomatic.
2 Fatigue.
3 Cardiac failure and/or dysrhythmias. These are the most common fatal complications of frequent transfusion.[13]
4 Endocrine organ damage causing diabetes mellitus (pancreas), hypogonadotropic hypogonadism (pituitary), hypothyroidism (thyroid) and hypoparathyroidism (parathyroid). This in turn can lead to osteopaenia/osteoporosis.
5 Liver damage.
6 Amenorrhoea.
7 Joint pain.
8 Abdominal pain.
9 Grey or bronze skin colour.
10 Possibly increased susceptibility to bacterial infection.

Diagnosis

Measure the serum ferritin level. A result of > 1000 mcg/L indicates iron overload.

Treatment

1 Therapeutic phlebotomy—this cannot be done in patients who are transfusion dependent.
2 Iron chelation therapy—these drugs actively remove iron from the plasma and liver but are less effective on the heart. They work by binding to free iron and enhancing its elimination in urine. An example is deferoxamine (also called desferrioxamine).
3 Minimise dietary intake of iron.

Anaesthesia and iron overload

1 These patients should be carefully screened for iron-induced organ damage, particularly cardiac impairment.
2 In patients having frequent transfusions, cross-matching blood may be difficult. **See Thalassaemia.**

◐ ISBAR

ISBAR is a standardised communication acronym to assist in the hand-over of vital patient information to another healthcare professional. It organises a conversation about a patient into essential elements so that vital information is not missed. The letters stand for:

I – **I**dentify—yourself, your role, the patient (name, sex, date of birth, age, medical record number), and check you are speaking to the correct person.

S – **S**ituation—what is happening with the patient/what triggered the conversation.

B – **B**ackground—what are the circumstances that led to the patient's situation/past medical history; what happened prior to the situation requiring review including medications and allergies.

A – **A**ssessment—what you think the problem is; use ABCDE (*see ABCDE assessment*). Other relevant information may include temperature, pain score etc.

R – **R**ecommendation—what do you think the patient requires? What do you recommend, and who will provide this treatment? Does the patient require transfer? When? Where? How?

◐ Ischaemic heart disease (IHD)

See Acute coronary syndrome and Intraoperative myocardial ischaemia.

Introduction

Ischaemic heart disease describes any disease resulting in inadequate oxygen supply to the myocardium. The causes are:

1 coronary artery disease (CAD)—the most important cause and the leading cause of death in most countries
2 coronary artery spasm
3 any other cause of insufficient oxygen delivery e.g severe anaemia, coronary artery dissection.

Pathophysiology

CAD is due to the formation of intra-arterial cholesterol plaques which cause progressive narrowing of the coronary arteries (atherosclerosis). The plaques can rupture, causing a blood clot and acute blockage of the coronary artery.

Clinical effects

1 Angina, pain in jaw, arms or shoulder.
2 Acute coronary syndrome (unstable angina, heart attack). *See Acute coronary syndrome.*
3 Shortness of breath.
4 Fatigue.
5 Weakness, light headedness.
6 Ischaemia that does not present with pain (silent ischaemia). This can occur in the heart transplant patient and diabetics. *See Heart transplant patient.*
7 Dysrhythmias.
8 Heart failure.

Causes

1 Family history.
2 Hypercholesterolaemia.

3 Smoking.
4 Hypertension.
5 Obesity/obstructive sleep apnoea (OSA).
6 Diabetes mellitus.
7 Lack of exercise.
8 Chronic kidney disease.
9 Stress.

Investigations

1 ECG.
2 Echocardiography.
3 Exercise stress test/dipyridamole-thallium scan.
4 Stress echocardiography.
5 CXR.
6 Coronary artery calcium score.
7 Coronary angiogram/cardiac catheterisation.

Treatment

Can be divided into:
1 Modification of lifestyle—diet, exercise, quit smoking.
2 Drug therapy.
3 Percutaneous coronary intervention—angioplasty, stents. **See Coronary artery stents.**
4 Coronary artery bypass grafting.
5 Enhanced external counterpulsation (EECP)—involves compressing blood vessels in the lower limbs, which results in coronary artery collaterals forming.

Drugs used to treat ischaemic heart disease

1 Statin therapy is used to lower cholesterol and stabilise plaques in coronary arteries. Statins are contraindicated in pregnancy.
2 Beta-adrenergic receptor blockers—reduce heart rate and therefore myocardial oxygen demand. **See Beta-adrenergic receptor blocker drugs.**
3 Aspirin and other antiplatelet drugs to reduce the risk of coronary artery thrombosis.
4 Calcium channel blocker drugs—used as an alternative to beta blocker drugs.
5 Optimal drug treatment of hypertension, diabetes mellitus and obesity.
6 Nitrates to vasodilate coronary arteries.
7 Ranolazine (Ranexa)—anti-anginal medication which inhibits persistent or late inward sodium current in heart muscle. This leads to reduced intracellular calcium levels and therefore reduced tension in the heart wall.
8 Nicorandil (Ikorel)—causes vasodilatation, particularly of veins. It is a nitrate derivative that forms nitric oxide (NO). It also opens potassium channels in arterial smooth muscle, leading to arterial dilatation. This drug therefore reduces end diastolic pressure and SVR.
9 Ivabradine. **See Ivabradine.**
10 Trimetazidine—this drug is a fatty acid oxidation inhibitor that improves myocardial glucose utilisation. It does this by inhibiting fatty acid metabolism. This means that ischaemic cells are more easily able to maintain cellular functions such as ion pumps.

❍ Isoflurane

Description

Obsolescent volatile anaesthetic drug. Halogenated methyl ether. MAC 1.15 vol %. *See Minimum alveolar concentration.*

Advantages

Potent anaesthetic suitable for most types of surgeries.

Disadvantages

1 Pungent odour makes it unsuitable for gaseous induction.
2 Significantly prolongs the QT interval. May precipitate torsades de pointes. *See Long QT syndrome (LQTS)* and *Torsades de pointes.*
3 Potent vasodilator—may cause coronary artery steal syndrome in the setting of coronary artery stenosis.

❍ Isoprenaline/isoproterenol (Isuprel)

Description

Synthetic catecholamine drug that acts on beta-adrenoreceptors, causing positive inotropy and chronotropy. There are no significant alpha-adrenoreceptors effects. It also dilates the bronchi and decreases diastolic blood pressure by lowering peripheral vascular resistance. *See Adrenoreceptors.* Indications for isoprenaline include:

1 Treating complete heart block or other causes of severe bradycardia. *See Heart block (HB).*
2 Inducing tachydysrhythmias during electrophysiological studies.
3 Treating asthma—but rarely used for this indication.

Preparation

Mix 2 mg of isoprenaline with 50 mL of 5% glucose, resulting in a concentration of 40 mcg/mL. Administer through a central venous access line only.

Dose for complete heart block

Adult

10–20 mcg IV, then an IV infusion run at 0.5–8 mcg/min (1–12 mL/h).

Child

0.4 mcg/kg IV bolus followed by an IV infusion 0.1–1 mcg/kg/min.

❍ Ivabradine (Corlanor)

Ivabradine inhibits the I_F or 'funny' channel (a mixed sodium/potassium channel) of the SA node. It slows the SA node pacemaker current, causing a decrease in heart rate. It is used to treat patients with stable angina and heart failure by slowing heart rate. It is used in patients intolerant of beta blockers. Used off-label to treat inappropriate sinus tachycardia. *See Postural orthostatic hypotensive syndrome (POTS).*

REFERENCES

1 Jain A, Sahni N, Banik S, Solanki SL. Accidental intraarterial injection of neostigmine with glycopyrrolate or atropine for reversal of residual neuromuscular blockade: a report of two cases. *Anesth Analg* 2012; 115: 210–211.

2 Gouny P, Gaitz JP, Vayssairat M. Acute hand ischaemia secondary to intraarterial buprenorphine injection: treatment with iloprost and dextran-40. *Angiology* 1999; 50: 605–606.

3 McGrath P. Accidental intra-arterial flucloxacillin: management using guanethidine. *Anaesth Intensive Care* 1992; 20: 518–519.

4 Iatrou C, Robinson S, Rosewarne F. Inadvertent intra-arterial midazolam (letter). *Anaesth Intensive Care* 1997; 25: 431.

5 Ohana E, Sheiner E, Gurman GM. Accidental intra-arterial injection of propofol. *Eur J Anaesthesiol* 1999; 16: 569–570.

6 DeLeon A, De Oliveira G, Kalayil M et al. The incidence of coagulopathy in pregnant patients with intrahepatic cholestasis: should we delay or avoid neuraxial analgesia? *J Clin Anesth* 2014; 8: 623–627.

7 Hansen E, Bechmann V. Intraoperative blood salvage in cancer surgery: safe and effective? *Transfus and Apher Sci* 2002; 27: 153–157.

8 National Blood Authority Australia. *Guidance for the provision of intraoperative cell salvage.* March 2014. Accessed online: www.blood.gov.au/ics, December 2022.

9 Alkhatib C, Rego-Cherian L, Cotter EK. Management of suspected intraoperative myocardial ischaemia. *Int Anesthesiol Clin* 2021; 59: 53–60.

10 Walsh M, Devereaux PJ, Garg AX et al. Relationship between intraoperative mean arterial pressure and clinical outcomes after noncardiac surgery: toward an empirical definition of hypotension. *Anesthesiol* 2013; 119: 507–515.

11 Velayudhareddy S, Kirankumar H. Management of foetal asphyxia by intrauterine foetal resuscitation. *Indian J Anaesth* 2010; 54: 394–399.

12 Kveraga R, Pawlowski J. Anaesthesia for the patient with myasthenia gravis. *UpToDate* May 2022. Accessed online: www.uptodate.com/contents/anesthesia-for-the-patient-with-myasthenia-gravis#!, July 2022.

13 Leung T, Lao T. Thalassaemia in pregnancy. *Best Pract Res Clin Obstet Gynaecol* 2012; 26: 37–51.

J

◗ Junctional tachycardia

See *Supraventricular tachycardia (SVT).*

◗ Jurnista

This is a trade name for hydromorphone used orally. *See* *Hydromorphone (Dilaudid, Jurnista).*

○ Kapanol

This is a trade name for oral morphine. **See Morphine.**

○ Ketamine (Ketalar)

Description

Ketamine is a non-competitive NMDA receptor antagonist and a sodium channel blocker. It may have an agonist effect at opioid receptors. It is useful for:

1 induction of anaesthesia—can be used as a sole agent in situations where resources are limited
2 analgesia for acute pain
3 treatment of chronic pain
4 treatment of depression
5 asthma treatment.

Dose for GA

For induction of anaesthesia—1.5–2 mg/kg IV. If no IV access, consider for the adult IM doses of 200 mg titrated to effect and for children use 4–6 mg/kg IM.

Ketamine for pain management

Brief painful procedures

For brief painful procedures, consider IV doses of 20–30 mg in the adult. Ketamine can also be given sublingually for this purpose at the same dose. Alternatively, oral ketamine 100–200 mg for adults or 6 mg/kg for children can be given.

Ketamine intraoperatively for reduction of intraoperative and postoperative opioid requirements

Bolus of IV ketamine 0.5 mg/kg then an infusion of 0.25 mg/kg/h. Cease the infusion 30–45 min before completion of surgery. 0.5 mg/kg/h is another suggested infusion rate.

Ketamine subcut or IV for postoperative analgesia

Used to treat opioid resistant acute pain and patients with, or at risk of, neuropathic pain. In adults, add 200 mg of ketamine to 50 mL N/S (4 mg/mL). Run the infusion at 1–2 mL/h. Adding 1 mg of haloperidol to the ketamine solution (200 mg in 50 mL N/S) may reduce ketamine induced dysphoria.

Advantages

1 Does not cause respiratory depression.
2 Causes cardiovascular stimulation via the sympathetic nervous system. This could also be a disadvantage in certain conditions such as hypertrophic cardiomyopathy.
3 Causes bronchodilation.
4 Airway reflexes are well preserved compared with other anaesthetic drugs. This increases the safety of ketamine when used in remote locations e.g. disaster zones.
5 Potent analgesic effects resulting in reduced opioid requirements.
6 Can be given IM or PO in uncooperative patients.

Disadvantages

1 Relatively slow onset.
2 Induction may be associated with involuntary movements.
3 Disturbing emergence and postoperative psychogenic reactions may occur, such as hallucinations and dysphoria.
4 There may be excessive salivation.
5 It may be associated with increased PONV.
6 Causes increased intraocular and intracranial pressure.
7 Has direct myocardial depressant effects.
8 Hepatic toxicity can occur with prolonged infusions.
9 Subject to addiction and recreational use. This can lead to bladder damage.
10 Patients on tacrolimus may become infused when receiving a ketamine infusion.

◑ Ketanserin

Antihypertensive drug used to treat pulmonary hypertension caused by protamine. It may also be helpful in treating carcinoid related hypertension. *See Carcinoid tumours and carcinoid syndrome*. It is a selective 5-HT$_{2A}$ receptor blocker. It is also used topically in the treatment of wounds/burns to promote epithelialisation.

◑ Ketorolac

Description
Potent non-selective NSAID. Available as an IV or IM injection or PO.

Dose—adult
IV/IM—10–30 mg q 4–6 h, maximum 90 mg/day (60 mg/day in the elderly).
PO—10 mg q 4–6 h, maximum 40 mg/day.

Special points

1 This is a potent NSAID and it may have significant side effects including:
  a) renal failure
  b) peptic ulcer
  c) GIT haemorrhage.
2 Do not use for more than 5 days by any route.
3 Do not use in patients with hypovolaemia, dehydration or renal dysfunction. *See Non-steroidal anti-inflammatory drugs (NSAIDS)*.

◑ Kidney transplant

See Renal transplant.

◑ Kinin-kallikrein system (KKS)

This system is another example of a metabolic cascade like the clotting system. It is a complex and poorly understood system that is involved in the inflammatory response, blood pressure, coagulation and pain. It is composed of kallikrein, kinins, kininase I and II and enkephalinase. Kinins are potent vasodilators and cause low blood pressure. They also promote natriuresis and diuresis and promote inflammation.

Bradykinin
The kinin-kallikrein system makes bradykinin by cleaving high-molecular-weight kininogen (HMWK) through the action of kallikrein. Plasmin can probably also generate bradykinin. *See Bradykinin*.

○ Labetalol (Trandate, Normodyne, Presolol)

Description
Labetalol is an alpha-1 and beta-adrenoreceptor receptor blocker. It is used to treat hypertension, hypertensive emergencies, chronic angina and heart failure. It is also used to treat hypertension in pregnancy. It is suitable for treating hypertension due to phaeochromocytoma. **See Phaeochromocytoma**. It decreases blood pressure by decreasing SVR.

Dose
Adult (to treat hypertensive emergency)
IV bolus 20 mg over 2 min followed by 40 mg then 80 mg × 3 at 10–20 min intervals as needed. IV infusion dose 20 mg/h increased at 20 min intervals to a maximum of 160 mg/h. No more than 300 mg/24 h by any route.

Advantages
1 Does not cause significant hypotension.
2 Can be used during pregnancy, for intracranial diseases requiring BP control and after MI.
3 Low doses can be used in patients with LV failure.

Disadvantages
1 Contraindicated in heart block and bradycardia.
2 Contraindicated in patients with asthma.

○ Lactate

NR 0.3–1.3 mmol/L. Lactate is produced by anaerobic metabolism, hence a rise in serum lactate reflects tissue hypoperfusion. Serum lactate correlates well with the degree of hypovolaemic shock due to haemorrhage. Elevated lactate levels improve as tissue oxygenation improves and there is increased liver perfusion (where lactate is metabolised).

○ Laparoscopic surgery

Creation of the pneumoperitoneum
A pneumoperitoneum is created by insufflating gas, usually CO_2, into the peritoneal cavity. The gas is insufflated at a rate of 4–6 L/min initially then at 200–400 mL/min to maintain the pneumoperitoneum. An intra-abdominal pressure (IAP) of 10–15 mmHg is sufficient for most procedures.

Physiological effects of pneumoperitoneum
Cardiovascular
1 Creation of a pneumoperitoneum can result in severe bradycardia or asystole due to vagal reflexes. In addition to releasing the gas, treatment includes:
   a) atropine 600 mcg IV
   b) circulating the atropine with CPR if asystole or severe bradycardia.

Do not give adrenaline 1 mg for this type of asystolic arrest.

2   Increased IAP causes autotransfusion of pooled blood in the gut, increasing venous return to the heart and cardiac output (CO). However, if IAP > 20 mmHg, the IVC is compressed, decreasing venous return and CO.

3   In the head-up reverse Trendelenburg position there may be venous pooling in the lower limbs with decreased venous return from the legs causing a reduced CO.

4   Increased IAP increases SVR by compressing the abdominal aorta. SVR is also increased by raised blood catecholamine levels. This maintains or increases mean arterial pressure (MAP), and causes tachycardia. This can lead to ischaemia in patients with ischaemic heart disease. *See Ischaemic heart disease (IHD)*.

5   Diaphragmatic elevation, due to increased IAP, leads to increased intrathoracic pressure, decreasing venous return via the IVC and SVC.

6   If the patient has impaired cardiac function or is hypovolaemic or IAP is too high, CO and MAP may decrease.

7   Venous gas embolism may occur, due to insufflation of gas directly into the venous system. Gas can also enter the circulation via a damaged blood vessel in the peritoneal space.

8   There is an increased risk of embolus (gas or blood clot) into the cerebral circulation via a patent foramen ovale (PFO). A PFO is present in about 25% of the population. IPPV, head-down positioning and pneumoperitoneum result in increased right atrial (RA) pressure which can exceed left atrial (LA) pressure. Therefore, an embolus in the RA can pass into the LA via the PFO. For the same reason, patients with cyanotic congenital heart disease may have increased shunting and worsening hypoxia with laparoscopic surgery. *See Congenital heart disease (CHD) overview*.

Respiratory

1   Elevation of the diaphragm due to pneumoperitoneum and head-down positioning causes reduced FRC and increased basal lung atelectasis. This leads to increased V/Q mismatching and can lead to hypoxia, particularly in the obese patient. Application of modest PEEP (e.g. 5 cm H_2O) may reduce this effect. In addition, ventilating with a large tidal volume (10–15 mL/kg ideal body weight) may also be helpful. *See Ideal body weight (IBW)*.

2   The tip of the ET tube may be displaced into a bronchus due to the raised diaphragm and head-down positioning.

3   Airway resistance increases and lung compliance decreases.

4   Increased IAP leads to increased intrathoracic pressure with lung compression and increased pulmonary vascular resistance. This may reduce cardiac output.

5   CO_2 is readily absorbed from the peritoneal cavity and may increase $PaCO_2$. This can lead to acidosis, increased catecholamine release, tachycardia and increased myocardial O_2 demand. Increasing the minute ventilation will 'breathe off' the excess CO_2.

6   Subcutaneous emphysema.

7   Pneumothorax or pneumomediastinum. *See Pneumothorax/tension pneumothorax*.

8   Prolonged head-down positioning and pneumoperitoneum may cause upper airway oedema and stridor post extubation.

Gastrointestinal

1   Raised IAP and head-down positioning may increase the risk of regurgitation and aspiration. Airway protection with a cuffed ET tube is recommended. This is not to say that supraglottic airways cannot be used in select patients who are having select procedures e.g. laparoscopic tubal ligation.

2 Laparoscopic gynaecological surgery is associated with a high incidence of postoperative nausea and vomiting. Administer prophylactic anti-nausea drugs and use propofol TCI rather than volatiles/N_2O. *See Postoperative nausea and vomiting (PONV).*

3 Excessive IAP can lead to gut and liver ischaemia.

4 The stomach may be injured or obscure surgical view/access during upper abdominal surgery. This risk can be reduced using an orogastric tube.

Renal

1 Excessive IAP may increase renal vascular resistance and decrease renal arterial flow, thus decreasing GFR and urine output. There may also be raised renal venous pressure.

2 The bladder may be injured or obscure surgical view/access. This risk can be reduced by emptying the bladder with a catheter.

3 Activation of the renin-aldosterone mechanism. *See Renin-angiotensin system.*

Neurological

1 Increased IAP increases ICP. In patients with elevated ICP (e.g. hydrocephalus), laparoscopic surgery is contraindicated.

2 Prolonged steep head-down positioning with pneumoperitoneum may increase the risk of cerebral oedema. Patients may have temporary neurological dysfunction after prolonged laparoscopic surgery in the head-down position.

Other effects

1 Prolonged steep head-down positioning with pneumoperitoneum may cause a form of compartment syndrome in the lower limbs. *See Well leg compartment syndrome.*

2 Distressing shoulder tip pain post procedure, possibly due to overstretching of the diaphragm by the pneumoperitoneum.

3 Risk of damage to blood vessels or organs from trocar insertion, or inadvertent inflation of a solid organ.

4 Risk of brachial plexus injury if extreme head-down positioning and shoulder braces are used to prevent patient slippage. Use a non-slip mat rather than shoulder bracing.

Contraindications to laparoscopic surgery

1 Hypovolaemia.

2 Cyanotic congenital heart disease.

3 Known patent foramen ovale.

4 Raised ICP.

⬦ Laryngeal anatomy

Laryngeal cartilages (see Figure L1)

The laryngeal cartilages are the:

1 *thyroid cartilage*—has the thyroid notch anteriorly

2 *cricoid cartilage*—shaped like a signet ring, with the narrowest part facing anteriorly. Between the thyroid and cricoid cartilages is the cricothyroid membrane

3 *arytenoid cartilages*—pyramidal in shape and articulate with the superolateral aspects of the cricoid cartilage

4 *epiglottis*—leaf-shaped cartilage attached at its lower end to the thyroid cartilage. The vocal cords run from the arytenoid cartilages to the posterior surface of the thyroid cartilage

5 *corniculate cartilages*—small nodules sitting on the arytenoid cartilages

6 *cuneiform cartilages*—flakes of cartilage within the aryepiglottic folds.

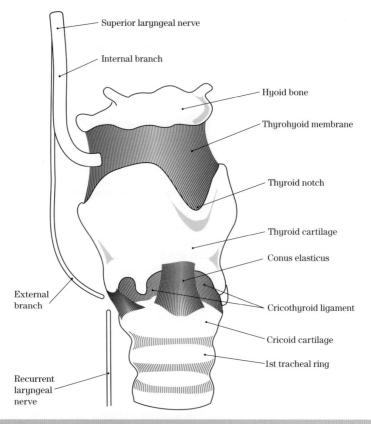

Figure L1 Laryngeal cartilages

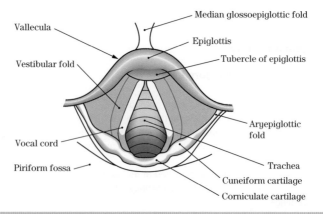

Figure L2 The laryngeal inlet

Innervation of the larynx

1 The larynx is innervated by the vagus nerve via the superior laryngeal nerve and the recurrent laryngeal nerve.
2 The superior laryngeal nerve supplies the interior of the larynx as far as the vocal cords (via its internal branch).
3 The recurrent laryngeal nerve supplies the intrinsic muscles of the larynx (apart from the cricothyroid) and sensory supply to the laryngeal mucosa inferior to the vocal cords.

▶ Laryngoscopy view grading, direct

*See **Direct laryngoscopy view grading.*** Figure L2 shows the anatomy of an ideal direct view of the laryngeal inlet.

▶ Laryngospasm

Description

Defined as the involuntary occlusion of the glottis and laryngeal inlet by contraction of the laryngeal muscles closing the true and/or false vocal cords. It can cause partial or total obstruction of the airway. Laryngospasm typically occurs when anaesthesia is light (i.e. induction or emergence) in patients without an ET tube in situ. Oral secretions or regurgitated fluid can irritate the vocal cords and produce laryngospasm.

Clinical effects

1 Stridor.
2 Respiratory distress (tachypnoea, chest retraction).
3 Negative pressure pulmonary oedema may occur. *See **Negative pressure pulmonary oedema (NPPO).***
4 Hypoxia, hypoxic arrest.

Prevention

1 Extubate patients when control of laryngeal reflexes is likely e.g. opening eyes, reaching for ET tube.
2 Suction oral secretions prior to extubation.

Treatment

1 Remove the stimulus causing laryngospasm if possible e.g. suction out oral secretions.
2 Try to 'break' the laryngospasm. Using bag-mask ventilation, attempt to augment the patient's inspiratory effort with positive pressure delivered in short, sharp squeezes of the bag. This may maintain SpO_2 long enough for the patient to regain control of laryngeal musculature. At the same time, optimise the airway (head tilt, jaw thrust).
3 Consider rapidly deepening anaesthesia with a bolus dose of IV propofol.
4 Applying bilateral pressure to the 'laryngospasm notch' by what is called the Larson manoeuvre. This 'notch' is between the mastoid process and the ramus of the mandible. Apply the middle finger to this notch bilaterally and pull the jaw forward.
5 If the laryngospasm is causing serious hypoxia, give suxamethonium or rocuronium and intubate the patient.
6 Ventilate with 100% O_2 until the patient is 'awake', then extubate.

⏵ Laser surgery

Introduction
Laser stands for **l**ight **a**mplification by **s**timulated **e**mission of **r**adiation. Photons are used to bombard the electrons of atoms. Electrons struck by photons enter a higher energy state (they are 'excited'). When an electron returns to its stable energy state, a photon is created. Under special conditions excited electrons go from a higher energy state to an in-between state called a metastable state, generating heat but no light. When a photon of a certain energy strikes an electron in a metastable state, the electron moves to a stable state and 2 photons of identical wavelengths are formed. These photon pairs strike more metastable electrons, setting up a chain reaction. Mirrors are used to focus these photons with identical wavelengths into an intense monochromatic beam—the laser beam.

Classes of lasers and safety advice for each class
- *Class 1*—do not look directly into the laser beam (but doing so will probably not damage eyes or skin).
- *Class 2*—like class 1 but not safe if viewed through lenses.
- *Class 2, 2M*—do not look directly into the laser beam/laser bar code scanner. Accidental flash probably okay but close eyes or look away. Not safe to shine the beam into eye.
- *Class 3R*—do not look directly into laser. Accidental flash view okay but staring into beam is hazardous e.g. laser pointer (1–5 mW power).
- *Class 3B*—hazardous to eyes and skin. **Must not be viewed directly.** Example—laser light show (5–500 mW).
- *Class 4*—hazardous to eyes and skin. Can cause fires. Even viewing diffuse reflection may be hazardous. Example—surgical laser (30–100 W).

Types of surgical laser
All surgical lasers use a second, low-powered laser (e.g. a helium-neon laser) for targeting. The medical laser beam may be visible or invisible. Types include the following:
1 **CO_2 laser**—causes massive heat and vaporisation of the first few layers of cells. Does not penetrate deeply. Beam is invisible. Destroys surface structures. Used for precise cutting as in ENT.
2 **Nd:YAG laser**—less intense heat but deep penetration, more thermal coagulation than vaporisation. Used for ENT, retina, anterior chamber eye surgery, dermatology. Also used for endobronchial pathology such as cancers.
3 **Ruby laser**—poorly absorbed except for pigmented cells. Used to treat pigmented cells and for tattoo removal.

Laser safety
Can be divided into engineering controls and administrative controls.

Engineering controls
These are controls built into the laser machine, including locks, automatic standby when laser is idle, foot pedal cover and audible and visible emission indicators when the laser is on.

Administrative controls

1 Warning signs that laser is in use on the outside of **all** doors, which must be **closed.**
2 No through traffic.
3 Appropriate protective safety goggles matched to the wavelength of the laser that is being used.
4 Presence of a Laser Safety Officer (LSO).
5 Appropriate training of all staff.
6 Fire-fighting equipment including a carbon dioxide fire extinguisher, a bucket of water to immerse small burning objects, and 50 mL syringes of sterile N/S for airway fires.
7 Non-flammable curtains over windows.
8 Non-shiny instruments to minimise laser reflection.
9 Wearing of special surgical masks to prevent the inhalation of laser plume, which can be hazardous e.g. aerosolised papilloma virus.
10 Laser plume evacuation device.

Anaesthetic considerations for laser surgery

The main risks to the patient are:

1 eye damage
2 skin damage
3 fire, especially airway fire.

General measures to protect the patient

1 Cover hair and face with a wet towel.
2 Cover the patient's exposed skin.
3 Place saline-soaked gauze around the surgical site.
4 Avoid alcohol-based preps which may catch fire. If they are used, make sure they are completely dry before draping.
5 If the patient is awake, they must wear appropriate laser-protection goggles.

Measures to protect the patient during laser airway surgery

1 Use laser-resistant ET tubes e.g. Mallinckrodt Laser-Flex.
2 Fill the ET cuff with saline and methylene blue to detect cuff rupture.
3 Minimise inhaled oxygen concentrations. Use air if possible; otherwise use the minimum effective inhaled concentration of O_2 in air. Do not use N_2O, which also supports combustion.
4 Consider suctioning O_2 in the oropharynx with a metal sucker before lasering. Flooding the surgical field with CO_2 is also effective.
5 Ensure the cuff of the ET tube is not leaking O_2 into the surgical field.
6 Ensure that the ET tube cuff is well below the cords **but** the tip of the ET tube is not in a bronchus.
7 After taping the eyes, place saline-soaked gauzes over the eyes. This will resist laser penetration.
8 Cover the face with a wet towel/gauze.
9 Ensure drapes do not have an oxygen-rich atmosphere pooled underneath them.
10 Prepare 50 mL syringes of sterile N/S to extinguish a fire in the surgical field.
11 The surgical laser power density and pulse duration should be at the minimum effective setting.
12 The tip of the laser should be visible at all times, deactivated before removal from the surgical site and placed in a sheath away from the patient when not in use.

Measures to protect the eye during laser surgery near the eye

For laser surgery near the eye, such as eyelid surgery, use stainless steel or lead eye-shields. Plastic eye-shields are unsuitable.

Management of airway fire

This is a crisis situation and can result in life-threatening airway injury.

1 Whoever sees the fire must alert all staff members that there is a **fire in the airway.**
2 Stop the ignition source (laser, diathermy, static electricity, argon beam coagulators).
3 Cease ventilation, disconnect the ET tube from the circuit and remove the ET tube from the airway.
4 Put the burning ET tube into the bucket of water preprepared for this purpose.
5 Extinguish visible airway fire with sterile N/S in 50 mL preprepared syringes.
6 Remove any foreign debris from the airway.
7 Only when the fire is extinguished and all smouldering debris is removed, commence mask ventilation with air. Titrate FiO_2 as necessary to maintain O_2 saturation. Continue anaesthesia with IV propofol.
8 If the fire has spread beyond the airway and is not extinguishable with the bucket of water or the N/S syringes, use the carbon dioxide fire extinguisher.
9 Examine the airway for injury with direct laryngoscopy. Remove any remaining debris.
10 Re-intubate the patient and perform flexible endoscopic bronchoscopy and saline lavage. Rigid bronchoscopy may be more effective for assessment and treatment.
11 Severe upper airway damage may necessitate low tracheostomy.
12 Assess the oropharynx and face for burns.
13 Arrange CXR and obtain ABG.
14 Consider IV steroids to reduce airway swelling.
15 Admit patient to ICU as the full extent of injury may not be evident for 48 h.

◐ Lateral femoral cutaneous nerve block/lateral cutaneous nerve of thigh block

See Fascia iliaca block.

◐ Lean body mass

This is defined as the mass of a body with fat mass excluded. It is calculated from body weight and the body fat percentage. Average body fat percentage for women is 25–31%, and for men is 18–24%. For fit people, the body fat percentage for women is 21–24% and for men it is 14–17%. In obese people, body fat percentage is > 32% for women and > 25% for men. Body fat calculators are available on the internet and use measurements of age, weight, height, neck circumference and waist circumference.

◐ Left-to-right shunt

See Congenital heart disease (CHD)—overview.

◐ Left ventricular ejection fraction (LVEF)

See Cardiac risk for non-cardiac surgery.

LVEF is defined as the fraction of volume of blood ejected in systole in relation to the end-diastolic LV volume. It is the central measure of LV systolic function. The NR is 50–70%. 40–49% is mildly abnormal and 30–39% moderately abnormal. LVEF < 30% is severe impairment. A hyperdynamic LVEF is > 70%.

�‌ Lepirudin

Description

This drug is a recombinant form of hirudin (a substance produced by leeches). It is an anticoagulant drug that acts as a direct and irreversible thrombin inhibitor. It binds to both free and clot-bound thrombin. It is used to prevent or treat DVT/PE/thromboemboli in patients that cannot have heparin due to heparin-induced thrombocytopenia type 2. **See Heparin-induced thrombocytopenia (HIT).**

Dose
Adult

IV bolus 0.4 mg/kg then IV infusion 0.15 mg/kg/h. If used for prophylaxis do not give a bolus dose. Treatment can be monitored with APTT. **See Activated partial thromboplastin time (APTT).**

Overdose/bleeding

There is no antidote but activated FVII may be helpful. Haemofiltration can remove the drug.

◌ Levobupivacaine (Chirocaine)

S-enantiomer of bupivacaine. It is used at the same doses as bupivacaine but has 30–50% less cardiotoxicity and neurotoxicity than racemic bupivacaine.

◌ Levosimendan

Description

Cardiotonic drug that increases myocardial contractility by enhancing the sensitivity of the heart muscle to calcium. There is no increase in myocardial O_2 consumption or effect on heart rhythm. It also has vasodilator properties by stimulating ATPIII channels. It is indicated for severe heart failure resistant to other therapies. With an infusion, the peak effect occurs after 10–30 min and the duration of action is 1–2 h.

Contraindications

1 Renal and liver failure.
2 Severe hypotension and tachycardia.
3 History of torsades de pointes.
4 LV outflow obstruction.

Dose
Adult

Mix 12.5 mg levosimendan with 250 mL 5% glucose (makes a solution of 0.05 mg/mL). Give a LD of 6–24 mcg/kg over 10 min–1 h (in a 70 kg patient = 8.4–33.6 mL). Then commence an IV infusion at a rate of 0.1 mcg/kg/min which equals 8.4 mL/h for a 70 kg patient. If after 30–60 min there is excessive hypotension or tachycardia, reduce the infusion rate to 0.05 mcg/kg/min. If the initial infusion rate is well tolerated, consider increasing it to 0.2 mcg/kg/min.

◌ Lignocaine (Lidocaine, Xylocaine)

Description

Amino amide-type LA and antiarrhythmic drug. Presented in strengths of 0.5–2% for local and regional anaesthesia and IV injection. There are also topical versions. Lignocaine is safer from a cardiotoxic perspective than bupivacaine or ropivacaine but is shorter acting.

Uses

1 Any type of local, regional or epidural anaesthesia but **not** subarachnoid block (SAB).
2 Antiarrhythmic drug (Class 1b) for shock-resistant VF, pulseless VT. **See Cardiac arrest.**
3 Reducing the stimulating effects of intubation and extubation.
4 Treatment of neonatal seizures.
5 Reduce the pain of IV propofol (add 30 mg lignocaine to 200 mg of propofol).
6 Intraoperative/postoperative analgesic effects.

Maximum doses for infiltration, topical and regional blocks

1 Lignocaine with adrenaline 7–8 mg/kg.
2 Lignocaine without adrenaline 4–5 mg/kg.
3 For effects of LA toxicity, **see Local anaesthetic (LA) toxicity.**

Reducing hypertensive/tachycardic effects of intubation and coughing on extubation

1 1.5 mg/kg 3 min before intubation.
2 1.5 mg/kg 2–3 min before extubation.

Infusion for pain management

1 Give IV bolus pre-induction of 1.5–2 mg/kg.
2 Run an infusion of 1–3 mg/kg/h intraoperatively and postoperatively with a reduced dose in liver disease.
3 Measure lignocaine levels every 8 h. Stop the infusion if lignocaine levels > 5 mcg/mL. Run the infusion for 24 h postoperatively.
4 Monitor the patient closely during the infusion, including continuous ECG monitoring.

◖ Lipid treatment of local anaesthetic toxicity

See Intralipid for treatment of ropivacaine/bupivacaine toxicity.

◖ Liver resection surgery

Introduction

The liver is the only human organ which can regenerate itself. A young fit patient with a healthy liver can survive after a 50–60% liver resection. Liver surgery has about a 3% mortality, and patients with cirrhosis are at particularly high risk. This is because of the difficulty of controlling intraoperative blood loss and the increased risk of postoperative liver failure.

Indications

1 Colorectal cancer metastases in the liver.
2 Primary liver cancer.
3 Benign liver tumours.
4 Liver cysts.
5 Donation of part of the liver for transplant.

Assessment

In addition to the routine investigations for major surgery it is especially important to evaluate:
1 liver function
2 coagulation status
3 presence of chronic liver disease such as cirrhosis and hepatitis
4 Child–Pugh score (see Table L1).

Table L1 Child–Pugh scoring system[1,2]

Points	1	2	3
Ascites	None	Some	Tense
Encephalopathy	Absent	Mild	Significant
Albumin (g/L)	> 35	28–35	< 28
Bilirubin (micromol/L)	< 34	34–50	> 50
INR	< 1.7	1.7–2.3	> 2.3

A patient: 5–6 points
B patient: 7–9 points
C patient: 10–15 points.
Surgery carries a greater risk in B and C patients and may be contraindicated.

Other preoperative issues

1 Heart disease—patients with liver disease/ascites may have a hyperdynamic circulation with reduced SVR and increased CO. This can lead to cardiac dysfunction (cirrhotic cardiomyopathy).
2 Renal function may progressively decline.

Surgical techniques

1 Parenchymal resection may be carried out using a Cavitron Ultrasonic Surgical Aspirator (CUSA), which disrupts the parenchyma and separates it from the bile ducts and blood vessels. Clamp crushing and the Hydrojet may also be used.
2 Electrocautery with bipolar forceps and cauterisation of the cut surfaces of the liver with argon beam coagulation may also be undertaken.
3 The Pringle manoeuvre involves temporary clamping of the hepatoduodenal ligament, thus occluding the portal vein and hepatic artery. The clamp is typically applied for 15–20 min.
4 Total vascular exclusion (TVE) is another option. This involves clamping the hilum of the liver and the IVC above and below the liver. It requires pre-procedure volume loading as profound hypotension may occur. Cardiac arrest is a risk of this manoeuvre.
5 Several other surgical manoeuvres can be used such as selective inflow occlusion.

Anaesthesia

The aims of liver surgery anaesthesia are:
1 keep CVP low to minimise blood loss from the cut surface of the liver
2 anticipate/treat problems associated with liver surgery (coagulopathy, hypoglycaemia, blood loss, gas embolism).
Towards these aims:
1 Invasive monitoring (central line, arterial line).
2 N/G tube, urinary catheter, temperature probe.
3 Be prepared for massive blood loss—IV transfusion pump set(s), warmed IV fluids, large-bore IV cannulas and current blood group and save.
4 Keep patient normothermic.
5 Do not use N_2O (worsens venous gas embolus if this occurs and increases gut distension).

6 Keep CVP low (< 5 mmHg) by:
   a) minimising IV fluids
   b) diuretic therapy
   c) GTN infusion to cause venodilation
   d) treating hypotension with vasopressors (metaraminol, phenylephrine) rather than IV fluids. A noradrenaline infusion may be required. Trendelenburg positioning may also help
   e) avoiding/minimising PEEP.

Note: The head-up position (reverse Trendelenburg) should **not** be used to reduce CVP because it will increase the risk of gas embolus.

7 If IV fluid loading is required, use intermittent boluses of 250 mL crystalloid and assess response.
8 Plasma-Lyte may be preferred to Hartmann's solution because the hepatic metabolism of lactate in Hartmann's may be impaired.
9 Consider 20% albumin solution if albumin is low or colloid is required.
10 Monitor BSL closely as hypoglycaemia may occur.
11 Consider tranexamic acid to reduce blood loss. **See *Tranexamic acid (TXA) (Cyklokapron).***
12 Avoid blood transfusion in patients with primary liver cancers as this may increase recurrence rates. **See *Onco-anaesthesia.***
13 After hepatic resection is completed, rehydrate the patient but do not over-hydrate.
14 Note that rocuronium is 50% metabolised by the liver so accumulation may occur.

Postoperative pain control

1 Thoracic epidural placement for postoperative pain relief may be effective but coagulopathy associated with liver disease/resection may increase the risk of epidural haematoma.
2 Wound catheters with LA infusions and PCA fentanyl is a useful approach.
3 Pre-anaesthetic intrathecal morphine can also be considered.
4 Do not use paracetamol until liver function has returned to normal.
5 Do not use NSAIDs.
6 Do not use morphine as it may precipitate encephalopathy in liver disease.

Postoperative care

Liver resection patients must be monitored in a high-dependency/ICU environment. They may suffer:

1 liver dysfunction/failure
2 hypoglycaemia—a glucose infusion may be required
3 coagulopathy
4 haemorrhage
5 renal dysfunction/failure (hepatorenal syndrome)
6 ascites/hypovolaemia.

◖ Local anaesthetic (LA) toxicity

Description

Systemic toxicity affecting the brain and the heart can occur with LA overdose. For the maximum safe dose of a selection of LA drugs, see the individual drug entries.

Effects of LA toxicity

1 Dysphoria, hearing changes.
2 Tingling in the lips and tongue, tongue numbness.
3 Visual disturbances.
4 Muscle twitching.
5 Severe agitation.
6 Decreased level of consciousness/loss of consciousness.
7 Convulsions.
8 Respiratory arrest.
9 Arrhythmias—sinus bradycardia, conduction blocks, ventricular tachyarrhythmias.
10 Cardiac arrest.

Treatment

1 General supportive measures for airway, breathing and circulation. Hyperventilation may be helpful by producing an alkalosis.
2 Control seizures with midazolam, thiopentone or propofol.
3 If cardiac arrest occurs, *see Cardiac arrest*. Do not use lignocaine as an antiarrhythmic. Use adrenaline cautiously in this situation at doses of < 1 mcg/kg.[3] Vasopressin may cause pulmonary haemorrhage and should be avoided.[3] Do not use calcium channel blockers or beta blockers.[3] Use amiodarone to treat ventricular arrhythmias.
4 Give intralipid 20% if risk of cardiac arrest or actual cardiac arrest. In the adult, give 100 mL IV over 1 min. Then run an intralipid infusion at 1000 mL/h. Repeat 100 mL bolus q 5 min × 2 if needed. *See Intralipid for the treatment of ropivacaine/bupivacaine toxicity.*
5 Increase intralipid infusion rate to 2000 mL/h if needed.
6 Maximum dose of intralipid is 12 mL/kg. In a 70 kg patient = 840 mL.
7 Children's doses are 1.5 mL/kg bolus over 1 min and infusion 15 mL/kg/h. Repeat bolus 1.5 mg/kg q 5 min × 2 and increase infusion rate to 30 mL/kg/h, if needed.
8 Cardiac arrest in this situation may be prolonged (> 1 h). Consider cardiopulmonary bypass if required.

◖ Long QT syndrome (LQTS)

Description

LQTS is a repolarisation disorder that may be inherited or acquired. It can result in serious, and even fatal, cardiac arrhythmias. It is a significant cause of sudden cardiac death in young people. There are about 15 known types of inherited LQTS. The syndrome may be an isolated defect or part of a more widespread inherited disorder involving deafness, periodic muscle weakness or other effects. Acquired LQTS can be due to medications, hypokalaemia or hypomagnesaemia. A slow heart rate can exacerbate this problem.

Inherited LQTS

There is an abnormality of potassium or sodium ion current channels leading to prolonged repolarisation. Either the repolarising potassium channel current is reduced or the depolarising late sodium channel is excessive.

The delay in repolarisation delays the inactivation of calcium channels, leading to early after-depolarisations which trigger the arrhythmia (R on T effect). There are many known genetic abnormalities leading to LQTS. Romano–Ward syndrome is the most common (30–35%), and only affects the heart. Jervell and Lange-Nielsen syndrome patients have LQTS and severe deafness. Andersen–Tawil syndrome patients have LQTS and hypokalaemic periodic paralysis.

Acquired LQTS

Some individuals may be predisposed to drug-induced LQTS due to a silent genetic predisposition. Types of drugs that can lead to acquired LQTS include:

1 antiarrhythmic drugs—amiodarone, sotalol, procainamide, disopyramide
2 antibiotics—erythromycin, azithromycin
3 antifungals (e.g. fluconazole), antivirals (e.g. nelfinavir) and antimalarials (e.g. chloroquine)
4 antidepressants—amitriptyline, imipramine, dothiepin
5 antipsychotics—risperidone, haloperidol, droperidol
6 antihistamines—terfenadine
7 methadone
8 volatile anaesthetic drugs, especially halothane. *See Halothane*
9 ondansetron
10 many others.

Acquired LQTS can also be due to:

1 metabolic abnormalities—hypokalaemia, hypomagnesaemia
2 anorexia nervosa
3 myocardial ischaemia.

Clinical effects

1 Asymptomatic.
2 Palpitations.
3 Syncope.
4 Seizures.
5 Sudden death.

Diagnosis

1 The QT interval varies with heart rate, so a corrected value is used (Q-Tc). Q-Tc equals the measured QT divided by the square root of the R-R interval measured in seconds. Q-Tc $= QT/\sqrt{R\text{-}R}$. The normal Q-Tc is 0.39 s $+/- 0.04$ s. Q-Tc > 0.44 s is prolonged, although in some LQTS patients the Q-Tc is normal.
2 T wave and U wave abnormalities. T waves may be large, bifid and/or there may be beat-to-beat variation in T wave amplitude.
3 Life-threatening arrhythmias include polymorphic VT and torsades de pointes.

Treatment

1 For treatment of torsades de pointes, *see Torsades de pointes.*
2 Avoidance of drugs which prolong the QT interval.
3 Aggressive treatment of electrolyte imbalances e.g. vomiting and diarrhoea.
4 Beta blockers—propranolol, nadolol. Mortality is greatly reduced with beta blocker therapy.
5 Mexiletine.
6 Left cardiac sympathetic denervation.
7 Placement of a pacemaker to allow intentional atrial pacing.
8 Implantable defibrillator.

Anaesthesia and LQTS

1 Discuss management with patient's cardiologist.
2 Baseline ECG prior to anaesthesia.
3 Continue beta blocker therapy up to the day of surgery.
4 Ensure serum electrolytes are optimised, especially potassium, calcium and magnesium.
5 If an AICD is present, **see** *Pacemakers*.
6 Consider invasive blood pressure monitoring.
7 Avoid increases in sympathetic activity.
8 Avoid hypoxia, hypocapnia, hypercapnia, high-pressure ventilation.
9 Maintain normothermia.
10 Midazolam, rocuronium, sugammadex and propofol (bolus and infusion) are safe. Volatile agents increase the QT interval but this is of doubtful significance.
11 Methadone increases the QT interval and should not be used. **See** *Methadone/ physeptone*.
12 Avoid using LA solutions containing adrenaline.
13 Restart beta blockers as soon as possible postoperatively.
14 If arrhythmias occur, **see** *Torsades de pointes*.
15 Dexamethasone, cyclizine and metoclopramide are safe. Do not use ondansetron or droperidol.

◗ Lorazepam (Ativan)

Long-acting benzodiazepine drug useful for the alleviation of anxiety preoperatively. Causes sedation with profound anterograde amnesia lasting up to 6 h. Also useful for the treatment of status epilepticus. **See** *Status epilepticus (SE)*.

Dose

For anxiety in the adult, give 2.5 mg PO. Give 4–8 mg IV for status epilepticus.

◗ Ludwig's angina

Description

Ludwig's angina is an extremely dangerous necrotising cellulitis of the floor of the mouth (submandibular space) and neck. It causes massive swelling displacing the tongue upwards and can cause airway obstruction. It is usually due to a tooth extraction or dental infection in the lower teeth (usually the lower second or third molars). Aspiration of pus into the airways can occur. Infection may spread to the mediastinum.

Presentation

The main symptoms and signs are:
1 trismus, pain, dysphagia
2 fever, septicaemia
3 sitting posture
4 inability to swallow secretions
5 upper airway obstruction with dyspnoea, stridor, cyanosis and asphyxiation.

Management

1 Antibiotic therapy. The usual causative organism(s) are *streptococci, staphylococci, Escherichia coli (E. coli), pseudomonas* or mixed infections. Recommended antibiotics (until the causative organism is known) are ampicillin-sulbactam or clindamycin. In immunocompromised patients add meropenem or piperacillin-tazobactam.[4]

2 CT or MRI to elucidate the extent of spread of the infection and the degree of airway obstruction.

3 If the patient does not respond adequately to antibiotics or the airway is threatened, intubation is required. This is usually achieved by awake nasal endoscopic intubation. *See Awake intubation.* Awake tracheostomy is another option.

4 There is a significant risk of intra-oral rupture of the abscess with aspiration of pus.

5 Surgical drainage of the infection is the next step.

◑ Lung disease

The respiratory system is made up of alveoli, airways, lung parenchyma containing elastic tissue, chest wall (ribs and muscles), pleura and diaphragm. The intercostal muscles and diaphragm contract to breathe in and relax to breathe out. Expiration is assisted by elastic tissue in the lung parenchyma. This elastic tissue helps keep the airways open. The 'stretchier' the elastic tissue is, the more compliant is the lung. The elastic tissue's ability to 'snap back' is called lung recoil. Recoil determines how much air is expired and how easily it is expired.

Classification

One classification is obstructive versus restrictive lung disease. There is also pulmonary vascular disease, which includes primary pulmonary hypertension and chronic thromboembolic disease. *See also Lung function tests.*

Restrictive lung disease

This means that a disease is restricting the ability of the lung to expand (its compliance). This could be due to diseases or conditions extrinsic to the lungs, such as:

1 innervation of the intercostal muscles and diaphragm is abnormal e.g. Guillain–Barré syndrome

2 diseases of the respiratory muscles e.g. muscular dystrophy

3 thoracic spine abnormalities—scoliosis, kyphoscoliosis

4 pleural effusion.

It could also be due to intrinsic diseases or conditions that cause restrictive lung diseases, including:

1 pneumonia

2 acute respiratory distress syndrome (ARDS)

3 pulmonary fibrosis/scarring.

Lung recoil is high with restrictive lung disease and the lungs are small. In addition:

1 Tidal volume (TV) is relatively normal.

2 Total lung capacity (TLC) is reduced.

3 Airway resistance is normal.

4 FEV_1 and FVC are both reduced but the FEV_1/FVC ratio will be > 80% as the decline in FVC is greater than the decline in FEV_1.

5 Flow volume loop looks normal but is shrunken in all directions.

6 There is no obstruction to expiration.

Obstructive lung disease

There is obstruction of the airways e.g. asthma, chronic bronchitis and emphysema. In emphysema there is destruction of lung elastic tissue which would normally hold the airways open. With loss of elastic tissue, compliance is increased but recoil is poor. Recoil helps expiration, which is therefore impaired.

1 TV is preserved.

2 TLC is increased, as is residual volume (RV).

3 FEV_1 is reduced.

4 FVC will also be reduced if there is significant disease but less than the reduction in FEV_1.

5 FEV_1/FVC will be < 70%.

6 The flow volume loop may show coving of the expiratory loop and a reduced PEFR.

Pulmonary vascular disease (PVD)

Lung mechanics are usually normal in PVD. Spirometry is usually not helpful.

◗ Lung function tests

Introduction

To interpret lung function tests, it is necessary to know the patient's height (which is related to lung size), age (lung function declines with age) and gender (males have larger lungs). From this information, predicted lung function test results can be derived. A patient's result is considered abnormal if it is < 80% of the predicted result. Abnormal lung function test results can be consistent with an obstructive lung pattern (asthma, chronic bronchitis) or a restrictive lung pattern (fibrosing alveolitis, chest wall abnormalities).

All results described below are for adults. The most basic tests are:

1 peak expiratory flow rate (PEFR)

2 spirometry

3 total lung capacity (TLC)

4 diffusing capacity of lungs for carbon monoxide (DLCO).

Peak expiratory flow rate (PEFR)

This is a measure of the maximum expiratory flow rate. It is measured with a peak flow meter. It should be about 440–550 L/min in males and 320–470 L/min in females. PEFR is reduced during an acute exacerbation of asthma.

Spirometry

1 FVC is forced vital capacity. The patient breathes in maximally, then breathes out as hard and as fast as possible. The measurement is made over 6 s. If the patient's FVC > 80% of the predicted value, the patient has no restriction of lung capacity. If FVC < 80% predicted, there is restriction **or** obstruction with air trapping, or both. The maximum slope of the expiration curve equals the peak expiratory flow rate (PEFR).

2 FEV_1 is the forced expiratory volume in 1 s. If the FEV_1/FVC > 0.7, there is no obstruction. If the FEV1/FVC < 0.7, there is obstruction.

3 Reactivity. Reactivity is present if there is an improvement in spirometry values after bronchodilator therapy. The change should be > 12% and > 200 mL in FEV1 or FVC.

4 Flow volume loop (FVL)—this is a graph of airflow (y axis) as a function of volume (x axis). The maximum volume in the lungs at the transition point from inspiration to expiration is the total lung capacity (TLC). TLC is increased in significant obstructive lung disease and reduced in restrictive lung disease. The total amount of air in the lungs at the transition point from expiration to inspiration is the residual volume (RV). The difference between TLC and RV is the FVC. However, where the x axis starts is unclear.

Diffusing capacity of lungs for carbon monoxide (DLCO)

The patient breathes in a maximal breath of a mixture of air, helium and 0.3% carbon monoxide (CO). The patient holds their breath for 10 s and some CO will enter the blood stream across the alveolar/capillary membrane. The patient then exhales and the first litre is discarded. The subsequent exhaled gas is analysed for CO concentration. This enables the calculation of the volume of CO that diffuses across the alveolar wall per minute per unit of pressure e.g. mL CO per minute per mmHg. If this is < 40% predicted, this is considered severe impairment. DLCO is decreased if the alveolar surface area is decreased (e.g. emphysema) or the alveolar/capillary membrane is thickened (e.g. interstitial lung disease).

◉ Lung volumes and capacities (adult)

Tidal volume (TV)
This is the amount of air breathed in or out during quiet respiration (normally about 500 mL or 6–8 mL/kg).

Inspiratory reserve volume (IRV)
The maximum amount of air that can be inspired in addition to the tidal volume. This is about 2–3 L on average.

Expiratory reserve volume (ERV)
The amount of air that can be expired on maximal effort after normal tidal expired volume. Normally about 700–1200 mL.

Residual volume (RV)
This is the volume of the lung that cannot be exhaled. Normally 1200 mL (20–25 mL/kg).

Inspiratory capacity (IC)
This is the sum of TV and IRV.

Functional residual capacity (FRC)
This is the sum of ERV and RV. It is normally 1800–2200 mL. The ratio of FRC to TLC is an index of hyperinflation. In COPD, FRC can be as high as 80% of TLC.

Vital capacity (VC)
This is TV + IRV + ERV. VC is about 4800 mL on average.

Total lung capacity (TLC)
This is the maximum volume of air the lungs can hold. TLC can be calculated by lung plethysmography, nitrogen washout and helium dilution techniques. In the average patient this is 6 L. TLC is reduced in patients with restrictive lung diseases.

REFERENCES

1 Child C, Turcotte J. The liver and portal hypertension. In: CI Child, ed. *Surgery and Portal Hypertension*. Philadelphia, USA: WB Saunders, 1964: 50–58.

2 Pugh R, Murray-Lyon I, Dawson J. Transection of the oesophagus for bleeding oesophageal varices. *Br J Surg* 1973; 60: 646–649.

3 Mahajan A, Derian A. Local anaesthetic toxicity. *StatPearls,* last updated October 2022. Accessed online: https://pubmed.ncbi.nlm.nih.gov/29763139/, March 2023.

4 An J, Madeo J, Singhal M. Ludwig angina. [Updated 2023 may 24]. In: StatPearls [Internet]. Treasure Island (FL): StatPearls publishing 2023 Jan- https://www.ncbi.nlm.nih.gov/books/NBK482354/#

⬤ MACE

An acronym for **M**ajor **A**dverse **C**ardiac **E**vent e.g. myocardial infarction, congestive cardiac failure, cardiac arrest. **See Cardiac risk for non-cardiac surgery**.

⬤ Magnesium

Magnesium is the second-most abundant cation in the body after potassium. The normal blood level of magnesium is 0.75–1.0 mmol/L (1.5–2 mEq/L). About 50% of the body's magnesium is in bone and the rest is in muscle and other tissues. Less than 1% of the body's magnesium is in blood.

Effects of hypomagnesaemia

1 Ventricular dysrhythmias.
2 May lead to intracellular potassium depletion.
3 Neuromuscular excitability, tetany, nystagmus and delirium.

Effects of hypermagnesaemia

1 somnolence
2 absent deep tendon reflexes, muscle paralysis, apnoea, respiratory arrest
3 heart block, cardiac arrest

⬤ Magnesium sulfate

Introduction

Magnesium sulfate ($MgSO_4$) is presented in 5 mL ampoules containing 2.465 g of magnesium sulfate, which equates to 10 mmol or 20 mEq of magnesium ions. This is a 50% w/v solution. Magnesium therapy has many pharmacologically useful effects. These include:

1 Antiarrhythmic effects—prolongs AV nodal conduction and suppresses conduction in accessory pathways.
2 Reduction of catecholamine release.
3 Antagonist at alpha-adrenergic receptors.
4 Potent arteriolar vasodilator.
5 Lung effects. $MgSO_4$ promotes bronchodilation and improved lung function in patients with asthma. It reduces lung hyperinflation and improves respiratory muscle strength in stable COPD.
6 Potentiates the effects of non-depolarising neuromuscular blocking drugs (NDNMBDs) and general anaesthetic drugs.
7 Analgesic-sparing effect.[1]
8 Uterine tocolytic drug.

In addition to hypomagnesaemia, indications for magnesium include:
• Cardiac rhythm disturbances
• Obstetric and asthmatic indications
• Anaesthetic indications, including anaesthesia for phaeochromocytoma
• Miscellaneous indications

- anaesthetic
- phaeochromocytoma
- miscellaneous.

Magnesium deficiency

Magnesium sulfate 5 g in 1 L N/S over 3 h.

Antiarrhythmic indications

Magnesium is used as adjunctive therapy for certain types of arrhythmias and as a first-line drug for torsades de points. *See Torsades de pointes.* Examples include:

1 Atrial fibrillation and multifocal atrial tachycardia.
2 Prevention of AF after cardiac surgery.
3 Refractory SVT, VT and VF. *See Cardiac arrest.*
4 Ventricular arrhythmias during acute myocardial infarction.

Obstetric indications

1 Preeclampsia/eclampsia. Magnesium therapy is used to prevent seizures and may assist in lowering blood pressure by reducing SVR. For dose *see Preeclampsia/eclampsia.*
2 Tocolytic drug for treatment of preterm labour.

Asthma

Magnesium is useful for treating asthma resistant to first-line drugs. *See Asthma.*

Anaesthetic indications

1 Intraoperative magnesium as an adjuvant to postoperative analgesia due to antagonist effects on N-methyl-D-aspartate (NMDA) receptors.[2] It is useful for opioid minimisation anaesthesia for indications such as bariatric surgery. *See Bariatric surgery.*
2 Reduction of the hypertensive response to intubation. *See Intubation—minimising hypertensive response.*
3 Decreases requirements for GA drugs.
4 Enhances the effects of NMBDs.

Phaeochromocytoma

Magnesium is useful for blood pressure control during this type of surgery. *See Phaeochromocytoma.*

Miscellaneous

1 Migraine.
2 Dyspepsia.

◐ Magnetic resonance imaging (MRI)

Basic principles of the MRI scanner

MRI scanning involves the use of high-strength magnetic fields to provide digitalised, tomographic, high-resolution images of tissues and organs. The device consists of:

1 Cryogenic magnet—a liquid nitrogen-cooled superconductor in an environment of liquid helium at a temperature of 4.22 K. This magnet produces a magnetic field which can be > 6 Tesla, although 1.5–3.0 Tesla is the usual. It takes about 72 h to establish this field. 1 Tesla (T) = 1000 Gauss (G). The earth's magnetic field is 5×10^{-5} T (about 0.5 G). A 1.5 Tesla magnet can lift a car.

2 Gradient coils—loops of wire that have gradient currents induced in them during the production of radiofrequency pulses. Torque in these wires results in the audible noise of the scanning process.

How the image is obtained

1 Atoms with net electrical charges from an odd number of protons and/or neutrons produce a randomly orientated magnetic field.

2 These magnetic fields are aligned by the static magnetic field of the MRI scanner.

3 A radiofrequency pulse produces a second magnetic field which deflects the orientation of these atoms. When the pulses cease, the atoms return to their aligned state in the static magnetic field (a process termed 'relaxation'), releasing energy.

4 These 'relaxation' rates vary between tissues and enable differentiation of structure. The energy released by realignment is detected by the receiver coil and is used to create the MRI image.

5 Hydrogen atoms are the most common type of atom used for imaging.

Contraindications to MRI scanning or proximity to MRI scanner

1 Cardiac pacemakers and implantable defibrillators. These may become reprogrammed, dislodged or inactivated. MRI-conditional pacemakers exist but, in terms of usage, are very much the exception.

2 Ferromagnetic intracerebral aneurysm clips.

3 Intraocular metallic foreign body. These can become dislodged and cause vitreous haemorrhage.

4 Other implanted devices that might be displaced by the magnetic field include cochlear implants, stents and coils.

5 Artificial heart valves may be unsafe and require cardiologist clearance.

6 If the implanted device is not ferromagnetic e.g. titanium, it does not pose a risk.

7 If the implanted object cannot move e.g. sternal wires, it does not pose a risk but it may degrade image quality.

8 MRI scanning in the first trimester of pregnancy is not associated with fetal risk.[3] However the use of gadolinium MRI at any time during pregnancy is associated with an increased risk of fetal inflammatory or infiltrative skin disease and an increased risk of fetal death.

9 If the patient is breast feeding, breast milk should be discarded for 24 h **only if Magnevist (gadopentetate) is used**. Other types of contrast media containing gadolinium are safe, and the discarding of breast milk is unneccessary.[4] However, always check with the radiologist/radiographer.

Hazards in the MRI scanning room

1 The scanning room is an austere environment that is often remote from the operating theatres and has limited resources.

2 Watches, credit cards and mobile phones may be damaged.

3 Ferromagnetic objects may become missiles and injure the patient and/or staff. Large objects may trap or crush patients or personnel.

4 Iron containing pigments in make-up or tattoos may become hot.

5 Gadolinium contrast can cause nausea, vomiting, anaphylaxis and nephrogenic systemic fibrosis in patients with impaired renal function.

6 The loud noise of the scanning process can damage hearing. Patients **must** have ear protection, including those who are anaesthetised.

7 The cryostat typically contains about 1000–2000 L of liquid helium at a few degrees above absolute zero temperature. The helium reduces the resistance of electrical current flow in the magnet to almost zero. If there is an emergency field shutdown due to the STOP button being pushed, the electromagnet starts to heat up. The liquid helium then expands and becomes gaseous and must be vented very quickly. This is termed a 'quench'. If venting to the outside fails or is inadequate, the MRI suite can fill with helium gas. Everyone must evacuate as soon as possible. Exposure to the helium gas may cause cold injuries and asphyxiation.

Anaesthesia and MRI

1 The patient is anaesthetised outside the MRI room.
2 The patient is transferred on a MRI-compatible trolley into the MRI room.
3 All equipment in the MRI suite must be MRI compatible. Outside equipment such as infusion pumps cannot be brought into the MRI room.
4 If infusions are needed, long infusion lines extending outside the room are required.
5 Volatile anaesthetic is probably less problematic than propofol TCI as it is not possible to monitor BIS/entropy and the propofol TCI pump must remain outside the room.
6 MRI safe pulse oximetry must be used. Standard pulse oximeters can cause burns.
7 MRI-compatible ECG monitoring may be available.
8 Capnography requires long sampling lines.

Points to note

1 'Magnetic resonance (MR) conditional'—refers to any device for which a specified MRI environment with specified conditions of use does not pose a known hazard.
2 'MR safe'—means no hazard in any MRI environment.
3 'MR unsafe'—any object that poses a hazard in the MRI room.

⦿ Major/massive haemorrhage

See *Blood loss—assessment, management and anaesthetic approach*.

⦿ Malignant hypertension

See *Hypertension*.

⦿ Malignant hyperthermia (MH)

Description and pathophysiology

MH is a catastrophic idiosyncratic reaction to suxamethonium or a volatile anaesthetic drug or both. It is due to an autosomal-dominant genetic disorder of skeletal muscle receptors, specifically the ryanodine receptor on the muscle sarcoplasmic reticulum (SR). As a result, on exposure to the 'trigger', there is uncontrolled release of calcium ions from the SR leading to inappropriate and severe muscle contraction. This leads to muscle rigidity, heat and CO_2 production, hyperkalaemia, hypoxia and acidosis. In some patients, exercise or exposure to hot environments may precipitate MH. Rarely, MH can occur in the minutes after cessation of volatile anaesthetic drug administration. MH affects about 1:100 000 people.

Clinical features

1 Hypercarbia—$ETCO_2$ > 60 mmHg during controlled ventilation or > 65 mmHg during spontaneous ventilation. This is often the first sign.
2 Tachypnoea—if the patient is breathing spontaneously.
3 Hypoxia.
4 Tachycardia.

5 Hyperthermia. Core body temperature can rise as fast as 1°C every few minutes. As the temperature rises above 41.5°C, vital organ dysfunction and damage will occur. A temperature rise occurring more than 1 h after cessation of triggering drugs, without any other MH manifestations, is very unlikely to be due to MH.

6 Muscle rigidity (may be masseter spasm or generalised). Generalised muscle rigidity in a paralysed patient is pathognomonic of MH.

7 Peaked T waves due to hyperkalaemia. *See Potassium*. Serum K^+ may be > 6 mmol/L.

8 Sweating.

9 Cutaneous vasoconstriction.

10 Rhabdomyolysis—muscle breakdown with release of myoglobin into the circulation. May cause serum myoglobin > 170 mcg/mL, urinary myoglobin > 60 mcg/mL, cola-coloured urine.

11 Kidney injury due to myoglobin causing effects such as acute tubular necrosis.

12 Metabolic and respiratory acidosis. The pH may be < 7.25.

13 Elevated creatine kinase (CK)—significant if > 20 000 units/L if suxamethonium used or > 10 000 units/L if volatile agent administered without suxamethonium.

14 Disseminated intravascular coagulation (DIC), which may be associated with very high body temperatures.

The syndrome can reoccur 2 or more hours after the initial event, termed 'recrudescence'. The incidence of this may be around 20%.[5]

Masseter muscle rigidity (MMR) and MH

It is normal to get increased masseter muscle tone after suxamethonium. Severe MMR ('jaws of steel') may indicate development of MH. *See Masseter spasm/masseter muscle rigidity (MMR)*. MMR is not of concern **if**:

1 it is easily overcome with normal efforts

2 it terminates within 60 s

3 it is not associated with generalised rigidity.

Differential diagnosis

1 Hypercarbia may be due to inadequate ventilation, exhausted soda lime.

2 Thyroid storm. *See Thyroid storm/thyrotoxic crisis*.

3 Fever due to infection.

4 Blood transfusion reaction.

5 Illicit drug reaction (cocaine, ecstasy).

6 Phaeochromocytoma. *See Phaeochromocytoma*.

7 Neuroleptic malignant syndrome. *See Neuroleptic malignant syndrome (NMS)*.

8 Intracerebral infection or bleeding.

9 Inadequate anaesthesia.

Treatment

This is a life-threatening crisis situation.

1 Declare a crisis. Notify the surgeon and ask the surgical team to expedite surgery.

2 Get sufficient numbers of skilled assistants.

3 Call for the 'MH box'. The MH box is a receptacle containing dantrolene, equipment for dissolving the dantrolene, treatment cards and other useful items as described below.

4 Change to a non-triggering anaesthetic (cease volatile, use propofol TCI).

5 Intubate the patient if not already intubated, using rocuronium as the muscle relaxant.

6 Administer 100% O_2 with a fresh gas flow of at least 10 L/min. Hyperventilate the patient.

7 Add activated charcoal filters to the inspiratory and expiratory limb of the circuit to remove volatile anaesthetic agent in the circuit.

8 Administer dantrolene 2.5 mg/kg IV. The older preparations of dantrolene are in 20 mg vials, which need to be mixed with 60 mL of sterile water. For a 70 kg patient, nine vials will be required, which will take precious minutes to prepare. A newer formulation is Ryanodex, which contains 250 mg dantrolene and requires only 5 mL of sterile water. It is prepared in seconds. Ryanodex is not currently available in Australia.

9 There should be reversal of clinical signs e.g. reducing expired CO_2, falling temperature. If this does not occur, repeat 2.5 mg/kg dantrolene as needed, up to a total dose of 10 mg/kg. Muscular patients may require more dantrolene.

10 Insert an arterial line and urinary catheter. Maintain urine output at 1–2 mL/kg/h.

11 Check ABGs and electrolytes and send blood for CK level.

12 Detect and treat hyperkalaemia. **See Potassium**. Although there are theoretical concerns about giving calcium chloride/gluconate, protection of the myocardium takes precedence. Do not give calcium in the same line as bicarbonate as this may cause calcium carbonate (a solid) to form.

13 Correct acidosis with sodium bicarbonate 1–2 mEq/kg IV over 5–10 min max 100 mEq/dose. Sodium bicarbonate will result in increased CO_2 production. Aim for a pH > 7.2.

14 Cool the patient if temperature is > 39°C. Aim for a core temperature of 38°C. Use surface cooling with ice. Also give IV fluids at 4°C if available. Consider cold saline peritoneal lavage if the peritoneum is accessible.

15 Treat cardiac arrhythmias using drugs other than verapamil and diltiazem. These drugs are contraindicated as they worsen hyperkalaemia, myocardial depression and hypotension when co-administered with dantrolene.

Ongoing management

1 Observe patient in ICU for at least 24 h.

2 Monitor patient closely for recrudescence.[5]

3 Check for disseminated intravascular coagulation (DIC) as this can occur in up to 7% of MH episodes.

4 Administer dantrolene 1 mg/kg q 4–6 h or an infusion of 0.25 mg/kg/h for at least 24 h.

5 Explain to the patient the significance of their condition and the ramifications for relevant family members.

6 The patient **must** have a muscle biopsy test to confirm the diagnosis of MH susceptibility. If positive, genetic testing can be done to look for a mutation. If a mutation is present and is also present in a family member, then that family member is considered MH susceptible. If the mutation is not present, the family member may still be MH susceptible.

Tests for MH

1 In vitro contraction test (IVCT)—a muscle biopsy specimen is exposed to caffeine and halothane and the contraction response measured. This test is considered definitive.

2 Genetic testing. If a diagnostic variant is found, treat the patient as MH susceptible. If genetic testing is negative, the patient may still be MH susceptible and should have a muscle biopsy.

Diseases associated with MH

1 Central core disease.
2 King–Denborough syndrome.
3 Multiminicore disease.
4 Certain forms of muscular dystrophy, although the relationship is very complex.
5 Carnitine palmitoyltransferase deficiency.
6 History of rhabdomyolysis e.g. after exercise in extreme heat or with statin therapy.
7 Periodic paralysis.
8 Other highly specific and rare diseases such as congenital myopathy with cores and rods.
Note: patients with osteogenesis imperfecta often develop a fever during GA.
See *Osteogenesis imperfecta (OI)*.

Anaesthesia for the MH susceptible patient

A patient is considered MH susceptible if:
1 they have had a previous MH reaction
2 they have positive IVCT
3 they have positive genetic testing
4 they have not been tested but a relative has a history of MH or positive IVCT.
When anaesthetising a MH susceptible patient:
1 Use a 'clean' anaesthetic machine (a machine not exposed to volatile agents). Alternatively remove the vaporiser and circuit and soda lime from an 'unclean' machine. Using a fresh circuit and soda lime, flush the machine for 10–30 min with 10 L/min O_2. Activated charcoal filters remove trace levels of volatile anaesthetic drugs. Only one on the inspiratory limb is required but they are packed in pairs so use both to avoid an error.
2 Use fresh gas flows of 10 L/min to avoid rebound increased release of volatile agent.
3 Use a non-triggering anaesthetic (no suxamethonium or volatile agent).
4 Monitor temperature in addition to other vital signs.

Obstetrics and MH

1 If the father of the baby is MH susceptible, there is a 50% chance the baby will also be MH susceptible. Treat the mother with a non-triggering anaesthetic (all agents are acceptable except suxamethonium and volatile agents).
2 If the mother develops MH and is treated with dantrolene, this will make the baby weak as dantrolene crosses the placenta. The baby could also potentially develop MH in this situation.

◗ Mallampati score (modified)

This test gives an indication of how much space there is between the tongue and the roof of the mouth. It is used to help predict a difficult airway. **See *Difficult airway management*.** The patient sits, opens their mouth widely and protrudes their tongue without phonation. The results can be graded as follows.
- Grade I—tonsillar pillars, soft palate and uvula are visible
- Grade II—tonsillar pillars and uvula partially obscured
- Grade III—hard and soft palate and base of uvula visible
- Grade IV—hard palate only visible.

◐ Mannitol

Description

Mannitol is a sugar alcohol. It is poorly metabolised by the body and rapidly excreted by the kidney, causing an osmotic diuresis. It does not cross the blood–brain barrier (BBB). It is presented as a 20% solution.

Uses

1 Decreasing ICP—mannitol increases the tonicity of plasma and cannot cross the BBB. Therefore, brain water is drawn out of the brain and into the plasma. Water and mannitol are then excreted by the kidneys.
2 Reduction of intraocular pressure—by drawing water out of the vitreous humor of the eye.
3 Kidney transplant surgery—mannitol increases renal blood flow due to the release of intrarenal vasodilating prostaglandins and atrial natriuretic polypeptide. *See Renal transplant*. It may also be an oxygen free radical scavenger. *See Oxygen free radicals*. Mannitol may impart some protection to the kidney allograft after reperfusion. Also, the osmotic diuretic effect may flush out cellular debris and prevent tubular cast formation in the renal graft.

Doses

See Renal transplant and *Intracranial pressure (ICP) and treatment of raised ICP*.

◐ Marfan syndrome

Description

Marfan syndrome is a genetic autosomal dominant connective tissue disorder with an incidence of 1:3000–5000. 30% of cases are due to mutations. It affects substrates of elastin. The Marfan patient typically has a tall and slender build, with long fingers, arms and legs.

Clinical picture

1 Eye problems, including myopia, lens dislocation, retinal detachment.
2 Aortic root dilatation with aortic regurgitation.
3 Aortic dissection at the aortic root and other regions of the aorta. *See Aortic dissection*.
4 Mitral valve prolapse with regurgitation.
5 Musculoskeletal abnormalities—kyphosis, scoliosis, pectus deformities. These can lead to restrictive lung disease. *See Lung disease*.
6 Increased risk of spontaneous pneumothorax.
7 Striae on skin.
8 Dural ectasia—increased diameter of the dural sac. This can cause back pain, headache, proximal leg and genital/rectal pain
9 High-arched palate, crowded teeth.
10 Joint laxity.
11 Increased risk of ventricular arrhythmias and coronary artery dissection.

Treatment

1 Beta blockers to reduce the rate of aortic dilatation.
2 Surgery such as aortic root replacement and thoracic aneurysm/dissection repair. An aortic root diameter of > 4 cm is associated with an increased risk of dissection.

3 If the aortic root diameter is $\geq$ 5 cm, elective aortic root replacement is recommended.

Anaesthesia
The main aim is to prevent a sudden increase in myocardial contractility and blood pressure, which may cause aortic dissection.
1 Continue beta blockers perioperatively.
2 Consider inserting an arterial line for significant surgery.
3 Blunt the haemodynamic response to intubation. *See Intubation—minimising hypertensive response.*
4 Intubation needs to be done carefully because of the risk of laxity of the temporomandibular joint and atlanto-occipital joint.
5 Do not use N_2O. Be aware that a pneumothorax can occur at any time.

Marfan syndrome and obstetrics
1 Imaging of the entire aorta before pregnancy is recommended.
2 There is an increased risk of aortic root dilatation and dissection during pregnancy, especially in the third trimester or early postpartum. Aortic root diameter should be monitored by echocardiography.
3 Dural ectasia may be present. Ask about relevant symptoms. There is an increased risk of dural puncture with epidural anaesthesia. Ligamentum flavum laxity may also increase the risk of dural puncture with epidural anaesthesia.
4 If Caesarean section (CS) is required, a single-shot spinal may be inadequate. A CSE may be more reliable.

◯ Masseter spasm/masseter muscle rigidity (MMR)

Description
Some increase in jaw muscle tone after suxamethonium is common. Masseter spasm can be defined as jaw tightness after suxamethonium that is severe enough to interfere with tracheal intubation. It most commonly occurs in children, but it can also occur in adults. It is hypothesised that masseter spasm may indicate malignant hyperthermia susceptibility and/or be the first sign of MH developing. Some patients who develop masseter spasm have an underlying muscle abnormality such as myotonia. *See Muscular dystrophy (MD).*

Treatment
Maintain oxygenation. Relaxation of the jaw usually occurs after a few minutes at most.
1 If surgery is elective, abandon surgery and allow the patient to wake up.
2 If surgery is urgent, change to a non-triggering anaesthetic and proceed with surgery.
3 Treat MH if this occurs. *See Malignant hyperthermia (MH).*
4 Check creatine kinase (CK) levels at the time of anaesthesia and at 6 h intervals until it is in the normal range (25–200 U/mL).
5 Observe for cola-coloured urine, indicating urinary myoglobin.
6 Observe the patient in hospital for at least 12 h.
7 Organise MH testing for the patient.

❍ Massive blood transfusion/massive transfusion protocol (MTP)

See Blood loss—assessment, management and anaesthetic approach.

❍ Mean arterial pressure (MAP)

Introduction

MAP is a very important concept because it is this pressure rather than systolic blood pressure (SBP) which determines organ perfusion. This is because SBP is affected by arterial wall compliance and distal pulse amplification (SBP higher peripherally than centrally). MAP is less affected by overdamping or underdamping of invasive arterial blood pressure measurement than the SBP. Non-invasive BP measurements give a more accurate measure of MAP than of SBP or DBP.

Defining and calculating MAP

MAP is defined as the average blood pressure throughout the cardiac cycle in the arteries. The cardiac cycle is made up of approximately two-thirds diastole and one-third systole. $MAP = (CO \times SVR) - CVP$. A simple formula is $MAP = DBP + \frac{1}{3}$ pulse pressure. Pulse pressure = SBP – DBP. *See Pulse pressure.* Normal MAP is 70–110 mmHg. MAP < 60 mmHg will likely lead to organ ischaemia.

❍ Mediastinal mass syndrome (MMS)

Description

The mediastinum is the region between the lungs, the diaphragm and the thoracic inlet. It contains many vital structures, including:

1 heart
2 great vessels
3 trachea and bronchi
4 oesophagus.

These vital structures may become compressed by a mediastinal mass, and this compression may worsen with GA. This can result in severe or even fatal cardiorespiratory compromise. This section does not cover anaesthesia for removal of a mediastinal mass.

Aetiology of mediastinal masses

The most common types are:

1 lymphoma
2 thymoma, thymic cyst
3 retrosternal thyroid mass
4 germ cell tumours and granulomas
5 lung cancers
6 bronchogenic cyst
7 vascular tumours
8 oesophageal cancer.

Clinical findings

A mediastinal mass may be asymptomatic or produce severe symptoms and signs. Always check if symptoms are worsened/improved by the patient being erect, supine, left and right lateral or prone. Symptoms may be worse when raising the arms above the head (this is called the Pemberton manoeuvre). A positive Pemberton's sign is facial congestion, cyanosis and dyspnoea after 1 minute due to superior vena cava (SVC) obstruction.

1 Respiratory—dyspnoea, wheeze and cough suggesting tracheal/bronchial compression/invasion.
2 Cardiovascular—dysrhythmias, paradoxical drop in BP when moving from erect to supine, dyspnoea with exercise. Ask the patient to perform a Valsalva manoeuvre. This may cause presyncope or syncope suggesting pressure on the right ventricle or pulmonary artery.
3 SVC obstruction—head and neck oedema, plethoric face, engorged neck veins, laryngeal oedema. *See Superior vena cava syndrome (SVCS).*
4 Effects of the tumour itself e.g. dysphagia with oesophageal cancer.

Effects of position/GA on the mediastinum

1 The transverse diameter of the mediastinum is decreased when moving from erect to supine due to the diaphragm being pushed cephalad by the abdominal contents.
2 Central blood volume increases in the supine position, which may increase the size of vascular tumours.
3 Muscle relaxants reduce chest wall tone, which also decreases the size of the mediastinum.
4 Effects of gravity on the tumour may cause pressure on vital structures.
5 The low-pressure SVC, RV and pulmonary artery system is much more vulnerable to mechanical compression than the higher-pressure system on the left side of the heart.
6 GA with IPPV increases airway compression by relaxing bronchial smooth muscle. In addition, the mechanics of spontaneous breathing with chest expansion splints the airways open, whereas IPPV is associated with increased airway compression.

Investigations

In addition to routine blood tests:

1 CXR—often the first test to reveal the mass
2 CT/MRI—essential to define the exact size and position of the mass and its interaction with surrounding structures. The combination of left mainstem bronchus and right pulmonary artery compression can lead to devastating ventilation perfusion mismatch under GA. Check tracheal diameter. A reduction of > 50% is predictive of respiratory complications under GA.[6]
3 Echocardiography—may indicate pericardial effusion or evidence of compression of heart chambers or great vessels. Compare sitting-up with lying-down views.
4 Lung function tests—may indicate airway obstruction. Look at flow volume loops erect and supine. *See Lung function tests.*
5 Bronchoscopy—required if there is a major concern regarding bronchial airway compression. Prophylactic airway stenting may be required.

Anaesthetic management

1 Consider LA or regional techniques to avoid GA.
2 Preoperative radiotherapy/chemotherapy may shrink the mass prior to GA.
3 Based on the above investigations, decide whether GA is likely to be safe, possibly unsafe or unsafe. GA is likely to be safe with a small mediastinal mass in an asymptomatic patient with no positional issues.

4 If SVC obstruction is present, the lower limbs must be used for IV access.
   See Superior vena cava syndrome (SVCS).

5 Consider an arterial line.

6 If there is tracheal compression, consider awake intubation with a reinforced tube.
   It may not be possible to push the reinforced tube past the obstruction. Consider
   rigid bronchoscopy performed by an ENT specialist to secure the airway. Another
   option is GA with insertion of a small-bore Teflon bougie past the obstruction.
   The reinforced ET tube is then passed over the bougie and through the area of
   compression with a rotational manoeuvre.

7 Spontaneous ventilation is preferred because the trans-pleural pressure
   gradient is maintained, splinting the airways open. Also, mediastinal pressures are
   lower.

8 For very high-risk cases, preparations should be made for emergency bypass or
   ECMO. Femoral access can be obtained under LA prior to GA.

Rescue measures for severe decompensation after induction of GA

1 Abandon procedure and wake patient up.

2 Change patient's position—left/right lateral, prone.

3 Rigid bronchoscopy to identify/relieve site of airway obstruction.

4 Treat severe hypotension with IV fluids and vasopressors. Consider pericardial
   tamponade as a cause.

5 Emergency sternotomy with elevation of the mass.

6 Emergency cardiopulmonary bypass/ECMO.

❍ Metabolic acidosis

See Arterial blood gas (ABG) interpretation for acidosis/alkalosis.

❍ Metabolic alkalosis

Description

Acid-base disorder due to plasma bicarbonate rising to an abnormally high level
(> 26 mmol/L) with blood pH > 7.45. *See Arterial blood gas interpretation for
acidosis/alkalosis.* Respiratory compensation involves hypoventilation to retain CO_2.

Causes

1 Exogenous bicarbonate—antacids, citrate in transfused blood.

2 Loss of hydrogen ions from the kidney or gut (vomiting, NG suction).

3 Hypokalaemia—hydrogen ions shift from the extracellular fluid into the cells.

4 Primary aldosteronism—*see Renin-angiotensin system* and *Conn's syndrome.*

5 Diuretic use.

The kidney and metabolic alkalosis

The kidney is very good at secreting bicarbonate but this can be impaired by:

1 chloride or potassium depletion

2 reduced GFR

3 hypovolaemia

4 renal impairment preventing bicarbonate excretion.

❍ Metabolic equivalent (MET)

See Cardiac risk for non-cardiac surgery.

◗ Metaraminol/Metaradine (Aramine)

Description
Alpha-adrenergic receptor agonist vasoconstrictive agent used for the treatment of hypotension. It also causes some stimulation of beta-1 receptors, thus increasing cardiac inotropy. It also causes some release of noradrenaline from sympathetic nerve endings. There is some uptake of metaraminol into adrenergic nerve endings, from which it is released as a weak neurotransmitter.

Dose

Adult
0.5–1 mg IV boluses q 2–5 min. Onset of effects occurs in 1–2 min and lasts 20–60 min. IV infusion—load 10 mg of metaraminol into 20 mL of N/S. Run at 1–10 mL/h titrated to effect.

Child
0.01 mg/kg IV boluses. IV infusion—0.1–1 mcg/kg/min. Titrate to BP.

Advantages
Fast, effective and convenient.

Disadvantages
1 Bradycardia may occur due to activation of the baroreceptor reflex in response to hypertension.
2 Monoamine oxidase inhibitors (MAOIs) may potentiate the effects of metaraminol because they inhibit the breakdown of noradrenaline. *See Monoamine oxidase inhibitors (MAOI)*.
3 Metaraminol effects may be potentiated by tricyclic antidepressants.
4 Digoxin's antiarrhythmic effects may be potentiated by metaraminol.

◗ Methadone/physeptone

Description
Synthetic opioid agonist with efficient oral absorption (> 80%), rapid onset (6–8 min if given IV) and long duration of action (24–36 h). It is used for:
1 postoperative pain and chronic pain management
2 the treatment of opioid addiction as a maintenance drug
3 cough suppression in terminal illness.

In addition to its effects on opioid receptors, methadone:
1 inhibits reuptake of serotonin and noradrenaline
2 blocks the NMDA receptor and is therefore effective in treating neuropathic pain.
   Its pharmacokinetics are complex, and methadone treatment requires expertise and experience.

Dose

Adult
Postoperative pain relief
Administer soon after induction of anaesthesia. Adult dose is 10–15 mg IV. 20 mg IV has been used in several clinical trials.[7] If used within 2 h of completion of surgery, emergence from GA may be slowed. Persistent drowsiness and respiratory depression may occur.

Chronic pain relief (oral dose)

A safe starting dose for opioid-naïve patients is 2.5 mg q 12 h. This can be increased weekly by increments of 2.5 mg q 12 h e.g. week two 5 mg q 12 h, week three 7.5 mg q 12 h.

Converting from oral morphine to oral methadone[8]

- If morphine daily oral dose 30–90 mg, use a methadone-to-morphine ratio 1:4 e.g. 22.5 mg methadone = 90 mg morphine.
- If morphine daily oral dose 90–300 mg, use a methadone-to-morphine ratio 1:8 e.g. 25 mg methadone = 200 mg morphine.
- If morphine daily oral dose > 300 mg, use a methadone-to-morphine ratio 1:12. 30 mg is the maximum dose as an outpatient.

Opioid dependence (oral dose)

Methadone is used as a daily dose to treat opioid dependence. The usual starting dose is 20–30 mg/day. It is rare that more than 40 mg/day is required.

Advantages

1 Has no active metabolite and is safe to use in kidney disease except for end-stage renal failure.
2 Long acting, therefore less frequent dosing required than other opioids. Acts about 10 × longer than morphine.
3 Highly lipophilic hence it is amenable to many routes of administration, including oral. Methadone has 3 × the bioavailability of morphine.
4 The clinical effectiveness of methadone increases with chronic dosing.
5 Can be used in patients with chronic liver disease.
6 Opioid-dependent pregnant patients can and should continue methadone throughout pregnancy. The dose may need to be increased as pregnancy progresses due to the physiological changes of pregnancy.
7 Breast feeding by patients stabilised on methadone can and should be continued. Abrupt cessation of breast feeding may result in withdrawal symptoms in the baby.

Disadvantages

1 If used intraoperatively its long duration of action means that side effects such as sedation will also be long acting.
2 May prolong the QT interval, leading to increased susceptibility to torsades de pointes. **See *Torsades de pointes*.**
3 Methadone can have a very long elimination time and may accumulate in the body.
4 Respiratory depression, as with other opioids, is the most life-threatening risk of methadone use.
5 Inhibits reuptake of serotonin and can contribute to the development of serotonin syndrome. **See *Serotonin syndrome/toxicity*.**

Anaesthetic implications of long-term methadone use[9]

1 Continue methadone therapy until the morning of elective surgery.
2 Continue the patient's usual dose of methadone throughout the perioperative period.
3 Give additional opioids for postoperative pain relief e.g. morphine PCA.
4 Giving the patient's usual maintenance daily dose of methadone divided into three doses may improve pain control e.g. if patient's daily oral dose is 30 mg, give 10 mg q 8 h.

5 If the patient is unable to take methadone orally, give IV but reduce the dose by between one-half to two-thirds and in divided doses q 6–8 h.

Methaemoglobin (MetHb)

Description

In this condition, ferrous iron in the haemoglobin molecule is oxidised to the ferric state. MetHb cannot bind O_2 and is brownish in colour. If more than 1% of the total haemoglobin (Hb) has become MetHb, methaemoglobinaemia is diagnosed. MetHb > 8% causes clinically significant effects. MetHb > 50% is severe and may be fatal.

Causes of MetHb

1 Inherited due to deficiency in the enzyme cytochrome b5 reductase.
2 Acquired due to drugs or other substances. These include:
  a) Prilocaine in doses > 600 mg in the adult.
  b) EMLA, topical benzocaine and tetracaine, topical lignocaine and teething medications in babies in sufficient doses may cause methaemoglobinaemia.
  c) Nitrates, nitrites and sodium nitroprusside.
  d) Dapsone.
  e) Trimethoprim, sulfonamides
  f) Some other substances such as diaspirin.
3 Patients with glucose-6-phosphate dehydrogenase deficiency are at increased risk of developing MetHb. ***See Glucose-6-phosphate dehydrogenase (G6PD) deficiency***.

Clinical effects

1 Cyanosis can occur when MetHb > 8–12%.
2 MetHb > 20–30% may cause headache, confusion, dyspnoea and increased respiratory rate.
3 MetHb > 50% may lead to decreased level of consciousness, seizures and coma.
4 MetHb > 70% is fatal.
5 Pulse oximetry will read 80–85% regardless of the true saturation.
6 The patient may appear a slate-grey colour.
7 MetHb is brownish and does not redden on exposure to O_2.
8 Arterial PaO_2 is normal despite cyanosis/hypoxia.

Diagnosis

1 Clinical grounds.
2 Co-oximeter calculation of MetHb levels.

Treatment

1 Cease the causative drug e.g. sodium nitroprusside.
2 Supplemental O_2 therapy.
3 Methylene blue—1–2 mg/kg IV infused as a 1% solution over 5 min. The response is usually rapid but it may need to be repeated after 1 h. Do not give methylene blue to patients with glucose-6-phosphate dehydrogenase deficiency. ***See Glucose-6-phosphate dehydrogenase (G6PD) deficiency***.
4 A blood transfusion or exchange transfusion may be required in severe cases.
5 Hyperbaric O_2 therapy.

⏵ Methoxyflurane (Penthrox) inhaler

Description
Used to provide analgesia for pain after trauma or prior to painful procedures. The inhaler contains 3 mL of methoxyflurane which is an obsolescent inhalational anaesthetic drug. To use the device, the patient breathes in and out through an inhaler and only the patient should hold the device. A higher dose of inhaled methoxyflurane can be achieved by occluding the diluter hole. The maximum daily dose is 6 mL. Do not use more than once per 48 h and no more than 15 mL/week, due to the risk of nephrotoxicity.

Contraindications
1 Malignant hyperthermia susceptibility.
2 Raised ICP.

⏵ Metoclopramide (Maxolon)

Description
Chlorinated procainamide derivative useful for the prevention and treatment of nausea/vomiting. It also increases the rate of gastric emptying. Acts mainly by antagonising central and peripheral dopaminergic (DA2) receptors. It has a direct stimulatory effect on gut smooth muscle.

Dose for nausea/vomiting

Adult
10 mg IV, IM, PO as required, up to 8 h.

Child
0.12 mg/kg/dose (max 10 mg/dose) as required, up to 8 h.

Disadvantages
1 Low efficacy.
2 Can cause dystonic reactions. **See *Dystonic reaction, acute*.**
3 Not suitable for patients with Parkinson's disease. **See *Parkinson's disease (PD)*.**
4 Its use is contraindicated in phaeochromocytoma and seizure disorders. **See *Phaeochromocytoma*.** Metoclopramide can provoke a severe hypertensive reaction in patients with phaeochromocytoma.

⏵ Metoprolol

Beta-1 selective adrenoreceptor blocker used to treat:
1 hypertension
2 angina
3 supraventricular tachycardias
4 premature ventricular ectopics
5 tremor
6 migraine.

Dose

Adult
1–2 mg IV q 1 min until desired effect to a maximum of 15–20 mg. PO 12.5–100 mg/dose q 6–8 h.

Child

0.1 mg/kg IV over 5 min (no more than 5 mg/dose). This can be repeated if needed at 5-minute intervals to a maximum of 3 doses.

Points to note

Compared with other beta-1 selective drugs (atenolol, esmolol), metoprolol is associated with an increased risk of cerebral strokes in patients undergoing non-cardiac surgery.[10]

▶ Metyrosine

This drug inhibits catecholamine synthesis. It may be useful in the management of phaeochromocytoma. *See Phaeochromocytoma.*

▶ Mexiletine (Mexitil)

Description

Class 1B antiarrhythmic drug structurally similar to lignocaine. It is used to treat ventricular dysrhythmias, such as sustained VT, that are considered life-threatening. It is also used to treat diabetic neuropathy.

Dose

Adult

200 mg q 8 h PO for initial control. Dose can be adjusted up or down in 2–3 days, depending on effect.

▶ Midazolam (Versed)

Description

Midazolam is a water-soluble benzodiazepine with a fast onset and short duration of action. It is used for:

1 anxiolysis
2 sedation
3 amnesia
4 seizure control in status epilepticus. *See Status epilepticus (SE).*

Dose for sedation

Adult

1–2 mg IV increments until patient is tolerant of procedure but still able to communicate meaningfully, up to 5–10 mg. For prolonged sedation, use an LD of 0.5–2 mg then 0.5–8 mg/hr.

Child

0.1–0.2 mg/kg IV increments up to 10 mg. Distressed children (and adults) can be given PO midazolam 0.5 mg/kg up to 15 mg mixed with a sweet drink 30–60 min before the procedure.

Points to note

1 When used with anti-emetic drugs, midazolam provides an additional anti-emetic effect.
2 Atorvastatin can prolong the effects of midazolam.

▶ Milrinone

Description

This drug is a phosphodiesterase III inhibitor used for the short-term treatment (≤ 48 h) of heart failure. *See Phosphodiesterase (PDE) III inhibitors*. It improves cardiac contractility and relaxation (lusitropy) and causes vasodilation, decreasing preload and afterload. It also reduces pulmonary hypertension and can be inhaled for this purpose. *See Pulmonary hypertension*. It is used IV preferably via a central line.

Dose

Start the infusion at 0.5 mcg/kg/min and assess response in 2 h. Increase or decrease dose by increments of 0.125 mcg/kg/min. The dose range is 0.125–0.5 mcg/kg/min and the maximum dose is 0.75 mcg/kg/min.

Advantages

1 May block platelet aggregation.
2 May attenuate the proinflammatory effects of cardiopulmonary bypass.

Disadvantages

1 HR increases, but less than with catecholamines.
2 Hypotension—noradrenaline may be required.
3 Arrhythmogenic.
4 Relatively contraindicated in severe CCF or severe pulmonary hypertension.
5 Reduce dose in renal failure.
6 Contraindicated in severe obstructive aortic or pulmonary valve disease and hypertrophic subaortic stenosis. *See Hypertrophic cardiomyopathy (HCM) and hypertrophic obstructive cardiomyopathy (HOCM)*.

▶ Minimum alveolar concentration (MAC)

Defined as the concentration of an inhalational anaesthetic agent in the lung alveoli (as a percentage) that will prevent movement in response to surgical stimulus in 50% of patients. Examples are sevoflurane 2.05, N_2O 104, desflurane 6.

▶ Minute ventilation (MV)

Defined as tidal volume × respiratory rate/min. Normal MV for a resting adult is 85–100 mL/kg. Normal MV for a resting child is 100–200 mL/kg.

▶ Mirror syndrome

Description

This illness may occur in pregnant patients when the fetus has hydrops fetalis. *See Hydrops fetalis* and *Thalassaemia*. It is also known as 'Ballantyne syndrome', 'triple oedema' and 'maternal hydrops pseudotoxaemia'. It is characterised by severe maternal oedema and a condition indistinguishable from preeclampsia (but the fetus is always hydropic). The mother's condition 'mirrors' the condition of the hydrops fetus. The cause is unknown.

Clinical picture

The following are typically seen:
1 Severe maternal swelling and weight gain.
2 Hypertension.

3 Proteinuria.

4 Elevated maternal uric acid levels.

5 Pulmonary oedema.

Management

1 Correction of the underlying fetal abnormality if possible.

2 Deliver the hydropic fetus and placenta.

3 If CS is required, oedema can make intubation and neuraxial anaesthesia more difficult.

4 Fetal mortality approaches 100%.

◐ Misoprostol (PGE1, Cytotec)

Description

Prostaglandin drug presented as 200 mcg tablets. Useful for the management of postpartum haemorrhage (PPH), and medical termination of pregnancy.

See Postpartum haemorrhage (PPH).

Dose

800 mcg PR.

◐ Mitochondrial disease (MD)

Description

Mitochondria are organelles in eukaryotic cells (cells with a nucleus) that use aerobic metabolism to make adenosine triphosphate (ATP). ATP is used by the cell as a source of chemical energy. In MD, the mitochondria are defective, and this can affect a wide range of organs and tissues. Mitochondria contain DNA from both parents and mitochondrial DNA (mtDNA) from the mother only. MD results from defects in the mitochondrial DNA but there can be a mixture of defective and normal mitochondria. In some people there is a threshold where this defect causes clinical problems.

Clinical features

These vary enormously among affected individuals and may include:

1 developmental delay, seizures, central hypoventilation, apnoea

2 weakness, fatigue, hypotonia, spasticity, ataxia

3 cardiomyopathy, conduction disorders

4 respiratory muscle weakness

5 dysphagia

6 eye problems—ophthalmoplegia, optic atrophy

7 deafness

8 diabetes mellitus, hypoparathyroidism

9 anaemia, low platelet count, neutropaenia

10 renal, liver impairment

11 intermittent or persistent lactic acidaemia.

There are many related syndromes such as MELAS (**m**itochondrial **e**ncephalopathy, **l**actic **a**cidosis, **s**troke-like syndromes) and MERRF (**m**yoclonic **e**pilepsy with **r**agged **r**ed **f**ibres). MD is associated with nearly 300 known mutations.[11]

Diagnosis

1 Genetic testing.
2 Muscle biopsy—if genetic testing is equivocal.

Treatment

1 Supportive.
2 Exercise.
3 Supplements such as vitamins, coenzyme Q10 and alpha-lipoic acid.

Anaesthetic implications

These patients may be under several different specialists and it may be helpful to consult with one or more of them. There is little evidence from the literature of harm due to anaesthetic drugs, as long as they are used thoughtfully and carefully. Considerations for the anaesthetic management include:

1 As with all serious illnesses and anaesthesia, the main concern with MD is its effects on the heart and respiratory system and the ability of the patient to swallow oral secretions.
2 Patients should not be fasted for prolonged periods of time as they are prone to hypoglycaemia and metabolic encephalopathy. Give clear apple juice up to 2 h before anaesthesia.
3 Measure BSL regularly.
4 Give IV glucose-containing solutions except in cases of patients with disorders of pyruvate metabolism or ketogenic diets for seizure control. These patients may develop hyperglycaemia or lactic acidosis.
5 Some MD patients do not metabolise lactate normally. Do not administer lactate-containing crystalloid fluids such as Hartmann's solution.[12]
6 Maintain core temperature.
7 There is no association between MD and malignant hyperthermia.[13]
8 Volatile agents are probably safe.
9 Boluses of propofol are probably safe but infusions may not be.[11, 12]
10 Suxamethonium may cause an exaggerated hyperkalaemic response and should be avoided. Rocuronium and sugammadex are probably safe.
11 LA and opioids are probably safe.
12 Barbiturates, ketamine, valproate and phenytoin should probably be avoided.
13 Dexmedetomidine and NSAIDs are safe.
14 Avoid repeated doses of paracetamol due to metabolic energy demands on the liver.
15 Use caution with postoperative opioids due to potential weakness of respiratory muscles.

◐ Mitral valve prolapse (MVP)

In this condition, part of a mitral valve leaflet projects above the annular plane during ventricular systole. The valve may be normal (functional prolapse, also called Barlow's syndrome) or diseased (anatomic prolapse). This is usually due to myxomatous degeneration leading to progressive mitral valve incompetence. *See Mitral valve regurgitation (MR), chronic*. Functional prolapse is almost always asymptomatic, with little or no regurgitation. It can however lead to mitral regurgitation.

▶ Mitral valve regurgitation (MR), acute

Description

Acute MR is a medical and surgical emergency. The patient will become gravely ill with acute heart failure. Only a brief description of this catastrophic event is provided in this manual. Mortality, even with mitral valve replacement, is very high.

Causes

1 Papillary muscle rupture due to myocardial infarction.
2 Ruptured mitral chordae tendineae due to causes such as myxomatous disease, infective endocarditis or chest trauma.
3 Iatrogenic e.g. insertion of a transcatheter aortic valve.
4 Malfunction of a mitral valve prosthesis.

Pathophysiology

1 Sudden increase in left atrial (LA) volume and pressure.
2 Sudden increase in pressure in the pulmonary circulation, resulting in acute pulmonary oedema.
3 Acute right-sided heart failure.
4 Reduced cardiac output.
5 Tachycardia and hypotension.
6 Cardiogenic shock.

Diagnosis

Emergency echocardiography will provide rapid diagnosis.

Treatment

1 Intra-aortic balloon counterpulsation and other circulatory assist devices.
2 Mitral valve repair or replacement.

▶ Mitral valve regurgitation (MR), chronic

Causes

This lesion can be caused by:
1 Rheumatic fever.
2 Dilated left ventricle (LV) causing dilatation of the annulus (secondary MR)—cardiomyopathy, ischaemic heart disease.
3 Papillary muscle dysfunction e.g. myxomatous disease, myocardial ischemia.
4 Congenital heart disease.
5 Marfan syndrome, Ehlers–Danlos syndrome. **See *Marfan syndrome*** and ***Ehlers–Danlos syndrome***.
6 Hypertrophic cardiomyopathy with mitral valve distortion.
   There may be mixed mitral valve disease (regurgitation and stenosis).

Pathophysiology

1 The LV pumps blood into both the left atrium (LA) and the aorta. This leads to increased LV end-diastolic volume.
2 LA becomes enlarged, which may lead to atrial fibrillation (AF).
3 LV wall thickens.
4 LV contractility begins to decline.
5 Cardiac output reduces.

6 Lungs become congested. There may be increased pulmonary venous pressure, pulmonary arterial pressure and increased RV load. This can cause RV enlargement, hypertrophy and eventual failure.

Clinical effects

These depend on the regurgitant fraction.

1 < 30%—mild symptoms.
2 30–60%—moderate symptoms.
3 > 60%—severe disease.

Clinical effects include:

1 easy fatiguability
2 dyspnoea
3 palpitations
4 symptoms of CCF
5 frequent chest infections (suggesting pulmonary hypertension)
6 raised JVP, peripheral oedema (suggesting RV failure)
7 atrial fibrillation may develop with the associated risk of thromboemboli.

Diagnosis

1 Pansystolic heart murmur.
2 Signs of CCF.
3 ECG—may show atrial fibrillation, P mitrale, LV hypertrophy.
4 CXR—LA, LV enlargement.
5 Echocardiography—will indicate nature and extent of valve abnormalities, cardiac chamber size and regurgitant fraction estimate.

Treatment

1 Medical treatment for CCF including ACE inhibitors, digoxin and calcium channel blockers. **See Congestive cardiac failure (CCF)—chronic.**
2 Mitral valve replacement.

Anaesthetic goals

Liaise with the patient's cardiologist and ensure medications are optimised. Keep the patient 'full, fast and forward'.

1 For major surgery, consider invasive monitoring (arterial line, CVP). TOE may be required.
2 Keep heart rate between 80–100 bpm. With slow heart rates the LV overfills, distending the annulus and making regurgitation worse. A higher heart rate reduces filling time of the LV, enhancing forward flow.
3 Avoid excess intravascular volume as this can also distend the LV. However also avoid hypovolaemia as the well-filled LA will lead to less blood regurgitating back into it.
4 An increase in SVR will increase the regurgitant fraction and should be avoided. Vasopressors should be used with caution. A carefully controlled decrease in SVR may improve CO.
5 Avoid factors that increase pulmonary vascular resistance such as hypoxia, hypercarbia and acidosis. **See Pulmonary hypertension.**
6 Maintain sinus rhythm. Acute AF must be treated promptly.
7 Dobutamine and milrinone may be required for inotropic support of LV failure.
8 Consider the need for bacterial endocarditis prophylaxis. **See Bacterial endocarditis (BE) prophylaxis.**

MR and pregnancy

1 Pregnancy is generally well tolerated because it is associated with hypervolaemia, fast heart rate and decreased peripheral vascular resistance.

2 If LV failure occurs, diuretics are usually helpful.

3 In labour a carefully administered epidural anaesthetic is usually well tolerated. Maintain adequate preload. Patients with MR should be encouraged to have an epidural because pain-related catecholamine release may increase SVR.

4 Ephedrine is preferable to metaraminol as a vasoconstrictor because heart rate is maintained and the vasoconstrictor effect is less.

5 For CS a carefully titrated epidural can be used. A CSE with a low-dose spinal component is probably acceptable.

6 GA for CS should follow the recommendations mentioned in 'Anaesthetic goals' above.

◑ Mitral valve stenosis (MS)

Patients with severe mitral stenosis are at increased risk for non-cardiac surgery. Mitral valve balloon commissurotomy may decrease risk. About 75% of patients will have other heart valve conditions.

Causes

1 Rheumatic fever is the most common cause, especially in developing countries.

2 Congenital.

3 Degenerative calcification.

4 Scarring due to endocarditis.

5 Infiltrative diseases.

6 Multisystem diseases such as sarcoidosis.

7 Calcium build-up on the valve.

Pathophysiology

The normal valve area is 4–6 cm^2 and the normal diastolic pressure gradient across the valve is < 5 mmHg. Grades of MS based on valve and pressure gradient across the valve are:

1 mild—1.5–2.5 cm^2, < 5 mmHg

2 moderate—1–1.5 cm^2, 6–10 mmHg

3 severe—< 1 cm^2, > 10 mmHg, may be > 25 mmHg.

As the valve stenoses:

1 The LA is initially able to compensate for the stenosis by dilating but eventually pressure in the LA becomes too high. LA dilatation may lead to AF with clot formation. AF worsens LV filling.

2 This leads to increased pressure in the pulmonary circulation, which can lead to RV hypertrophy, dilatation and failure.

3 Reactive pulmonary vasoconstriction may occur, leading to pulmonary hypertension.

4 LV filling is compromised leading to a decreased, 'fixed' CO.

5 LV dysfunction can also be due to muscle atrophy and inflammatory myocardial fibrosis.

6 There may also be mitral regurgitation (MR) due to thickened/scarred leaflets not being able to oppose correctly. Mixed mitral disease is common.

Clinical features

1 Dyspnoea can occur when valve area is 2.5 cm^2 or less, especially with stressors such as exercise, pregnancy, anaemia or onset of AF.
2 Thromboembolic disease.
3 Fainting, dizziness, tiredness.
4 Haemoptysis.
5 Chest pain.
6 Palpitations.

Diagnosis

1 Typical heart murmur. There is usually an 'opening snap' at the beginning of diastole and a mid-diastolic murmur with pre-systolic accentuation.
2 Evidence of RV failure—elevated JVP, peripheral oedema, liver distension.
3 ECG—atrial fibrillation, P mitrale.
4 CXR—left atrial enlargement.
5 Echocardiography—will show severity of MS and cardiac chamber effects.
6 Cardiac catheterisation.

Treatment

1 Beta blockers to control heart rate.
2 Diuretics.
3 Cardioversion of AF.
4 Anticoagulants for persistent AF.
5 Percutaneous techniques—balloon valvuloplasty.
6 Open mitral valve commissurotomy—the surgeon uses a scalpel to free up the mitral valve leaflets under direct vision while the patient is on bypass.
7 Closed mitral valve commissurotomy—an operation performed on the beating heart. The surgeon introduces a transvalvular dilator either through the LA or LV. This is rarely done now.
8 Mitral valve replacement.

Anaesthesia

Involvement of the cardiologist and optimisation of the patient's medical management are both vitally important. Aim to keep the patient euvolaemic with a slow heart rate—'slow and tight'. If the patient is on anticoagulants, *see Anticoagulant and antiplatelet drugs and surgery/neuraxial anaesthesia*.

1 Mitral valve replacement, commissurotomy or balloon valvuloplasty should be considered before non-cardiac surgery if MS is severe.
2 Tachycardia must be avoided as it is poorly tolerated. It reduces the time available for LV diastolic filling, leading to decreased stroke volume and CO. It can also cause a rise in LA pressure, which can lead to pulmonary oedema. Therefore, avoid all drugs that can cause tachycardia such as atropine, glycopyrrolate, ephedrine, ketamine and hyoscine.
3 Tachycardia on intubation can be attenuated with an appropriate dose of fentanyl and a bolus of esmolol—1–2 mg/kg 4 min before intubation.
4 Preserve SR—treat new-onset AF promptly with cardioversion.
5 For moderate-to-severe MS, consider invasive monitoring (arterial line, CVP, TOE).
6 Hypotension is poorly tolerated as CO is fixed. Maintain SVR with metaraminol (not ephedrine) and replace fluid losses promptly.
7 Hypervolaemia is also tolerated poorly and must be avoided.
8 If the patient has pulmonary hypertension, avoid all factors that may exacerbate this (e.g. hypoxia, hypercarbia and acidosis). *See Pulmonary hypertension*.

9 Provide thromboembolic prophylaxis.

10 Avoid the Trendelenburg position, which might cause pulmonary oedema.

11 Avoid high inflation pressures as they may decrease venous return to the heart.

12 Use sugammadex to reverse rocuronium to avoid tachycardia from atropine or glycopyrrolate.

13 Consider the need for bacterial endocarditis prophylaxis. *See Bacterial endocarditis (BE) prophylaxis.*

Mitral stenosis and pregnancy

Severe MS is a high-risk lesion in pregnancy. Asymptomatic patients without pulmonary hypertension, a valve area > 1.5 cm^2 and a gradient < 5 mmHg are at low risk.

Pregnancy physiology and MS

1 Heart rate goes up in pregnancy and this results in less time for LV filling.

2 As CO is fixed, the heart may not able to increase to meet the demands of pregnancy.

3 There is an increased risk of pulmonary oedema. 'Flash' pulmonary oedema may occur immediately after delivery due to:[14]

  a) sudden release of aortocaval compression

  b) autotransfusion from uterine contraction

  c) tachycardia or atrial arrhythmia.

4 The onset of atrial fibrillation worsens this scenario and increases the risk of thromboembolic disease.

5 Be aware of the risk of aortocaval compression.

Treatment of MS in pregnancy

1 Treatment includes bed rest, oxygen, diuretics and beta blockers.

2 If AF occurs, cardioversion, digoxin and anticoagulation may be required. *See Anticoagulation and pregnancy.*

3 Percutaneous balloon mitral valvuloplasty should be considered in women with severe disease and a valve area < 1 cm^2.

4 Mitral valve replacement may need to be considered but is associated with a fetal loss rate of up to 30%.[15]

Labour

1 Patients with significant MS should be encouraged to have an epidural in labour. It reduces the incidence of tachycardia associated with labour pain.

2 It is of utmost importance to avoid overfilling or underfilling the patient with IV fluid during epidural anaesthesia. Small incremental boluses of Hartmann's 100–200 mL are suggested.[16]

3 Use assisted delivery in the second stage (low forceps, vacuum) to avoid Valsalva/extreme pushing effort.

4 Patients may go into pulmonary oedema post delivery. See the description of 'flash' pulmonary oedema above. Treat with head-up position, oxygen therapy and invasive ventilation with PEEP if severe.

Caesarean section

1 A carefully titrated epidural or CSE with a low-dose spinal component can be considered.

2 A SAB may cause a catastrophic decrease in SVR with hypotension and impaired myocardial perfusion. This might lead to a spiral of worsening cardiac function.

3 Oxytocin should be used very cautiously as it is vasodilating.

4 Ergometrine is contraindicated due to its pulmonary vasoconstrictive effects.

○ Mivacurium

Description

Benzylisoquinolinium diester non-depolarising neuromuscular blocking drug (NMBD) with a short duration of action. It is metabolised primarily by pseudocholinesterase. It is cleared from the plasma but the duration of its effects is variable. It is intended for use during procedures that require a short period of muscle relaxation.

Dose

Adult

0.2–0.25 mg/kg IV. Top-up dose 0.1 mg/kg at 15 min intervals. Infusion dose 0.36–0.42 mg/kg/h.

Advantages

1 It was used in the past for short procedures such as ECT in patients who could not have suxamethonium for reasons other than sux apnoea.
2 It may not require reversal drugs if sufficient time has passed—check with nerve stimulator.
3 It can be used in patients with renal or liver failure.

Disadvantages

1 Causes significant histamine release, which can cause flushing and hypotension.
2 Relatively slow onset to paralysis.
3 Recovery time will be delayed if a patient has inadequate or abnormal pseudocholinesterase.
4 Neostigmine may not effectively reverse mivacurium as it may impair pseudocholinesterase.

Comment

1 Mivacurium is still available in developed countries that have access to rocuronium and sugammadex. Why this is so is unclear.
2 It perhaps has a role in countries or areas without access to sugammadex or in patients that cannot have suxamethonium, rocuronium and/or sugammadex.

○ Monoamine oxidase inhibitor (MAOI) drugs

Description

These drugs are used in the treatment of severe depression and Parkinson's disease. Monoamine oxidase breaks down monoamines, which include serotonin, dopamine, adrenaline and noradrenaline. This substance is found in the CNS and many other parts of the body. There are two types:

1 MAO-A (liver, gastrointestinal tract, pulmonary vascular endothelium)
2 MAO-B found mainly in platelets.
  MAOIs may be selective (A or B) or non-selective. Inhibition of MAO-A is responsible for the antidepressant effect.

Non-selective MAOIs

These include phenelzine and tranylcypromine. Non-selective MAOIs cause irreversible inhibition of MAO. These drugs are associated with a high risk of a hypertensive crisis occurring if foods containing tyramine or phenethylamine are ingested (aged cheese, aged meats, fermented foods). Drug interactions include the following:

1 Indirect acting sympathomimetic drugs that cause endogenous release of noradrenaline (NA) can cause profound hypertension. Examples include ephedrine, metaraminol and amphetamines.

2 Direct-acting sympathomimetics can be used e.g. adrenaline, noradrenaline, phenylephrine. **However, they must be used with extreme caution.**

3 Use of pethidine, methadone, tramadol or tapentadol may result in a sudden increase in serotonin levels, causing confusion, hypertension, tremor, hyperactivity, coma and death. Fentanyl and morphine can be used safely.

4 Methyldopa may precipitate hypertension.

5 Levodopa and imipramine are contraindicated.

Consideration should be given to ceasing non-selective MAOI drugs for 2 weeks prior to anaesthesia.

Selective MAOIs

These drugs reversibly inhibit either MAO-A (e.g. moclobemide) or MAO-B (e.g. selegiline). There is much less potential for hypertension with ingestion of tyramine or phenethylamine. These drugs have a short half-life and can be stopped the day before surgery. If not ceased:

1 pethidine is contraindicated

2 indirect-acting sympathomimetics should not be used with moclobemide.

◖ Morphine

Description

Morphine is an alkaloid of opium and is the 'prototype' opioid against which other opioids are measured.

Dose

Adult

1 IV: 2–2.5 mg q 5 min up to 10–15 mg.

2 IM/subcut: 5–10 mg q 4 h.

3 IV infusion: 10–40 mcg/kg/h.

4 PCA: 1–2 mg boluses with a 5 min lockout.

5 Intrathecal: 100–150 mcg (preservative free).

6 Epidural: 3 mg (preservative free).

7 PO: some average starting doses for adults are: Kapanol capsules, sustained release 20 mg q 12–24 h; MS Contin, controlled release 30 mg q 12 h; MS Mono, controlled release 60 mg q 24 h; Sevredol, immediate-release tablets 20–40 mg q 4 h. There are many other formulations.

Child

1 IM/subcut: 0.1–0.15 mg/kg (preferably via subcut cannula placed intraoperatively).

2 IV: 0.15 mg/kg in 10 mL N/S in a syringe. Give 1 mL q 5 min until pain controlled.

3 Infusion: load 1 mg/kg morphine in 50 mL of 5% glucose. Run infusion at 0.5–2.5 mL/hr = 10–50 mcg/kg/hr.

Advantages

1 Long acting—about 4 h.

2 Reasonably fast onset 15–30 min.

3 Potent.

4 Less addictive than many other opioids (e.g. pethidine, fentanyl, oxycodone).

5 May be more effective than fentanyl for PCA use in opioid-dependent patients due to high potency and longer duration of action.
6 Long acting when used intrathecally or epidurally (about 12 h).
7 Can be safely used in patients taking monoamine oxidase inhibitor (MAOI) drugs. *See Monoamine oxidase inhibitor (MAOI) drugs.*
8 Useful for cough suppression and treating diarrhoea.

Disadvantages
1 Causes histamine release. This can cause a rash and, in asthmatic patients, bronchospasm.
2 Readily crosses the placental barrier, which can result in respiratory depression in the newborn.
3 Has an active metabolite morphine-6-glucuronide, which can accumulate in patients with renal disease. This metabolite can result in respiratory depression.
4 Less suitable than fentanyl for use in PCA for OSA patients due to its slower onset of action and longer-lasting effects.
5 Poor oral absorption—about 30% of ingested morphine reaches target receptors.

Oral forms of morphine
These can be divided into sustained-release (SR) and immediate-release (IR) forms.
SR oral morphine includes:
1 MS Contin (tablets and suspension) used q 12 h
2 Kapanol, which is given **once** daily.
IR oral morphine preparations include Ordine syrup.

▶ Motor neurone disease (MND)

Description
MND is a disease of the upper or lower motor neurones or both. It is probably due to a combination of genetic and environmental factors, but the actual cause is unknown. It is progressively debilitating and usually fatal in 3–5 years. Upper motor neurones originate from the motor region of the cerebral cortex. They synapse with lower motor neurones in the brainstem and spinal cord in the ventral horns. The lower motor neurones continue out of the spinal cord to the target muscle. There are four main types of MND:
1 Amyotrophic lateral sclerosis (ALS)—patients may present with limb weakness, dysarthria, dysphagia, emotional lability, respiratory weakness and hyperreflexia. Muscle cramps and twitching may occur. It is also called Lou Gehrig's disease. Stephen Hawking had ALS.
2 Progressive muscular atrophy—progressive flaccid paralysis, muscle wasting, hyporeflexia/areflexia, fasciculations. It presents as mainly a lower motor neurone disease.
3 Progressive spinal muscular atrophy—a lower motor neurone form of MND marked by muscle wasting, weakness and fasciculations.
4 Primary lateral sclerosis—affects upper motor neurones, causing limb stiffness, spasticity, balance difficulties, hyperreflexia, dysphagia and dysarthria. There may be hoarseness, chewing problems and drooling. It can be extremely disabling but may not shorten life expectancy.

Diagnosis

MND is a diagnosis of exclusion. It involves painless progressive weakness without any sensory effects, distinguishing it from multiple sclerosis. The usual tests undertaken include:

1 cerebral and spinal MRI imaging
2 lumbar puncture
3 nerve conduction studies.

Treatment

1 Supportive measures.
2 Drugs that reduce the rate of neuronal death e.g. sodium phenylbutyrate/ taurursodiol, riluzole, edaravone.

Anaesthesia and MND

1 MND patients may be at increased risk of regurgitation and aspiration.
2 Suxamethonium is contraindicated. *See Suxamethonium*.
3 NDNMBDs should be used carefully in reduced doses with neuromuscular monitoring. The combination of rocuronium and sugammadex is efficacious.
4 Respiratory complications are common and there may be a need for post-procedure ventilation with subsequent weaning problems.

▷ Moyamoya disease

Introduction

Moyamoya disease is a type of cerebrovascular occlusive syndrome affecting the internal carotid arteries and their branches at the skull base. Friable collateral vessels develop which look like a 'puff of smoke' ('moyamoya' in Japanese) on cerebral angiography. Patients are at risk of both haemorrhagic and ischaemic stroke. Other manifestations include headache, TIAs and seizures. It is probably genetic and more common in females. There may also be intracranial aneurysm(s).

Treatment

The main treatment option is superficial temporal artery to middle cerebral artery anastomosis, to bypass the stenosed segment. Alternatively, the superficial temporal artery can be laid upon the cortical surface, resulting in neo-vascularisation over months or years.

Anaesthetic aims (non-neurosurgical procedures)

Haemodynamic stability is the main aim, to avoid both hypertension and hypotension.
1 Pre-induction arterial line.
2 TIVA to avoid cerebral steal with inhalational agents. This is a theoretical suggestion.
3 Phenylephrine infusion—target BP to pre-operative baseline or slightly higher.
4 Maintain normocapnia.

Obstetric anaesthesia

A suggested approach to neuraxial anaesthesia for CS is a carefully titrated epidural. Use IV crystalloid fluid loading and a phenylephrine infusion and invasive arterial monitoring. Avoid/detect/treat hypertension or hypotension, the aim being to maintain the patient's normal blood pressure. SAB anaesthesia is probably best avoided due to the risk of hypotension. A CSE with a low-dose spinal component can be considered with the above precautions.

❍ MS Contin (MR)

This is a brand name for modified-release oral morphine in tablet form. *See Morphine.*

❍ MS Mono (MR)

This is a brand name for modified-release oral morphine in capsule/pellet form.
See Morphine.

❍ Multifocal atrial tachycardia (MAT)

Description

In this condition the heart rate (HR) is > 100 bpm, P waves vary in morphology and the PP, PR and RR intervals vary. If the HR is between 60–100, the condition is termed 'wandering atrial pacemaker'.

Cause

It may result from right atrial hypertension and distension, and can occur during exacerbations of chronic obstructive pulmonary disease (COPD). It is often associated with elderly patients with severe health problems. Other causes include hypokalaemia, hypomagnesaemia, CKD, sepsis and some drugs e.g. isoproterenol.

Treatment

Correct the underlying cause.

❍ Multiple sclerosis (MS)

Description

MS is a progressive autoimmune inflammatory demyelinating disorder affecting the central nervous system axons. There are usually symptomatic episodes that occur months or years apart (relapsing, remitting pattern), affecting different anatomical locations. Some patients experience steady neurological decline. The cause is unknown but is thought to relate to an interaction of genetic and environmental factors.

Clinical presentation

1 Sensory loss.
2 Muscle cramping/spasticity.
3 Bladder, bowel and/or sexual dysfunction.
4 Cerebellar effects—Charcot's triad of scanning speech, nystagmus and intention tremor.
5 Optic neuritis—loss of vision, loss of colour vision.
6 Nonspecific symptoms—fatigue, dizziness, sleep disturbance.
7 Cognitive impairment—memory, planning, problem solving.
8 Psychiatric issues—euphoria, bipolar disorder.
9 Acute transverse myelitis—usually partial.
10 Many other neurological issues.

Diagnosis

1 Clinical history.
2 Plaque lesions on MRI of brain and/or spinal cord, cerebral atrophy and 'black holes' indicating axonal death.
3 Oligoclonal bands and intrathecal immunoglobulin production in CSF.
4 Evoked potentials abnormalities.

Treatment

1 Immunotherapies—aim to reduce the frequency and severity of attacks. These drugs include interferon, Copaxone and dimethyl fumarate.

2 Corticosteroids—used in high dose to treat the symptoms of an acute attack.

3 Plasmapheresis—for acute severe attacks not responding to steroids.

4 Targeted treatments for MS complications—e.g. botox for spasticity, oxybutynin for bladder problems.

5 Stem cell therapy.

Anaesthesia

There is no evidence that general anaesthesia exacerbates MS in any way.

1 Do not use suxamethonium due to the risk of hyperkalaemia.

2 Stress steroids may be required in patients that have received high-dose steroid therapy. **See *Stress steroids*.**

Obstetric anaesthesia

1 Pregnancy is associated with a decrease in relapse rates of MS, with a return to pre-pregnancy relapse rates after three months.[17] Some studies suggest an increase in relapse rates after pregnancy.

2 Epidural anaesthesia has no impact on MS.[17]

3 There is concern that LA may have a direct toxicity effect on demyelinated axons, and there is some clinical data to support this view. Spinal anaesthesia is probably safe in MS patients, but this area remains controversial and definitive advice cannot be given.[18]

4 It is very important that pre-procedure neurological assessment is undertaken and the patient is made fully aware of any potential risks.

◐ Muscular dystrophy (MD)

Description

This is a vast topic, and only a brief coverage is provided in this manual. MD describes a group of more than 30 inherited disorders that cause progressive weakness and breakdown of skeletal muscle. There is variation between the disorders in terms of:

1 severity

2 pattern of muscle impairment

3 effects on other organs.

The most common types are:

1 Duchenne muscular dystrophy (DMD).

2 Becker muscular dystrophy.

3 Facioscapulohumeral muscular dystrophy.

4 Myotonic dystrophy.

There is typically progressive muscular wasting, scoliosis, gait disorders, respiratory difficulty, muscle spasms and cardiomyopathy.

Duchenne muscular dystrophy (DMD)

Affects mainly boys, although mild symptoms may occur in female carriers.

There is progressive muscle weakness and wasting, starting distally and progressing proximally. By age 12, most patients are unable to walk and respiratory muscle paralysis eventually occurs. Lifespan ranges from 15–45 yrs.

1 Suxamethonium is contraindicated. Hyperkalaemia and rhabdomyolysis may occur.

2 There may be difficulty with intubation due to macroglossia and limited mobility of the jaw and cervical spine.

3 **Do not use volatile anaesthetics.** Episodes of rhabdomyolysis, hyperkalaemia and hyperthermia have been reported in DMD patients receiving volatiles.[19]

4 There is **no association** between DMD and malignant hyperthermia.

5 TIVA can be used safely.[19]

6 Respiratory muscle involvement may lead to postoperative ventilation problems.

7 Paracetamol may lead to liver injury and failure despite use within therapeutic guidelines. This may be due to reduced muscle mass resulting in decreased glutathione stores in skeletal muscle.[20]

Becker muscular dystrophy

A less severe variant of DMD. Life expectancy can be normal, but patients can develop a severe dilated cardiomyopathy in adulthood. Do not use suxamethonium or volatile anaesthetic drugs.

Congenital muscular dystrophy (CMD)

There is generalised weakness and muscle degeneration, resulting in impairment ranging from mild to severe. Lifespan is shortened.

Myotonic dystrophy (also called dystrophia myotonica)

This disease causes myotonia, muscle weakness and cardiomyopathy. Myotonia is a condition in which muscles are unable to relax after they contract. Patients will develop muscle rigidity with exposure to suxamethonium, which is contraindicated. They are sensitive to NDNMBDs. Anticholinesterase drugs such as neostigmine may cause a myotonic crisis and severe bradycardia.[21] Use rocuronium and sugammadex if muscle paralysis is required.

▶ Myasthenia gravis (MG)

Description

MG is an autoimmune neuromuscular junction disorder in which there is destruction of the post-synaptic nicotinic acetylcholine receptors by autoantibodies made in the thymus (80–90% of patients). 50% of patients who do not have anti-acetylcholine receptor antibodies have antibodies to muscle-specific receptor tyrosine kinase. These antibodies result in skeletal muscle weakness and fatiguability with exertion. Only skeletal muscle is affected. Most patients have thymus abnormalities (e.g. hyperplasia or thymoma).

Clinical effects

There are two clinical forms.

1 Ocular myasthenia—only eyelids and extraocular muscles are involved. 50% of these patients will go on to develop generalised disease.

2 Generalised disease—ocular, bulbar, limb and respiratory muscle involvement to varying degrees.

As the disease progresses:

- weakness tends to worsen through the day
- bulbar involvement may result in weakness of chewing, dysarthria, dysphagia and aspiration. Nasal regurgitation of liquids may occur
- respiratory muscle weakness can lead to respiratory failure
- most patients reach a peak in their weakness after two years.

Diagnosis

1 Serological tests for autoantibodies.
2 Electrophysiological studies.
3 Ice pack test—in patients with ptosis, the ptosis improves after placing an ice pack on the closed eyelid for two minutes.
4 The 'Tensilon test' is no longer done due to the lack of availability of edrophonium (Tensilon).

Treatment

1 Thymectomy for patients with autoantibodies to the nicotinic acetylcholine receptor.
2 Acetylcholinesterase inhibition—pyridostigmine.
3 Immunosuppressive drugs—azathioprine, mycophenolate or methotrexate.
4 Glucocorticoids.
5 Plasma exchange.
6 IV immune globulin (IVIG).
7 Monoclonal antibody therapy—rituximab and eculizumab.
8 Propantheline or glycopyrrolate to block the muscarinic effects of acetylcholinesterase inhibition.

Myasthenic crisis

This is a life-threatening exacerbation of MG (respiratory failure, often with oropharyngeal muscle weakness). Myasthenic crisis can be precipitated by stressors such as infection, surgery or pregnancy. Treatment includes:
1 respiratory support, including invasive ventilation
2 cessation of anticholinesterase medication to reduce secretions
3 treating the cause e.g. infection
4 plasma exchange or IV immune globulin
5 glucocorticoids e.g. prednisone 60–80 mg/day.

Cholinergic crisis

Cholinergic crisis is due to excessive acetylcholinesterase inhibition medication. It is very rare and unlikely if the pyridostigmine dose is < 120 mg q 3 h. Treatment is supportive. Atropine will help treat the muscarinic effects of acetylcholine excess. Cholinergic crisis can also occur with poisoning from organophosphate or nerve gas/toxin. Pralidoxime is used to treat organophosphate poisoning by reactivating acetylcholinesterase.

Drugs which may worsen MG

Many drugs—too many to list in full—can worsen MG. They include gentamicin and other aminoglycosides, ampicillin, erythromycin, beta blockers, quinidine, calcium channel blockers, magnesium, metronidazole, anti-epileptics and steroids.

Anaesthesia and myasthenia gravis

The main concerns with MG are respiratory impairment and bulbar symptoms, with an increased risk of aspiration. There is also the risk of precipitating a myasthenic crisis. Patients with a thymic mass may be at risk of tracheal compression. *See Mediastinal mass syndrome (MMS)*. The worse the MG, the more likely post-procedure invasive ventilation will be required. Lung function tests may be helpful and may give an indication of baseline function.

In general:

1 Continue pyridostigmine up to the time of surgery.
2 Consider alternatives to GA e.g. neuraxial anaesthesia, regional anaesthesia. Caution must be used with any block that may paralyse the diaphragm e.g. supraclavicular brachial plexus block. This may not be tolerated by the MG patient. Also, any neuraxial block which impairs the respiratory muscles may also be poorly tolerated.
3 When GA is required, use short-acting agents e.g. alfentanil, remifentanil.
4 If muscle relaxation is required, use rocuronium reversed by sugammadex. Use neuromuscular blocker monitoring.
5 MG patients are resistant to suxamethonium and require a higher dose. The suxamethonium may last longer than in normal patients due to the effects of pyridostigmine.
6 Use amide rather than ester LA agents.
7 Patients on high-dose steroid therapy will require stress steroid cover. **See Stress steroids**.
8 Patients with MG should be carefully monitored for deterioration postoperatively in a high-dependency area as late-onset respiratory depression may occur. Caution must be used with postoperative opioids. Consider other analgesics that do not cause respiratory depression.

Obstetric anaesthesia and MG

1 About 30% of pregnant patients with MG experience a worsening of their condition.
2 Newborns can have congenital myasthenic syndrome due to transfer of antibodies from a mother with MG which lasts for about 18 days. **See Myasthenic syndromes**.
3 Magnesium for preeclampsia can greatly exacerbate MG.
4 Avoid a high epidural block in labour as it may impair respiratory function.
5 A carefully titrated epidural or CSE with low-dose spinal component may be better tolerated for CS than a SAB.
6 GA may be required for patients with severe bulbar palsy or respiratory compromise to better prevent aspiration, deal with secretions and control ventilation.

◗ Myasthenic syndromes

Lambert–Eaton syndrome

Weakness in this syndrome is due to antibodies to presynaptic calcium channels at the neuromuscular junction (NMJ). Unlike the situation with MG, patients may show an increase in muscle strength with repeated effort and proximal muscles are affected more than distal muscles. It is usually associated with small-cell lung cancer or lymphoproliferative disorders. These patients may be resistant to NMBDs.

Penicillamine-induced myasthenia

Penicillamine (which is used to treat conditions such as rheumatoid arthritis and Wilson's disease) can cause the production of acetylcholine nicotinic receptor antibodies.

Congenital myasthenic syndromes

Congenital myasthenic syndromes include:

1 several types of rare NMJ abnormalities
2 antibodies from a MG mother affecting the newborn. **See Myasthenia gravis**.

❍ Myocardial ischaemia/infarction

See Acute coronary syndrome, Ischaemic heart disease (IHD) and *Intraoperative myocardial ischaemia.*

❍ Myotonic dystrophy/myotonia

See Muscular dystrophy.

REFERENCES

1   Do S-H. Magnesium: a versatile drug for anaesthesiologists. *Korean J Anesthesiol* 2013; 65: 4–8.

2   Dubé L, Granry J-C. The therapeutic use of magnesium in anesthesiology, intensive care and emergency medicine: a review. *Neuroanesth Intens Care* 2003; 50: 732–746.

3   Ray JG, Vermeulen M, Bharatha A et al. Association between MRI exposure during pregnancy and fetal and childhood outcomes. *JAMA* 2016; 316: 952–961.

4   Health, Western Sydney Local Health District Fact Sheet. *Breastfeeding your baby after MRI or CT scan.* May 2019. Accessed online: www.wslhd.health.nsw.gov.au/ArticleDocuments/1122/Breastfeeding%20after%20MRI%20CT%20scans%20V4_21-05-2019.pdf.aspx, September 2022.

5   Rosenbaum HK, Rosenberg H. Malignant hyperthermia: diagnosis and management of acute crisis. *UpToDate* March 2022. Accessed online: www.uptodate.com/contents/malignant-hyperthermia-diagnosis-and-management-of-acute-crisis, July 2022.

6   Bechard P, Letournea L, Lacasse Y. Perioperative cardiorespiratory complications in adults with mediastinal mass. *Anesthesiol* 2004; 100: 826–834.

7   Murphy GS, Szokol JW. Intraoperative methadone in surgical patients: a review of clinical investigations. *Anesthesiology* 2019; 131: 678–692.

8   Manfred PL, Houde RW. Prescribing methadone, a unique analgesic. *J Support Oncol* 2003; 1: 216–220.

9   Harrison TK, Kornfeld H, Aggarwal AK, Lembke A. Perioperative considerations for the patient with opioid use disorder on buprenorphine, methadone or naltrexone maintenance therapy. *Anesthesiology Clin* 2018; 36: 345–359.

10 Mashour GA, Sharifpour M, Freundlich RE et al. Perioperative metoprolol and risk of stroke after non-cardiac surgery. *Anesthesiol* 2013; 119: 1340–1346.

11 Desai V, Salicath J. Mitochondrial disease and anaesthesia. *WFSA Paediatric Anaesthesia Tutorial 436.* Published November 2020. Accessed online: https://resources.wfsahq.org/atotw/mitochondrial-disease-and-anaesthesia, October 2022.

12 Hsieh V, Krane EJ, Morgan PG. Mitochondrial disease and anaesthesia. *J Inborn Errors Metab Screen* 2017; 5: 1–5.

13 Malignant Hyperthermia Association of the United States. *Does mitochondrial myopathy (MM) increase an individual's susceptibility to malignant hyperthermia (MH)?* December 2019. Accessed online: www.mhaus.org/mhau001/assets/File/Recommendations/Does%20Mitochondrial%20Myopathy%20Increase%20an%20Individual%27s%20Susceptibility%20to%20MH(1).pdf, October 2022.

14 Arendt KW. Anesthesia for labor and delivery in high-risk heart disease: specific lesions. *UpToDate* July 2022. Accessed online: www.uptodate.com/contents/anesthesia-for-labor-and-delivery-in-high-risk-heart-disease-specific-lesions, December 2022.

15 Reimold SC, Rutherford JD. Valvular heart disease in pregnancy. *N Eng J Med* 2003; 349: 52–59.

16 Burt CC, Durbridge J. Management of cardiac diseases in pregnancy. *Cont Educ Anaesth, Crit Care & Pain*. 2009; 9: 44–47.

17 Varytė G, Zakarevičienė J, Ramašauskaitė D et al. Pregnancy and multiple sclerosis: an update on the disease modifying strategy and review of pregnancy's impact on disease activity. *Medicina (Kaunas)* 2020; 56: 49.

18 Gerhart C. Use of regional anaesthesia in patients with multiple sclerosis. *Global J Anaesth Pain Med* 2020; 3: 251–255.

19 Muenster T, Mueller C, Forst J et al. Anaesthetic management in patients with Duchenne muscular dystrophy undergoing orthopaedic surgery; a review of 232 cases. *European J Anaesthesiol* 2012; 29: 489–494.

20 Yin JL, Teo KS, Phillipose Z. Normal dose paracetamol in muscular dystrophy patients— is it normal? *J R Coll Physicians Edinb* 2020; 50: 411–413.

21 Gupta N, Saxena KN, Panda AK et al. Myotonic dystrophy: an anaesthetic dilemma. *Indian J Anaesth* 2009; 53: 688–691.

⬧ Nadolol (Corgard)

Description

Non-selective beta blocker drug used to treat:

1 Hypertension.
2 Angina.
3 Atrial fibrillation.
4 Some inherited arrhythmic syndromes such as catecholaminergic polymorphic ventricular tachycardia (CPVT) and long QT syndrome. *See **Catecholaminergic polymorphic ventricular tachycardia (CPVT)** and **Long QT syndrome (LQTS)**.*
5 Migraine.

Nadolol is also used to reduce the risk of variceal bleeding in patients with portal hypertension.

Dose

Adult

PO 40–80 mg/day (max dose 240 mg).

Special points

Sudden cessation of nadolol may result in rebound effects such as heart attack, CVA, severe hypertension or arrhythmia. It should be weaned over a 1–2 week period.

⬧ Nalbuphine (Nubain)

Opioid agonist-antagonist drug. This drug is used to treat pain and, unlike pure opioid agonists, has little to no potential to cause euphoria or respiratory depression.

⬧ Naloxone (Narcan)

Description

Opioid antagonist drug, used to reverse the effects of opioids, including respiratory depression and pruritis. It acts by competitively blocking the opioid receptors. High-dose naloxone given to an opioid-dependent person can result in acute withdrawal with nausea and vomiting, sweating, tachycardia, hypertension and seizures.

Dose

Adult

For respiratory depression/excessive sedation—IV boluses 50–100 mcg. Acts within 2 min and effects last about 20 min. Repeat doses or an infusion may be required. IV infusion dose 4–5 mcg/kg/h titrated to effect. Nyxoid is a nasal spray version of naloxone. Administer 1 spray every 2–3 min.

For opioid-induced pruritis—40 mcg IV every 5 min to a maximum dose of 240 mcg.

Child—for opioid intoxication

5–10 mcg/kg IV every 2–3 min until desired response achieved.

▶ Naltrexone

Description

Long-acting opioid antagonist drug used to treat alcohol or substance abuse. It reduces cravings for opioids in patients who have undergone detoxification.

Implications

1 While on naltrexone, patients will be resistant to the effects of opioids.
2 After ceasing naltrexone, patients may have greatly increased sensitivity to the effects of opioids and be at increased risk for respiratory depression.
3 Naltrexone should be ceased for 3 days before surgery.
4 Use non-opioid pain treatment strategies. *See Bariatric surgery*.
5 If patients require PCA, monitor them closely for respiratory depression.

▶ Nausea and vomiting

See Postoperative nausea and vomiting (PONV).

▶ Neck haematoma management

Description

Haematoma after neck surgery or neck trauma can lead to airway obstruction and death. Surgery that has the potential to cause neck haematoma includes:

1 Thyroid resection, or parathyroidectomy. 50% of neck haematomas after thyroid surgery occur within 6 h of surgical completion.[1]
2 Carotid endarterectomy.
3 Neck dissection for cancer.
4 Cervical spine surgery.

In addition to the physical pressure of the haematoma, patients may also develop peri laryngeal oedema which will not be relieved by clot evacuation. Unfortunately, there is no 'one size fits all' approach to this highly stressful crisis situation and an abundance of caution is required.

Presentation

1 Agitation, anxiety.
2 Difficulty swallowing (dysphagia).
3 Painful swallowing (odynophagia).
4 Difficulty breathing, stridor.
5 Pain.
6 Neck swelling.
7 Desaturation.

Treatment

1 Notify the surgical team and source a second anaesthetist if possible. Organise immediate transfer to an operating theatre.
2 If the airway is immediately threatened post-surgery, open the wound (cut sutures, remove staples), open superficial and deep layers of muscles, scoop out haematoma and pack the wound. The haematoma causing airway compression is a greater threat to the patient than the blood loss.

3 Sit the patient up and provide supplementary O_2 (by face mask or high-flow nasal prongs).
4 Consider immediate nasal endoscopic inspection of the larynx to assess difficulty of intubation.
5 Consider IV hydrocortisone and nebulised adrenaline to reduce swelling.[1,2]
6 Alternatively, consider spraying the tongue, pharynx and larynx with LA and performing video laryngoscopy awake. If the airway looks reasonable to intubate, proceed with anaesthesia and intubation.
7 If the airway looks difficult, perform an awake intubation if possible. *See Awake intubation*. Consider the option of awake tracheostomy.
8 If the patient is uncooperative, or the situation is rapidly deteriorating, induce anaesthesia with IV propofol and fentanyl, administer rocuronium and use a video laryngoscope. This is to ensure your first attempt at intubation is your best attempt. *See Difficult airway management*. If the airway cannot be intubated and the patient is desaturating, use the Vortex implementation tool (best attempt at bag-mask ventilation and supraglottic airway). If the situation becomes a 'can't intubate, can't oxygenate' scenario (CICO), obtain a surgical airway. *See Difficult airway management*.

◑ Negative pressure pulmonary oedema (NPPO)

NPPO is divided into type 1 and type 2.

Type 1 NPPO

In type 1 NPPO, pulmonary oedema results from the generation of high negative intrathoracic pressure in an attempt by the patient (while anaesthetised) to overcome upper airway obstruction. The high negative airway pressure (50–140 cm H_2O) results in increased pulmonary vascular volume, increased capillary transmural pressure and transudation of intravascular fluid into the alveoli. Causes include forceful inspiratory effort:

1 during laryngospasm
2 while biting the ET tube or supraglottic airway
3 during asynchrony with a ventilator.

In addition, there may be activation of the sympathetic nervous system due to the perceived need to breathe in maximally. This leads to peripheral vasoconstriction, which in turn can cause increased preload and subsequent enhanced blood flow to the lungs.

Type 2 NPPO

In type 2 NPPO, pulmonary oedema is due to the relief of chronic upper airway obstruction e.g. large tonsils. With chronic upper airway obstruction, there is a significant level of auto-PEEP and increased end expiratory lung volume. When the obstruction is released, the lung volumes return to normal. This sudden loss of PEEP leads to interstitial fluid transudation and pulmonary oedema. Cardiac abnormalities, such as cardiomyopathy, may increase the risk of type 2 NPPO.

Prevention of type 1 NPPO

1 Extubate the patient when they have control of their airway, as suggested by the patient opening their eyes or demonstrating purposeful movement.
2 Use a bite-block (e.g. a roll of gauze) on emergence, if the patient's ET tube or supraglottic airway can be obstructed by biting.

Clinical effects

1 Hypoxia.
2 Pink frothy sputum.
3 Restlessness/agitation.
4 Tachycardia.
5 Crackles/wheezes on chest auscultation.
6 CXR findings consistent with pulmonary oedema—diffuse interstitial and alveolar infiltrates, Kerley B lines, air bronchograms.

Treatment[3]

1 Relieve the upper airway obstruction due to causes such as laryngospasm or biting on the ET tube. This is rapidly and effectively achieved with IV suxamethonium or rocuronium.
2 High-concentration O_2 therapy.
3 Use of CPAP in the conscious patient.
4 In severe cases of NPPO, provide GA, intubation and IPPV with PEEP.
5 There is **no** good evidence for the use of diuretics or morphine.

◐ Neonatal resuscitation

Introduction

About 85% of newborns will commence spontaneous respiration within 30 s of birth. Another 10% will start to breathe with drying and other stimulation. Heart rate (HR) should be > 100 bpm. Some newborns will be more at risk of needing resuscitation than others e.g. premature babies or those whose mothers have preeclampsia. Effective ventilation is the key to successful newborn resuscitation.[4] Resuscitation should occur under a pre-heated radiant heater.

Initial assessment

The initial assessment should be targeted at:

1 Tone and response to stimulation—a baby moving all limbs and with a flexed posture is unlikely to need resuscitation, whereas a floppy infant is more at risk. Dry the baby with a towel to stimulate him/her.
2 Breathing—if the HR < 100 bpm, the tone is low and the newborn is not breathing, commence positive pressure ventilation. If the respiratory effort is present but poor (grunting, indrawing of lower ribs and sternum), provide CPAP. Attach a pulse oximeter as soon as possible. The target range of pulse oximetry is:[3]
   • 1 min – 60–70%
   • 2 min – 65–80%
   • 4 min – 75–90%
   • 5 min – 80–90%
   • 10 min – 85–90%.
3 HR should be > 100 bpm within 2 min of birth. An accelerating HR is reassuring. If HR < 100 bpm, initiate CPAP or IPPV.
4 Keep body temperature between 36.5–37.5°C.

Face-mask ventilation of the newborn

1 Place the newborn on his/her back, with the head in a neutral or slightly extended position. A 2 cm thickness of blanket or towel between the shoulder blades may help head positioning.
2 Do not suction the airway unless airway obstruction is suspected (meconium, blood clots).

3 Use a T-piece resuscitator device if available. Otherwise use a self-inflating bag device (about 240 mL capacity).

4 Use an oropharyngeal or nasopharyngeal airway if airway obstruction is due to anatomical features such as a small jaw or large tongue.

5 For IPPV of newborns, use a T-piece resuscitator device. An example of such a device is the Neopuff™ by Fisher & Paykel Healthcare. This device consists of:

  a) A pressure gauge in the upper centre of the interface.

  b) A gas-out port on the lower left of the interface.

  c) A gas-in port in the lower right of the interface.

  d) The Peak Inspiratory Pressure (PIP) control above the gas-out port.

  e) A Maximum Pressure Relief (MPR) control above the gas-in port. This control sets a maximum inflation pressure and acts as a 'pop off' valve.

  f) A Neopuff circuit. This has an inspiratory line which connects the gas source to the gas-in port. The gas source should preferably have an O_2 blender so FiO_2 can be adjusted. It also has the patient circuit which connects to the 'gas-out' port. The patient circuit has an integral PEEP valve.

6 Set the gas flow to 15 L/min (range 5–15 L/min). Turn the MPR and PIP controls fully clockwise.

7 Occlude the PEEP valve and mask connector. The pressure gauge should read > 70 cm H_2O.

8 Adjust the MPR control by turning it anti-clockwise until the pressure gauge reads 30 cm H_2O. This is the maximum pressure the newborn's lungs can be exposed to.

9 While still occluding the circuit, turn the PIP control anti-clockwise until the pressure gauge reads 20 cm H_2O. This the inflation pressure.

10 Next adjust the PEEP valve while still occluding the mask connector orifice. This should be set to 5–8 cm H_2O.

11 Begin ventilating the infant with a gas flow of 10 L/min. Use air initially in term or near term infants, and a $FiO_2 < 0.3$ in preterm babies < 35 weeks' gestation. Set the PIP to 30 cm H_2O for term newborns and to 20–25 cm H_2O for premature babies. Ventilation is achieved by intermittently occluding the PEEP valve orifice at a rate of 40–60 breaths/min with an inspiratory time of 0.3–0.5 s.

12 Higher PIP than 30 cm H_2O may be required temporarily.

13 Adjust FiO_2 as required. Reduce FiO_2 and inflation pressures as the baby begins to respond favourably to ventilation. Aim for an O_2 saturation of 90%.

Intubation and chest compression

1 If HR remains low, or O_2 saturation is falling or failing to rise, consider intubation. Use:

  a) 2.5 mm ETT for an infant weighing < 1 kg

  b) 3 mm ETT for 1–2 kg

  c) 3.5 mm ETT for larger infants.

2 For a term baby, insertion depth for the ET tube is about 8–8.5 cm at the lips. Make sure the chest moves with each inflation and use a CO_2 detector if available. If unable to intubate, insert a size 1 LMA.

3 If the HR < 60 bpm despite persistent effective ventilation, commence chest compressions. Compress over the lower third of the sternum, just above the xiphisternum and just below the nipples.

4 Position the hands with the fingers around the thorax and the thumbs providing the compression.

5 Compress one-third the AP diameter of the chest at a rate of 90 compressions per minute with a ventilation after every three compressions. Pause compressions for 0.5 s to allow ventilation.

6 Ventilate using 100 % O_2.

7 Continue compressions until signs of life or spontaneous HR > 60 bpm. Gradually reduce the inspired concentration of O_2 as the newborn's condition improves.

Medications, fluids and umbilical vein catheter

1 An umbilical vein catheter is the preferred IV access. To insert an umbilical vein catheter:

   a) Use a sterile technique.

   b) Attach a three-way tap to a 5 Fr umbilical vein catheter and prime with N/S.

   c) Sterilise the umbilical cord and surrounding skin with chlorhexidine and cover the periumbilical area with a fenestrated drape.

   d) Pass an umbilical tie around the base of the cord.

   e) The umbilical vein will be at the 12 o'clock position, is thin walled and larger than the two umbilical arteries, which will pout slightly.

   f) An assistant holds the cord up by grasping the cord clamp.

   g) Using a sterile scalpel, cut the cord horizontally just above the skin so the stump is 1–1.5 cm long. Use the umbilical tie to control bleeding. Blot away blood rather than wiping. Identify the vein.

   h) Use forceps to hold the stump.

   i) Insert the umbilical vein catheter to a depth of 3–5 cm below the skin of the abdominal wall. Ensure blood can be aspirated.

   j) Secure the catheter with a suture.

   k) Loop the catheter and place a Tegaderm over the loop to secure it against the baby's skin but leave the stump exposed.

   l) Place a sterile dressing over the stump.

2 Alternatively, use a peripheral line or intraosseous route.

3 If the HR is still < 60 bpm after chest compressions and adequate ventilation, give adrenaline 10–30 mcg/kg (0.1–0.3 mL/kg of 1:10 000 solution) followed by a saline flush. Repeat the dose every 3–5 min as needed. For a 2.5 kg baby, this is 0.25–0.75 mL of 1:10 000 adrenaline.

4 If unable to achieve IV access, give adrenaline 50–100 mcg/kg down the ET tube.

5 If hypovolaemia is suspected, give 10 mL/kg N/S over several minutes. Repeat this dose as needed.

6 If blood loss is suspected, give O negative blood 10 mL/kg and assess response.

7 Treat hypoglycaemia (BSL < 2.5 mmol/L) with IV 10% glucose 5mL/kg.

○ Neostigmine

Description

Quaternary amine that acts as a reversible, acid-transferring inhibitor of acetylcholinesterase. It binds to acetylcholinesterase and prevents it from binding to acetylcholine and breaking it down. Used to reverse the effects of a non-depolarising neuromuscular blocking drug (NDNMBD) by increasing the availability of acetylcholine.

Dose

For reversal of NDNMBD administer 50 mcg/kg IV. Max 60–80 mcg/kg. Note that neostigmine will be ineffective if the residual concentration of NDNMBD is too high. Neostigmine causes side effects due to excess acetylcholine at sites other than the neuromuscular junction. *See Acetylcholine receptors (cholinergic receptors).* These side effects include:

1 bradycardia
2 excess salivation
3 abdominal cramps
4 bronchoconstriction
5 nausea and vomiting.

For this reason, neostigmine is given with an anticholinergic drug such as atropine or glycopyrrolate. In an adult give IV neostigmine 2.5 mg + glycopyrrolate 400 mcg **or** atropine 1.2 mg.

◗ Neuraxial anaesthesia

See Epidural anaesthesia/analgesia, Subarachnoid block (SAB) and *Ultrasound-assisted neuraxial anaesthesia.*

◗ Neuro-anaesthesia

Description

This section is intended for the anaesthetist who may occasionally be required to provide neuro-anaesthesia. Only a brief overview of this highly complex subspeciality can be provided in this manual.

Indications

1 Brain tumour surgery. The tumour may be a primary or a metastatic tumour. Common primary tumours are astrocytoma, glioblastoma multiforme, meningioma and pituitary adenoma. There may be associated seizures, headaches and neurological deficits. Patients must have their regular steroid and anticonvulsant medication on the morning of surgery.
2 Cerebral aneurysm and arteriovenous malformation surgery. *See Cerebral aneurysm and subarachnoid haemorrhage (SAH).*
3 Evacuation of intracerebral, extradural or subdural haematoma.
4 Insertion of ICP monitoring/management devices (e.g. extra-ventricular drain, Rickham reservoir, V-P shunt).

Anaesthetic goals

1 Provide the best possible operating conditions for the neurosurgeon by controlling intracranial pressure, optimising brain blood flow and prevention of patient movement.
2 Enable fast wake-up of the patient for a rapid neurological assessment postoperatively.
3 There may be a requirement for neurophysiological monitoring. Types of monitoring include:
   a) motor evoked potentials (MEPs)
   b) somatosensory evoked potentials (SSEPs)
   c) brainstem auditory evoked potentials (BAEPs).
4 Electromyography and associated techniques.
5 EEG.

Preoperative preparation and monitoring

1 Large-bore IV access.
2 Arterial line.

3 Consider central venous access, although internal jugular vein cannulation should be avoided. Multi-lumen PICC insertion is often convenient and appropriate. *See **Peripherally inserted central catheter (PICC)**.*

4 Urinary catheter if a long procedure or if mannitol/hypertonic saline will be given.

5 Temperature probe.

6 Peripheral nerve stimulator for neuromuscular block monitoring.

7 Entropy or BIS monitoring contralateral to surgical site if possible.

8 Calf compressors and compression stockings.

9 Monitoring for venous air embolism is important in tumours abutting venous sinuses or in craniotomy approaches in the region of the sinuses. Options include precordial Doppler or stethoscope, or an oesophageal stethoscope. End tidal CO_2 should be closely monitored. A sudden decrease in $ETCO_2$ may be indicative of decreased pulmonary blood flow due to a gas embolism. *See **Gas embolism**.*

Intraoperative management up until pin placement

1 Aim for a smooth induction with minimal haemodynamic effects e.g. give fentanyl 3 mcg/kg IV +/− lignocaine 2 mg/kg 2 min before propofol TCI. *See **Propofol (Diprivan)**.*

2 Rocuronium 0.6 mg/kg IV. Ensure the patient is completely paralysed before laryngoscopy.

3 Spray the cords with 1% lignocaine, especially for neurovascular procedures.

4 Intubate using a reinforced ET tube. Tape the tube—**do not tie the tube** as this will compress the neck veins. If motor evoked potentials (MEPs) are to be used, insert a soft bite-block.

5 Cover the eyes with occlusive dressings and pad the eyes carefully. **Do not allow surgical prep to come into contact with the eyes.**

6 Administer mannitol 20% 0.5 g/kg IV over 15 min. *See **Mannitol** and **Intracranial pressure (ICP) and treatment of raised ICP**.*

7 Maintain anaesthesia with propofol/remifentanil infusions. Use O_2 and air as the ventilating gas mixture. Do not use N_2O. Propofol reduces ICP and cerebral blood volume while preserving autoregulation.[5] The next-best option is sevoflurane. It affects cerebral vasodilation and autoregulation the least of the volatile agents. In practice, many procedures such as subdural haematoma evacuation and V-P shunt or reservoir insertion can easily be performed with volatile anaesthetic. If raised ICP is an issue, or if neurophysiological monitoring is being used, or if cerebral dehydration with mannitol is required, it is preferable to use propofol TCI.

8 Commence a rocuronium infusion 0.3–0.6 mg/kg/h. **The patient must not move.**

9 Ventilate with IPPV using minimal PEEP. PEEP may increase intracranial pressure and decrease mean arterial pressure (MAP). Aim for modest hypocapnia 30–35 mmHg.

10 Give prophylactic antibiotic cover e.g. cefazolin 2 g IV.

11 Maintain MAP within 20% of preoperative values.

12 Give dexamethasone 8 mg IV.

13 The neurosurgeon may request anticonvulsant therapy. Levetiracetam and phenytoin are common first-line agents.

Placement of pins and opening the dura

1 Mayfield pin placement can be extremely stimulating—consider a bolus of remifentanil 2 min before pin placement. Also consider LA with adrenaline infiltration at the pin insertion sites.[6] Do not give metaraminol to treat hypotension in the few minutes prior to pin placement as profound hypertension may occur. Expedite pin placement, if required, to 'treat' hypotension.

2 Before opening the dura, the neurosurgeon may request:
  a) head-up elevation 10° (reverse Trendelenburg) positioning
  b) frusemide 0.5–1 mg/kg IV if the response to mannitol is inadequate.
3 Give intraoperative parecoxib and paracetamol.
4 Use Plasma-Lyte for IV fluids.
5 Maintain normothermia.
6 Give prophylactic anti-nausea medication e.g. ondansetron, droperidol.
7 If the patient becomes hypertensive, consider:
  a) increasing propofol and/or remifentanil infusion rates
  b) clonidine 50 mcg increments IV (max 300 mcg)
  c) beta blocker e.g. metoprolol, esmolol
  d) hydralazine 5–10 mg IV boluses
  e) clevidipine infusion. **See *Clevidipine (Cleviprex)*.**
  For a one-off rapid treatment of severe hypertension, consider 10 mmol magnesium sulfate IV bolus.
8 Cease the rocuronium infusion once the dura is closed, but do not reduce the propofol/remifentanil infusion, or sevoflurane, at this time.
9 If the patient coughs or moves while the Mayfield pins are still in situ, serious injury may occur.

Emergence

Aim for smooth emergence with minimal coughing and the facilitation of rapid neurological assessment. Measures that should be taken include:
1 Judicious dose of fentanyl.
2 Ensure rocuronium is fully reversed prior to 'wake-up'.
3 Lignocaine 1–2 mg/kg IV at least 2 min before extubation.
4 Cease propofol but continue a low-dose remifentanil infusion.
5 Extubate the patient when they are is responding purposefully.

Recovery and ward

1 Cautious fentanyl bolus dosing until comfortable.
2 Oral immediate-release opioids on the ward e.g. oxycodone.
3 Chart regular paracetamol.

❍ Neuroendocrine tumours

These include:
1 Carcinoid tumours. **See *Carcinoid tumours and carcinoid syndrome*.**
2 Phaeochromocytoma. **See *Phaeochromocytoma*.**
3 Gastrinoma.
4 Insulinoma.
5 Glucagonoma.

❍ Neurokinin-1 (NK1) receptors and antagonists

These are also called tachykinin receptor 1 or substance P receptors. They are found in the central and peripheral nervous systems. They are also found in many other types of tissues. NK1 receptor blockers provide treatment for:
1 Nausea and vomiting e.g. aprepitant, rolapitant and casopitant. **See *Aprepitant (Cinvanti)*.**
2 Migraine.
3 Anxiety.
4 Depression.

◗ Neuroleptic malignant syndrome (NMS)

Description

This syndrome occurs as an idiosyncratic reaction to major neuroleptic drugs including thioridazine, haloperidol, chlorpromazine and perphenazine. It may be due to D-2 receptor antagonism. It can also occur with the withdrawal of levodopa in Parkinson's disease. *See Parkinson's disease (PD)*. This illness is similar to, but in no way related to, malignant hyperthermia.

Clinical features

This is a very serious condition with a high mortality rate that tends to develop over days to weeks. With treatment it tends to resolve over about 9 days. Clinical features include:

1 High fever.
2 Muscle stiffness.
3 Altered mental state such as paranoid behaviour.
4 Autonomic dysfunction—swings in blood pressure, tachycardia, sweating.
5 Muscle damage—increased CPK, urinary myoglobin.
6 Dyspnoea/respiratory failure.
7 DIC.

Treatment

1 Stop the neuroleptic drug.
2 Supportive—ensure adequate airway and ventilation. Intubate if needed.
3 Support the circulation (pulse rate, blood pressure).
4 Ensure hydration is optimal; give IV fluids.
5 Cool the patient (cooling blanket, cool IV fluids, ice).
6 Dantrolene to treat muscle rigidity. *See Malignant hyperthermia (MH)*.
7 Dopamine receptor agonists such as bromocriptine or amantadine. *See Parkinson's disease (PD)*.
8 Plasmapheresis.
9 Levodopa/carbidopa, anticholinergics, calcium channel blocker drugs.
10 ECT may be helpful.

◗ New York Heart Association (NYHA) functional classification of patients with heart failure

Table N1 NYHA classification of heart failure

Class	Description
1	Asymptomatic at rest, symptoms with heavy exercise
2	Symptoms with ordinary activity but comfortable at rest
3	Symptoms with minimal activity but comfortable at rest
4	Symptoms at rest

◗ Nicardipine (Cardene)

Description

Dihydropyridine-type calcium channel blocker drug used to treat hypertension and chronic stable angina. It can also be used to treat Raynaud's phenomenon.

Dose

Adult

Oral dose 20 mg q 8 h to a maximum of 40 mg q 8 h. IV infusion—start at 1–5 mg/h, increase or decrease rate by 0.5 mg/h depending on clinical effect, to a maximum dose of 15 mg/h.

◗ Nifedipine (Adalat)

Dihydropyridine-type calcium channel blocker drug with the same indications as nicardipine—treatment of chronic stable angina and hypertension.

Dose

Adult

Oral dose 10–20 mg q 12 h, max 40 mg q 12 h.

◗ Nimodipine (Nimotop)

Description

Nimodipine is a dihydropyridine calcium channel blocker drug that preferentially causes smooth muscle relaxation in the cerebral arteries. It is used to treat and prevent cerebral artery vasospasm after subarachnoid haemorrhage (SAH). It decreases the incidence of cerebral infarction by one-third. **See Cerebral aneurysm and subarachnoid haemorrhage (SAH).**

Dose

Adult

60 mg PO q 4 h started within 4 h of SAH. If given IV, use a central line. Administer 1 mg/h IV for 2 h with a co-infusion of N/S running at 20 mL/h (e.g. using a three-way tap). Increase to 2 mg/h with a 40 mL/h co-infusion of N/S if MAP is well maintained. Continue for 5–14 days and for at least 5 days after cerebral aneurysm surgery.

◗ Nitrate drugs

Description

Nitrates are used to treat and prevent angina. They act by relaxing blood vessel walls by conversion to nitric oxide. They act mainly on venous vessels, coronary arteries and small arterioles. In addition to relaxing coronary arteries, the venodilation caused by nitrates decreases preload. This in turn decreases LV end diastolic pressure and decreases LV workload and oxygen demand. They can be short acting or long acting. Other indications include the treatment of severe hypertension and for uterine relaxation.

Short-acting nitrates

These include glyceryl trinitrate (GTN), also called nitroglycerin, which can be used as sprays or tablets, and isosorbide dinitrate sprays or tablets. **See Glyceryl trinitrate (GTN).**

Long-acting nitrates

Include isosorbide mononitrate and all other nitrates in special, long-acting preparations such as patches.

Important points

Nitrates cannot be used in patients that have recently taken sildenafil (Viagra), tadalafil (Cialis) or vardenafil (Levitra). This is because of the risk of severe hypotension. Nitrates can be used 24 h after the last dose of Viagra or Levitra and 48 h after Cialis. These drugs are phosphodiesterase 5 (PDE5) inhibitors. *See Phosphodiesterase (PDE) and phosphodiesterase inhibitors.*

⊙ Nitric oxide (NO)

Nitric oxide is a potent vasodilator of arteries and veins. It acts by activating guanylate cyclase in vascular smooth muscle. This increases cGMP production in the smooth muscle cells, which activates protein kinase G. This in turn activates phosphatases which inhibit myosin light chains, causing relaxation of smooth muscle.

⊙ Nitrous oxide (N₂O)

Description

Gas at room temperature. Stored in cylinders as a liquid at pressures > 71.7 atm. It is used for:

1 analgesia (it may also be associated with euphoria)
2 anaesthetic properties, but it cannot be used as a sole anaesthetic agent at atmospheric pressure.

Advantages

1 Useful for short, painful procedures, labour pain.
2 Rapid recovery with no hangover effect. Patient can drive the same day.
3 Does not depress respiration.
4 Safe in MH susceptible patients. *See Malignant hyperthermia (MH).*
5 Extremely safe drug overall. It has been in continuous use for over 150 years.

Disadvantages

1 Increased incidence of postoperative nausea and vomiting.
2 N_2O inactivates vitamin B12, preventing it from functioning as a co-factor for methionine synthase. This can lead to megaloblastic anaemia and subacute combined degeneration of the spinal cord with chronic use. This risk is probably only significant in patients who abuse N_2O or who are vitamin B12 deficient.
3 Worsens pulmonary hypertension. *See Pulmonary hypertension.*
4 Exacerbates elevated ICP. *See Intracranial pressure (ICP) and treatment of elevated ICP.*
5 Supports combustion as much as oxygen.
6 Contributes to greenhouse gas emissions and the destruction of the ozone layer. About 96% of N_2O emissions come from microbial action on nitrogenous fertilisers.
7 Can rapidly increase the size of gas-filled spaces such as a pneumothorax or gas embolus, making the clinical effects worse. *See Gas embolism.*

⊙ Non-invasive ventilation (NIV)

Only a very brief description of NIV is provided. There are two basic types:

1 continuous positive airway pressure (CPAP)
2 bi-level positive airway pressure (BiPAP).

CPAP

CPAP is used to treat type I respiratory failure (hypoxia without CO_2 retention). It is helpful by causing recruitment of collapsed alveoli and splinting them open and improving lung compliance. This also increases FRC and decreases the work of breathing. Oxygenation is mainly determined by the amount of CPAP and the FiO_2. CPAP is a very helpful treatment for CCF by increasing intrathoracic pressure and reducing preload. This reduces cardiac distension, enabling the heart to operate at a more favourable part of the Frank–Starling curve. CPAP also reduces pulmonary interstitial fluid, improving alveolar gas exchange. CPAP can also be used to treat OSA, by splinting open the upper airway. *See Obstructive sleep apnoea (OSA)*. Aim for SpO_2 88–92%.

Settings
5–25 cm H_2O. Caution must be used with higher settings, as the decrease in preload, due to elevated intrathoracic pressure, may lead to significantly reduced CO. Also, higher pressures may result in gastric distension, leading to vomiting.

BiPAP

BiPAP is used to treat type 2 respiratory failure ($PaCO_2 > 45$ mmHg ± hypoxia). There are two pressure settings:

1 IPAP—inspiratory positive airway pressure
2 EPAP—expiratory positive airway pressure.

The IPAP minus the EPAP is the amount of pressure support. The greater the pressure support, the higher the TV. The aim of BiPAP is to increase minute ventilation by increasing tidal volume ($MV = TV \times RR$), thus decreasing $PaCO_2$. The EPAP also acts in the same way as CPAP (recruits collapsed alveoli and splints them open, increasing FRC and decreasing the work of breathing).

Settings
EPAP acts like CPAP. It can be set to 0 cm H_2O if oxygenation is not the problem. Set to a number less than the IPAP. Start at 4 cm H_2O. IPAP starts when the ventilator senses inspiratory effort. The IPAP supports inspiration. Settings range from 5–30 cm H_2O. Start IPAP at 10–15 cm H_2O. A back-up respiratory rate can be set if the patient becomes apnoeic. The inspiratory time can also be set (time allowed for patient to inspire). Start with an I:E ratio of 1:2. Rise time, i.e. how quickly the breath is delivered to the patient, can also be set (1–5 = faster to slower). Start with 1–2.

Contraindications to NIV
1 Claustrophobia.
2 Vomiting.
3 Pneumothorax—perform CXR before NIV.
4 Excessive sputum.

◑ Non-steroidal anti-inflammatory drugs (NSAIDs)

Description
NSAIDs act by inhibiting cyclo-oxygenase 2, which is found in inflammatory cells. They may also inhibit cyclo-oxygenase 1, which is involved in maintaining the lining of the stomach and small intestine, platelet function and kidney function. NSAIDs are divided into selective (COX-2 inhibition) and non-selective (COX-1 and COX-2) inhibition.

Non-selective NSAIDs
These include diclofenac, ketorolac and indomethacin. They are effective anti-inflammatory drugs but may cause:

1 bleeding due to platelet inhibition
2 renal impairment
3 peptic ulcers.

Selective COX-2 inhibitors

Examples include celecoxib and parecoxib. These drugs are less likely to cause peptic ulcers and platelet dysfunction.

Adverse effects of NSAIDs

1 Increased risk of thrombotic events (CVA, MI), especially COX-2 inhibitors. Risk profiles differ between individual drugs e.g. etoricoxib and diclofenac are more prothrombotic than naproxen and ibuprofen.
2 Association with anastomotic leak in GIT surgery.
3 NSAIDs should not be used in patients with a history of peptic ulcer disease, GIT bleeding or renal disease.
4 NSAIDs should not be used in patients with bleeding disorders, preeclampsia, hypovolaemia or uncontrolled hypertension.
5 Non-selective NSAIDs are contraindicated in patients with aspirin-sensitive asthma. Other asthmatics are not affected.
6 Patients on ACE inhibitors may be at increased risk of renal failure if given NSAIDs.
7 Celecoxib, apricoxib and parecoxib are contraindicated in patients with a sulfonamide allergy.
8 NSAIDs should not be taken by pregnant women after 38 weeks' gestation. They can cause premature closure of the ductus arteriosus, with potentially fatal effects on the fetus.[7]
9 NSAIDs taken during pregnancy can cause fetal renal failure.[8]

◖ Noonan syndrome (NS)

This is a common autosomal-dominant disorder characterised by:
1 Facial abnormalities—hypertelorism, low-set ears, down-slanting eyes, low hairline.
2 Webbed neck.
3 Intellectual impairment.
4 Short stature.
5 Chest deformity such as an enlarged thorax.
6 Spinal abnormalities.
7 Congenital heart disease (CHD), especially pulmonary valve stenosis and atrial septal defect (ASD). Hypertrophic cardiomyopathy may also be present. **See Hypertrophic cardiomyopathy (HCM) and hypertrophic obstructive cardiomyopathy (HOCM).**
8 Airway abnormalities, dysarthria.
9 Absent or small abdominal wall muscles.
10 Haematological problems such as myeloproliferative disorders, increased bleeding tendency.

It affects males and females in equal proportions and has an incidence of 1:1000–2500 live births.

Anaesthesia and NS

1 Check coagulation profile and platelet function.
2 Airway management may be challenging due to a webbed neck.
3 Management of cardiac abnormalities such as pulmonary valve stenosis are described under the relevant entries in this manual.

◖ Noradrenaline (NA)/norepinephrine (Levophed)

Description

Noradrenaline is a catecholamine hormone and neurotransmitter released by the adrenal medulla and sympathetic nerves. In the brain, it causes increased alertness. It is a neurotransmitter in the sympathetic ganglia and is secreted in response to the 'fight or flight' response. It acts mainly on alpha-1 and -2 receptors and beta-1 receptors. **See *Adrenergic receptors*.** It is a potent vasoconstrictor with some direct inotropic effect but little effect on heart rate. It improves cardiac and cerebral perfusion by beta-1 effects but may cause ischaemia in the gut and kidney.

Use as a drug

NA is used for the treatment of refractory hypotension due to decreased peripheral vascular resistance as occurs with septic shock, post phaeochromocytoma resection and total spinal anaesthesia. It is useful in the management of anaphylaxis unresponsive to adrenaline. **See *Anaphylaxis*.**

Dose

Adult

Prepare by mixing 6 mg NA (3 mL of 2 mg/mL solution) with 97 mL 5% glucose (60 mcg/mL). Administer by a central line (or a large peripheral vein in an emergency). Start at 2–10 mL/h and titrate by 1 mL/h every 15 min, depending on response. In terms of mcg/min, start the infusion at 2–10 mcg/min = 2–10 mL/h. Titrate to desired blood pressure. The usual dose range is 0.5–30 mcg/min = 0.5–30 mL/h.

Child

Mix 0.15 mg/kg NA with 50 mL 5% glucose. Run at 0.1–2 mcg/kg/min = 2–40 mL/h.

Special points

1 NA is inactivated by alkaline solutions such as sodium bicarbonate.
2 NA half-life is only 1–2 minutes—caution with line changes.

◖ Normal saline (0.9% saline)

Crystalloid IV solution containing:
1 sodium 150 mmol/L
2 chloride 150 mmol/L
3 pH 4.0–7.0
4 osmolarity 308 mosm/L.

Comparison with other IV crystalloids

1 Contains no calcium (unlike Hartmann's solution). It will not cause blood being transfused to clot.
2 Most commonly used crystalloid world-wide.
3 Can treat mild sodium depletion.
4 Suitable for patients with net chloride loss.
5 Infusion of large volumes can result in hyperchloraemic metabolic acidosis, which will also cause potassium ions to come out of the cells and enter the intravascular fluid in exchange for hydrogen ions.
6 When N/S is compared with Plasma-Lyte 148, there is an increased risk of adverse renal outcomes with N/S. It is thought that hyperchloraemia may cause kidney damage.[9]
7 Does not contain potassium so patients may become hypokalaemic.

⊙ Norspan

Norspan is the trade name for transdermal buprenorphine patches.
See Buprenorphine.

⊙ NSQIP

NSQIP stands for **N**ational **S**urgical **Q**uality **I**mprovement **P**rogram. Of particular use to the anaesthetist is the NSQIP surgical risk calculator. It is used to calculate the complication risk across a range of operations based on patient factors such as age and co-morbidities. It can be very useful to help communicate to patients, surgeons and anaesthetists the risk of an adverse outcome if a particular surgery is undertaken. Also *see POSSUM scoring*.

NSQIP MICA (myocardial infarction or cardiac arrest within 30 days after surgery)[10]

This model was built in 2007 and has five predictors:

1 type of surgery
2 functional status
3 creatinine > 133 mmol/L
4 ASA class
5 age.

⊙ N-terminal pro b-type natriuretic peptide (NTproBNP)

See *B-type natriuretic peptide (BNP) and N-terminal-proBNP (NT-proBNP)*.

REFERENCES

1 Lliff HA, El-Boghdadly K, Ahmad I et al. Management of haematoma after thyroid surgery: systematic review and multidisciplinary consensus guidelines from the Difficult Airway Society, the British Association of Endocrine and Thyroid Surgeons and British Association of Otorhinolaryngology, Head and Neck Surgery. *Anaesthesia* 2022; 77: 82–95.

2 Gerasimov M, Lee B, Bittner EA. Postoperative anterior neck haematoma (ANH): timely intervention is vital. *Anaesthesia Patient Safety Foundation Newsletter* 2021; 36: 44–47.

3 Bhaskar B, Fraser J. Negative pressure pulmonary edema revisited: pathophysiology and review of management. *Saudi J Anaesth* 2011; 5: 308–313.

4 The Australian and New Zealand Committee on Resuscitation (ANZCOR). *ANZCOR Guideline 13.4 – Airway Management and Mask Ventilation of the Newborn,* April 2021.

5 Sanders B, Catania S, Luoma AMV. Principles of intraoperative neurophysiological monitoring and anaesthetic considerations. *Anaesth Intensive Care Med* 2020; 21: 39–44.

6 Arshad A, Shamin MS, Waqas M et al. How effective is local anaesthetic infiltration of pin sites prior to application of head clamps: a prospective observational cohort study of haemodynamic response in patients undergoing elective craniotomy. *Surg Neurol Int* 2013; 4: 93.

7 Vermillion ST, Scardo JA, Lashus AG et al. The effect of indomethacin tocolysis on fetal ductus arteriosus constriction with advancing gestational age. *Am J Obstet Gynecol* 1997; 177: 256–259.

8 Phadke V, Bhardwaj S, Sahoo B et al. Maternal ingestion of diclofenac leading to renal failure in newborns. *Pediatr Nephrol* 2012; 27: 1033–1036.

9 Weinberg L, Collins N, Van Mourik K et al. Plasma-Lyte 148: a clinical review. *World J Crit Care Med* 2016; 5: 235–250.

10 Lobo S, Fischer S. *Cardiac risk assessment.* StatPearls Publishing 2022. Last updated July 2022. Accessed online: https://www.statpearls.com/articlelibrary/viewarticle/131/, March 2023.

O

▶ Obesity

See *Body mass index (BMI) and obesity.*

▶ Obstetric cardiac arrest

See *Resuscitative hysterotomy.*

▶ Obstetric cholestasis

See *Intrahepatic cholestasis of pregnancy (ICP).*

▶ Obstructive lung disease/chronic obstructive pulmonary disease

In obstructive lung disease, there is difficulty with expiration (air trapping). There is poorly reversible airflow obstruction and an abnormal lung inflammatory response. Types of obstructive lung disease include:

1 asthma
2 COPD
3 chronic bronchitis
4 bronchiectasis
5 cystic fibrosis
6 emphysema.
      See *Lung function tests.*

▶ Obstructive sleep apnoea (OSA)

Description

OSA is defined as a sleep-related breathing disorder in which the airway is intermittently partially or fully obstructed by soft tissues above the larynx.
This leads to episodes of apnoea, hypopnoea and hypoxaemia. This can cause severe and potentially fatal physiological effects. There is often associated obesity.

Long-term clinical effects

These may include:

1 daytime sleepiness
2 morning headaches
3 snoring
4 fatigue, tiredness, lack of energy
5 pulmonary and systemic hypertension
6 right and left ventricular hypertrophy and failure
7 dysrhythmias
8 polycythaemia
9 respiratory failure.

Diagnosis

The best test for OSA is the overnight polysomnography. This provides an apnoea-hypopnoea index (AHI). This number is the average number of apnoeas/hypopnoeas per h of sleep. AHI 5–15 is mild, 15–30 moderate and > 30 severe.

OSA can be inferred from the 'STOP-BANG' score:

S – do you **S**nore loudly?

T – do you often feel **T**ired, fatigued or sleepy during the daytime?

O – has anyone **O**bserved your breathing stop during sleep?

P – do you have high blood **P**ressure?

B – do you have a **B**MI > 35?

A – are you **A**ged > 50 years?

N – do you have a **N**eck circumference > 40 cm?

G – **G**ender—are you male?

Five or more 'yes' answers indicates increased probability of moderate to severe OSA.

Other simple tests are:[1]

1 FBC.
2 Check renal function.
3 HbA1c.
4 Venous bicarbonate 27 mmol/L or greater.
5 ECG—looking for abnormalities such as LVH, RVH, right heart strain and dysrhythmias.

Anaesthetic concerns

OSA may be associated with:
1 difficult mask ventilation
2 difficult intubation
3 increased risk of aspiration.

Anaesthetic approach

Minimise opioids—**see Bariatric surgery**. Use alternative forms of analgesia e.g. paracetamol, NSAIDs or nerve blocks.

Postoperative concerns

The main concern is postoperative respiratory depression and hypoxia. The highest-risk patients have severe OSA, significant co-morbidities and major surgery under GA. The following is recommended for such patients.[1]

1 The patient should remain in the post-anaesthetic care unit (PACU) for 60 min after PACU criteria are met.
2 If the patient has had a SAB, they should stay in PACU until SAB has regressed below surgical incision.
3 They should stay in PACU if recurrent hypoxaemia < 90% or $PaCO_2$ > 50 mmHg.
4 The patient may require their own CPAP machine in PACU. The AIRVO 2 high-flow nasal oxygen/air device may also be effective for maintaining adequate oxygen saturation.
5 The patient should go from PACU to a high-dependency unit with the following explicit instructions:
   a) Nurse patient sitting up, not supine.
   b) Give supplementary O_2 unless the patient relies on hypoxic drive for ventilation.
   c) Continuous pulse oximetry with alarms switched on and set to < 90%.
   d) Explicit instructions to obtain review if SpO_2 < 92% or increasing O_2 requirements.
   e) Patient to use their own CPAP machine when asleep +/− supplementary O_2.

▷ Octreotide (Sandostatin)

This drug is a synthetic version of the inhibiting hormone somatostatin. Somatostatin is also known as 'growth hormone inhibiting hormone' (GHIH). Its actions include reduced acid secretion in the stomach, inhibiting the release of thyroid-stimulating hormone (TSH) and reduced contractions and blood flow in the small intestine. Octreotide is used for the treatment of:

1 Carcinoid syndrome/crisis. *See Carcinoid tumours and carcinoid syndrome.*
2 Acromegaly, TSH-secreting tumours and glucagonoma.
3 Bleeding oesophageal varices by reducing portal venous pressure.

▷ Oculogyric crisis

See Dystonic reaction, acute.

▷ Onco-anaesthesia

Description

Onco-anaesthesia is an emerging subspecialty of anaesthetics which aims to optimise long-term cancer outcomes by anaesthetic interventions during the perioperative period. This is a massive and evolving area of study, and only a brief overview can be offered in this manual. The basic premises of onco-anaesthesia are:

1 Interventions which boost the body's defences against cancer cells, in particular natural killer (NK) cells, are beneficial. These cells play an important role in destroying residual cancer cells after cancer surgery.
2 Interventions which reduce the inflammatory response and other activators of macrophages may improve cancer outcomes.
3 The physiological stress response of surgery releases factors which support tumour cell growth and suppress NK cells and T-lymphocytes.

Anaesthetic interventions that may be associated with poorer outcomes

1 Inhalational anaesthetic drugs such as sevoflurane. These may inhibit NK cells. Inhalational agents may promote tumorigenic growth factors such as hypoxia-inducible factors (HIFs) and insulin-like growth factor (IGF).[2]
2 Opioid drugs. These may promote tumour growth, angiogenesis (cancer blood supply) and increase rates of metastases.

Anaesthetic interventions that may be associated with reduced cancer recurrence

1 Propofol TCI—*see Propofol (DIPRIVAN)*. Propofol has the opposite effect on tumorigenic growth factors compared with volatile anaesthetic drugs and may inhibit tumour cell growth.[2]
2 Opioid-free/minimised anaesthesia. However, ketamine should be avoided as it suppresses NK cells.
3 Use of neuraxial/regional anaesthesia—partly due to a reduction in opioid requirements and partly because of a reduction in sympathetic activation.
4 IV lignocaine peri-operatively. *See Lignocaine (Xylocaine)*. Lignocaine may enhance NK cell function and have some direct cancer cell cytotoxicity.[2]
5 NSAIDs—these may be beneficial by reducing the inflammatory response and the activation of macrophages. COX-2 inhibitors may be particularly beneficial.[3]
6 Beta blockers may be of benefit by reducing the activation of the sympathetic nervous system.[4]

◗ Ondansetron

Ondansetron is a $5\text{-}HT_3$ receptor antagonist. $5\text{-}HT_3$ stands for 5-hydroxytryptamine and these receptors are also called serotonin 3 receptors. It is used for the prevention and treatment of postoperative nausea and vomiting (PONV). *See Postoperative nausea and vomiting (PONV).*

Dose for PONV

Adult

Prevention of PONV 4 mg IV. For treatment of PONV 4–8 mg IV. Can give up to 16 mg in 24 h. If IV access not available use disintegrating tablets PO.

Child

0.1 mg/kg IV maximum 4 mg/dose.

Adverse effects

1 Headache.
2 Elevated liver enzymes.
3 Constipation.
4 May decrease efficacy of tramadol.
5 QT segment prolongation

◗ One-lung ventilation (OLV)

Introduction

One-lung ventilation is usually achieved by inserting a double lumen tube (DLT) or using a bronchial blocker. A left-sided DLT is usually adequate for left or right lung ventilation and is easier to insert than a right-sided DLT. Indications include:

1 Lung surgery e.g. lobectomy.
2 Haemoptysis from one lung. *See Haemoptysis, life-threatening.*
3 Bronchopleural fistula. *See Bronchopleural fistula (BPF).*
4 Prevention of spillage of pus from one lung to the other lung.
5 Unilateral bronchopulmonary lavage e.g. cystic fibrosis, pulmonary alveolar proteinosis.
6 Split-lung ventilation
7 Provide surgical exposure for certain operations e.g. cervical sympathectomy, thoracic aortic surgery.
  Only the left-sided DLT will be covered in this manual due to content restrictions.

DLT sizes

Seven sizes are available from 26–41 Fr. The usual size selection is adult male 39 Fr; adult female 37 Fr.

Preparation of the left-sided DLT

1 Inside the box is a DLT with stylet in situ, two tube connectors, a Y connection port and two catheter mount connectors with caps. There is also a clamp and two suction catheters.
2 Remove the bronchial tube stylet and attach the tube connectors. Reinsert the bronchial tube stylet.
3 Attach the Y connection port to the two catheter mount connectors. Make sure the caps are closed.

Insertion technique

A flexible small-bore bronchoscope should be available. A 3.6–4.2 mm external diameter scope will fit down all sizes of DLT. A 4.9 mm external diameter scope will fit down a size 39–41 Fr DLT. Another option is to use a disposable slim bronchoscope such as the Ambu aScope. The disposable left-sided DLT has two curves—a distal curve for insertion into the left main bronchus and a proximal curve. Ensure the cuffs are well lubricated and tested before insertion.

1 Induce anaesthesia.
2 Insert the DLT with the distal curve concave anteriorly.
3 Once the distal curve has passed the cords, remove the stylet.
4 Then, during insertion, rotate the tube 90° counter-clockwise. The proximal curve is now concave anteriorly.
5 Advance the DLT until slight resistance is felt, usually at a depth of 27–31 cm.
6 Inflate the tracheal cuff with 5–10 mL air and the blue bronchial cuff with 2–3 mL air.
7 Ventilate the patient and listen and look for bilateral lung inflation.
8 Clamp the bronchial lumen tube Y connector tubing and open the top cap so the bronchial lumen is open to air. Ventilate the patient. Only the right lung should inflate.
9 Unclamp the bronchial lumen and close the bronchial lumen cap. Clamp the tracheal lumen Y connection tubing and open the tracheal lumen cap to air, then check inflation. Only the left lung should inflate. The air in the bronchial cuff can be adjusted by deflating the cuff, then slowly inflating it during ventilation until there is no leak.
10 If both lungs inflate, deflate both cuffs and insert the DLT further into the trachea/bronchus and repeat steps 5–7.
11 Alternatively pull the DLT back and insert the bronchoscope through the bronchial lumen. Identify the left main bronchus and insert the bronchoscope into this. Then railroad the bronchial lumen into the left main bronchus. Repeat steps 5–7.
12 Ensure that the left lung apex is being inflated as the bronchial lumen may obstruct the left upper lobe bronchus.
13 Confirmation of correct placement can be obtained by inserting the bronchoscope into the tracheal lumen. Identify the carina and the trachealis muscle, a smooth sheet of muscle in the posterior trachea. The blue cuff should be just visible in the left main bronchus. The right main bronchus can be identified by inserting the bronchoscope into it and seeing the unique right upper lobe bronchus with three divisions.
14 A useful innovation is the VivaSight™-DL. This system has a chip camera and light in the tracheal lumen to enable accurate placement.

Physiology of one-lung ventilation (OLV)

In the left lateral position:
1 Blood flow to the dependent lung is 60% of the total pulmonary blood flow. When the patient is breathing spontaneously, more ventilation goes to the dependent lung, matching perfusion.
2 With IPPV to both lungs, ventilation preferably goes to the non-dependent lung, which is receiving about 40% of the total pulmonary blood flow (ventilation/perfusion mismatch).
3 When the chest is open and the non-dependent lung is collapsed, hypoxic vasoconstriction increases blood flow to the dependent lung by about 80%.

4 Volatile anaesthetic drugs decrease hypoxic vasoconstriction so that the blood flow to the dependent lung is about 75%.

5 Some atelectasis of the dependent lung will occur due to the weight of the mediastinum and compression of the diaphragm by the abdominal contents.

Optimising oxygenation during OLV

1 Start with a tidal volume (TV) of 10 mL/kg and limit plateau airway pressure to 25 cm H_2O. Increase the TV incrementally to a max of 15 mL/kg but keep plateau airway pressure < 30 cm H_2O.

2 Set the respiratory rate so the $ETCO_2$ is maintained at 40 mmHg. Consider permissive hypercapnia if barotrauma is a risk.

3 Use TCI propofol as this has no effect on hypoxic vasoconstriction.

4 Do **not** use N_2O, which can increase dependent lung atelectasis.

5 If hypoxia still occurs:

   a) Use a separate T piece circuit to apply CPAP 5–10 cm H_2O to the non-dependent lung. Allow the non-dependent lung to inflate to a size that does not interfere with surgery.

   b) CPAP is most effective if commenced before the lung is deflated or after a large volume inflation of the non-dependent lung to overcome critical opening pressures.

   c) Alternatively insufflate O_2 into the collapsed lung via the suction catheter provided.

6 If hypoxia is still a concern, consider applying 5 cm PEEP to the dependent lung. Although this will reduce some dependent lung atelectasis, it may also divert blood to the non-dependent lung, worsening hypoxia.

7 Other strategies to reduce hypoxia include:

   a) increasing FiO_2

   b) intermittent reinflation of the non-dependent lung

   c) temporarily returning to two-lung ventilation

   d) clamping the pulmonary blood flow to the non-dependent lung

   e) excluding other causes of hypoxia e.g. bronchospasm

   f) maintaining adequate cardiac output.

◗ Opioid dependence and anaesthesia

See Opioid-tolerant patients.

◗ Opioid-free/minimised anaesthesia

See Bariatric surgery.

◗ Opioid-induced hyperalgesia

This phenomenon occurs when prolonged opioid administration leads to abnormal and increased sensitivity to painful stimuli. It is thought to be due to activation of N-methyl-D-aspartate (NMDA) receptors by mu receptor agonists such as remifentanil. *See Opioid receptors*.

Treatment

1 Drugs that reduce this effect include clonidine and ketamine.

2 Opioid switching—replace current opioid with a different agent e.g. substituting methadone for oxycodone.

3 Non-opioid analgesics such as NSAIDs.

◑ Opioid potencies compared

Morphine 10 mg IV is equivalent to:
- Alfentanil   500 mcg
- Diacetylmorphine (heroin)   5 mg
- Fentanyl   100 mcg
- Hydromorphone   2 mg
- Oxycodone   10 mg
- Pethidine   100 mg
- Remifentanil   100 mcg
- Sufentanil   5–10 mcg
- Tapentadol   100 mg

Morphine 10 mg PO is equivalent to:
- Buprenorphine (sublingual)   166 mcg
- Codeine   80 mg
- Dextropropoxyphene   100 mg
- Hydrocodone   5 mg
- Hydromorphone   2 mg
- Methadone   3 mg
- Oxycodone   7 mg
- Tapentadol   30–50 mg
- Tramadol   50 mg

Transdermal patch conversions
- Fentanyl 12 mcg/h patch is equivalent to 12 mg morphine PO/day.
- Buprenorphine 5 mcg/h patch is equivalent to 30–45 mg morphine PO/day.

Lozenge conversion
Fentanyl lozenge 200 mcg has no direct conversion to oral morphine.

Methadone PO and heroin addiction
Initial starting dose is usually 10–15 mg daily. This can be increased by increments of 5–10 mg. 80–100 mg/day may be required. **See Methadone.**

◑ Opioid receptors

These are categorised as:
1 **Mu (μ) receptors**
   a) Mu-1—stimulation causes miosis, euphoria, supraspinal analgesia, NMDA receptor activation leading to hyperalgesia.
   b) Mu-2—stimulation causes respiratory depression, inhibition of gut motility and bradycardia.
2 **Kappa (κ) receptors**
   Stimulation causes respiratory depression, sedation and spinal anaesthesia.
3 **Sigma (σ) receptors**
   Stimulation causes dysphoria, hallucinations, mydriasis, respiratory stimulation and tachycardia.
4 **Delta (δ) receptors**
   Stimulatory effects include ventilatory depression and modification of mu receptor activity.

○ Opioid-tolerant patients

Description

Opioid-tolerant patients are those who use opioids regularly in significant dosages. It is essential to prevent opioid withdrawal and provide adequate postoperative pain relief. A plan aimed at reducing and eventually stopping inappropriate opioid use should be considered. A multidisciplinary approach involving the GP, patient, pain specialist, psychologist and other services is desirable. Postoperative pain can be very difficult to treat in these patients.

General approach

1 If the patient is on methadone, continue this up to the time of surgery and recommence postoperatively when practical.
2 If the patient is on transdermal opioids, continue these throughout the peri-operative period at their baseline dose. Note that the opioid delivery rate from patches is increased by inadvertently warming the patch e.g. contact between the patch and a warming blanket.
3 Use non-opioid analgesic drugs—paracetamol, NSAIDs, ketamine and gabapentinoids.
4 Intraoperative methadone IV may be a good choice of opioid for tolerant patients. In contrast, a remifentanil infusion may lead to acute tolerance and hyperalgesia.[5]
5 Use of regional and neuraxial analgesic techniques when indicated. Consider LA infusions for ongoing pain management. Note that some opioid will still be required to prevent withdrawal.
6 Use of intraoperative lignocaine, magnesium and dexmedetomidine—**see Bariatric surgery**.
7 Patients on buprenorphine patches (any dose) should continue to use the patches uninterrupted. **See Buprenorphine**.
8 Use PCA morphine with an initial bolus of 1.5–2 mg.

○ Opioid withdrawal

This is characterised by:
1 anxiety, fear, restlessness
2 diarrhoea, abdominal pain
3 delirium, convulsion
4 dysphoric mood
5 lacrimation
6 rhinorrhoea
7 pupillary dilation
8 piloerection
9 sweating
10 yawning
11 fever
12 insomnia.

Treatment

Pharmacological therapy may include:
1 agonists such as methadone
2 partial agonists—buprenorphine is very useful in this situation
3 alpha-2 adrenergic receptor agonist e.g. clonidine and lofexidine.

◐ Ordine

This is a brand name for oral morphine. *See Morphine.*

◐ Osteogenesis imperfecta (OI)

Description

OI is due to a genetic defect in type I collagen synthesis. There are many types of OI, the most common types being:

- Type I—the mildest and most common form, with blue sclera and 50% incidence of deafness.
- Type II—the severest form: lethal.
- Type III—normal sclera but severe disease with fractures at birth. Death usually occurs in childhood or adolescence, usually due to cardiopulmonary complications.
- Type IV—normal sclera and moderately severe disease. Hearing is not affected.

Clinical manifestations

1 Short stature and short neck.
2 Blue or grey sclera.
3 Poor dentition, with brownish opalescent teeth.
4 Hypermobile joints with brittle bones, osteoporosis and craniovertebral junction abnormalities. There may be basilar invagination (where the top of the spine gets pushed into the base of the skull).
5 Coagulopathy with increased risk of haemorrhage, due to impaired platelet function.
6 Restrictive pulmonary disease.
7 Scoliosis.
8 Hearing loss (in some types).
9 OSA due to pharyngeal abnormalities.
10 Hypermetabolism with heat intolerance, sweating, tachycardia, tachypnoea.
11 Fragile skin.
12 Cardiac valve abnormalities.
13 50% or more of OI patients have increased serum thyroxine levels.[6]

Diagnosis

1 Clinical presentation.
2 Family history.
3 Genetic testing.

Treatment

1 Treatment is supportive with prompt surgical correction of fractures.
2 Bisphosphonates can be used to increase bone density.
3 Growth hormone.
4 Denosumab is used to inhibit osteoclast formation. Osteoclasts are large cells that break down bone.
5 Surgery to fix and/or prevent bone fractures.

Anaesthesia and OI

1 Identify all risk factors such as cardiac abnormalities and respiratory compromise due to skeletal deformity. Consider echocardiography to evaluate heart function. Check platelet count and clotting studies.

2 Neuraxial anaesthesia may have increased risk in OI, but this has to be balanced against the risk of GA. Both GA and neuraxial anaesthesia have been used successfully in case reports.[6] There may be compression fractures, disc degeneration, deformities and spinal canal stenosis. It is difficult to estimate the dose required for SAB due to the short stature of some patients.

3 Bleeding is more likely, due to fragile capillaries and decreased ability of blood vessels to constrict.

4 Use regional anaesthesia if possible.

5 Position the patient very carefully with generous padding. Consider a mattress that moulds to the patient's shape. Limb joints must not be overextended.

6 Consider using an arterial line as the BP cuff may cause a fracture.[6]

7 Intraoperative bleeding due to platelet dysfunction may be significant.

8 The patient may have a difficult airway for the reasons described above. *See Difficult airway management.* Do not overextend the head on the cervical spine. Awake intubation may be required.

9 Kyphoscoliosis is almost inevitable with OI, restricting lung function. *See Lung function tests.* Severe dysfunction is suggested by a VC < 15 mL/kg (normal is 70 mL/kg). FEV_1 and FVC are both reduced and the ratio may be greater than 80%, supporting a diagnosis of restrictive lung disease.

10 Suggested ventilation strategies are TV 4–8 mL/kg, RR titrated to expired CO_2 and plateau airway pressures kept below 30 cm H_2O.[7]

11 Suxamethonium-induced fasciculations may cause fractures. Use NDNMBDs instead.

12 Hyperthermia due to a hypermetabolic state which is not malignant hyperthermia may occur. The cause is unknown. It can be treated in a similar way to MH, with cooling, increased O_2, sodium bicarbonate for acidosis and IV dantrolene. Use a non-triggering anaesthetic (no suxamethonium or volatile) to prevent any confusion with MH.

Obstetrics and OI

As stated above, these patients are highly complex, and there is little guidance from the literature. In a retrospective cohort study, 75% of parturients had a CS.[8]

◐ Oxycodone

Description
Synthetic opioid used for pain relief. Analgesia lasts 4–6 h. If used in patients with renal impairment, the dose should be reduced and dosing interval increased.

Forms of oxycodone

1 Endone 5 mg tablets, an immediate-release form of oxycodone.

2 OxyNorm capsules 5 mg, 10 mg, 20 mg (also an immediate-release form).

3 Oxycodone syrup 1 mg/mL.

4 OxyContin—oxycodone modified release (MR) in 5 mg, 10 mg, 15 mg, 20 mg, 30 mg, 40 mg, 80 mg strengths.

5 Oxycodone IV solution 10 mg in 1 mL.

6 Targin—this drug is a combination of oxycodone SR and naloxone for oral use. *See Targin.*

Dose

Adult

For acute pain, give oxycodone IR (immediate release) 5–10 mg PO up to every 4 h to a maximum of 50–60 mg/day. Reduce this dose in the elderly or patients with significant co-morbidities. For Caesarean section patients who are breast feeding, use a maximum daily dose of 40 mg. IV oxycodone—give 2–5 mg up to 10 mg up to every 4 h.

Dose

Child

For acute pain give oxycodone IR 0.1–0.2 mg/kg PO (maximum 10 mg/dose) up to every 4 h as needed. Can also be used by IV infusion. Add 0.5 mg/kg IV oxycodone to N/S to make a total volume of 50 mL. Infuse at 0–4 mL/h. If an initial bolus is required, give 5 mL of this solution.

▷ OxyContin (MR)

This is a brand name for oral oxycodone. *See Oxycodone*.

▷ Oxygen content of the blood

This is calculated from the equation: O_2 content (mL) per 100 mL $= 1.34 \times O_2$ saturation $\times$ Hb concentration per 100 mL $+ 0.003 \times PaO_2$. The normal value is 16–22 mL/100 mL arterial blood.

▷ Oxygen free radicals

These are very reactive molecules containing oxygen that can cause cell damage. The main types are single oxygen, superoxide anion, hydroxy, peroxy and alkoxy radicals. They contain an unpaired electron and avidly bind with another atom or molecule to stabilise themselves.

▷ OxyNorm

This is a brand name for oral oxycodone. *See Oxycodone*.

▷ Oxytocin

See Syntocinon (Oxytocin).

REFERENCES

1 ANZCA. *Guidelines to manage patients at risk of complications of obstructive sleep apnoea (OSA) developed by Dr Pippa Jerram and Dr Leesa* 2022. Accessed online: www.anzca .edu.au/getattachment/3ef16306-770b-4d74-93ca-baaef1e0e6a8/OSA-cards-CDHB, October 2022.

2 Evans MT, Wigmore T, Kelliher LJS. The impact of anaesthetic technique upon outcome in oncological surgery. *BJA* 2019; 19: 14–20.

3 Heaney A, Buggy DJ. Can anaesthetic and analgesic techniques affect cancer recurrence or metastases? *BJA* 2012; 109: 117–128.

4 Zhou L, Li Y, Li X et al. Propranolol attenuates surgical stress-induced elevation of the regulatory T cell response in patients undergoing radical mastectomy. *J Immunol* 2016; 196: 3460–3469.
5 Coluzzi F, Bifulco F, Cuomo A et al. The challenge of perioperative pain management in opioid-tolerant patients. *Ther Clin Risk Manag* 2017; 13: 1163–1173.
6 Gupta D, Purohit A. Anesthetic management in a patient with osteogenesis imperfecta for rush nail removal in femur. *Anest Essays Res* 2016; 10: 677–679.
7 Oakley I, Pilleteri Reece L. Anaesthetic implications for the patient with osteogenesis imperfecta. *AANA J* 2010; 78: 47–53.
8 Ruiter-Ligeti J, Czuzoj-Shulman, Spence AR et al. Pregnancy outcomes in women with osteogenesis imperfecta: a retrospective cohort study. *J Perinatol* 2016; 36: 828–831.

◍ PACE

This is a graded assertiveness tool that can be used when faced with challenging behaviour from other health care professionals. The letters stand for:

    P – **P**robe—this means, in a non-critical situation, obtain the person's attention and ask probing or clarifying questions. Use questions beginning with 'I'.

    A – be more **A**ssertive—means making 'we' statements and stating specific concerns.

    C – express **C**oncern—direct statements; state your concerns outright and the need to discuss them with higher authorities.

    E – use **E**mergency language—'stop'; 'no'; 'cease and desist'; 'you are wrong'.

◍ Pacemakers

There are three types of pacemakers:
1. Implanted pacemakers—these may or may not have defibrillation/cardioversion capabilities.
2. Transcutaneous pacing.
3. Transvenous pacing.

Pacemaker technology is constantly evolving, and the anaesthetist will be exposed to multiple generations and types of pacemakers.

Implanted pacemakers/defibrillators

Indications
1. Bradycardia due to various causes e.g. complete heart block, sick sinus syndrome.
2. Overdrive pacing to treat some tachyarrhythmias.
3. Cardioversion of malignant arrhythmias/anti-tachycardia pacing. This type is termed an automatic implantable cardioverter defibrillator (AICD).
4. Cardiac resynchronisation therapy (CRT) for heart failure.

Components
1. Pulse generator and battery.
2. Lead to right ventricle (RV). If this is the only lead, this is termed a single-chamber pacemaker.
3. Lead to RV and right atrium (RA). This is termed a dual-chamber pacemaker.
4. Biventricular pacemakers have a third lead planted in the coronary sinus, allowing pacing of the left ventricle.
5. AICDs have defibrillator electrodes. These are visible on the CXR as thick, opaque sections terminating in the RV.

Modes
Modes of pacing are described by 3, 4 or, rarely, 5 code letters. These code letters stand for:
- *Position 1* – the chamber paced—**A**-atrium, **V**-ventricle, **D**-dual.
- *Position 2* – the chamber sensed—**A, V, D** or **O** (O means the pacemaker paces without sensing).

- *Position 3* – the response to sensing—**T**-triggered, **I**-inhibited, **D**-dual (pacemaker pulses can be inhibited or triggered) or **O**-nil.
- *Position 4* – indicates programmability/rate modulation—either **O**-nil or **R**-rate modulation. The rate changes on the basis of perceived physiological need e.g. movement of an accelerometer in the pacemaker.
- *Position 5* – indicates multisite pacing capability—either **O**-nil, **A**-atrial (one or both atria), **V** – one or both ventricles or **D** – combination of A and V. This is almost never used.

Common terms used to describe pacing modes

1 Asynchronous e.g. VOO. The RV is paced and there is no sensing or inhibition. This is wasteful of the pacemaker's battery and can cause competition with the patient's intrinsic rhythm, leading to pacemaker syndrome (see below). Almost every pacemaker will revert to asynchronous mode if a pacemaker magnet is placed over it.

2 Single-chamber demand pacing e.g. AAI, VVI. The device paces unless it senses intrinsic activity. The sensed and the paced chambers are the same in the examples given.

3 Sequential/dual chamber e.g. VAT, VDD. This type maintains the atrio-ventricular contraction sequence. Universal (DDD) senses the patient's P and R waves and paces the atria and ventricle sequentially.

4 Rate modulation—uses sensors to determine whether the patient is exercising to increase heart rate e.g. sensing respiratory rate.

Pacemakers (not AICDs) and elective surgery

1 The patient should have a pacemaker check within 12 months of surgery to ensure that the pacemaker is functioning properly and battery life is adequate.[1]

2 Discuss management of the pacemaker with the cardiologist and pacemaker technician, unless surgery is too far away from the pacemaker to affect function. This means below the umbilicus. In addition, surgery that does not involve diathermy will generally be safe.

3 It is important to know whether the patient is pacemaker dependent (paced 40% of the time or more). Examine the preoperative ECG for pacing spikes. If the patient is pacemaker dependent, transcutaneous pacing should be rapidly available, in the event of pacemaker malfunction.

4 If the patient is pacemaker dependent and monopolar diathermy is necessary, the technician should change the mode to asynchronous. The pacemaker will pace the patient at a set rate, no matter what else happens.

5 Consider invasive arterial monitoring if significant surgery.

6 The filter of the ECG monitor should be set to 'diagnostic' so that pacing spikes are displayed.

7 The cautery pad should be positioned so that diathermy current does not pass across the pacemaker or pacing wires.

8 Use bipolar rather than monopolar diathermy if possible. With bipolar diathermy, the 2 electrodes are located on the instrument tip. The current passes between the electrodes. With monopolar diathermy, the current passes through the body from the surgeon's electrode to the grounding plate, which is usually on the patient's leg.

9 If inserting a central line, the anti-tachyarrhythmia function should be switched off and asynchronous mode initiated. There is a risk of displacing a lead, especially in the first three months after pacemaker surgery.[1]

10 The patient may not be able to respond to hypovolaemia with increased heart rate—treat hypovolaemia and hypotension with IV fluid therapy and vasopressors.

11 Shivering, seizures and fasciculations can interfere with some pacemakers.

12 Antibiotic cover is not required.

Magnet and non-AICD pacemaker

Application of a magnet will usually cause the pacemaker to pace in asynchronous mode.

AICD and surgery involving diathermy

1 The AICD should be checked within 6 months of surgery.

2 The anti-tachycardia function, if available, should be switched off by the pacemaker technician. The AICD should be set to asynchronous mode and the rate-responsive sensor switched off.

3 Transcutaneous pacing pads should be applied, but not over the device. Usually, an anterior-posterior placement is used. The same pads can be used for defibrillation or cardioversion.

Magnet and AICD

1 Applying a magnet to AICD will disable anti-tachycardia and defibrillation functions.

2 It **will not** suspend pacing capabilities. This means diathermy may cause bradycardia or asystole.

3 There may be difficulty maintaining magnet position if the patient is lateral or prone.

4 For emergency surgery requiring monopolar diathermy without time for pacemaker technician involvement, apply a magnet to the pacemaker. Also, consider the application of transcutaneous pacing/defibrillation pads.

Postoperative period

If the pacemaker has been reprogrammed preoperatively, the original settings should be restored by the pacemaker technician.

Pacemaker syndrome

Pacemaker syndrome is defined as new or worsened dyspnoea, orthopnoea, elevated JVP, dizziness, fatigue and hypotension during single-chamber ventricular pacing. It is due to loss of atrio-ventricular synchrony during pacing. The haemodynamic effects are due to loss of atrial 'kick' for ventricular filling and atrial stretch (due to atrial contraction at the same time as ventricular contraction), causing reflex vasodilation. Pacemaker syndrome can be treated by upgrading to a dual-chamber pacemaker (atrial and ventricular leads), with sequential pacing.

Special circumstances

1 Extracorporeal shock wave lithotripsy can result in bradycardia/asystole if the patient is pacemaker dependent and the pacemaker has a sensing mode. Switch these pacemakers to fixed rate only.

2 For patients having ECT, deactivate an AICD device during therapy (either with a magnet or by programming).[2] The risk of inappropriate shock from an AICD during ECT is probably very low.[3] Discuss with the cardiologist and programming technician.

3 MRI is usually contraindicated but discuss with the cardiologist. **See Magnetic resonance imaging (MRI).** MRI-conditional pacemakers do exist but are rare.

Transvenous pacing

The indications for transvenous pacing are bradycardia and/or overdrive pacing. Transvenous pacing is achieved by inserting a temporary pacing wire and attaching this to a pacing device such as a Medtronic 5392. There are two cables—blue for the right atrium and white for the right ventricle. Only ventricular pacing will be described. The steps are:

1 Using a sterile technique, insert a central venous sheath as described for internal jugular vein catheterisation. *See **Internal jugular vein (IJV) central line.*** A suitable device is the Arrow percutaneous sheath introducer kit, which contains a 6 Fr sheath and a 5 Fr pacing catheter/wire.

2 Prior to inserting the wire, attach the protective plastic cover to the sheath.

3 Insert a pacing wire through the sheath towards the apex of the right ventricle, either under X-ray guidance or by using a flotation balloon.

4 Attach the two pins to the D and P sockets on the proximal end of the wire. 'D' stands for distal. It is the negative electrode. 'P' stands for proximal; it is the positive electrode.

5 Attach the pins to the ventricular lead (white) into the corresponding P and D channels.

6 Attach the ventricular lead to the impulse generator.

7 The default settings on the impulse generator are a rate of 80 beats per min, atrial electrical output of 10 milliamps and ventricular electrical output of 10 milliamps. The default mode is VVI. Set the atrial output to zero.

8 Look for capture on the ECG—there should be a QRS complex following every pacing spike. Keep increasing ventricular output until this occurs. Note that the controls are locked. Push the green key icon to unlock the controls for adjustment.

9 The Medtronic device is capable of sensing intrinsic beats, and if this occurs pacing is suspended briefly. Adjust the sensitivity so that this occurs. The usual sensitivity required is between 1.5 and 3 mV.

10 Put a sterile dressing over the insertion area.

Transcutaneous pacing

1 The optimal pad positioning is anterior/posterior. Apply the anterior pad to the left of the sternum, over the precordium. Apply the posterior pad immediately behind the anterior pad on the back to the left of the spine.

2 Connect the pads to the defibrillator and turn on the pacing function.

3 The default settings are a rate of 80 bpm. The default mode is 'fixed'. There will be 80 impulses per min without regard to the patient's intrinsic cardiac activity. You do not need ECG monitor leads in fixed mode.

4 For conscious patients, gradually increase the strength of the pacing signal until capture occurs, usually between 50–90 milliamps. Another approach is to start with 1 milliamp/kg. If capture does not occur with maximum output (usually 140 milliamps), reposition the pads.

5 For unconscious or very unstable patients, start with maximum milliamps output to ensure capture occurs as soon as possible. Then titrate this down until capture is lost.

6 Pace the patient with a current that is 10% above the capture threshold.

7 There is also a demand mode. The pacemaker will sense the patient's intrinsic rate. However, ECG leads must be attached to do this. They can be attached to the defibrillator or there can be a 'slave' cable between the monitor and the defibrillator.

8 Sedate and analgese the conscious patient.

▶ Palexia

See Tapentadol.

▶ Palliative shunts

Due to space constraints, only a brief description of these shunts is provided.

Blalock–Taussig shunt

Connection of a subclavian artery to a pulmonary artery. It is performed to increase pulmonary blood flow, in conditions such as pulmonary valve atresia and tetralogy of Fallot. In a modified Blalock–Taussig shunt, a graft is placed between the subclavian artery and the pulmonary artery.

Bidirectional Glenn procedure (also called the Hemi–Fontan procedure)

The superior vena cava (SVC) is attached to the right pulmonary artery. This shunt is used in the treatment of single ventricle congenital heart disease (CHD) such as hypoplastic left heart syndrome (HLHS).

Fontan procedure/Fontan completion

The inferior vena cava (IVC) is disconnected from the right atrium and attached to the pulmonary artery. It is used to treat single ventricle lesions such as HLHS. In the lateral tunnel Fontan, a baffle is placed in the right atrium to link the IVC and SVC and exclude most of the RA.

▶ Palonosetron (Aloxi)

Second-generation 5-HT$_3$ antagonist which also inhibits the neurokinin 1 (NK1) receptor and is used to treat nausea and vomiting. It is more effective than other 5-HT$_3$ antagonists and is as effective as aprepitant. It has a 40 h half-life. *See Aprepitant (Cinvanti).*

Dose

Adult

For prevention of postoperative nausea and vomiting (PONV)—0.075 mg IV over 10 s, immediately before anaesthesia.

▶ Panadeine

This drug is a combination of paracetamol 500 mg and codeine 8 mg per tablet. *See Codeine* and *Paracetamol/Acetaminophen (Panadol, Tylenol).*

▶ Panadeine Forte

This drug is a combination of paracetamol 500 mg and codeine 30 mg per tablet. *See Codeine* and *Paracetamol/Acetominophen (Panadol, Tylenol).*

▶ Pancreatectomy and pancreatic islet cell auto-transplantation

Introduction

Chronic severe pancreatitis, causing disabling intractable pain, may be treated with total pancreatectomy. Often the spleen is also removed. Consider the need for post-splenectomy *pneumococcal, H. influenzae type B, meningococcal* and influenza immunisations. Pancreatic islet cell auto-transplantation may prevent diabetes mellitus from occurring, or make this condition less severe. There is a reduced risk of death from hypoglycaemia in patients who have pancreatic islet cell auto-transplantation, compared to those that do not, after total pancreatectomy.[4]

Anaesthetic technique

As for any type of major surgery, the patient requires:

1 large-bore IV access, warmed IV fluids
2 arterial and central line
3 temperature probe and urinary catheter.

A thoracic epidural is avoided because the pancreatic islet cells are intensely thrombogenic and the patient requires therapeutic anticoagulation for 48 h post-transplant.

The surgeon may choose an upper midline laparotomy. Once the pancreas is devascularised:

1 The patient is commenced on an insulin/glucose infusion as per local protocols. The BSL should be kept between 4 and 8 mmol/L. This range is critical to the survival of the islet cells (when they are transplanted).
2 Isolation of the islet cells can take 4 h or more and involves a process of mechanical and enzymatic digestion in a sterile lab.
3 The islets are then infused into the portal circulation via the colic vein or recanalised umbilical vein. Heparin 2500 units is mixed with the islets prior to transfusion.
4 An additional 2500 units of heparin is given to the patient IV by the surgeon.
5 For paediatric patients, the equivalent dose of heparin is 35 units/kg mixed with the islets, and 35 units/kg injected IV by the surgeon.
6 When the islet cells are being infused IV, the catheter pressure is measured every 5 min. The pressure should be around 13 mmHg. Pressures higher than this suggest that the infusion is not entering the portal vein circulation **or** portal vein thrombosis is occurring.

Patient management during and after islet cell transfusion

1 Measure BSL every 5 min during the islet cell infusion, which takes 15–20 min.
2 A sudden drop in BSL may indicate beta cell lysis.
3 After the infusion, measure BSL every 15 min for 1 h then every 30 min for 2 h.
4 2 h after completion of the surgery, commence a heparin infusion, aiming for full heparinisation. **See *Heparin (unfractionated and low-molecular-weight heparins)*.** Do not give a LD of heparin.
5 Consider advanced pain control techniques such as wound infusion catheters, PCA and a ketamine infusion. These patients are frequently on very high doses of opioids preoperatively, making postoperative pain management challenging. **See *Opioid-tolerant patients*.**
6 Do not give the patient steroids as this will make diabetic management more difficult.
7 The efficiency or otherwise of the islets at making insulin is usually clear within the next 30 days. In one series, 22% of patients were insulin free at 10.7 months.[5]

❯ Pancuronium

Description

Long-acting non-depolarising neuromuscular blocking drug (NDNMBD). It is a bis-quaternary aminosteroid.

Dose

0.1 mg/kg IV. Effects last 45–50 min. Top-up doses are 0.03 mg/kg.

Advantages

Its long duration of action is convenient for long operations.

Disadvantages

1 Causes increased heart rate, blood pressure and cardiac output via a vagolytic action and enhanced sympathetic activity.
2 Metabolised in the liver and excreted in the urine. The dose should therefore be reduced if there is liver or renal impairment.

◑ Paracetamol/Acetaminophen (Panadol, Tylenol)

Description

Acetanilide-derivative analgesic and anti-pyretic drug used orally, PR and IV. Its mechanism of action is complex and may involve:
1 Inhibition of cyclo-oxygenases.
2 An active metabolite stimulating cannabinoid receptors.
3 Activation of descending serotonergic pathways.
Paracetamol has minimal anti-inflammatory effects.

Indications

1 Treatment of mild to moderate pain.
2 Anti-pyretic.

Dose

Adult

500–1000 mg q 4–6 h max 4 g/day.

Child

Child > 5 kg, give 15 mg/kg PO/PR/IV up to q 6 h, to a maximum of 60 mg/day.

Advantages

1 Highly safe if used as directed. Most commonly used analgesic world-wide.
2 Often combined with other drugs to improve efficacy such as ibuprofen, codeine or caffeine.

Disadvantages

1 Hepatotoxicity—this is due to the limited ability of hepatic glutathione to conjugate the toxic metabolite of paracetamol, N-acetyl-p-benzoquinone imine. Paracetamol overdose can cause liver injury over 2–4 days and fulminant liver failure may occur. Treatment should be initiated within 8 h of overdose if possible. The main drugs used are N-acetyl cysteine or methionine. Paracetamol should be used cautiously in patients with liver impairment.
2 Fulminant liver failure may occur in patients with muscular dystrophy treated with paracetamol. This may be due to the smaller muscle mass of these patients resulting in reduced glutathione stores in skeletal muscle. *See Muscular dystrophy (MD)*.
3 Very rarely, thrombocytopenia or neutropenia may occur with chronic use.

◑ Paravertebral block

Anatomy

This technique involves blocking the nerve roots as they leave the intervertebral foramina. These foramina are situated midway between the adjacent transverse processes and 2 cm anterior to the plane of the transverse processes.

Indications

For postoperative pain relief after chest or abdominal surgery.

Thoracic paravertebral block technique (ultrasound guided)

Anatomy

1 The rib articulates with the vertebral body and the transverse process.
2 Overlying the transverse processes are the erector spinae muscles. **See Erector spinae plane (ESP) block.**
3 Between the ribs there is the internal intercostal muscle, which terminates as the internal intercostal membrane.
4 Between the transverse process and rib is the superior costotransverse ligament.
5 The nerve rami split to pass in front of and behind the costotransverse ligament through slits.
6 The medial boundary of the paravertebral space is the intervertebral foramen and the body of the vertebrae.
7 The pleura makes up the anterolateral boundary of the space.

Technique

1 Sit the patient up. Use a fully sterile technique. With the ultrasound probe oriented parallel to the spine, place the probe over the transverse processes corresponding to the desired level of block.
2 Tilt the probe slightly laterally so the transverse processes/ribs and pleura are in view.
3 Insert the block needle out-of-plane between the transverse processes/ribs until the tip is just above the pleura.
4 Aspirate for blood, cerebrospinal fluid (CSF) or air before injecting.
5 Inject 5 mL of ropivacaine 0.5% at each level to be blocked e.g. breast surgery T2–T6. The pleura should be seen to be pushed down.

Risks

The main risks are pneumothorax and accidental epidural or subarachnoid injection.

Lumbar paravertebral block technique (non-ultrasound guided)

Use a fully aseptic technique.

1 Identify the spinous process at the level of the nerve to be blocked.
2 The needle entry point is 3 cm lateral to the spinous process on the side to be blocked.
3 Insert the block needle and contact the transverse process at a depth of about 2.5–5 cm.
4 Walk the needle tip off the lower medial edge of the transverse process, then advance the needle 2 cm.
5 After careful aspiration for blood and CSF, inject 5–10 mL of ropivacaine 0.5%.

◐ Parecoxib (Dynastat)

Description

Parenteral COX-2 selective NSAID used for treating acute pain. It is a pro-drug of valdecoxib and can be given IV or IM.

Dose

Adult

40 mg IV or IM. Approved for single dose use only. Reduce dose to 20 mg in elderly patients < 50 kg, and patients with moderate hepatic impairment. Effects last up to 24 h.

Advantages

As for other COX-2 selective NSAIDs. *See Non-steroidal anti-inflammatory drugs (NSAIDs).*

Disadvantages

1 Contraindicated in patients with sulfonamide allergy.
2 Contraindicated in cardiac surgery, severe unstable IHD and major vascular surgery.
3 Do not administer to patients with renal impairment.
4 Not approved for children.
5 Category C drug in pregnancy—potentially harmful to fetus.

◗ Parkinson's disease (PD)

Description

This illness is a progressive neurodegenerative disorder caused by dopamine (DA) depletion from the basal ganglia, including the substantia nigra. The dopamine depletion is due to a reduction in the number of dopamine-producing neurones. The cause of this illness is unknown. Age and family history are the most important risk factors.

Clinical features

1 Tremor—resting, 'pill rolling', usually not present with intentional movement.
2 Bradykinesia—decreased ability to initiate voluntary movement, masked facial expression, micrographia.
3 Rigidity—'cog-wheel' type.
4 Postural instability.
5 Many other non-specific manifestations.

Parkinson's disease can be a feature of many types of more generalised neurodegenerative disorders.

Treatment

1 Monoamine oxidase B inhibitors to prevent the breakdown of dopamine in the basal ganglia, increasing dopamine levels. These drugs also inhibit dopamine reuptake, further increasing dopamine levels. Examples are selegiline, rasagiline and safinamide.
2 Anticholinergic drugs that act centrally. These include benztropine and procyclidine. These help because dopamine depletion leads to increased cholinergic sensitivity. Blocking acetylcholine improves PD symptoms.
3 Amantadine—a tricyclic amine derivative dopamine agonist. Amantadine increases dopamine release and inhibits reuptake.
4 Levodopa—a precursor of dopamine. This drug can cross the blood–brain barrier. It increases dopamine levels in the substantia nigra. Dopamine cannot cross the blood–brain barrier. To increase the bio-availability of levodopa, a dopamine carboxylase inhibitor can be given, such as carbidopa or benserazide. These drugs therefore decrease the peripheral conversion levodopa to dopamine. Examples include carbidopa and benserazide.
5 Non-ergot dopamine agonists e.g. pramipexole and ropinirole. Apomorphine is another example of a drug that can be used for rescue therapy in patients having an akinetic episode. These drugs have largely replaced ergot-derived dopamine agonists such as bromocriptine and pergolide.
6 Catechol-O-methyltransferase (COMT) inhibitors e.g. entacapone. These drugs prolong and potentiate the levodopa effect.
7 Surgical treatments—deep brain stimulation, ablative therapy and stem cell transplantation.

Syndromes associated with PD and its treatment

1 Parkinsonian hyperpyrexia syndrome. PD patients who have withdrawal of their medication, especially levodopa, may develop neuroleptic malignant syndrome, which can be fatal. This condition overlaps with acute akinesia that can also occur in PD patients. *See Neuroleptic malignant syndrome (NMS).*

2 Dopamine agonist withdrawal syndrome can also occur with withdrawal of PD medication. This syndrome consists of anxiety, panic attacks, suicidal ideation and many other unpleasant features.

3 Dopamine blocking drugs such as metoclopramide can cause a severe exacerbation of PD.

Secondary Parkinsonism

This can be due to:

1 drugs such as atypical antipsychotic agents, metoclopramide, prochlorperazine and reserpine

2 trauma—e.g. repeated head trauma from boxing

3 brain diseases such as hydrocephalus, tumour and chronic subdural haematoma

4 Wilson's disease. *See Wilson's disease/hepatolenticular degeneration.*

5 cerebrovascular Parkinsonism

6 carbon monoxide poisoning. *See Burns.*

Anaesthesia and Parkinson's disease

Patients with PD may have orthostatic hypotension, difficulty with temperature control, pharyngeal muscle dysfunction and respiratory muscle impairment. There may be excessive salivation and many other issues.

PD drugs

1 Continue PD medication until the last possible moment before anaesthesia. Restart medication as soon as possible after surgery e.g. by nasogastric tube if necessary. Try to adhere to the patient's medication schedule rather than the hospital's medication schedule.

2 Parenteral PD treatment agents can be considered in exceptional circumstances under the guidance of a neurologist. These include benztropine, diphenhydramine and apomorphine. Apomorphine is very emetogenic and use with domperidone is recommended. *See Domperidone.*

Awake surgery

Diphenhydramine can be useful for sedation in patients having awake operations such as cataract surgery. It may also reduce tremor. *See Diphenhydramine.*

Induction drugs for GA

1 Propofol is probably the safest drug.

2 Ketamine and thiopentone have been used without complications.[6]

Opioids

1 In PD patients, fentanyl may result in muscle rigidity, which resolves with NDNMBDs.

2 Do not use pethidine in patients taking MAO type B inhibitors. *See Monoamine oxidase inhibitors (MAOI).* This may result in agitation, muscle rigidity and hyperthermia.

3 Acute dystonia after alfentanil has been described.[6]

4 Morphine inhibits dyskinesia at lower doses and increases it at higher doses.

Inhalational agents

Sevoflurane is safe.

Anti-emetics

1 Domperidone is a useful anti-nausea drug in PD. It is a dopamine receptor blocker, but minimal amounts cross the blood–brain barrier.

2 Metoclopramide, droperidol and prochlorperazine must not be used to treat nausea and vomiting, as they are antidopaminergic.

3 Ondansetron, cyclizine and dexamethasone can be used.

Neuromuscular blocker drugs

1 Theoretically, suxamethonium might raise concerns of inducing hyperkalaemia but this is not supported by the literature.[6] It is easily avoided by using rocuronium.

2 Reverse rocuronium with sugammadex. Neostigmine may increase the risk of bronchospasm.[7]

Postoperative

Consider benzodiazepines used carefully for postoperative confusion and agitation.

◖ Paroxysmal supraventricular tachycardia (PSVT)

See Supraventricular tachycardia (SVT).

Description

These are regular, narrow complex (usually) tachycardias that start and stop abruptly. The most common type is atrioventricular nodal re-entrant tachycardia (AVNRT). *See Atrioventricular nodal re-entrant tachycardia (AVNRT).* Other causes include:

1 Wolff–Parkinson–White syndrome. *See Wolff–Parkinson–White (WPW) syndrome.*

2 Atrial tachycardia. *See Atrial tachycardia.*

3 Atrioventricular re-entrant tachycardia (AVRT). *See Atrioventricular re-entrant tachycardia (AVRT).*

◖ Patent ductus arteriosus (PDA)

Description

The ductus arteriosus (DA) is part of the fetal circulation. It connects the trunk of the pulmonary artery to the proximal descending aorta. It allows most of the blood from the right ventricle to bypass the lungs and enter the systemic circulation. The DA is kept open by prostaglandins produced by the placenta and the DA itself. NSAIDs taken after the 28th week of pregnancy can cross the placenta and cause premature closure of the DA. *See Non-steroidal anti-inflammatory drugs (NSAIDs).* After birth, the DA closes over 18–24 h and forms the ligamentum arteriosum.

Patent ductus arteriosus effects

Prematurity increases the risk of PDA. PDA results in a left-to-right shunt due to blood from the aorta entering the pulmonary artery. This in turn results in:

1 Pulmonary hypertension.

2 RV failure (LV failure can also occur).

3 Dysrhythmias, especially atrial fibrillation.

4 Recurrent pneumonia.

5 PDA is not in itself a risk for endocarditis, but there may be an increased risk in the first 6 months after catheter repair.

6 Fluid overload.

7 Long-standing pulmonary hypertension can result in a reversal of shunt (right-to-left shunt) with cyanosis (Eisenmenger syndrome). *See Eisenmenger syndrome/ Eisenmenger complex.*

Treatment

1 Surgical closure of the PDA.
2 NSAIDs are helpful in premature babies to constrict the PDA but are not effective in full-term babies, children or adults.
3 Catheter procedure to close the ductus using a plug or coil.

Keeping the ductus open

This may be required to provide a pulmonary blood flow in conditions such as pulmonary atresia. This can be achieved with prostaglandin therapy—either alprostadil (prostaglandin E1) or dinoprostone (prostaglandin E2).

PDA and anaesthesia

Patients may be extremely unwell with an unrepaired PDA (pulmonary hypertension, CCF) or asymptomatic or somewhere in between. They require the usual extensive cardiac workup—ECG, CXR, cardiac echo and cardiologist input. If pulmonary hypertension is present, *see Pulmonary hypertension.*

▶ Patent foramen ovale (PFO)

Description

The foramen ovale is an important part of the fetal circulation, allowing oxygenated venous blood to bypass the RV and enter the LA, LV and systemic circulation. A persistent PFO is probably quite common and can vary in size from 1 to 19 mm.[8] The most important clinical effect of a PFO is that it can allow a paradoxical embolus to occur if the pressure in the right atrium (RA) exceeds the pressure in the left atrium (LA), as may occur with laparoscopic surgery in Trendelenburg positioning. PFOs do not permit a left-to-right shunt. Scuba divers with PFO are at increased risk of decompression sickness.[8]

Diagnosis

1 Transoesophageal echo showing venous injected air bubbles travelling from the right atrium to the left atrium.
2 A large PFO may act as an atrial septal defect and produce a heart murmur. *See Atrial septal defect (ASD).*

Treatment

1 Usually indicated if a paradoxical embolus has occurred.
2 PFO closure as a percutaneous procedure is the treatment of choice.

Anaesthesia and PFO

Take extra care not to introduce any air into venous lines as this can embolise to the systemic arterial circulation.

▶ Patient-controlled analgesia (PCA)

Description

With this technique, the patient is able to self-administer an intravenous analgesic drug at a set dose and a set minimum time interval between doses. The following must be considered:

1 Patients must receive supplementary O_2 therapy and regular observations while on PCA.
2 Respiratory depression and excessive sedation are the main risks.
3 Only the patient can press the button, except in very exceptional circumstances such as a developmentally delayed patient, in which case the nurse can push the button.

Adult dosage regimes

1 **Fentanyl**—2000 mcg in 100 mL N/S—start with a bolus 10–20 mcg with a 5 min lockout.
2 **Morphine**—200 mg in 100 mL N/S—start with 1–2 mg boluses with a 5 min lockout. Morphine must not be used in patients with renal failure due to its metabolites.
3 **Hydromorphone**—50 mg in 50 mL N/S—start with a bolus of 0.2 mL (200 mcg) with a 5 min lockout. Can be used in patients with renal failure.
4 **Tramadol**—300 mg in 60 mL N/S—start with a 10–20 mg bolus with a 5 min lockout.
5 **Oxycodone**—120 mg in 60 mL N/S—start with a 1 mg bolus with a 5 min lockout.

Child dosage regimes

Do not use PCA in children < 5 yrs.
1 **Fentanyl**—50 mcg/kg in 50 mL 5% glucose. 0.5 mL bolus (0.5 mcg/kg) with a 5 min lockout.
2 **Morphine**—1 mg/kg in 50 mL 5% glucose. 1 mL bolus (20 mcg/kg) with a 5 min lockout.

◗ PECS 1 and 2 blocks

Introduction

The lateral and medial pectoral nerves lie between pectoralis major and pectoralis minor muscles. The lateral pectoral nerve arises from the lateral cord of the brachial plexus (BP) and carries fibres from the C5–7 cervical nerves. It supplies motor and some sensory innervation to pec major. The medial pectoral nerve arises from the medial cord of the BP and carries fibres from C8 and T1. It innervates pec major and pec minor. The pectoral branch of the thoracoacromial artery also lies in this plane between pec major and pec minor and must be avoided.

These blocks are used for:
1 PECS 1 block—blocks the lateral and medial pectoral nerves. Used for surgery such as breast surgery and insertion of pacemaker devices. Use 20 mL of 1% ropivacaine.
2 PECS 2 block—blocks the lateral and medial pectoral nerves and the intercostobrachial nerve and the lateral cutaneous branches of the intercostal nerves. Useful for surgery covered by PECS 1 block but also covers the axilla for e.g. axillary clearance, mastectomy. Use 25 mL of 0.75% ropivacaine.

Technique PECS 1 block

1 Position patient sitting up comfortably on the bed. The block arm is abducted 90° and the elbow flexed to 90°.
2 Observe the usual precautions (cannula in contralateral limb, full sterile technique).
3 The probe is positioned in a similar position to the infraclavicular BPB (Figures P1 and P2). **See Brachial plexus block (BPB)**. Visualise pec major and pec minor. Pec minor overlies the axillary artery and vein and the BP.
4 Slide the probe caudally to identify the second and third ribs.
5 Slightly rotate the probe and move it laterally to identify the plane between pec major and pec minor and the thoracoacromial artery (use colour Doppler).
6 Insert the block needle in-plane from cranial to caudal so that the tip lies in the fascia between pec major and pec minor. After negative aspiration and a 2 mL test dose, inject 18 mL of LA.

Technique PECS 2 block

1 Perform PECS 1 block with 10 mL of ropivacaine 0.75%.
2 Slide transducer laterally to identify fourth, fifth and sixth ribs and the serratus anterior muscle (Figures P1 and P2).
3 Advance the needle tip to the plane between the serratus anterior and pec minor.
4 After negative aspiration, inject a 2 mL test dose, then inject 13 mL of 0.75% ropivacaine.

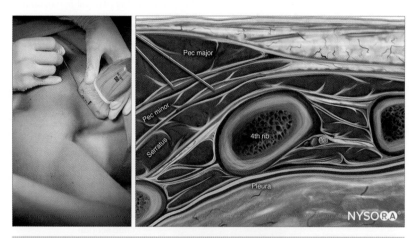

Figure P1 Probe position and anatomy for PECS 1 and PECS 2 blocks
Image courtesy of NYSORA

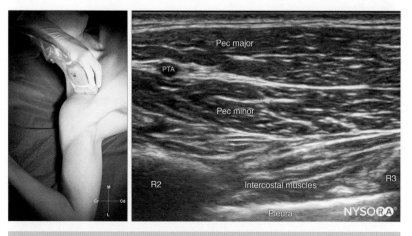

Figure P2 Probe position and sonoanatomy for PECS 1 and PECS 2 blocks
Image courtesy of NYSORA

▶ Penetrating eye injury

See *Eye injury, penetrating.*

▶ Penile block/dorsal penile nerve block

This block is useful for analgesia after penile surgery, such as circumcision, correction of paraphimosis and repair of penile trauma.

Anatomy

The penis is innervated by the dorsal nerve of the penis and the perineal nerve, both of which are branches of the pudendal nerve (S2–S4). The pudendal nerve runs in the pudendal canal. It divides in the canal, into the dorsal nerve of the penis and the perineal nerve on each side. The dorsal nerves pass under the pubic ramus deep to Buck's fascia, which is the deep fascia of the penis. It covers the corpus cavernosum and splits to encircle the corpus spongiosum. It also splits dorsally to surround the dorsal nerve of the penis and the deep dorsal vein (which is in the midline).

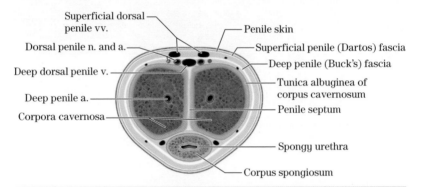

Figure P3 Anatomy of the base of the penis

Reproduced with permission from DA Morton, KB Foreman, KH Albertine. The Big Picture: Gross Anatomy, Medical Course & Step 1 Review, 2nd Ed. NY:McGraw Hill, 2019.

Procedure

1 Use a 50:50 mix of 2% lignocaine and 0.5% bupivacaine. For the adult, inject 3–4 mL on each side of the midline (as described below). For a child, inject 1 mL + 0.1 mL/kg of the mix on each side.
2 Sterilise the skin over the symphysis pubis and at the base of the penis.
3 Stand on the left side of the patient and use two fingers of the left hand to displace the penis downwards.
4 Insert a 23 g × 32 mm sharp needle in the midline just deep enough to touch the lower edge of the symphysis pubis.
5 Redirect the needle in the 10 o'clock direction (facing the base of the penis) and insert the needle 3–5 mm deeper under the symphysis pubis. The aim is to be in the space deep to the fascia which contains the dorsal nerve of the penis. However, there is usually no 'pop' sensation.

6 Aspirate carefully for blood (to ensure there is no penetration of the dorsal vein, dorsal artery or corpus cavernosum).

7 Inject LA. The injection should meet with little or no resistance.

8 Withdraw the needle partially then redirect it to the 2 o'clock position and proceed as for the 10 o'clock position.

9 Inject a bleb of LA at the penile scrotal junction, extending a few millimetres to each side of the midline to block the branches of the perineal nerve that supply the frenulum.

10 **Do not use adrenaline-containing solutions.**

Complications

1 Haematoma deep to Buck's fascia causing compression of the dorsal veins and arteries with penile ischaemia.

2 Intravascular injection of LA.

Penile block using ultrasound

1 Using sterile technique, place the probe transversely over the base of the penis. The corpus cavernosum on each side and corpus spongiosum in the midline should be clearly seen.

2 The vessels and nerves will be in the position illustrated in Figure P3.

3 Use an in-line approach, bilaterally aiming to deposit LA beneath Buck's fascia near the nerves.

4 Always aspirate for blood prior to injecting.

Ring block of the penis

Simply inject LA subcutaneously around the base of the penile shaft. Do not use adrenaline-containing solutions.

◗ Pentazocine

Opioid agonist-antagonist drug. Its antagonist properties are weak. It is used to treat moderate to severe pain.

◗ Perfusion pressure

Perfusion pressure is the pressure gradient required to drive blood through a specific vascular bed or organ. Cerebral perfusion pressure is equal to mean arterial pressure minus the intracranial pressure or jugular venous pressure (whichever is higher). *See Cerebral perfusion pressure (CPP).* Coronary perfusion pressure (CPP) equals aortic diastolic pressure minus LVEDP. *See Coronary perfusion pressure (CPP).*

◗ Pericardial effusion

This term describes a fluid build-up in the pericardium. If the build-up is gradual, the pericardium can stretch to accommodate more fluid. For a description of the causes, *see Cardiac tamponade.*

◗ Pericardial tamponade

See Cardiac tamponade.

◗ Pericardiocentesis

See Cardiac tamponade.

◖ Perimortem Caesarean section (CS)

See *Resuscitative hysterotomy*.

◖ Peripartum cardiomyopathy

Introduction

Peripartum cardiomyopathy is defined as an idiopathic cardiomyopathy, presenting with heart failure secondary to LV systolic function, occurring towards the end of pregnancy or up to 5 months postpartum. Incidence is about 1:3000–1:10 000 pregnancies.

Defining features include:

1 It is a diagnosis of exclusion of other causes.
2 There is LV dysfunction, defined as LVEF < 45%.
3 The disease is usually a dilated cardiomyopathy type, but the LV may not be dilated.

Risk factors

These are many and are not particularly helpful. They include:

1 Previous peripartum cardiomyopathy.
2 Age > 30.
3 Multiparity, multiple pregnancy.
4 Hypertension including essential/pregnancy associated.
5 African descent.
6 Tocolytic therapy with beta agonists.

The cause is unknown but is thought to be related to an interaction between pregnancy-induced immune function changes and viral myocarditis.

Presentation

See *Congestive cardiac failure (CCF)—chronic*.

Diagnosis

Diagnosis is made on clinical grounds supplemented by CXR and echocardiography. Other causes of heart failure must be excluded. See *Congestive cardiac failure (CCF)—chronic*.

Treatment of mild to moderate heart failure

1 Rest, fluid and salt restriction.
2 Diuretics—frusemide is useful for reducing pulmonary and peripheral oedema and is safe in pregnancy and lactation.
3 Hydralazine is useful for afterload reduction.
4 ACE inhibitors can be used postpartum but are contraindicated during pregnancy due to fetal toxicity. They are safe to use during breast feeding.
5 Beta blockers are used for second-line treatment, but prolonged use in pregnancy can result in low birth weight. Carvedilol has been shown to reduce mortality in patients with dilated cardiomyopathy.
6 Digoxin is useful and safe in pregnancy.
7 Calcium channel blocker drugs, except amlodipine, should be avoided due to negative inotropic effects.
8 Antithrombotic drugs are indicated if LVEF < 35% or there are other complications such as AF. Warfarin can be used between 12 and 36 weeks and postpartum. LMWH should be used after 36 weeks. See *Anticoagulation in pregnancy*.

Treatment of severe heart failure
See Cardiogenic shock. These patients need to be managed in a high-dependency/ICU environment with invasive monitoring. Treatment includes:

1 O_2 therapy (facemask, CPAP, BiPAP, intubation and ventilation).
2 Position the patient sitting up.
3 Frusemide to decrease preload.
4 If SBP > 110 mmHg, use GTN to decrease afterload. *See Glyceryl trinitrate (GTN).* Sodium nitroprusside (SNP) is relatively contraindicated due to the risk of accumulation of thiocyanate and cyanide in the fetus.
5 Inotropic support may be required with dobutamine, dopamine, milrinone and/or levosimendan.
6 Mechanical assist devices may be required (intra-aortic balloon pump/ventricular assist device). ECMO may be required.
7 Heart transplant/artificial heart implant.
8 Intensive fetal monitoring, with a decision made about the optimal delivery time.

Anaesthetic approach
A multidisciplinary approach is required involving the anaesthetist, obstetrician, cardiologist, intensivist and patient. The type of anaesthesia chosen will depend on the anaesthetist's experience and the severity of the situation.

Epidural anaesthesia for labour
Should be titrated slowly and carefully with appropriate monitoring, which may include an arterial line. Beneficial effects include reduced preload and afterload. Instrumental delivery may reduce myocardial workload and the adverse haemodynamic effects of pushing. Avoid fluid overhydration.

Caesarean section
Epidural or carefully performed CSE can be used in patients with mild to moderate heart failure. Single-shot spinal should not be used.
GA may be required for:
• emergency CS
• patients with severe heart failure
• anticoagulated patients.
Patients with severe heart failure are at high risk for morbidity/mortality. Therefore, in addition to all other usual precautions with CS anaesthesia:

1 Insert an arterial line and central line prior to GA.
2 Use a carefully titrated anaesthetic based on the skill and experience of the anaesthetist involved.
3 Inotropic support may be required with dobutamine, levosimendan or a phosphodiesterase inhibitor. *See Cardiogenic shock.*
4 Caution should be used with oxytocin—administer by infusion rather than a bolus dose.

◖ Peripherally inserted central catheter (PICC)

Description
PICCs can have 1–3 lumens and can be used for short-term or long-term IV therapy.

Technique
1 Perform a pre-procedure ultrasound scan of the upper limb proximal to the antecubital fossa with a tourniquet applied.

2   Select a suitable vein. The PICC can be placed in the brachial, cephalic or basilic vein. **See *Veins of the upper limb*.** The basilic vein is preferred. Mark the insertion point and release the tourniquet.

3   With a tape measure, calculate the distance from the third or fourth intercostal space on the right side of the sternum, up to the sternal notch, then to the axillary crease and finally to the arm insertion point. This will be the length of catheter insertion.

4   Use full sterile precautions. Wear sterile gloves and gown. Prep and drape the site of insertion.

5   The assistant will then open the PICC set, which contains the PICC, echogenic access needle, guide wire, peel-away introducer, syringe, stiffening wire (in the PICC), caps, sterile measuring tape, scalpel and a StatLock securing device. Cut the PICC to the required length, using the sterile scissors or the scalpel. Make the sure the stiffening wire is pulled back sufficiently before cutting the distal end of the PICC.

6   Flush all the lumens of the PICC and clamp them.

7   The tourniquet is reapplied, and the target vein again imaged on ultrasound. Use LA to anaesthetise the insertion site.

8   Insert the access needle using an out-of-plane approach.

9   Insert the guide wire through the access needle into the vein and remove the needle. Check with the ultrasound that the wire is in the vein.

10 Nick the skin at the guide wire insertion point. Insert the peel-away introducer and dilator over the guide wire and advance the introducer and dilator into the vein.

11 Remove the guide wire and dilator. Loosen the tourniquet.

12 Insert the PICC through the peel-away introducer. Ask the patient to take deep, regular breaths during insertion. Insert the PICC during each inspiration. If fluoroscopy is available, the position of the PICC can be confirmed. The tip should be in the lower third of the SVC.

13 Remove the peel-away introducer incrementally while advancing the PICC with alternant movements.

14 Insert the PICC to its final insertion position, remove the stiffening wire, then check blood can be aspirated from each lumen. Flush each lumen with N/S and cap each lumen.

15 Secure the catheter with a StatLock and cover with a sterile dressing.

16 Check the position of the tip of the PICC with a chest X-ray.

Using ECG attachment for PICC positioning

1   After inserting the PICC a short distance, attach the red ECG wire to the proximal end of the PICC. This will show the intracavity ECG when the PICC is inserted into the heart.

2   Look for an increase in the size of the P waves, suggesting the tip is in the SVC. A P wave with a negative deflection. This suggests optimal PICC tip positioning. A biphasic P wave suggests the tip is well into the RA.

3   Pull the catheter back slightly to see a maximally tall positive P wave without any negative deflection.

◖ Peritonsillar abscess/quinsy

Description

This disease is a complication of acute tonsillitis. The most common causative bacterium is *beta-haemolytic streptococcus*.

Clinical presentation

1 Dysphagia/sore throat/dehydration.
2 Fever.
3 Facial swelling.
4 Limited mouth opening.

Treatment

1 IV antibiotics—penicillin G 2 million units IV q 6 h or clindamycin 600 mg IV q 8 h +/− metronidazole 500 mg IV q 8 h.
2 Intraoral incision of the abscess with a scalpel or aspiration of pus with a needle and syringe may be possible with LA +/− sedation. Topical anaesthesia can be provided by gargling viscous lignocaine.

Anaesthesia for surgical drainage

1 Mouth opening may be restricted and airway anatomy distorted.
2 Inspect the airway nasally with nasal endoscopy.
3 If the patient has good mouth opening, oral intubation may be possible. Otherwise, awake nasal intubation will be the safest option. **See *Awake intubation*.**
4 Topicalisation of the oral airway and airway inspection awake with a videolaryngoscope can also be considered.

◗ Pethidine/meperidine

Description

Fully synthetic opioid drug used IM, IV and epidurally. It is one-tenth as potent as morphine. Useful for the treatment of pain and postoperative shivering. It is disappearing from use.

Dose

Adult

25–100 mg IM up to q 3 h as required. For IV analgesia give 20–25 mg increments q 5 min to a maximum dose of 150 mg.

Child

1 mg/kg/dose IM. For IV dosing—add 1 mg/kg to N/S to a total volume of 10 mL, and give 1 mL increments up to every 5 min until pain controlled.

Advantages

1 Fast onset of action.
2 Less histamine release than morphine, so may be safer for use in asthmatic patients.
3 Effective for relieving/reducing postoperative shivering.

Disadvantages

1 Inferior to morphine for analgesia at equivalent doses.
2 Causes stinging when injected subcut.
3 Cannot be used in renal failure due to the accumulation of norpethidine, which can cause tremors, twitches, seizures and myoclonus.
4 Large doses can cause norpethidine accumulation in patients without renal impairment.
5 More addictive than morphine.
6 Shorter duration of action than morphine (2–3 h).
7 Contraindicated in patients taking monoamine oxidase inhibitor (MAOI) drugs, both non-selective and selective. **See *Monoamine oxidase inhibitor (MAOI) drugs*.**

▶ Phaeochromocytoma

Description

This is a neuroendocrine tumour of chromaffin tissue that synthesises catecholamines (adrenaline, noradrenaline and dopamine). About 90% arise from the adrenal medulla, about 10% are bilateral and about 10% are malignant. A catecholamine-secreting paraganglioma can present in the same way as a phaeochromocytoma, and may be referred to as an 'extra-adrenal phaeochromocytoma'. Phaeochromocytomas may be sporadic or genetic.

Presentation

Symptoms and signs are present in 50% of patients with phaeochromocytoma and are typically paroxysmal. They include:

1 Sustained or paroxysmal hypertension. Episodes of severe hypertension can be initiated by many factors including induction of anaesthesia, ingestion of food/drinks containing tyramine and certain drugs such as metoclopramide and beta blockers. Monoamine oxidase inhibitor (MAOI) drugs can also cause a hypertensive crisis in a patient with a phaeochromocytoma. Glucagon is also contraindicated.
2 Headache, which is often associated with nausea and vomiting and bradycardia.
3 Generalised sweating.
4 Palpitations/arrhythmias.
5 Tremor, generalised weakness, panic attacks.
6 Pallor.
7 Dyspnoea.
8 Phaeochromocytoma crisis—hypertension or hypotension, hyperthermia, mental state changes and other organ dysfunction.
9 Postural hypotension due to volume depletion.
10 Hyperglycaemia due to alpha-2 adrenoreceptor stimulation decreasing insulin release and promoting glycogenolysis. Patients may require peri-operative insulin.
11 Catecholamine-induced cardiomyopathy/cardiac failure. Patients may present with pulmonary oedema, then deteriorate on commencement of beta blocker therapy.
12 Death.

Associated conditions

1 Multiple endocrine neoplasia type 2 (MEN 2)—an autosomal dominant condition causing medullary thyroid cancer and hyperparathyroidism.
2 Neurofibromatosis.
3 Von Hippel–Lindau syndrome (cerebral haemangiomas, renal cell cancer).

Diagnosis

1 Measurement of catecholamines in a 24 h urine sample.
2 CT/MRI.
3 PET scan.
4 Selective adrenal venous sampling is **not** recommended.

Treatment

Surgical resection is the only curative treatment. At least 7 days of pharmacological preparation are required.

1 Cease all interfering medications—these include beta blockers without alpha blockade, glucagon, high-dose steroids and metoclopramide.
2 Alpha-adrenergic blockade—phenoxybenzamine. **See Phenoxybenzamine.** Give 10 mg PO q 12 h, increase by 10–20 mg in divided doses every 2–3 days to

a final dose of 20–100 mg per day. The aim of treatment is to prevent blood pressure rises greater than 165/90 and to have a mild postural hypotension (SBP > 90 mmHg on standing). Cease the drug 24–48 h before surgery. An alternative is prazosin. Give 1 mg PO q 8 h, gradually increasing to 12 mg daily. Another alternative is doxazosin. Give 2–8 mg PO daily.

3 A high sodium diet started on day 2 or 3 of phenoxybenzamine treatment to increase intravascular volume, unless heart failure is also present.

4 Beta blocker drugs, to control tachycardia. **Never give beta blockers before alpha blockade.** This is because unopposed beta blockade will block beta-2-mediated vasodilation of splanchnic and muscle vascular beds, leading to severe hypertension. In addition, beta blockade may result in cardiac failure and pulmonary oedema due to myocardial depression coupled with high SVR. Drugs that can be used include metoprolol 12.5 mg PO q 12 h, gradually increased to a maximum of 200 mg/day.

5 Calcium channel blockers can be used to help control blood pressure or as an alternative to peri-operative alpha-adrenergic blockade. Nicardipine and amlodipine are the most commonly used drugs. Nicardipine may be used as an intravenous infusion perioperatively. *See Nicardipine.*

6 Metyrosine. This orally administered drug inhibits catecholamine synthesis. It is used when other drugs are ineffective or not tolerated or are contraindicated. Metyrosine may also be used when tumour destruction by means such as radiofrequency ablation is considered. A suggested dosage regime is 250 mg q 6 h on day 1; 500 mg q 6 h on day 2; 750 mg q 6 h on day 3; 1000 mg q 6 h on the day before the procedure. Give the last dose of 1000 mg on the morning of surgery.[9]

Anaesthesia

If the lesion is solitary and in the adrenal gland, usually the whole gland is removed. This can be done open, laparoscopically or robotically. The main issue is to avoid blood pressure surges.

1 Insert an arterial line with liberal LA plus midazolam IV.

2 Establish large-bore IV access.

3 It is very important to minimise the hypertensive effects of intubation. A useful technique is to induce anaesthesia with fentanyl 250–350 mcg, propofol and magnesium 40–60 mg/kg (before intubation). Then run an infusion of magnesium at 1–2 g/h.[10] Repeated boluses of magnesium can be given, if required. *See Intubation-minimising hypertensive response.* Magnesium reduces catecholamine release and is an antagonist at alpha-adrenergic receptors. Use rocuronium for muscle relation. **Do not use suxamethonium.**

4 Insert a CVP line, urinary catheter and temperature probe.

5 Do not use ketamine, desflurane or N_2O.

6 Morphine and hydromorphone can cause histamine release which increases catecholamine release from the tumour, so avoid these drugs.

7 Do not give metoclopramide as it can cause catecholamine release from the tumour and precipitate a hypertensive crisis.

8 A clevidipine infusion will usually provide excellent blood pressure control. *See Clevidipine.* If the response to clevidipine is inadequate consider:

a) Sodium nitroprusside (SNP) infusion. *See Sodium nitroprusside (SNP).*

b) Esmolol infusion. *See Esmolol.* Patient must be on an alpha blocker before commencing esmolol.

c) Phentolamine is an excellent drug for BP spikes but has very limited availability.

d) Glyceryl trinitrate infusion—*see Glyceryl trinitrate (GTN).*

9 Remifentanil is **not** helpful for phaeochromocytoma BP control.[11]

10 Fluid load the patient before tumour venous ligation and treat hypotension with IV fluid boluses after ligation.

11 After venous ligation, reduce or cease antihypertensive infusion(s).

12 Post tumour resection hypotension may occur for many reasons, including persistent effects of alpha and beta blockade and downregulation of adrenoreceptors. If IV fluids and metaraminol boluses are inadequate, commence a noradrenaline infusion. If ineffective, commence a vasopressin infusion (0.5–4 units/h). **See Vasopressin.**

13 Consider hydrocortisone if hypoadrenalism is suspected.

14 Monitor BSL as hypoglycaemia may occur.

Postoperative care

These patients require ongoing monitoring in a high-dependency unit.

◐ Phenoxybenzamine

A non-selective adrenergic receptor blocker. It is used to reduce bladder sphincter tone and for control of blood pressure associated with phaeochromocytoma. **See Phaeochromocytoma.** Other uses include treating hypoplastic left heart syndrome and managing complex regional pain syndrome. This drug has many side effects, including retrograde ejaculation, somnolence, headache and nasal congestion.

◐ Phentolamine

Extremely useful anti-hypertensive imidazoline agent. Acts by alpha adrenoreceptor-1 blockade with some alpha-2 blockade. Causes arterial vasodilation with little venous dilation. Unfortunately, it is very difficult to source.

Dose for hypertension

Adult

5–10 mg IM or 1 mg boluses IV. Can also be given by infusion at a rate of 1–20 mcg/kg/min.

◐ Phenylephrine/Neo-Synephrine

Description

Phenylephrine is an alpha-1 adrenergic agonist used to treat hypertension. It is 10 × more potent than metaraminol. It is also used as a nasal decongestant, for dilating the pupil and for topical haemorrhoid treatment. It causes reflex bradycardia due to stimulation of the baroreceptor reflex.

Dose

For the treatment of hypotension in adult: IV bolus dose 50–100 mcg. Infusion—add 2 mg phenylephrine to a 20 mL syringe of N/S. Titrate rate to desired blood pressure.

◐ Phenytoin (Dilantin) and fosphenytoin

Description

Phenytoin is a barbiturate-like hydantoin derivative. Fosphenytoin is a phosphate ester prodrug for phenytoin. Both drugs are used to prevent epileptic seizures and to treat status epilepticus. Phenytoin is also a class 1 antiarrhythmic drug that is useful for treating dysrhythmias associated with digoxin toxicity.

Phenytoin dose for rapid seizure control

1 LD 10–15 mg/kg IV in N/S (**not glucose**). Give no faster than 50 mg/min with ECG monitoring. Hypotension, bradycardia and QT prolongation may occur. Effects are decreased by slowing the infusion rate.

2 If the patient is already taking oral phenytoin, halve the LD.

3 Maintenance IV dose 100 mg q 6–8 h.

4 Severe tissue necrosis can occur if the drug extravasates.

5 TR 10–20 mcg/mL.

Dose for cardiac dysrhythmias

May be used when dysrhythmia is unresponsive to other drugs and cardioversion. Give 3–5 mg/kg IV.

Fosphenytoin

This drug is water soluble and can be given IM. Doses are the same as for phenytoin but it can be infused faster (150 mg/min) and may have fewer haemodynamic side effects.

Phenytoin and NMBDs

Regular phenytoin use results in a shorter duration of action of vecuronium and rocuronium. Cisatracurium is not affected. Acute phenytoin administration results in increased potency of rocuronium.[12]

◖ Phosphodiesterase (PDE) and phosphodiesterase inhibitors

A phosphodiesterase (PDE) is a substance which breaks a phosphodiester bond. In cells PDE breaks down cAMP and cGMP, which decrease intracellular calcium levels by driving calcium into the sarcoplasmic reticulum. Inhibitors lead to an increase in cAMP and cGMP in cells, making less calcium available for contraction. Phosphodiesterase III, IV and V inhibitors are discussed below.

Phosphodiesterase III (PDE III) inhibitors

Phosphodiesterase III is found in vascular smooth muscle and cardiac myocytes. Inhibitors of PDE III result in venous and arterial vasodilation, decreasing preload and afterload. This is beneficial in the treatment of heart failure. PDE III inhibitors increase myocardial contractility and improve lusitropy (myocardial relaxation). The mechanism for this is complex—inhibition of cAMP breakdown increases protein kinase A, which improves Ca^{2+} inward current. This leads to calcium-induced calcium release from the sarcoplasmic reticulum, leading to increased contractility. Examples include dipyridamole, amrinone and milrinone. **See *Amrinone/inamrinone (inocor)* and *Milrinone*.**

Phosphodiesterase IV (PDE IV) inhibitors

These drugs increase levels of cAMP in the smooth muscle of the airways, decreasing intracellular calcium. This leads to smooth muscle relaxation, hence PDE IV drugs are useful for treating asthma and chronic airflow limitation (CAL). They are also useful for treating psoriasis, atopic dermatitis, inflammatory bowel disease and rheumatoid arthritis. Examples include roflumilast and apremilast.

Phosphodiesterase V (PDE V) inhibitors

PDE V degrades cGMP levels in vascular smooth muscle, leading to contraction. PDE V inhibitors cause vascular smooth muscle to relax, targeting the penis and the lungs. They include sildenafil (Viagra) and tadalafil (Cialis). Nitrate drugs are contraindicated if PDE V drugs have been recently ingested. **See *Nitrate drugs*.**

○ Physiology of term pregnancy

Cardiovascular

1 Blood volume increases by 35% (plasma 45% and RBC 20%, leading to a physiological anaemia).
2 Cardiac output (CO) increases by 40–50%. Heart rate increases by 15–20% and stroke volume (SV) by 25–30%. CO reaches maximal at about 28 weeks' gestation but increases again during labour.
3 Systemic vascular resistance (SVR) decreases by 15–40% due to the effects of progesterone on vascular tone. Pulmonary vascular resistance (PVR) also decreases. There is a state of arterial underfilling, with most of the circulation in the venous system.
4 SBP and DBP blood pressure decreases by an average of 10–15 mmHg but increases to normal towards term.
5 Central venous pressure (CVP) decreases by about 5 mmHg.
6 The heart is shifted upwards and leftwards by the elevated diaphragm.
7 A systolic ejection murmur (SEM) may occur due to increased blood flow. A third heart sound may be heard.
8 Supine hypotension (supine hypotensive syndrome) may occur due to pressure of the gravid uterus on the IVC, reducing venous return to the heart.
9 Colloid osmotic pressure/pulmonary capillary pressure gradient is reduced by about 30%, increasing the risk of pulmonary oedema.
10 Peripheral oedema is common.
11 ECG changes may include left axis deviation and Q waves in leads II, III, and aVF. There may also be T wave changes (such as flat or inverted T waves) in leads III and V1–V3.[13]

Respiratory

1 Increased minute ventilation (MV) up to 50%, mainly due to increased tidal volume (TV). Arterial $PaCO_2$ decreases, leading to a respiratory alkalosis compensated for by renal bicarbonate excretion.
2 Capillary engorgement of the mucosa of the respiratory tract with swelling of the larynx and pharynx, nasal mucosa and trachea. There is an increased risk of difficult intubation and mucosal bleeding.
3 Elevation of the diaphragm due to increased intra-abdominal pressure and enlarging uterus.
4 Decreased functional residual capacity (FRC) by about 20%. **See *Lung function tests***. FRC is further decreased in the supine position by another 25%.
5 Oxygen consumption is increased by 20% due to the metabolic needs of the fetus, uterus and placenta. CO_2 production is also increased by 20%. The metabolic rate is increased by 15%.

Haematological

1 Platelet count decreases during pregnancy due to haemodilution, increased breakdown in peripheral tissues and increased aggregation due to increased levels of thromboxane A2.[14] A pregnant patient is not considered thrombocytopenic unless the platelet count is less than $100\,000/mm^3$.
2 RBC volume is increased less than plasma volume, leading to a physiological anaemia. Mean corpuscular volume and mean corpuscular haemoglobin concentration are unchanged. However, there is an increased requirement for dietary iron and folate.

3 There is a physiological hypercoagulable state with elevated levels of certain clotting factors and fibrinogen. Although tests of clotting remain normal, there is an increased risk of thromboembolic disease (DVT/PE).

4 Decreased venous flow in the lower limbs, especially the left leg, further increasing the risk of DVT.

Renal

1 Renal blood flow is increased.

2 The renin-angiotensin-aldosterone mechanism is activated but a resistance to angiotensin II occurs.

3 GFR rises and serum creatinine and urea levels fall.

Gastrointestinal

1 Appetite is increased with a tendency to gain weight. The fetus, placenta, uterus, membranes and amniotic fluid weigh about 5 kg.

2 Increased propensity to reflux, regurgitation and aspiration due to progesterone effects and increased intra-abdominal pressure.

Endocrine

1 Pregnancy is a diabetogenic state, with insulin resistance in the mother late in pregnancy. Glucose levels are reduced due to uptake by the fetus, decreased glucose production by the liver and increased storage as glycogen.

2 Gestational diabetes may occur, particularly if the parturient is overweight, older or from south-east Asia. There are several other risk factors. The cause may be increased insulin resistance due to the effects of placental hormones in some parturients.

⊙ Physostigmine

Alkaloid anticholinesterase drug which crosses the blood–brain barrier. Used to treat central anticholinergic syndrome. **See *Central anticholinergic syndrome*.** Also used to treat glaucoma, delayed gastric emptying and tricyclic antidepressant poisoning.

⊙ Placenta accreta spectrum

In this rare (1:1000 live births) and extremely serious condition, the chorionic villi of the placenta attach to the uterine myometrium or invade the myometrium. The placenta, or part of the placenta, cannot separate from the uterine wall after delivery, and attempts to do so will result in catastrophic haemorrhage. Postpartum hysterectomy, which is technically challenging anyway, may be further complicated by invasion of the placenta into other organs.

Types

Three types of placenta accreta form the placenta accreta spectrum. These are:

1 Placenta accreta—placental chorionic villi attach to the myometrium.

2 Placenta increta—chorionic villi invade into the myometrium.

3 Placenta percreta—chorionic villi invade through the myometrium into the serosal layer of the uterus or beyond into other organs such as the bladder.

Note: henceforth only the term 'placenta accreta' will be used in this section.

Causes

Placenta accreta is thought to be due to uterine decidual damage/scarring. The most important risk factor is previous Caesarean section(s). Previous gynaecological uterine surgery is also a risk. Placenta praevia after previous Caesarean section is associated with a high risk of placenta accreta. In 20% of cases, there is no identifiable risk factor.[15]

Diagnosis

1 Prenatal ultrasound.
2 MRI scan.
3 If undiagnosed before birth there will be an inability to manually deliver the placenta, associated with catastrophic bleeding.

Planned management

If diagnosed before delivery, the options for treatment are:

1 Caesarean section with peripartum hysterectomy
2 Caesarean section with the uterine wound closed and the placenta left in situ.
   There should be a multidisciplinary team approach that involves an obstetrician, anaesthetist, maternal-fetal medicine specialist, radiologist and a surgeon with extensive experience in complex gynaecological surgery (usually a gynaecological oncology surgeon). Consider the preoperative insertion of endovascular balloon-tipped catheters into both internal iliac arteries to help control intraoperative haemorrhage. Uterine artery embolisation with a substance such as Gelfoam® may also be considered. This is a highly controversial area of management.

Anaesthesia for Caesarean section

1 Prepare for catastrophic blood loss—2 large-bore IV cannulas/RIC, arterial line, blood cross-match and a rapid infusion system e.g. Belmont Rapid Infuser. *See Rapid infusion catheter (RIC) exchange set.* Consider cell salvage—*see Blood salvage, intraoperative.*
2 Many/most anaesthetists prefer general anaesthesia as surgery may be very prolonged and associated with massive blood loss. Also, a vertical abdominal incision may be used and intraoperative coagulopathy may occur.
3 Administer tranexamic acid 1 g. *See Tranexamic acid (TXA) (cyklokapron).*
4 Neuraxial blockade can be considered in cases of suspected or minimal placenta accreta.
5 SAB for delivery of the baby followed by GA for peripartum hysterectomy has also been described.[15]
6 Uterotonics are not used for either peripartum hysterectomy or if the placenta is left in situ.

Anaesthesia for placenta accreta diagnosed at delivery

Management is the same as for any other cause of massive haemorrhage. *See Blood loss—assessment, management and anaesthetic approach.*

◑ Placental abruption (PA)/abruptio placentae

Description

PA is the separation of the placenta from its decidua basalis after 20 weeks' gestation and prior to delivery of the fetus. This results in maternal haemorrhage between the placenta and uterine wall. About 90% of cases are mild to moderate and well tolerated by mother and fetus. The cause is often unknown.

Risk factors

1 Smoking, alcohol and/or cocaine use.
2 Maternal age > 35 yrs.
3 Hypertension.

4 Previous PA.

5 Trauma.

Clinical presentation

1 Severely painful, unrelenting uterine contractions with incomplete uterine relaxation.

2 Tetanic contractions.

3 Uterine tenderness.

4 Uterus feels hard to palpation.

5 Non-reassuring fetal heart trace, fetal death.

6 Concealed or revealed blood loss, which may cause varying degrees of shock.

7 Coagulopathy, DIC.

Diagnosis

1 This is based on clinical signs and physical examination.

2 Ultrasound examination is useful for excluding planta praevia but has low sensitivity for visualising PA.

Anaesthesia

1 PA can range in its presentation from asymptomatic to profound maternal shock and/or a severely compromised or dead fetus.

2 Vaginal delivery may be appropriate in mild cases or in some cases of fetal death.

3 Epidural or subarachnoid block (SAB) can be considered if the patient has been fully resuscitated, is haemodynamically stable and there is no coagulopathy or fetal distress.

4 For patients who are haemodynamically compromised or coagulopathic or where there is significant fetal distress, GA will be required.

5 For management of the shocked patient **see Blood loss—assessment, management and anaesthetic approach.**

◐ Placenta praevia (PP)

Description

In this condition, the placenta is situated over, or near, the internal os of the uterus. This means that cervical dilatation will result in catastrophic bleeding and the fetus **cannot** be delivered vaginally. A low-lying placenta is a placenta that has an edge within 2–3.5 cm of the uterine os. Most of these placentas will 'migrate' away to a safe distance from the os as pregnancy progresses.

There are four grades of PP:

- Grade 1—placenta is in the lower uterine segment but does not touch the os (the placental edge is within 2 cm of the internal os).
- Grade 2—placenta is at the uterine os but does not cover it.
- Grade 3—placenta partially covers the os.
- Grade 4—placenta completely covers the os.

Placenta praevia occurs in about 0.5% of deliveries. There is an increased risk of associated placenta accreta. **See Placenta accreta spectrum.**

Risk factors

1 Previous PP.

2 Smoking, cocaine use, advanced maternal age, multiparity.

3 Assisted reproductive technology.

4 Previous CS.

5 Previous uterine curettage.

Clinical presentation

1 Painless vaginal bleeding.
2 Diagnosis is usually by ultrasound.
3 Speculum examination may enable visualisation of the placenta if the cervix is dilated.
4 **Digital examination may cause catastrophic bleeding and must not be done.**

Anaesthetic management

1 Preparation should be made for massive blood loss (two large-bore IV cannulas/ RIC, blood group and hold). *See Rapid infusion catheter (RIC) exchange set.*
2 Neuraxial anaesthesia is appropriate and safe.
3 It may be necessary to cut through the placenta if it is anterior.
4 If massive blood loss occurs, *see Blood loss—assessment, management and anaesthetic approach.*

◗ Plasma exchange/plasmapheresis

Plasma exchange is a technique used to remove circulating harmful substances such as antibodies, immune complexes and poisons. Conditions which may be treated this way include:

- Guillain–Barré syndrome
- Myasthenia gravis
- Wilson's disease.

One total plasma volume is replaced with albumin solution. RBC, WBC and platelets are returned to the patient. Other solutions that can be used as patient plasma replacement are FFP and Gelofusine® or combinations of these.

◗ Plasma-Lyte 148

Description

This is an isotonic crystalloid that has some advantages over Hartmann's solution and N/S.

Contents

The contents of this solution are meant to mimic plasma. They include:

- sodium 140 mmol/L
- chloride 98 mmol/L
- gluconate 23 mmol/L
- potassium 5 mmol/L
- acetate 27 mmol/L
- magnesium 1.5 mmol/L
- pH range 6.5–8.0 (adjusted with sodium hydroxide).

Comparison with other crystalloids

1 Unlike Hartmann's solution, Plasma-Lyte 148 does not contain calcium hence it will not cause citrated blood in the same line to clot.
2 Unlike N/S, it contains potassium so it is unsuitable for patients with hyperkalaemia.
3 It is not suitable for patients with hypermagnesaemia due to its magnesium content.
4 Acetate in Plasma-Lyte 148 and lactate in Hartmann's solution are both metabolised to bicarbonate, but this occurs at a faster rate in Plasma-Lyte 148. Acetate metabolism is not affected by liver function or severe shock. Plasma-Lyte 148 is an alkalinising solution and should not be used in patients with a metabolic alkalosis.

5 Acetate has no effect on blood glucose levels, unlike lactate. Therefore Plasma-Lyte 148 is preferred to Hartmann's solution in patients with brittle diabetes.[16]

▶ Plasminogen and plasminogen activator inhibitor (PAI)

Plasminogen is converted to plasmin by tissue plasminogen activator (tPA). *See Tissue plasminogen activator (tPA).* Plasmin dissolves clots. Plasminogen activator inhibitor (PAI) inhibits activation of plasminogen. Deficiency in PAI can result in thrombogenic disease.

▶ Plateau pressure

Plateau pressure is the pressure that is applied by a mechanical ventilator to the small airways and alveoli. It is measured by maintaining inspiratory pressure at the end of inspiration for 0.5–1 s. There is no flow of gas during the measurement of plateau pressure. The plateau pressure should not exceed 30 cmH$_2$O due to the risk of barotrauma.

▶ Platelet adenosine diphosphate (ADP) receptor antagonists/ PY$_{12}$ receptor antagonists

See Anticoagulant and antiplatelet drugs and surgery/neuraxial anaesthesia.

Description

These are thienopyridine drugs that are potent inhibitors of platelet adhesion and aggregation. Examples include clopidogrel (Plavix), ticlopidine (Ticlid) and prasugrel. Ticagrelor (Brilinta) is a non-thienopyridine ADP receptor antagonist. These drugs act irreversibly on platelet ADP receptors and their effects take 24–48 h to manifest. The effects of these drugs on platelets act synergistically with aspirin.

Uses

1 Post coronary artery stenting.
2 Ischaemic heart disease without stents.
3 Acute coronary syndromes.
4 Cerebrovascular disease.

Anaesthesia/surgery

Patients who have had recent coronary artery stent insertion may be at high risk of stent thrombosis if their antiplatelet drugs are stopped. *See Coronary artery stents (CAS).*

In general:
1 Clopidogrel—cease for 5 days (7 days if neuraxial block).
2 Ticlopidine—cease for 14 days.
3 Prasugrel—cease for 7 days.
4 Ticagrelor—cease for 5 days.

Emergency surgery/haemorrhage

Consider desmopressin for minor bleeding, and platelet transfusion for major bleeding.

▶ Platelet glycoprotein IIb/IIIa receptor antagonists

Description

These drugs are used IV during percutaneous coronary artery interventions or acute coronary syndromes (or both). They include abciximab (ReoPro), tirofiban (Aggrastat) and eptifibatide (Integrilin). They are always used with other anti-clotting drugs such as heparin or aspirin. *See Anticoagulant and antiplatelet drugs and surgery/neuraxial anaesthesia.*

Elective surgery

These drugs are used in patients who would be inappropriate for elective surgery due to high MACE risk. *See MACE.*

Emergency surgery

Cease the drug as soon as possible. These drugs are short acting and their effects will wear off as follows:

1 Abciximab—48 h.
2 Tirofiban—8 h.
3 Eptifibatide—8 h.

Platelet transfusion can be considered if abciximab is ceased < 12–24 h before surgery. Platelet transfusion is not effective if the patient has received recent tirofiban or eptifibatide.[17]

◑ Platelet therapy

A whole blood donation unit has its platelets extracted and these are suspended in 35–60 mL of plasma. This is called a 'unit of platelets' or 'a random donor platelet unit'. Alternatively, blood is taken from the donor, platelets are removed and then the blood is returned to the donor. This is known as 'single donor platelets' or 'apheresis platelets'. Apheresis platelet units have 5–8 × more platelets than a random donor platelet unit. The platelets are stored in a mixture of platelet additive solution (PAS) and plasma. One unit of 'pooled platelets' contains the platelets from 4 units of donated whole blood. These platelets are suspended in PAS.

Indications for platelet transfusion

1 Reduce/prevent bleeding in patients with a low platelet count (< 5000–10 000 per mm^3).
2 Reduce/prevent bleeding in patients with dysfunctional platelets e.g. patient on aspirin.
3 Prevention of spontaneous bleeding in patients with a very low platelet count (< 5000–10 000 per mm^3).

Dose

Adult

This is a controversial area. 1 unit of platelets/10 kg body weight is recommended (about 5 units). If apheresis platelets are used, the dose is 1 unit (198 mL). If a pool of platelets is used, the dose is 1 pool ($\approx$ 326 mL). 1 unit of apheresis platelets or 1 unit of pooled platelets is expected to increase the platelet count by 20 000–40 000 per mm^3.

Child

All children should receive apheresis leukocyte-depleted platelets. For neonates give 10 mL/kg. For older children give 1 unit. In an 18 kg child, this should increase platelet count by 20 000 per mm.^{3}

Platelets and blood groups

Platelets should preferably be of the same ABO/RhD type as the recipient, but matching blood group type is more important than RhD type. If this is not possible, the order of preference is shown in Table P1.

Table P1 Preferred donor platelet blood group based on recipient's blood group

Recipient's ABO group	Platelet product ABO group—first choice	Platelet product ABO group—second choice	Platelet product ABO group—third choice
O	O	A	B
A	A	B or O	AB
B	B	A or O	AB
AB	AB	A or B	O
Unknown	A or O		

Practical aspects of platelet transfusion

1 All platelets are leukocyte depleted and irradiated.
2 Use a new blood administration filter (containing a 170–200 micron filter).
3 Platelets should be transfused before red cells because red cell debris may trap platelets in the filter.
4 Platelets are stored at room temperature and last one week.
5 Unless in critical situations, transfuse platelets over 1–2 h and no longer than 4 h.
6 HLA matched platelets may be required for patients with HLA alloimmunisation.
7 HPA matched platelets may be required for patients with fetal maternal alloimmune thrombocytopenia (FMAIT) or post-transfusion purpura (PTP).

Risks of platelet transfusion

1 Transfusion reactions—platelet transfusions account for more reactions than blood transfusions.[18]
2 Transfusion-related acute lung injury (TRALI).
3 Circulatory overload.

⊙ Pneumothorax/tension pneumothorax

Description

A pneumothorax is the presence of air between the chest wall and the lung in the pleural space (between the parietal and visceral pleura). This can partially or fully collapse the lung. A tension pneumothorax is the accumulation of air under pressure in the pleural space and is a life-threatening emergency that can cause sudden cardiac arrest. *See Cardiac arrest.*

Classification and causes

A pneumothorax may be traumatic or atraumatic. An atraumatic pneumothorax can be primary or secondary. A pneumothorax can also be simple, tension or open. A tension pneumothorax shifts the mediastinal structures.

Traumatic pneumothorax

Can be due to blunt or penetrating trauma. An open wound traumatic pneumothorax can result in air moving in and out of the chest—a 'sucking chest wound'. A traumatic pneumothorax can also be due to barotrauma e.g. high-pressure ventilation, rapid ascent while scuba diving. Traumatic pneumothorax may be iatrogenic due to procedures such as:

• surgery
• subclavian central line insertion

- supraclavicular brachial plexus block
- intercostal nerve block
- pleural biopsy
- tracheostomy.

Primary spontaneous pneumothorax

The pneumothorax occurs without a known cause. It is more likely to occur in tall, thin people.

Secondary spontaneous pneumothorax

This is due to lung disease, including:

1 asthma
2 cystic fibrosis
3 emphysema
4 cancer
5 pneumonia.

Systemic disease may be associated with pneumothorax e.g. Marfan syndrome, Ehlers–Danlos syndrome. **See *Marfan syndrome* and *Ehlers–Danlos syndrome (EDS)*.**

Clinical effects of simple pneumothorax

1 Chest pain.
2 Dyspnoea.
3 Asymmetrical lung expansion.
4 Hyper-resonant percussion note and reduced breath sounds over the pneumothorax.
5 Subcutaneous emphysema.

Clinical effects of tension pneumothorax

All the above can occur plus:

1 displacement of mediastinal structures
2 severe shortness of breath/respiratory failure/cyanosis
3 hypotension
4 tachycardia
5 elevated JVP
6 cardiovascular collapse/cardiac arrest.

Diagnosis

1 Clinical history and examination.
2 CXR—erect. There are absent lung markings lateral to the lung edge. A 2.5 cm width of airspace on CXR correlates with a 30% pneumothorax. A supine CXR makes detecting a pneumothorax much more difficult.
3 Ultrasound:
   - Place the linear probe orientated parallel to the ribs on the anterior chest wall in the third intercostal space in the midclavicular line.
   - The visceral and parietal pleura are seen as shimmering white lines that slide against each other.
   - One can imagine shiny 'ants' moving along this line.
   - One may also see 'comet tails', which are streaks of white at right angles to the pleura that rapidly appear and disappear.

- If there is a pneumothorax, there is a shiny white line (the parietal pleura) but no sliding or shimmering. There are also no comet tails.
- The probe can be placed on the lateral chest wall to get an idea of the size of the pneumothorax.

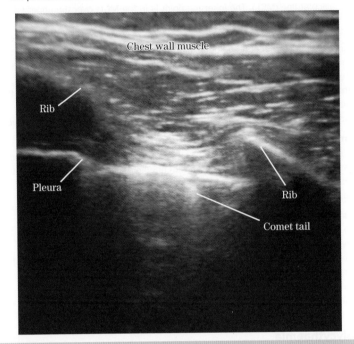

Figure P4 Comet tail artefact seen with ultrasound in normal lung

4 M-mode ultrasound can be used. It will show the 'seashore' sign if a pneumothorax is not present. The chest wall shows no motion and is the 'waves' whereas the moving lung makes the 'sand'. With a pneumothorax there is no 'sand', just 'waves' (called the 'barcode' sign).

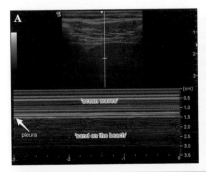
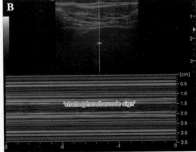

Figure P5 Ultrasound images of 'seashore sign'—the normal lung is on the left (sand and waves). The lung with a pneumothorax is on the right 'barcode sign'.
Image courtesy of Matt Doane

Treatment of tension pneumothorax

A tension pneumothorax is a crisis situation that requires immediate decompression. To do this:

1 Identify the second intercostal space (between the second and third rib) in the midclavicular line (MCL). The insertion point is in the MCL, over the upper edge of the third rib (lateral to the nipple in men).
2 Using sterile precautions, remove the plug from a 16 or 14 G IV cannula. Insert the cannula fully, in a direction perpendicular to the skin.
3 A 'hiss' of air should be heard and the patient's condition should improve. After 5 seconds, remove the cannula needle but leave the cannula in place.
4 If the above site is compromised, use the fourth or fifth intercostal space in the anterior axillary line.
5 Following this emergency procedure, insert a chest drain. *See Chest drain/tube.*

Treatment of other types of pneumothorax

1 A small, asymptomatic pneumothorax (< 2 cm width on erect CXR) can be observed.
2 A larger pneumothorax can be treated with needle aspiration, a pleural catheter or a chest drain. *See Chest drain/tube.*
3 Supplementary O_2 will increase the absorption rate.

Anaesthesia and pneumothorax

1 N_2O will make the pneumothorax bigger and must not be used.
2 IPPV may cause a pneumothorax to become a tension pneumothorax.
3 A known pneumothorax should have a chest tube inserted before induction of anaesthesia.
4 If this is not possible due to patient refusal or inability to cooperate, induce anaesthesia and use a spontaneous breathing technique, if possible, until a chest drain can be inserted.

◐ Polycythaemia

Description

Polycythaemia is defined as a Hb level > 170 g/L (Hct > 0.52) in males and > 160 g/L (Hct > 0.48) in females. This condition can be classified as:

1 *Apparent or stress polycythaemia*—due to causes such as smoking, obstructive sleep apnoea (OSA), alcohol excess, obesity, medications such as diuretics. RBC mass is normal.
2 *Relative polycythaemia*—RBC mass is normal but there is a reduction in plasma volume due to e.g. dehydration, fluid loss from burns.
3 *Absolute polycythaemia*—RBC mass is increased. This may be due to a primary process such as overproduction in the bone marrow (a myeloproliferative syndrome) or secondary to chronic hypoxia e.g. high altitude or cyanotic congenital heart disease. Over-transfusion is another cause.

Types of absolute polycythaemia

1 Primary polycythaemia is due to overproduction of red cells by the bone marrow. Polycythaemia vera (polycythaemia rubra vera) is a type of blood cancer. There may also be overproduction of white cells and platelets. There is also a primary familial polycythaemia which is not malignant.
2 Secondary polycythaemia—this can be a physiological adaption to low O_2 availability e.g. high altitudes, cyanotic heart disease and chronic lung disease. Secondary polycythaemia can be non-physiological and due to causes such as erythropoietin-producing cancers.

Polycythaemia vera (PV)

This disease is due to a mutation of the JAK-2 gene. It is a myeloproliferative disorder of the haemopoietic stem cells. This results in issues with vascular occlusion and haemorrhage. Above a Hct of 0.55–0.6, blood viscosity increases exponentially.

Clinical effects

1 Headaches, cortical venous sinus thrombosis.
2 Dizziness, fatigue.
3 Nosebleeds, gastric bleeding, bleeding from other sites—due to thrombocytopenia, platelet dysfunction and sometimes abnormal fibrinolysis. Patients may be deficient in von Willebrand factor.[19] *See Von Willebrand disease (VWD).*
4 Itchiness.
5 Pain, numbness or tingling in different parts of the body (Mitchell's disease/ erythromelalgia).
6 Phlebitis.
7 Vision problems.
8 Cyanosis.
9 Gout.
10 Kidney stones.
11 Enlarged spleen.
12 Thromboembolic disease—CVA, heart attack.
13 Heart failure.
14 Pulmonary hypertension.
15 Budd–Chiari syndrome—occlusion of hepatic veins.
16 Eventual myelofibrosis.
17 Acute myeloid leukaemia.

Diagnosis

1 Bone marrow biopsy.
2 Genetic testing for mutation of JAK-2 gene.
3 Normal or reduced erythropoietin level.
4 Absence of another cause e.g. cyanotic heart disease.

Treatment

Once polycythaemia vera becomes symptomatic, the mortality rate is about 50%, if it is left untreated. Treatment options include:

1 Weekly phlebotomy until RBC mass is reduced to Hct < 0.5, then phlebotomy as needed.
2 Medical therapy to reduce RBC production (interferon, hydroxyurea).
3 Blood 'thinners' e.g. aspirin, warfarin.

Anaesthesia and polycythaemia vera

1 Discuss management with the patient's haematologist.
2 Prevent/treat any situation which may decrease plasma volume such as prolonged fasting, dehydration, vomiting and/or diarrhoea.
3 Phlebotomy should be undertaken if Hct > 0.65. If removing blood urgently replace each unit removed with 500 mL N/S.
4 Aim for a preoperative Hct of < 0.45 in males and < 0.42 in females.

◑ Polymorphic ventricular tachycardia

This is a lethal arrhythmia requiring immediate defibrillation. The QRS pattern changes over time and deteriorates to VF. Long QT syndrome leads to a type of polymorphic VT called torsades de pointes. *See Torsades de pointes.* Other causes include organic heart disease such as ischaemic heart disease, Brugada syndrome, short QT syndrome, drug-induced and catecholaminergic polymorphic VT.

◑ Popliteal sciatic nerve block

See Sciatic nerve block.

◑ Porphyria

Description

Only a brief outline of this broad spectrum of illnesses is provided here.

1 Porphyria describes a group of inherited metabolic disorders involving the process of haem synthesis. Haem is the iron-containing ring structure in haemoglobin but it is also found in many other compounds. 80% of haem is made in the bone marrow and most of the rest in the liver, although all tissues make it.
2 The symptoms and signs of porphyria are due to overproduction of different haem precursors.
3 Porphyria can be divided into acute and non-acute forms.
4 All acute forms can develop into a neurovisceral crisis.
5 Non-acute forms of porphyria do not cause a neurovisceral crisis and are of much less concern to the anaesthetist.
6 Inheritance is usually autosomal dominant with variable expression.
7 There is an increased risk of hypertension, liver cancer and renal impairment.
8 Urine may turn red/purple on exposure to light.

Classification

Acute forms of porphyria (of concern to anaesthetists)

1 Acute intermittent porphyria (AIP)—the most common of the acute types. It is a hepatic porphyria.
2 Variegate porphyria (VP).
3 Hereditary coproporphyria (HCP).
4 5-aminolevulinic acid dehydratase deficiency (ALA dehydratase deficiency)—extremely rare.

Non-acute forms of porphyria (of much less concern to anaesthetists)

These porphyrias cause chronic skin problems due to the accumulation of porphyrins. This group includes:

1 Porphyria cutanea tarda (PCT)—the most common form of porphyria. It is the only porphyria not caused by a gene mutation. It is associated with light sensitivity (burning pain, blisters), and has been referred to as 'the vampire disease'.
2 Congenital erythropoietic porphyria.
3 Erythropoietic protoporphyria.

Precipitating events for a neurovisceral crisis

1 Fasting.
2 Dehydration.

3 Infection.
4 Drugs/alcohol.
5 Smoking.
6 Stress—emotional or physical.
7 Endogenous hormones e.g. progesterone, oestrogen.

Neurovisceral crisis features

These are 5 × more common in women. Pregnancy may exacerbate or provoke an acute attack.

1 Abdominal pain which can be mistaken for an acute abdomen e.g. appendicitis.
2 Nausea and vomiting.
3 Tachycardia/hypertension/postural hypotension/autonomic instability.
4 Weakness due to nerve effects—especially proximally and upper limbs. This can be very severe with respiratory failure. Bulbar paresis can occur.
5 Psychiatric features—anxiety, confusion, psychosis.
6 Pain in the back, chest and extremities and sensory disturbances.
7 Seizures.
8 Hyponatraemia/hypomagnesaemia/hypercalcaemia.

There is no fever or elevated WCC. Cutaneous features such as blistering skin lesions can occur with VP and HCP. CSF is usually normal.

Diagnosis

Porphyria can mimic many other illnesses, including an acute psychiatric episode. Diagnosis can be made by:

1 Detection of porphobilinogen in a fresh urine sample protected from light. A normal level rules out AIP, VP and HCP. ALA dehydratase deficiency will not be ruled out.
2 An EDTA blood sample protected from light should be taken to determine the type of porphyria.
3 Stool samples also show increased porphyrin levels.

Treatment of a neurovisceral crisis

1 Remove the cause.
2 Avoid a catabolic state by providing 200 g of glucose/day (PO, NG tube or IV).
3 Avoid/treat hyponatraemia.
4 IV haem arginate. This drug suppresses hepatic production of 5-aminolevulinic acid (ALA) dehydratase and other porphyrin precursors while replenishing haem. Give 3 mg/kg to a maximum of 250 mg daily for 4 days. Give via a large-bore IV cannula or central line.
5 Supportive measures such as analgesia, anti-emetics and anxiolytics. Check which drugs are safe and which are unsafe (see below).
6 Treat convulsions with diazepam (despite reports of porphyric crisis with this drug).

Safe drugs—the literature may be contradictory

1 Haloperidol—useful for delirium.
2 Zopiclone—useful for insomnia.
3 Prochlorperazine, ondansetron.
4 Lorazepam, midazolam.
5 Beta blockers.
6 Safe anticonvulsants include benzodiazepines, levetiracetam, gabapentin, vigabatrin, magnesium.
7 Propofol.

8 Alfentanil.

9 Clonidine is probably safe.

10 Omeprazole.

11 LMWH.

12 Paracetamol.

Unsafe drugs—the literature may be contradictory

1 Some anticonvulsants such as phenytoin.

2 Thiopentone, ketamine, etomidate, other barbiturates.

3 Oxycodone may be unsafe.

4 Ephedrine.

5 Some antibiotics e.g. rifampicin, erythromycin.

6 Alpha-methyldopa.

7 Alcohol.

8 Ergot derivatives.

9 Oestrogens.

10 Hydralazine.

11 Nifedipine.

Anaesthetic approach

1 Minimise fasting times.

2 Administer 4% glucose/0.18% NaCl solution to avoid calorie restrictions.

3 Regional anaesthesia can be used. Bupivacaine is safe and lignocaine is probably safe.

4 Propofol can be used but not thiopentone, ketamine or etomidate. A propofol infusion may be safe or unsafe.

5 Sevoflurane is probably safe.

6 Opioids are safe except for oxycodone.

7 Diclofenac, ibuprofen and fenoprofen should not be used.

8 Indomethacin is safe.

9 Suxamethonium, cisatracurium and vecuronium are safe. Pancuronium is unsafe.

10 Keep the patient in hospital at least overnight in case there is a delayed reaction.

◗ POSSUM scoring

POSSUM stands for **P**hysiological and **O**perative **S**everity **S**core for the en**U**meration of **M**ortality and morbidity. There are various forms of these calculator tools, including Vascular (V-POSSUM) and Portsmouth (P-POSSUM). They are intended to enable direct comparisons of outcomes of surgeons and institutions, taking into account population differences. This information can also be used to calculate an individual patient's risk of morbidity or mortality. The V-POSSUM calculator and other versions of POSSUM are available online.

◗ Post dural puncture headache (PDPH)

Description

This type of headache typically follows a recognised or unrecognised dural 'tap' during attempted epidural anaesthesia/analgesia. Less commonly, it can occur after a lumbar puncture. It occurs within 5 days (usually within 72 h) of the procedure and is due to leakage of CSF through the breach in the dura. The cause of the headache may be due to traction on pain-sensitive structures in the skull due to CSF volume loss and/or reflex cerebral vasodilation.

Symptoms

1 Frontal or occipital headache.
2 Postural component—the headache is usually worse on sitting/standing.
3 Headache worse on coughing or sneezing/straining.
4 Neck stiffness.
5 Hearing disturbance—e.g. tinnitus and/or deafness.
6 Abducens nerve palsy may occur—eye cannot turn outward.
7 A subdural haematoma may occur due to stretching and rupturing of bridging veins.

Differential diagnosis

1 Meningitis.
2 Cerebral vein/sinus thrombosis.
3 Migraine.
4 Preeclampsia.

Treatment

1 Bed rest with adequate hydration.
2 Analgesia—paracetamol, NSAIDs, oxycodone.
3 Blood patch after 24–48 if conservative measures fail.

Blood patch

1 Explain all the risks of the procedure to the patient, including the potential for arachnoiditis.
2 Perform an epidural at the same level as the causative procedure or one level below as blood tends to track up in a cephalad direction.
3 Once the epidural space is identified, an assistant, using aseptic technique, obtains 20 mL of venous blood from the patient. This is handed to the neuraxial anaesthetist.
4 The blood is then injected slowly through the epidural needle. The patient may complain of back pain or leg pressure. Stop injecting then recommence. Stop if symptoms become significant. Inject up to 20 mL of blood.
5 The patient should lie flat for 2 h after the procedure.
6 The success rates are 30–50% for one blood patch, increasing to 90% for a second blood patch.

Patient who declines, or is unsuitable for, blood patch

Treatment options include:

1 Drugs such as PO caffeine (maximum 900 mg in 24 h or 200 mg if breast feeding), sumatriptan 6 mg subcut or pregabalin 50 mg PO q 8 h.
2 Bilateral sphenopalatine block. *See Sphenopalatine ganglion (SPG) block.*

◖ Postoperative nausea and vomiting (PONV)

Risk factors

1 History of PONV.
2 Female.
3 Non-smoker.
4 History of motion sickness.
5 Age < 50 years.
6 Use of volatile anaesthetics/N_2O.
7 Use of opioids.
8 Laparoscopic surgery.
9 Prolonged fasting.
10 Length of surgery > 60 min.

Risk reduction strategies

1 Avoiding GA e.g. brachial plexus block for upper limb surgery.
2 Total intravenous anaesthesia (TIVA).
3 Avoiding/minimising opioids. Intrathecal opioids may increase PONV.
4 Preoperative paracetamol/peri-operative NSAIDs.
5 Alpha-2 agonists such as clonidine and beta blockers reduce PONV.
6 Nerve blocks/wound catheters to reduce opioid requirements.
7 Sugammadex may be less likely to produce nausea and vomiting than neostigmine.[20]

Drug prophylaxis

Patients with one or two risk factors should receive dual anti-emetic drugs from different classes. A suitable combination is dexamethasone 4–8 mg IV on induction and ondansetron 4 mg IV towards the end of the procedure. If more than two risk factors consider three agents such as ondansetron, dexamethasone and droperidol 0.625 mg.

Treatment of PONV

Use an agent from a different treatment class if prophylaxis was given. Options for adults include:

1 Ondansetron—4–8 mg IV or dolasetron, granisetron, palonosetron, tropisetron.
2 Droperidol—0.625 mg IV.
3 Cyclizine—50 mg IV.
4 Aprepitant—130 mg IV over 2 min.

Paediatric anti-emetic drugs and dosages

1 Ondansetron—50–100 mcg/kg up to 4 mg.
2 Dexamethasone—150 mcg/kg up to 5 mg.
3 Aprepitant—3 mg/kg up to 125 mg.
4 Droperidol—10–15 mcg/kg up to 1.25 mg (only if other therapy has failed and patient is being admitted to hospital).

◖ Postoperative shivering

Prevention

Prevent the patient from becoming cold with strategies such as forced-air warmers and warmed IV fluids. Check for hypoglycaemia and fever.

Treatment

In addition to warming the patient up, consider for the adult:

1 Pethidine—0.5 mg/kg IV.
2 Clonidine—1.5 mcg/kg IV.
3 Tramadol—1 mg/kg IV.

◖ Postpartum haemorrhage (PPH)

Definition

Defined as > 500 mL blood loss after vaginal delivery, or > 1000 mL after CS. Blood loss of 500–1000 mL is considered minor PPH and is easily dealt with. Major PPH is defined as > 40% total blood volume (TBV) lost ≈ 2000 mL.

Causes

Think of 'the 4 Ts':

1 Tone—uterine atony (causes 70% of PPH)
2 Tissue—retained placenta or products (causes 10% of PPH), uterine inversion, placenta accreta.
3 Trauma—to the uterus or birth canal (causes 20% of PPH).
4 Thrombin—coagulation issues (< 1% of PPH).

Treatment

For general management of massive blood loss, **see Blood loss—assessment, management and anaesthetic approach.**

Prevention of uterine atony

1 Vaginal delivery—10 units of oxytocin IM with delivery of anterior shoulder.
2 Elective uncomplicated CS—carbetocin 100 mcg IV.
3 All other CS—oxytocin 3 units IV then infusion 40 units in 1000 mL Hartmann's over 4 h.

Treatment of uterine atony

1 Uterine massage, ensure bladder is empty, oxytocin bolus IV.
2 If under GA ensure that excess volatile is not being used.
3 Syntometrine (oxytocin 5 units + ergometrine 500 mcg in 1 mL of solution). Give 0.5 mL IV and 0.5 mL IM.
4 Give a bolus of Hartmann's IV 500 mL.
5 Misoprostol 400–600 mcg sublingual, oral, PV or rectal. Repeat after 15 minutes if required. The maximum dose is 800 mcg.
6 Carboprost (15-methyl prostaglandin F2-alpha) 500 mcg in 20 mL N/S injected into the myometrium at several sites. Carboprost can also be given IM 250 mcg repeated 15 minutely up to eight doses. Carboprost can cause systemic and pulmonary hypertension, pulmonary oedema, bronchospasm and coronary artery spasm. GA may be required due to severe patient distress.
7 Sulprostone 500 mcg given as an infusion at 100 mcg/h to a maximum dose of 1500 mcg.
8 Ensure the uterus is empty (retained products, clots). Identify/treat uterine inversion.
9 Insertion of a Bakri balloon.
10 Uterine packing.
11 Aggressive surgical management, including hysterectomy.

Tissue

For management of retained placenta, **see Retained placenta**. Re-examine the placenta for completeness. Other products that may be retained include an accessory placental lobe and membranes. Manual evacuation will be required. For management of uterine inversion, **see Uterine inversion**. For management of placenta accreta, **see Placenta accreta spectrum**.

Trauma

Requires surgical repair.

Coagulation abnormalities

See Blood loss—assessment, management and anaesthetic approach.

◑ Postural orthostatic tachycardia syndrome (POTS)

Description
Afflicted patients suffer from tachycardia, dizziness and fatigue when transitioning from lying down to standing up. It is a type of orthostatic intolerance and it affects mainly women of child-bearing age. It may follow a significant illness or surgery, pregnancy or other trauma. The cause is unknown but is thought to be a disorder of the autonomic nervous system.

Diagnosis
Heart rate should increase by > 30 bpm from supine baseline or exceed 120 bpm when moving from lying to standing within the first 10 min, in the absence of orthostatic hypotension.

Treatment
1 Non-specific treatments (yoga, diet, exercise, meditation).
2 Increasing fluid and salt consumption.
3 Beta blockers e.g. propranolol.
4 Clonidine, desmopressin, fludrocortisone and ivabradine, among other drugs, may be helpful.

Anaesthesia and POTS
It is difficult to make any specific recommendations regarding the anaesthetic management of these patients. It is not a fatal condition.

◑ Potassium

Description
Potassium is the major intracellular cation and is integral to the function of excitable tissue such as nerve conduction and cardiac myocytes. Plasma levels of potassium are rigidly controlled between 3.5–5 mmol/L. 98% of potassium in the body is intracellular, especially muscle cells.

Hyperkalaemia
Causes are many and include:
1 Decreased excretion due to kidney disease or adrenal mineralocorticoid insufficiency (hypoaldosteronism) as occurs with Addison's disease.
2 Shift of potassium from the inside to the outside of cells due to acidosis e.g. lactic acidosis, DKA.
3 Destruction of cells—haemolysis, rhabdomyolysis, malignant hyperthermia, burns.
4 Exogenous source—diet (excessive bananas, honeydew melon), massive blood transfusion, iatrogenic.
5 Drugs e.g. suxamethonium, K^+ sparing diuretic e.g. spironolactone.
Hyperkalaemia is severe if > 6.5 mmol/L and very severe if > 7.0 mmol/L.

Clinical effects of hyperkalaemia
1 ECG changes including peaked T waves, flattened P waves and widening of the QRS complex and PR interval. Development of deep S waves, sinus arrest with nodal rhythm, sine wave ECG pattern and asystole may occur.
2 Cardiac arrhythmias such as ventricular ectopics, atrial arrest, atrio-ventricular block, VT and VF.

3 Antagonism of NDNMBDs.
4 Tingling, weakness, flaccid paralysis.
5 Hypotension.
6 Dyspnoea, hyperventilation.
7 Nausea and vomiting, ileus.

Treatment

Adult

1 Stop any exogenous potassium administration.
2 Calcium chloride 5–10 mL 10% solution IV or calcium gluconate 15–30 mL 10% solution IV. *See Calcium.* This is to stabilise the myocardium against the effects of hyperkalaemia.
3 Glucose 50% 50 mL IV + 10 units Actrapid (to cause cellular uptake of potassium).
4 Salbutamol nebulised 15 mg over 30 min.
5 Calcium resonium 15 g PO q 6 h or PR 30 g q 8 h.
6 Treat the cause e.g. acute renal insufficiency.
7 Haemodialysis.
8 Sodium bicarbonate 8.4% solution 1 mL/kg IV if there is a co-existing metabolic acidosis e.g. malignant hyperthermia. **Do not mix calcium and sodium bicarbonate as calcium bicarbonate (a solid) may be formed.**
9 Consider hydrocortisone 1–2 mg/kg if suspicion of adrenal insufficiency.

Treatment

Child

1 Stop any exogenous K^+ intake.
2 Calcium chloride 10% 0.5 mL/kg IV over 2–5 min.
3 Glucose 50% 1 mL/kg + Actrapid 0.1 unit/kg (max 10 units).
4 Salbutamol nebulised 2.5 mg.
5 Sodium bicarbonate 8.4% solution 1 mL/kg IV **if** there is co-existing metabolic acidosis.
6 Resonium 0.3–1 g/kg PO or PR 6 h.
7 Haemodialysis.

Hypokalaemia

There are many causes, including:
1 vomiting, diarrhoea
2 diuretic therapy
3 transient redistribution of potassium into cells, as occurs with hypokalaemic periodic paralysis or metabolic or respiratory alkalosis
4 low potassium intake (rare)
5 hypothermia
6 dialysis
7 mineralocorticoid excess (**see Conn's syndrome**)
8 drugs such as insulin, catecholamines (adrenaline, beta-adrenergic agonists such as salbutamol)
9 excessive sweating.

Clinical effects of hypokalaemia

This is severe if $K^+ < 2.5$ mmol/L.
1 Characteristic ECG changes—atrial ectopics, prolongation of the PR interval, T wave inversion and prominent U waves.

2 Dysrhythmias such as atrial and ventricular tachycardias and torsades de pointes.
3 Weakness, hypotonicity, ventilatory failure.
4 Increased duration of effect of NDNMBDs.
5 Rhabdomyolysis if prolonged severe hypokalaemia.

Treatment (adult)

1 IV potassium chloride. For rapid correction give 10 mmol in 100 mL N/S over 30 min–1 h, preferably in a large peripheral vein or central vein. Check the serum K^+ each h and repeat this dose until serum K^+ is 4 mmol/L.
2 In less urgent situations, add 40 mmol K^+ to a 1000 mL bag of N/S and administer no faster that 250 mL/h.
3 Serum magnesium is often low as well and should also be corrected.
4 Patients with hypokalaemic periodic paralysis may suffer rebound hyperkalaemia with replacement therapy.
5 Oral potassium replacement can be used for mild hypokalaemia.
6 Treat the underlying cause.

◗ Praxbind

See *Idarucizumab (Praxbind)*.

◗ Precedex

See *Dexmedetomidine (Precedex)*.

◗ Preeclampsia/eclampsia

Introduction

Preeclampsia is a multisystem disorder unique to pregnancy, occurring after the 20th week. It occurs in up to 7% of deliveries and can occur up to 6 weeks post-delivery. The most common feature is hypertension defined as SBP > 140 mmHg and DBP > 90 mmHg. The second most common feature is proteinuria, which is an indicator of kidney damage. It is the fourth most common cause of direct maternal death in Australia. If 1 or more seizures occur, the condition is termed 'eclampsia'. Risk factors are multiple and varied and include first pregnancy, obesity, twin pregnancy and diabetes mellitus. In women with pre-existing chronic hypertension, aspirin 81 mg/day from the 12th week of pregnancy, reduces the risk of developing preeclampsia.

Aetiology

The cause of the condition is unknown but thought to be related to an abnormal uterine/placental interaction. There is inadequate cytotrophoblastic uterine invasion (abnormal placentation). This results in failure of the uterine spiral arteries to transform into low-resistance, large-calibre vessels as the pregnancy progresses. In preeclampsia, the spiral arteries become high-resistance vessels responsive to vasomotor stimuli, leading to placental ischaemia and infarction. The placenta responds by releasing pro-inflammatory substances such as soluble endoglin and soluble endothelial growth factor that cause endothelial cell dysfunction in the mother. This leads to:
1 vasoconstriction
2 salt retention by the kidney
3 hypertension due to **1** and **2** above.

Effects of preeclampsia on organ systems

Cardiovascular
1 Hypertension.
2 Hypovolaemia due to arterial vasoconstriction and capillary leakage.
3 Increased SVR causing increased LV workload.
4 Myocardial dysfunction may occur with cardiogenic pulmonary oedema.

Respiratory
1 Increased pulmonary capillary permeability and decreased plasma oncotic pressure (due to proteinuria) may cause non-cardiogenic pulmonary oedema.
2 Pharyngeal and laryngeal oedema.

Neurological effects
1 Headache due to hypertension ± brain oedema.
2 Visual disturbances such as flashing lights due to retinal ischaemia secondary to vasospasm.
3 Hyperreflexia with sustained clonus.
4 Seizures (eclampsia).
5 Intracranial haemorrhage.

Renal effects
1 Proteinuria (spot urine protein/creatinine ratio > 30 mg/mmol).
2 Oliguria (< 80 mL/4 h).
3 Serum creatinine > 90 μmol/L.
4 Serum urate is not included in the diagnostic criteria but may be a marker of increased fetal risk. A rapidly rising urate level may suggest worsening preeclampsia. Normal urate levels are 0.15–0.40 mmol/L.

Hepatic/gastrointestinal effects
1 Hepatocellular damage with raised serum transaminases and liver swelling, which may lead to liver pain/rupture.
2 Nausea and vomiting.

Haematological
1 Thrombocytopenia (platelet count < 100 000/mm^3).
2 Haemolysis causing a rising bilirubin and lactate. Urine can become red or black. There may be decreased haptoglobin.
3 Coagulopathy/DIC.
4 Increased blood viscosity.

Utero/placental/fetal
1 Intrauterine growth retardation/fetal death.
2 Placental abruption.
3 Oligohydramnios.
4 Abnormal umbilical artery Doppler flows.

Multifactorial
1 Hyperkalaemia due to haemolysis and renal failure.
2 Generalised oedema.

HELLP syndrome

This syndrome describes a combination of **H**aemolysis, **E**levated **L**iver enzymes, **L**ow **P**latelet count and preeclampsia/eclampsia. Up to 15% of patients are not hypertensive. Laboratory findings suggestive of HELLP syndrome are:

1 lactate dehydrogenase (LDH) > 600 U/L. LDH NR 140–280 U/L.
2 aspartate aminotransferase (AST) > 2 × normal. The normal range is 8–33 U/L.
3 platelet count < 100000/mm^3.

Classification of preeclampsia

1 **Early onset vs late onset.** Early onset occurs before 34 weeks' gestation, comprises about 20% of cases and is associated with an 8 × greater cardiovascular morbidity. Risk of recurrence in subsequent pregnancies is high. Late onset (after 34 weeks) tends to be a milder disease and is less likely to occur in subsequent pregnancies.
2 **Severity of illness.**
   • Mild disease—SBP 140–159 mmHg, DBP 90–110 mmHg, proteinuria < 300 mg/24 h (spot urine protein/creatinine ratio > 30 mg/mmol).
   • Severe disease—SBP > 160 mmHg, DBP > 110 mmHg, evidence of major systemic illness e.g. thrombocytopenia, deranged LFTs.
There is no moderate category.

Management

The only definitive management is removing the placenta. Otherwise, treatment aims at alleviating the effects of preeclampsia. The main aims of treatment are:

1 Blood pressure control.
2 Seizure prevention/management.
3 Fluid management.
4 Management of other complications such as thrombocytopenia.
5 Optimising delivery time depending on maternal and fetal well-being.

Hypertension control

The blood pressure target is SBP 140–150 mmHg and DBP 90–100 mmHg. If hypertension is severe (SBP > 160 mmHg, DBP > 110 mmHg), treat with:

1 Nifedipine 5–20 mg PO, repeat after 30 min if needed. If the patient is on a magnesium infusion, giving nifedipine may cause marked hypotension.
2 Labetalol—20 mg IV over 2 min. Repeat 20–50 mg doses after 10–20 min up to four doses. The maximum cumulative dose is 300 mg/day. Do not use this drug if the patient has asthma, heart block or bradycardia.
3 Hydralazine—5 mg IV over 2 min. Repeat dose after 30 min up to 3 doses. Give a 250 mL IV bolus of crystalloid.
4 Diazoxide—30 mg IV. Repeat dose q 5 min to a maximum of 300 mg.
If more aggressive management is required, insert an arterial line. Consider:
1 Labetalol infusion—20–160 mg/h IV.
2 Hydralazine infusion—0.5–10 mg/h IV.
3 Sodium nitroprusside should be considered for severe refractory hypertension. This may result in fetal cyanide and thiocyanate toxicity. Urgent delivery should be organised. **See *Sodium nitroprusside (SNP).***
4 Clevidipine, a calcium antagonist hypotensive agent, may have a role in this situation. However, there is little information in the literature so no guidelines can be offered. **See *Clevidipine.***
5 If there is associated pulmonary oedema, consider a GTN infusion 5 mcg/min, increasing every 3–5 min to a maximum of 100 mcg/min. **See *Glyceryl trinitrate (GTN).***

For milder hypertension consider:

1 Methyldopa—250–750 mg PO q 8 h. If inadequate add:
2 Labetalol—100–400 mg PO q 8 h. If inadequate add:
3 Nifedipine—20 mg PO q 12 h, max 40 mg q 12 h.

Other drugs to consider are oral prazosin 20–50 mg q 8 h and oral hydralazine 25–50 mg q 8 h.

Seizure prevention/treatment

Eclamptic seizures are an obstetric emergency and may be preceded by headache and/or visual disturbances. The seizures are usually self-limiting. Treatment includes:

1 Declare an emergency, activate the emergency response system.
2 A, B—ensure patent airway and adequate oxygenation.
3 Diazepam IV 2 mg/min to a maximum of 10 mg or clonazepam IV 1–2 mg over 2–5 min.
4 Magnesium therapy. 4 g IV over 10 minutes. If pre-prepared bags are available these contain 40 g of magnesium in 500 mL. Administer 50 mL then commence an infusion of 1 g/h (12.5 mL/h).

To prevent seizures, commence a magnesium infusion using the pre-prepared bags (40 g in 500 mL). Give a loading dose of 4 g over 20 min (50 mL) then an infusion of 1 g/h (12.5 mL/h). If a patient has a seizure while on magnesium therapy, give a bolus of 2–4 g over 10 minutes (25–50 mL). Monitor deep tendon reflexes to identify magnesium toxicity. *See Magnesium.*

Fluid management

Pulmonary oedema is a life-threatening complication of preeclampsia.

1 A general guideline is to administer fluid at a rate of 1 mL/kg/h ≈ 80 mL/h.
2 A urine output of > 80 mL/4 h is acceptable.
3 If urine output is less than this and renal function is normal and there is no evidence of pulmonary oedema, a bolus of 250 mL Hartmann's can be given. Assess the response over the next 4 h. Aggressively chasing urine output with IV fluids may precipitate pulmonary oedema.
4 If pulmonary oedema occurs, treat with:
   a) Non-invasive ventilation. *See Non-invasive ventilation.*
   b) Urgent reduction of elevated BP—GTN is the drug of choice (**see** *Hypertension control* above).
   c) Frusemide 20–40 mg IV over 2 min. Give a second dose of 40–60 mg after 30 min if response inadequate.
   d) Fluid restriction.
   e) Sit patient up.

Neuraxial anaesthesia

1 Obtain a FBC—if platelet count > 100 000/mm^3, proceed.
2 If platelet count > 75 000/mm^3 and coagulation tests are normal, proceed.
3 A FBC within 24 h is acceptable in mild disease. A FBC < 6 h before neuraxial anaesthesia is acceptable for severe disease.
4 If the platelet count < 50 000 mm^3 and/or coagulation studies are abnormal, neuraxial anaesthesia is contraindicated. Correct abnormalities with platelets and FFP and proceed to CS under GA.
5 A platelet count between 50 000 and 75 000 mm^3 is a grey area and a risk/benefit analysis must be made.

6 Do not fluid preload the patient.

7 Treat hypotension with IV fluid boluses of 250 mL unless pulmonary oedema is present.

8 Use vasoconstrictor drugs very cautiously.

9 The use of a combination of 2% lignocaine + adrenaline for epidural boluses for CS is probably safe but a hypertensive crisis due to absorbed adrenaline is possible.[21] Observe the patient carefully.

General anaesthesia for CS

1 Correct low platelets and coagulation abnormalities (see *Neuraxial anaesthesia* above).

2 Sudden severe rises in blood pressure must be avoided. The target SBP is < 160 mmHg and DBP is < 110 mmHg.

3 Consider a bolus of magnesium 2–4 g IV over 30 min prior to induction. This may increase the patient's sensitivity to NDNMBDs.

4 Insert an arterial line. Pre-oxygenate the patient. Prepare for a difficult intubation due to airway oedema. **See Difficult airway management.**

5 Commence a remifentanil infusion 1–1.5 mcg/kg/min and/or a bolus of 1 mcg/kg 60–90 s before induction.

6 Modified rapid sequence induction with propofol and rocuronium.

7 If hypertension persists, give boluses of esmolol 1–2 mg/kg IV.

8 Subsequent management as per the section on anaesthesia for Caesarean section earlier in this chapter, but do not give NSAIDs.

9 If postpartum haemorrhage occurs, do not give ergometrine, as severe hypertension may occur. Use misoprostol or carboprost. **See Postpartum haemorrhage (PPH).**

◖ Pre-excitation

Pre-excitation describes the situation in which impulses from the SA node are able to pass from the atria to the ventricles through an accessory pathway (AP), in addition to the AV node. Conduction through the AP is much faster than through the AV node. Therefore, the ventricles depolarise much sooner than normal, manifesting on the ECG as:

1 Short PR interval (< than three small squares, < 120 ms).

2 A slurred upstroke of the QRS (delta wave).

3 Widened QRS due to the addition of the delta wave.

Pre-excitation is usually intermittent. There will also be ST and T wave changes. This is because pre-excitation causes abnormal depolarisation of the ventricles leading to abnormal repolarisation. A positive delta wave leads to a ST segment depression and T wave inversion.

◖ Pregnancy and non-obstetric surgery

See Physiology of term pregnancy.

Introduction

About 1–2% of pregnancies are complicated by the need for non-obstetric surgery, most commonly appendicectomy and biliary disease.

Elective surgery

1 Elective surgery should be avoided during pregnancy, due to the perceived increased risk of miscarriage, fetal abnormalities and premature labour.

2 Whether all women of child-bearing age should be screened for pregnancy prior to elective surgery is a highly complex issue and beyond the focus of this manual.

3 Non-elective surgery is ideally performed between gestational age 13–26 weeks (small uterus, lowest risk of preterm delivery).[22]
4 Elective surgery should be delayed until 6 weeks postpartum.[22]
5 Giving corticosteroids to accelerate fetal lung maturity should be considered if major surgery is required after 32 weeks' gestation.

Anaesthesia and the unborn child

1 Although anaesthetic drugs in high doses have been shown to be teratogenic in animals, there is no evidence of teratogenicity in humans. A possible exception is sugammadex. Progesterone is critical for pregnancy maintenance and sugammadex encapsulates progesterone, so this drug should be avoided in early pregnancy.[23]
2 It is unknown whether anaesthetics affect fetal brain development. Repeated anaesthetics and surgery > 3 h may be harmful.
3 Although diazepam was thought to be associated with increased risk of cleft palate, no issues have been identified with the use of midazolam.
4 N_2O inhibits methionine synthetase and impairs DNA production. Use during the first and second trimester should be avoided.
5 Document fetal heart rate before and after anaesthesia and surgery.

General maternal issues

1 Regional and neuraxial anaesthesia are preferred to general anaesthesia to minimise fetal exposure to drugs.
2 Sedation should be used cautiously because of an increased risk of aspiration and respiratory depression.
3 Pregnant patients will desaturate faster than non-pregnant patients, due to the increased O_2 requirements of pregnancy and the reduction in FRC.
4 BIS/entropy monitoring may allow for titration of GA agents to avoid excessive dosages.

Cardiovascular issues

1 Aortocaval compression (supine hypotensive syndrome) may occur after 20 weeks' gestation. Consider 15° left lateral tilt.
2 Pregnant patients are at increased risk of thromboembolism.
3 It is imperative to maintain adequate blood pressure to avoid compromised uterine blood flow. Adequate maternal blood pressure is the most significant determinant of utero-placental perfusion. Maintain SBP > 100 mmHg and MAP > 65 mmHg.
4 Phenylephrine or metaraminol are reasonable vasopressors to use. Ephedrine is also safe.

Respiratory issues

1 Pregnancy is associated with an increased aspiration risk from as early as the 12th week, and especially after the 20th week. A rapid sequence induction and intubation should be performed after 20 weeks' gestation and considered before this time. Sodium citrate prior to induction should be considered.
2 There is increased vascularity and oedema of the airway. This may make intubation more difficult, as may breast enlargement and weight gain. Nasal intubation is likely to cause epistaxis. Use a smaller ET tube than usual and videolaryngoscopy is recommended. *See Difficult airway management.*
3 Pregnant women will desaturate faster than those in the non-pregnant state due to increased oxygen consumption and reduced FRC.

4 IPPV should aim to maintain the physiological respiratory alkalosis of pregnancy with an $ETCO_2$ of 30–32 mmHg during the last half of pregnancy.[24] Both hypercarbia and hypocarbia can be deleterious to the fetus. Hypercarbia can cause fetal acidosis and myocardial depression. Hypocarbia can cause decreased uterine blood flow.

Postoperative care

NSAIDs should **not** be used, especially in the early first trimester and after 30 weeks' gestation. There is an increased risk of miscarriage and fetal abnormalities in early pregnancy. After 30 weeks' gestation there is increased risk of premature closure of the ductus arteriosus and oligohydramnios. A single dose in mid-gestation is probably safe.

Radiological issues and pregnancy

See also Radiation dangers. The effects of X-rays on the fetus depends on the dose of radiation exposure. This may be measured in rad, roentgen (R), gray (Gy), roentgen equivalent man (rem) and Sievert (Sv). 1 Sv = 1 Gy = 100 rem = 107.2 R.

1 The risk of adverse fetal outcome begins to rise above a threshold of 50 mGy (50 mSv).

2 The most dangerous period for malformations is between 4 and 17 weeks.

3 Prior to 4 weeks, the fetus is either destroyed or no malformation occurs (all or nothing).

4 There may be a slightly increased risk of childhood cancers. Use fetal shielding if possible.

Table P2 Estimated radiation exposure to the fetus from procedures involving X-rays

Procedure	Fetal exposure (mSv)
CXR	up to 0.01
Ventilation scan	0.01–0.1
Pulmonary angiography	> 0.5
Cervical spine 3 views	0.001
CT head	0.5
Abdo X-ray	2
Pelvic X-ray	3
Abdo CT	26–90

◗ Pregnancy, physiological changes

See Physiology of term pregnancy.

◗ Pre-oxygenation

See Rapid sequence induction.

◗ Prochlorperazine (Stemetil)

Description

Phenothiazine of the piperazine subclass, acts by a central anti-dopaminergic receptor effect. Used to treat:

1 nausea and vomiting

2 vertigo.

Dose

Adult

5–20 mg PO q 8–12 h, IM 12.5 mg up to q 6 h.

Note:

1 Cannot be used in patients with Parkinson's disease. *See Parkinson's disease.*
2 Can cause neuroleptic malignant syndrome. *See Neuroleptic malignant syndrome (NMS).*
3 Can cause dystonic reaction. *See Dystonic reaction, acute.*
4 Not licensed for IV use.

◐ Proladone

This drug is oxycodone used as a suppository. It has the same potency as oral oxycodone.

◐ Promethazine (Phenergan)

Description

Promethazine is a phenothiazine antihistamine drug with sedative and anti-emetic properties. Its main actions are:

1 H_1 histaminergic receptor blocker.
2 Has anticholinergic and antidopaminergic effects.
3 Has antiserotonergic properties.

It is useful for the treatment of:

• allergic reactions
• pruritus
• nausea and vomiting.

Dose

Adult

25–50 mg IV or 25–75 mg PO daily in divided doses.

Child

0.2–0.5 mg/kg/dose q 6–8 h IV, IM or PO.

Precautions

1 If given IV, promethazine can leach from the vein and cause severe tissue damage.
2 Intra-arterial injection can result in gangrene peripherally. *See Intra-arterial injection.*
3 If used parenterally, injection should be deep IM or in a well-functioning drip in a concentration of at least 25 mg/mL and no faster than 25 mg/min.

◐ Propafenone (Rythmol)

Class 1c antiarrhythmic drug. Also has beta blocker effects. Used to treat rapid arrhythmias (atrial and ventricular). Can cause bradycardia and bronchospasm.

◐ Propofol (Diprivan)

Description

Propofol is an intravenous anaesthetic agent and one of the most important advances in anaesthetic care in the last 200 years. This drug is a 2,6-diisopropyl phenol (a hindered phenol). It is used for induction of anaesthesia, maintenance of anaesthesia and for sedation. It can also be used to treat status epilepticus when other drugs have not worked. *See Status epilepticus (SE)*. In Canada it is used for medically assisted death. The use of propofol for the execution of criminals is banned by the manufacturer.

Mechanism of action

It is thought to work in part by interaction with GABA-mediated chloride channels in the brain.

Propofol formulations

Propofol formulations are made up of the active drug propofol, mixed with a lipid base.

1 Fresofol 1% has a lipid base of soya oil.
2 Fresofol 1% MLT/LCT has a lipid base of coconut oil, palm kernel oil and soya oil.
3 Fospropofol is a water-soluble prodrug.
4 Propofol-Lipuro—this formulation of 1 or 2% propofol uses medium- and long-chain fatty acids and may produce less pain on injection.
5 Aquafol—uses surfactants and co-surfactants to emulsify the propofol in water. It avoids the use of animal products (eggs) but is very painful on injection.

Dose for induction of anaesthesia

Adult
2.5–3.5 mg/kg.

Child
2–2.5 mg/kg.

Dose for maintenance of anaesthesia

Use a target-controlled infusion (TCI) with BIS or entropy monitoring. TCI dose for maintenance of anaesthesia is about 3–5.3 mcg/mL.

Dose for sedation

Using TCI—0.5–2 mcg/mL.

Advantages

1 Propofol is the only practical safe drug for total intravenous anaesthesia (TIVA). Rapid redistribution and elimination result in short duration of action, even after prolonged use.
2 Less hangover effect and less nausea and vomiting than thiopentone.
3 TCI with propofol is less likely to cause nausea and vomiting than volatile anaesthesia.
4 Propofol has anticonvulsant properties and is useful for treating status epilepticus. *See Status epilepticus (SE)*.
5 Propofol is probably safe as a single dose for patients with porphyria but it may not be safe to administer a propofol infusion. *See Porphyria*.
6 It has anxiolytic effects.
7 Allergic reactions are extremely rare. Adult patients with egg or soy allergy can have propofol safely.[25] A more cautious approach in children may be justified.[26]

Disadvantages

1 Propofol may cause pain on injection. This can be prevented by mixing 30 mg lignocaine with 20 mL of propofol.
2 TCI propofol anaesthesia for children aged between 1 month and 3 years should not be used for longer than 60 min.

3 Propofol has abuse potential due to it causing mild euphoria, hallucinations and disinhibition. Several deaths have resulted.

4 It may cause seizure-like movements on induction. Some clinicians avoid its use in epileptics.

5 Propofol sedation is contraindicated for children in ICU. Propofol infusions in ICU in children and young adults have been associated with rhabdomyolysis, metabolic acidosis, cardiac dysrhythmias and death. This is called propofol infusion syndrome and may be due to propofol-induced disruption of fatty acid metabolism, leading to cardiac and skeletal muscle death.

6 There are animal studies suggesting that propofol may be harmful to the fetus. Its use in pregnancy and obstetric anaesthesia is **not supported** by the manufacturer. However, there is no human data suggesting harm. The safety of sedating pregnant patients with propofol in the ICU is unknown.

7 Propofol supports bacterial growth. It should be used promptly after drawing up into the syringe.

8 Although TIVA is felt to be more environmentally friendly than volatile drugs, propofol is not completely environmentally innocent. Propofol is very toxic to aquatic life and does not break down easily. Propofol needs to be incinerated to be destroyed.[27]

○ Propranolol (Inderal)

Non-selective beta blocker drug. **See Beta-adrenergic receptor blocker drugs.** Used to treat:
- angina
- tachyarrhythmias
- thyrotoxicosis
- hypertrophic cardiomyopathy
- tremors
- migraine
- phaeochromocytoma (with an alpha receptor blocker)
- acute exacerbations of porphyria.

Dose

Adult

1–10 mg IV titrated to desired clinical response. 40 mg PO q 8–12 h.

Note:

1 Not recommended for the treatment of hypertension because of an increased risk of adverse outcomes.[28]

2 Do not cease abruptly as angina or myocardial infarction may result.

○ Prostaglandin F2-alpha (Carboprost)

Carboprost is a synthetic form of prostaglandin F2-alpha. It is used to cause uterine contraction for therapeutic abortion and for the treatment of postpartum haemorrhage due to uterine atony. **See Postpartum haemorrhage (PPH).**

○ Prostate surgery

See Trans-urethral resection of prostate (TURP).

◑ Prosthetic joints, infection prophylaxis

There is concern that bacteraemia from surgical sources could result in infection in a prosthetic joint.[29] Many orthopaedic surgeons advise:
1 Avoiding non-urgent dental treatment for 3 months post joint replacement
2 Having amoxicillin 2 g PO 1 h before a dental procedure. If penicillin allergic, have clindamycin 600 mg PO 1 h before the procedure.

Other experts feel this advice is unnecessary.[30] Other factors may influence the decision to give antibiotics or not. These factors include:
1 the orthopaedic surgeon's expressed wishes
2 patient distress if antibiotics are not given
3 significant dental infection e.g. dental abscess
4 an immunocompromised patient.

◑ Protamine

Description
Protamine is a mixture of cationic proteins from fish sperm. It is used to reverse the anticoagulant effect of heparin.

Dose for reversal of unfractionated heparin
1 mg of protamine IV neutralises 100 U of heparin. However, over time less protamine is required. After 30–60 min since heparin administration, give 0.5–0.75 mg/100 U. If greater than 2 h since heparin administration, give 0.25–0.375 mg/100 U heparin.

Give the drug slowly as it can cause hypotension, bradycardia, bronchospasm, pulmonary oedema, pulmonary vasoconstriction, pulmonary hypertension and allergic reactions. Do not exceed 50 mg.

Dose for reversal of fractionated heparin
- **Dalteparin (Fragmin)**—1 mg protamine neutralises 100 U dalteparin. If bleeding continues or APTT remains prolonged 2–4 h after protamine, give 0.5 mg protamine/100 U dalteparin.
- **Enoxaparin (Clexane)**—If < 8 h after last dose of enoxaparin, give protamine 1 mg/1 mg enoxaparin. If 8–12 h after last dose of enoxaparin give protamine 0.5 mg/1 mg enoxaparin. If bleeding continues or APPT remains high, give protamine 0.5 mg/1 mg enoxaparin. If > 12 h since enoxaparin dose, protamine is not indicated.

Protamine allergic reactions
These are most likely in patients with:
1 fish allergy
2 vasectomy
3 insulin exposure
4 previous protamine exposure.

◑ Protein C and protein S

Protein C is an anticoagulant protein that acts by inactivating FVa and FVIIIa. It also stimulates plasminogen activator. Normal levels are 70–164%. Protein S enhances the action of protein C. Normal levels are 63–160%. Deficiency in either or both results in a prothrombotic state. Note that the factor V Leiden mutation also results in a thrombogenic state. This is because it prevents protein C from inactivating FVa.

◖ Prothrombin complex concentrate (PCC)

These drugs bypass the effects of certain types of anticoagulant drugs such as warfarin and apixaban.
See Prothrombinex®-VF.

◖ Prothrombinex®-VF

This drug is a type of four-factor prothrombin complex concentrate (PCC). It contains factors II, IX and X and low levels of VII. It is used to reverse the effects of warfarin in emergency settings. Four-factor PCC can also be used to treat patients that are haemorrhaging while on some anti-factor Xa drugs. These include apixaban, rivaroxaban and endoxaban. However, adexanet alfa is preferred. *See Adexanet alfa (andexXa).* Prothrombinex®-VF is contraindicated in patients with thrombosis or DIC. The vials contain heparin so do not use this drug in patients with HITTS. *See Heparin-induced thrombocytopenia (HIT).*

Dose for warfarin reversal

30–50 IU/kg IV infused over 20–30 min. The actual dose used depends on the initial INR and the target INR. The drug takes 15 min to work and effects last 12–24 h. To prevent a rebound in INR values, give with vitamin K. *See Warfarin.*

◖ Prothrombin time

Prothrombin time (PT) is a measure of the extrinsic and common clotting pathways. *See Clotting pathways.* It measures the activity of clotting factors fibrinogen, prothrombin, V, VII and X. It is performed by adding tissue factor to a plasma specimen after citrate has been reversed with calcium. The clotting time is then measured. NR for PT is 10–12 s. *See International normalised ratio (INR).*

◖ Pseudocholinesterase deficiency

See Suxamethonium/succinylcholine and sux apnoea.

◖ Pulmonary artery stenosis

See Pulmonary stenosis.

◖ Pulmonary atresia

This is total obstruction of the right ventricular outflow tract. Postnatal survival is impossible without a patent ductus arteriosus or major collaterals from the aorta to the pulmonary arteries.

◖ Pulmonary embolism (PE)

Description

PE is a life-threatening emergency and is one of the causes of sudden cardiac arrest. It may be due to blood clot, gas embolism, amniotic fluid, bone marrow (fat) or bone cement. *See Amniotic fluid embolism (AFE), Fat embolism syndrome (FES) and bone cement implantation syndrome (BCIS)* and *Gas embolism.* The rest of this section is concerned with blood clot pulmonary embolism. PE is the occlusion of pulmonary arteries by thrombus or thrombi that originate from elsewhere, usually the legs or pelvis.

Causes/predisposing factors

Conditions that predispose to deep venous thrombosis also predispose to PE. *See Deep venous thrombosis (DVT) prophylaxis.* The most common risk factors in general terms are:

1 obesity
2 smoking
3 hypertension
4 long-haul air travel
5 surgery
6 trauma
7 immobilisation
8 pneumonia
9 COVID-19
10 CCF
11 genetic factors
12 oral contraceptive pill.

Pathophysiology

The pathophysiology of PE centres on mechanical obstruction of the pulmonary arteries and release of humoral substances by the tissues, platelets and other sites. Effects include:

1 sudden increase in pulmonary vascular resistance
2 ventilation/perfusion mismatch
3 reduced cardiac output
4 impaired RV function, which can be profound
5 hypotension
6 lung ischaemia/infarction.
   Organised persistent emboli may cause pulmonary hypertension over time.

Clinical presentation

1 Acute dyspnoea/tachypnoea/hypoxia.
2 Pleuritic chest pain.
3 Cough.
4 Haemoptysis.
5 Tachycardia.
6 Hypotension.
7 Distended internal jugular veins.
8 RV heave.
9 Presyncope/syncope.
10 Confusion.
11 Cardiac arrest.
12 Presence of a DVT.

Diagnosis

1 Clinical presentation in the context of predisposing factor(s) e.g. long-haul flight.
2 CXR—atelectasis, focal infiltrates, elevated hemidiaphragm, pleural effusion, loss of vascular markings, peripheral wedge-shaped density, enlargement of right descending pulmonary artery.
3 ECG—tachycardia, prominent S wave in I, Q wave in III and inverted T wave in III (S1Q3T3). There may be RV strain pattern with RBBB, right axis deviation and P pulmonale.

4 ABG—hypoxia, hypocapnia, increased alveolar to arterial O_2 gradient (**see A-a gradient**).

5 D-dimer test—elevated levels suggest recent thrombus.

6 CT pulmonary angiography.

7 Ventilation/perfusion (V/Q) scanning—useful if renal insufficiency or CT contrast contraindicated. Can be done as a bed-side test.

8 Duplex ultrasonography to detect leg or arm thrombus.

9 Elevated troponins—suggesting RV ischaemia.

Treatment

1 If cardiac arrest, **see Cardiac arrest**.

2 Oxygen therapy.

3 Treat hypotension with crystalloid boluses and vasopressors. Noradrenaline may be required.

4 Anticoagulation—heparin or fractionated heparin:
   a) Heparin—LD 5000 IU IV then infusion 18 U/kg/h. Aim for APPT 1.5–2.5 × control (i.e a target APTT of 50–90 s).
   b) Fractionated heparin e.g. enoxaparin 1 mg/kg q 12 h or 1.5 mg/kg/day subcut.

5 In more critical situations (e.g. patients with persistent hypotension) consider:
   a) Systemic thrombolytic therapy with alteplase (tissue plasminogen activator).
   b) Catheter-directed therapy—thrombolytics or embolectomy.
   c) Surgical embolectomy, especially in patients who are not candidates for thrombolytic therapy or who fail this therapy.

6 ECMO may be lifesaving as a bridge to the therapies described above. **See Extracorporeal membrane oxygenation (ECMO)**.

7 Placement of an IVC filter in patients who cannot be anticoagulated to protect them from subsequent emboli.

◖ Pulmonary function tests

See Lung function tests.

◖ Pulmonary hypertension

Introduction

Pulmonary hypertension is a vast and complex spectrum of disease processes. Only a very brief overview of this topic can be provided here. The gold standard for diagnosing pulmonary hypertension (PH) is by right heart catheterisation and measurement of mean pulmonary artery pressure (NR 12–15 mmHg). Pulmonary hypertension can be categorised as:

- **mild**   20–40 mmHg
- **moderate**   41–55 mmHg
- **severe**   > 55 mmHg.

Echocardiographic studies can be used to infer the presence of pulmonary hypertension.

Classification

Pulmonary hypertension has been placed into five groups by the World Health Organization:

1 Pulmonary arterial hypertension not due to lung disease or pulmonary emboli. This can be due to many causes, including idiopathic, inherited, drugs (e.g. fenfluramine), toxins and, in association with many other diseases such as HIV, connective tissue disorders and congenital heart disease (CHD). Examples of CHD that can cause pulmonary hypertension include atrial septal defect, ventricular septal defect and patent ductus arteriosus.

2 Left heart disease associated PH (LV failure, valvular heart disease).

3 PH due to lung disease and/or hypoxia e.g. due to OSA.

4 Chronic thromboembolic pulmonary hypertension (CTEPH).

5 PH with unclear multi-factorial mechanisms.

Pathophysiology

Pulmonary vascular resistance (PVR) is normally very low and constant, even with exercise, unless the exercise is beyond the anaerobic threshold. The right ventricle (RV) is normally a low-pressure, low-resistance pump. In patients with pulmonary hypertension the following features are seen:

1 Pulmonary vasoconstriction.

2 Cellular proliferation in the intima and adventitial layers of the pulmonary vasculature.

3 Localised thrombi formation, which adds to the obstruction of capillary blood flow.

4 RV hypertrophy and stiffening, with diastolic dysfunction, elevated filling pressures and right atrial (RA) distension leading to elevated CVP.

5 Tricuspid valve regurgitation due to tricuspid annulus dilatation.

6 Bulging of the intraventricular septum into the LV reducing LV filling and cardiac output (CO).

7 Impaired venous return and intermittent reversal of flow in the SVC and IVC. This leads to hepatic congestion, decreased renal perfusion and peripheral oedema.

8 A mild tachycardia helps the situation by reducing the time for regurgitation to occur and reducing RV distension, by shortening the filling time. Bradycardia has the opposite effect.

9 The RV becomes increasingly hypertrophied resulting in right coronary artery (RCA) blood flow only occurring in diastole (as occurs with the LV). A fall in SVR may result in inadequate RCA blood flow, leading to RV ischaemia and failure in a downward spiral.

10 Pulmonary valve dysfunction may occur.

11 RV failure may result in a fall in PAP.

Clinical picture

1 Asymptomatic.

2 Dyspnoea.

3 Chest pain.

4 Syncope.

5 Haemoptysis.

6 Arrhythmias e.g. AF.

7 Clinical signs such as RV heave, TR murmur, loud second heart sound with increased splitting, evidence of RV failure (elevated CVP, hepatomegaly), hoarse voice due to left main pulmonary artery enlargement stretching the left recurrent laryngeal nerve.

8 Evidence of the causative disease such as pulmonary interstitial fibrosis.

WHO PH functional class

1 Class 1—asymptomatic.
2 Class 2—dyspnoea, chest pain or near syncope with ordinary activity.
3 Class 3—marked limitation of ordinary activity but comfortable at rest.
4 Class 4—all symptoms present at rest and worsen with activity.

Investigations

1 ECG—RV strain pattern. *See Electrocardiography (ECG)—a brief guide.*
2 CXR—may show enlarged heart, prominent pulmonary arteries and evidence of causative lung disease.
3 Right heart catheterisation—this is the most diagnostic test and enables pressure measurements to accurately grade the severity of the PH.
4 Transthoracic or transoesophageal echocardiography is extremely helpful and may be diagnostic. RV hypertrophy, right atrial dilatation, tricuspid regurgitation and ventricular septal displacement will typically be seen.
5 MRI scanning of the heart.
6 Six-minute walk test. Less than 300 m correlates with increased morbidity and mortality while > 500 m is reassuring.
7 Brain natriuretic peptide (BNP)—if significantly elevated is suggestive of severe disease. *See Cardiac risk for non-cardiac surgery.*

Treatment

1 Endothelin receptor antagonists. These include bosentan, ambrisentan and macitentan. Unfortunately, they are contraindicated in pregnancy due to teratogenicity.
2 Phosphodiesterase type 5 inhibitors. These drugs increase nitric oxide in the pulmonary vascular bed and include sildenafil and riociguat. *See Phosphodiesterase (PDE) and phosphodiesterase inhibitors.*
3 Prostacyclin analogues—these can be administered continuously IV e.g. epoprostenol or inhaled e.g. iloprost. There is a subcutaneous drug also available called treprostinil.
4 Soluble guanylate cyclase stimulants.

Anaesthesia

'Keep them where they live.' Aim to maintain the same haemodynamic parameters for the awake non-sedated patient while anaesthetised. CO tends to be fixed due to inability of the RV to increase its output. An arterial line should be placed in most cases and a central venous catheter should also be considered.

1 Avoid any factors that will increase PVR. These are:
   a) hypoxia
   b) hypercarbia
   c) acidosis
   d) N_2O
   e) adrenaline, dopamine and other alpha agonists
   f) PEEP, large tidal volumes
   g) cold, anxiety, stress—keep the patient warm
   h) sympathetic stimulation e.g. pain.
2 PVR can be reduced by:
   a) hypocarbia.
   b) inhaled nitric oxide or inhaled iloprost, or inhaled or IV prostacyclin (also called prostaglandin I2 or PGI2 or epoprostenol).
   c) isoprenaline may be beneficial.

3 To maintain haemodynamic stability:
   a) Avoid marked decreases in venous return. This will result in decreased RV filling with decreased RV output. Correct fluid and blood loss rapidly.
   b) Avoid marked decreases in SVR. The patient will be unable to maintain BP by increasing CO. Treat hypotension with boluses of phenylephrine or an infusion. Metaraminol, vasopressin and noradrenaline can also be considered. SAB is strongly not recommended for these patients. A slowly titrated epidural block or low-dose spinal component CSE, with invasive monitoring, are preferred options.
   c) Avoid drugs that cause myocardial depression.
   d) Maintain HR. Bradycardia may result in RV failure for the reasons described above.
   e) IPPV may cause severe hypotension due to decreased venous return. PEEP and large tidal volumes should be avoided for the same reasons.
   f) Milrinone can be useful for increasing cardiac output but causes vasodilation, so should be infused with vasopressin or noradrenaline. Give an LD of 50 mcg/kg over 10 min then an infusion of 0.25–0.75 mcg/kg/min.
   g) Frusemide may be required to reduce RV overload.
   h) Dobutamine may be helpful for heart failure.
4 NSAIDs are contraindicated.

Specific pulmonary vasodilator therapy for peri-operative use
1 Nebulised iloprost 10 mcg (a synthetic analogue of epoprostenol), 6–9 doses per day. Effects last 1–2 h. This can be administered using a PARI nebuliser.
2 IV epoprostenol. This can also be nebulised with an ultrasonic nebuliser.[31]
3 Subcut treprostinil.
4 Bosentan and ambrisentan are endothelin receptor antagonists used orally.
5 Riociguat is a guanylate cyclase stimulator oral medication.
6 Sildenafil is a PDE V inhibitor used orally.
7 Inhaled nitric oxide 20–40 ppm.

Patient in extremis/peri-arrest
1 Prostacyclin IV 25–50 mcg × 3 doses.
2 Epoprostenol given by Aeroneb® if patient intubated, given at a rate of 5–10 mL/h.
3 Consider ECMO.

Obstetrics
Maternal mortality is about 30%. Women with significant pulmonary hypertension should be advised against pregnancy. Prior to labour, the most hazardous period is between 20 and 30 weeks.[31] Death is most likely to occur soon after delivery from RV failure or thromboembolic disease. Invasive arterial BP monitoring should be used. Thromboembolic prophylaxis should be initiated as soon as it is safe to do so. Prostaglandin F2 alpha is contraindicated.

Epidural for labour
1 Epidural anaesthesia should be established slowly and carefully.
2 Forceps or vacuum extraction should be used during the second stage to avoid the effects of pushing/Valsalva.

Caesarean section under neuraxial anaesthesia
1 Epidural anaesthesia as described above can be used or CSE with a low-dose spinal component. For CSE, a spinal component of 0.5 mL heavy bupivacaine 0.5% is suggested plus cautious titration of the epidural component with ropivacaine 0.75%.
2 Single-shot SAB is contraindicated.

Caesarean section under general anaesthesia

GA should be performed following the principles described in *Caesarean section under neuraxial anaesthesia* above.

1. Carboprost (prostaglandin F2 alpha) causes intense pulmonary vasoconstriction and is contraindicated. Ergometrine may also be unsafe.[31] Misoprostol can be used.
2. Oxytocin should be given cautiously e.g. 0.1 unit boluses at delivery and 10 units/h of 40 units in 40 mL.
3. If cardiac arrest or patient in extremis, give prostacyclin IV 25–50 mcg × 3 doses. Epoprostenol (Flolan) can be given by Aeroneb® if the patient is intubated. Use a 500 mcg 50 mL solution nebulised at 5–10 mL/h.

Postop care

Monitor in a high-dependency/ICU environment for 48–72 h post surgery.

Pulmonary oedema

See Acute pulmonary oedema (APO) and ***Negative pressure pulmonary oedema (NPPO).***

Pulmonary stenosis (PS)

Description

This term refers to any lesion causing obstruction to RV outflow. The lesion may be valvular, subvalvular, supravalvular or in the pulmonary artery tree. These lesions produce a similar clinical picture.

Pulmonary artery stenosis

Pulmonary artery narrowing leads to an increased workload for the RV. If mild, it is often asymptomatic.

Causes

The narrowing may be in the pulmonary artery or the right and/or left branch.

1. It may be a birth defect associated with other congenital heart abnormalities.
2. It may develop after certain heart surgeries.
3. It can result from congenital rubella.
4. It may be part of certain syndromes such as Alagille syndrome.
5. Takayasu's arteritis may cause this lesion.

Pulmonary valve and subvalvular stenosis

This can be a congenital condition or can develop later in life. It is the most common congenital heart defect associated with Noonan syndrome. ***See Noonan syndrome (NS).***

Pathophysiology

1. Increased workload leads to RV hypertrophy and failure.
2. RA may enlarge with dysrhythmias.
3. Reduced pulmonary venous return to the LA and LV leads to reduced CO.

Grading of severity

Severity is based on the peak systolic RV pressure gradient across the obstruction:

1. Trivial < 25 mmHg.
2. Mild 25–49 mmHg.
3. Moderate 50–79 mmHg.
4. Severe > 80 mmHg.

Clinical effects

1 SEM heard best at the left sternal edge, widely split second heart sound, third heart sound (gallop).
2 Precordial heave.
3 Dyspnoea.
4 Fatigue.
5 Chest pain.
6 Tachycardia.
7 Light-headedness.
8 Syncope.
9 Cyanosis may occur in very severe disease due to right-to-left shunting through a patent foramen ovale or ASD.

Diagnosis

1 ECG—RV hypertrophy, P pulmonale, right axis deviation.
2 CXR—prominent pulmonary artery, dilated RA and RV.
3 Echocardiography.
4 Cardiac magnetic resonance imaging.

Treatment of PS

1 Pulmonary artery stenosis can be treated with balloon dilatation $+/-$ stent, surgical repair and beta blockers to control heart rate.
2 Pulmonary valve stenosis can be treated surgically or trans-venously using devices such as the Melody valve or the SAPIEN XT valve.

Anaesthesia and PS

Patients with mild PS do not require any special measures. With more significant lesions the aims are to avoid excessively fast or slow heart rates, maintain preload and afterload and avoid increases in pulmonary vascular resistance. To achieve these aims:

1 Invasive arterial BP monitoring should be used if significant surgery. Also consider a central line.
2 Maintain RV filling pressures by maintaining venous return. Avoid hypovolaemia and replace fluid losses promptly.
3 A modest tachycardia is helpful but marked tachycardia reduces the time for RV filling and decreases cardiac output.
4 Excessive hydration can result in acute right heart failure and AF due to RA distension.
5 Pulmonary vascular resistance should be kept low as elevated PVR reduces RV output and may precipitate acute RV failure. Factors which increase PVR include acidosis, hypercarbia, hypothermia, hypoxia, N_2O and high inflation pressures. **See Pulmonary hypertension.**
6 A fall in SVR may result in severe hypotension due to an inability of the heart to increase CO. SVR must be defended.
7 Consider the need for endocarditis prophylaxis. **See Bacterial endocarditis (BE) prophylaxis.**
8 Cardiac arrhythmias must be treated promptly due to their effects on CO.
9 CPR may be ineffective due to the RV outflow tract obstruction.
10 Consider a dobutamine infusion if RV failure is suspected e.g. rising CVP.

Obstetrics and PS

Labour

If an epidural is required, it should be titrated slowly and carefully, with consideration for invasive BP monitoring, careful attention to preload and maintenance of SVR with a vasopressor.

Caesarean section

1 Epidural anaesthesia can be considered with the same precautions as described for labour.

2 CSE with a low-dose spinal component (e.g. 0.5 mL heavy bupivacaine 0.5%) can be considered with the same precautions as for epidural anaesthesia.

3 Single-shot spinal anaesthesia is contraindicated.

4 GA for CS should follow the recommendations for anaesthesia discussed above.

See also Caesarean section (CS).

◗ Pulmonary valve stenosis

See Pulmonary stenosis (PS).

◗ Pulse pressure

This is the difference between systolic blood pressure and diastolic blood pressure. The normal range is 40–60 mmHg. A widened pulse pressure can be due to such causes as aortic incompetence. A narrow pulse pressure occurs in the early stages of hypovolaemic shock and severe aortic stenosis.

REFERENCES

1 Chakravarthy M, Prabhakumar D, George A. Anaesthetic consideration in patients with cardiac implantable electronic devices scheduled for surgery. *Indian J Anaesth* 2017; 61: 736–743.

2 Lapid MI, Rummans TA, Hofmann VE et al. ECT and automatic internal cardioverter-defibrillator. *J ECT* 2001; 17: 146–148.

3 Bryson E, Popeo D, Briggs M et al. Automatic implantable cardioverter defibrillator in electroconvulsive therapy. *J ECT* 2015; 31. Accessed online: https://journals.lww.com/ectjournal/Abstract/2015/03000/Automatic_Implantable_Cardioverter_Defibrillator.27.aspx, January 2023.

4 Billings BF, Christen JD, Harmsen WS et al. Quality-of-life after total pancreatectomy: is it really that bad on long-term follow-up? *J Gastrointest Surg* 2005; 9: 1059–1067.

5 Farnell M. Islet cell autotransplantation and chronic pancreatitis—still options. *HPB* (Oxford) 2011: 13: 596.

6 Nicholson G, Pereira AC, Hall GM. Parkinson's disease and anaesthesia. *BJA* 2002; 89: 904–916.

7 Shaikh S, Verma H. Parkinson's disease and anaesthesia. *Indian J Anaesth* 2011; 55: 228–234.

8 Sukernik M, Mets B, Bennett-Guerrero E. Patent foramen ovale and its significance in the perioperative period. *Anaesth Analg* 2001; 93: 1137–1146.

9 Steinsapir J, Carr AA, Prisant LM et al. Metyrosine and pheochromocytoma. *Arch Intern Med* 1997; 157: 901.

10 Watson VF, Vaughan RS. Magnesium and the anaesthetist. *Br J Anaesth CEPD reviews* 2001; 1: 16–20.

11 Baraka A, Siddik S, Alameddine M. Remifentanil for modulation of haemodynamics in a patient undergoing laparoscopic resection of pheochromocytoma. *Middle East J Anaesthesiol* 2004; 17: 585–592.

12 Lee YK, Park SK, Kim JW et al. The effect of phenytoin on rocuronium-induced neuromuscular blockade using rat phrenic nerve-hemidiaphragm preparation. *Korean J Anesthesiol* 2003; 45: 244–250.

13 Sunitha M, Cahandrasekharappa S, Brid SV. Electrocardiographic Qrs axis, Q wave and T wave changes in 2nd and 3rd trimester of normal pregnancy. *J Clin Diagn Res* 2014; 8: BC17–BC21.

14 Ciobanu AM, Colibaba S, Cimpoca B et al. Thrombocytopenia in pregnancy. *Maedica* 2016; 11: 55–60.

15 Snegovskikh D, Clebone A, Norwitz E. Anaesthetic management of patients with placenta accreta and resuscitation strategies for associated massive haemorrhage. *Curr Opin Anesthesiol* 2011; 24: 274–281.

16 Weinberg L, Collins N, Van Mourik K et al. Plasma-Lyte 148: a clinical review. *World J Crit Care Med* 2016; 5: 235–250.

17 Tcheng JE. Clinical challenges of platelet glycoprotein IIb/IIIa receptor inhibitor therapy: bleeding, reversal, thrombocytopenia and retreatment. *Am Heart J* 2000; 139: S38–S35.

18 Redding N, Plews D, Dodds A. Risks of perioperative blood transfusions. *Anaesth Intens Care Med* 2022; 23: 80–84.

19 Rottenstreich A, Kleinstern G, Krichevsky S et al. Factors related to the development of acquired von Willebrand syndrome in patients with essential polycythemia vera. *Europ J Int Med* 2017; 41: 49–54.

20 Koyuncu O, Turhaoglu S, Akkurt CO et al. Comparison of sugammadex and conventional reversal on postoperative nausea and vomiting: a randomized, blinded trial. *J Clin Anesth* 2015; 27: 51–56.

21 Dennis AT. Management of preeclampsia: issues for anaesthetists. *Anaesthesia* 2012; 67: 1009–1020.

22 Sviggum H. Anesthesia for nonobstetric surgery during pregnancy. *UpToDate* May 2022. Accessed online: www.uptodate.com/contents/anesthesia-for-nonobstetric-surgery-during-pregnancy, October 2022.

23 Society of Obstetric Anesthesia and Perinatology. *SOAP Statement on Sugammadex during pregnancy and lactation.* Ad Hoc task force Willett, Butwick, Togioka et al. April 22, 2019. Accessed online: www.soap.org/assets/docs/SOAP_Statement_Sugammadex_During_Pregnancy_Lactation_APPROVED.pdf, October 2022.

24 Haggerty E, Daly J. Anaesthesia and non-obstetric surgery in pregnancy. *BJA* 2021; 21: 42–43.

25 American Academy of Allergy Asthma & Immunology. *Soy-allergic and egg-allergic patients can safely receive anaesthesia.* Reviewed September 2020. Accessed online: www.aaaai.org/Tools-for-the-Public/Conditions-Library/Allergies/soy-egg-anesthesia, September 2022.

26 Harper NJN. Propofol and food allergy. *BJA* 2016; 116: 11–13.

27 Naggs T. Pick your poison. *Australian Anaesthetist* 2022, September; 10–12.

28 James PA, Oparil S, Carter BL et al. 2014 evidence-based guideline for the management of high blood pressure in adults: report from the panel members appointed by the Eighth Joint National Committee. *Jama* 2014; 311: 507–520.

29 McNally C, Visvanathan R, Adams R. Antibiotic prophylaxis for dental treatment after prosthetic joint replacement: exploring the orthopaedic surgeon's opinion. *Arthroplasty Today* 2016; Sept 2(3): 123–126. Accessed online: www.arthroplastytoday.org/article/S2352-3441(15)00110-7/fulltext, January 2023.

30 Legout L, Beltrand E, Migaud H et al. Antibiotic prophylaxis to reduce the risk of joint implant contamination during dental surgery seems unnecessary. *Othop Traumatol Surg Res* 2012; 98(8): 910.

31 Kariyawasam S, Brown J. Pulmonary arterial hypertension in pregnancy. *BJA* 2023; 23: 24–31.

▶ Quadriplegia

See Spinal cord injury (pre-existing) and anaesthesia.

QUICK FLICK

Q

R

◐ Radiation dangers

This is a highly complex and important safety issue. **See also Pregnancy and non-obstetric surgery.** Ionising radiation consists of either subatomic particles or electromagnetic waves that have sufficient energy to remove electrons from molecules, thus 'ionising' them. Ionising electromagnetic waves are X-rays, gamma rays and the higher-energy ultraviolet part of the electromagnetic spectrum. Ionising subatomic particles are alpha and beta particles and neutrons, which are typically created by radioactive decay. There are also cosmic particles produced by cosmic rays interacting with earth's atmosphere.

Radiation activity

This is how much radiation is being emitted. It is measured in the SI unit becquerel (Bq). One Bq is defined as the activity of a quantity of radioactive material in which one nucleus decays per s.

Units of exposure

The amount of radiation a person or object is exposed to.
1 The SI unit of exposure for ionising radiation is the coulomb per kg (C/kg).
2 The older unit is the roentgen (R). 1 R = 2.58×10^{-4} C/kg.

Units of absorbed dose

This is the amount of radiation absorbed by a person or object.
1 The SI unit is the gray (Gy) and has units of joules/kg.
2 The rad is an older term: 100 rad = 1 Gy.

Table R1 Radiation risks compared

Radiation dose (mrems)	Exposure source
20 000	Radioactive iodine treatment
5000	Maximum yearly exposure permitted for workers in the radiation industry
810	Abdominal CT scan
500	Maximum permissible exposure for a pregnant person over 9 months of pregnancy
300	Normal background radiation at sea level per year
200	Head CT
2	CXR

Units of equivalent dose

This is a measure of the biological effect on tissue of the radiation dose weighted for harmful effects of different types of radiation. The units are:
1 Roentgen equivalent man (rem): 1 rem = 1 rad.
2 The sievert (Sv) is the SI unit of equivalent dose and effective dose: 1 Sv = 1 Gy. Although highly oversimplified, from the above 1 Sv = 1 Gy = 100 rad = 100 rem.

Radiation risk

6 000 000 mrems exposure has a 100% mortality rate and 450 000 mrems has a 50% mortality rate. Table R1 shows the radiation risks of various exposure sources.

◐ Raised intracranial pressure

See Intracranial pressure (ICP) and treatment of raised ICP.

◐ Ramosetron

Anti-emetic second-generation 5-HT$_3$ blocker that is more effective than ondansetron in preventing PONV. It is also used to treat diarrhoea-predominant irritable bowel syndrome.

Dose for nausea and vomiting

Adult 0.3 mg IV.

◐ Rapid infusion catheter (RIC) exchange set

Description

This device is designed to provide the largest bore IV access commercially available. The set contains a 7.5 Fr, 5 cm catheter, or an 8.5 Fr, 6.4 cm catheter. There is also a dilator, a 0.64 mm diameter guide wire and a scalpel.

Technique

1 Apply a tourniquet and select a suitable large vein in the arm or use the internal jugular vein.
2 Sterilise the skin over the selected vein and ideally drape the area.
3 Use LA if the patient is awake.
4 Insert a 20 G cannula (preferably one without a reflux valve).
5 Release the tourniquet and insert the guide wire.
6 Remove the 20 G cannula and nick the skin with the scalpel at the wire insertion point.
7 Insert the RIC with dilator over the guide wire. Once the RIC is well into the vein, slide it off the dilator.
8 Remove the guide wire and dilator.
9 Cap and secure the RIC with a suture and adhesive clear dressing.

◐ Rapid sequence induction (RSI)

Description

RSI is used to decrease the risk of aspiration circumstances such as:
1 inadequate fasting or unknown fasting status
2 bowel obstruction
3 injury soon after eating
4 acute abdomen
5 Caesarean section (CS) under GA
6 severe reflux
7 high BMI in some cases
8 surgery during pregnancy other than CS.

QUICK FLICK R

Technique

Make all necessary preparations, including:

- appropriate monitoring
- suction
- presence of a skilled assistant
- availability of alternative airway devices such as an LMA
- a videolaryngoscope
- a CICO kit
- availability of another anaesthetist if possible.

There must be a plan B and a plan C in case intubation fails, and these plans must be discussed with the airway team prior to induction. *See **Difficult airway management**.* The suggested steps are:

1 Preoxygenate the patient in an upper body ramped position. The aim of preoxygenation is to replace nitrogen in the patient's lungs with oxygen, particularly in the FRC. This will increase the safe apnoea time. *See **Safe apnoea time**.* Evidence of optimal preoxygenation is end tidal expired $O_2 > 90\%$. Techniques include:

   a) Breathing 100% O_2 with a tight-fitting face mask for 3 min.
   b) As above but ask the patient to take eight deep vital capacity breaths in 60 s. Push the O_2 flush button during inspiration.
   c) Addition of CPAP or PEEP. An easy technique is to set the ventilator to PSVPro with 10 cm H_2O pressure support and 100% O_2. (*See **Ventilator settings and modes**.*) Hold the mask on the patient's face tightly with two hands for 2 minutes. It is very important to explain this technique to the patient prior to its application as the patient may find it unpleasant.
   d) High-flow nasal oxygen/trans-nasal humidified rapid-insufflation ventilatory exchange (HFNO/THRIVE) may provide an effective alternative form of preoxygenation.

2 Ensure the patient is in the ideal 'sniffing' intubating position (neck flexed, head extended). Ask the patient to keep their eyes open.

3 Administer an appropriate dose of opioid and then an appropriate dose of propofol or thiopentone.

4 As the patient's eyes begin to close, apply cricoid pressure. *See **Cricoid pressure**.*

5 Administer suxamethonium 1.5 mg/kg or rocuronium 1–1.2 mg/kg (termed 'modified rapid sequence induction').

6 Mask ventilation during RSI has traditionally been avoided. However, the Difficult Airway Society guidelines since 2015 have recommended low-pressure mask ventilation while waiting for the muscle relaxant to take effect.[1]

7 Intubate the patient after 60 s.

8 Inflate the ET tube cuff. Once correct placement of the ET tube is confirmed (by $ETCO_2$), the anaesthetist asks the assistant to release the cricoid pressure.

◐ Recombinant activated factor VII/rFVIIa/Eptacog alfa-activated (NovoSeven RT)

Description

Made from baby hamster kidney cells genetically engineered to make the product. Each vial when reconstituted contains 1 mg/mL (50 000 IU/mL rFVIIa).

Indications

Indicated for control of bleeding in the following situations:

1 Inhibitors to FVIII or FIX in people with haemophilia A or B. **See Haemophilia.**
2 Congenital FVII deficiency.
3 Glanzmann thrombasthenia.
4 Warfarin overdose.
5 To treat severe refractory haemorrhage unresponsive to all other measures.
   See Blood loss—assessment, management and anaesthetic approach. This is an off-license use.

rFVIIa for severe haemorrhage

There is a lack of high-level evidence of efficacy for treating severe haemorrhage with rFVIIa. To give rFVIIa the best chance of being effective, aim for:

- pH > 7.1
- platelet count > 50 000/mm³.

Administer

1 90 mcg/kg over 3–5 min rounded to the nearest vial.
2 Repeat dose in 30 min if needed.

▶ Recombinant tissue plasminogen activator (rtPA)/alteplase (Activase)

Description

Alteplase is a thrombolytic drug that acts by selectively binding to fibrin and converting plasminogen to plasmin, which dissolves the fibrin matrix of clots. It is used for the treatment of:

1 Myocardial infarction. **See Acute coronary syndrome.**
2 Pulmonary thromboembolism with haemodynamic instability. **See Pulmonary embolism (PE).**
3 Ischaemic acute stroke. **See Acute stroke.**
4 Occlusive iliac venous thrombosis.

Contraindications

These are relative and include:

1 Bleeding disorder/thrombocytopenia.
2 Anticoagulation.
3 Prolonged CPR.
4 Recent surgery.
5 Rapid resolution of stroke symptoms.
6 SBP > 185 mmHg, DBP > 110 mmHg.
7 Seizure.

Dose (adult)

1 Myocardial infarction—bolus and infusion depending on timeframe.
2 PE—IV bolus 10 mg over 1–2 min then 90 mg IV infusion over 2 h. If patient is < 65 kg give a maximum total dose of 1.5 mg/kg.
3 Ischaemic stroke—total dose 0.9 mg/kg with 10% of this amount administered as a bolus and the rest IV over 60 min. Do not exceed a total dose of 90 mg.

▶ Recruitment manoeuvres

These are deliberate and transient elevations in airway pressure in patients being mechanically ventilated. The aim is to reopen collapsed lung units to increase the number of alveoli participating in gas exchange. An example is to set the ventilator to CPAP mode and increase the pressure to 30–40 cm H_2O for 30–40 s. Monitor the patient for haemodynamic compromise during the manoeuvre. Not all patients will be responsive to recruitment manoeuvres.

▶ Rectus sheath block

Indication

This block is used for midline and paramedian abdominal surgical wounds such as midline incisional hernia repair. The aim is to block the terminal branches of T9–T11 intercostal nerves which run between the internal oblique and transversus abdominis muscles and then penetrate the posterior wall of the rectus abdominis muscle. The area covered is from the symphysis pubis to the xiphisternum.

Anatomy

The rectus abdominis muscles are paired muscles that lie on either side of the midline of the abdomen, separated by a midline band of connective tissue called the linea alba. The paired muscles are crisscrossed by transverse fibrous bands forming the 'six pack'. On the lateral side of each rectus abdominis is the linea semilunaris, which joins the rectus abdominis muscles to the lateral muscles of the abdomen.

The rectus sheath is a tendon sheath which encloses the rectus abdominis and pyramidalis muscles. It is an extension of the aponeuroses of the external and internal oblique muscles and the transversus abdominis muscles.

Technique

Use a short-bevelled 50 mm block needle and 40 mL of ropivacaine 0.5%.

1 Using the usual precautions (aseptic technique and inserting an IV access cannula), place the probe in the midline orientated at right angles to the long axis of the body at the level of the umbilicus (Figures R1 and R2).

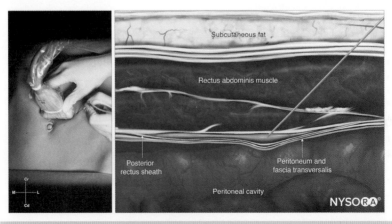

Figure R1 Probe position and anatomy for the rectus sheath block
Image courtesy of NYSORA

2 The linea alba and the bellies of the rectus abdominis muscles will be clearly seen.

3 Use an in-plane approach to pass the needle through the rectus abdominis muscle from lateral to medial. The target is when the needle tip touches the posterior rectus sheath, but does not pierce it. Use caution, because the transversalis fascia and peritoneum are just below the rectus sheath. The posterior rectus sheath and the fascia transversalis/peritoneum layer give the appearance of 'train tracks' or parallel lines. The needle tip should be just touching the 'train tracks' but not be between them. By sliding the probe caudally below the umbilicus there comes a point where the 'train tracks' disappear and only one line is seen. This is the arcuate line and the point where the rectus sheath terminates. A block can only be achieved above the arcuate line.

4 After negative aspiration and a 2 mL test dose, inject 20 mL of ropivacaine 0.5%, which should be seen to spread along the posterior aspect of the rectus abdominis muscle, forming an ellipse.

5 Repeat the block on the other side.

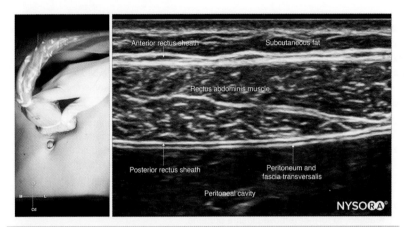

Figure R2 Probe position and sonoanatomy for the rectus sheath block
Image courtesy of NYSORA

○ Red cells/packed cells

Description

Red cells (or packed cells) are the red cell component of a unit of whole blood with most of the plasma removed and the unit reconstituted with saline. All units of packed cells and platelets are leukocyte depleted by the Australian Red Cross Blood Service. Leukocyte depletion filters are not required.[2]

Storage/contents

Packed cells are stored at 2–6°C for up to 42 days. The unit contains glucose, mannitol, adenine, N/S, sodium citrate and phosphate. As stored blood ages, it becomes more acidic and the potassium concentration increases.

Administration

1 Once the unit is opened, it is considered expired in 4 h.
2 Administer the unit over 1–3 h.
3 The infusion set must have an approved filter (170–200 micron) to remove clots and debris.
4 Transfusion should be commenced within 30 min of removal from cold storage.

Table R2 Blood group transfusion compatibility

Recipient group	Donor group
O	O
A	A or O
B	B or O
AB	AB, B, A or O

Rh (D) matching

1 Rh (D) positive patients can have Rh (D) positive or negative blood.
2 Rh (D) negative patients should have Rh (D) negative blood.
3 In extenuating circumstances, Rh (D) negative patients may be allocated Rh (D) positive blood if these patients are men or post-menopausal women.

Special circumstances

1 Cytomegalovirus (CMV) negative blood may be indicated for immunosuppressed patients, pregnant patients, intrauterine transfusions and neonatal transfusion.
2 Irradiated red cells may be required for neonates in ICU, directed donations from relatives, bone marrow transplant, stem cell transplants and intrauterine transfusion. This is to prevent foreign T-cells engrafting and causing graft vs host disease.
3 Washed red cells may be indicated in patients with a history of transfusion reaction, to further remove plasma proteins.

Risks of red cell transfusion

See Blood transfusion reactions/adverse events.

◖ Red person syndrome

Description

This is an infusion-related reaction that can occur with vancomycin. It consists of pruritis, a diffuse burning sensation, rash and, less frequently, hypotension and angioedema. It is due to giving IV vancomycin rapidly, resulting in histamine release.

Treatment

1 Discontinue the vancomycin infusion.
2 Oral diphenhydramine 50 mg.
3 Resume the vancomycin infusion at a slower rate once the rash resolves.

Prevention

Infuse vancomycin over 60 min.

▷ Reflexes

Table R3 Nerve roots involved in upper and lower limb reflexes

Reflex	Nerve roots
Plantar	S1
Ankle	S1, 2
Knee	L3, 4
Biceps	C5, 6
Triceps	C7, 8

▷ Remifentanil

Description
4-anilidopiperidine ultra-short-acting selective mu receptor agonist opioid with a similar potency to fentanyl. It is rapidly metabolised by non-specific plasma esterases, resulting in an elimination half-life of 8 minutes.

Uses
1 By infusion during GA and sedation.
2 Bolus dose for ultra-short procedures such as electroconvulsive therapy (ECT) and awake laryngoscopy.
3 Intubation without muscle relaxation.

Dose (effect site concentration and mcg/kg/min)
1 Intraoperative nociceptive stimulation control—2–8 ng/mL (maximum 12 ng/mL) **or** 0.05–0.5 mcg/kg/min (maximum 2 mcg/kg/min).
2 Prevention of hypertensive response to intubation—1 mcg/kg IV over 2 minutes during induction then an IV infusion run at 0.05 mcg/kg/min. **See Intubation-minimising hypertensive response.**
3 Bolus dose adult 100–200 mcg IV.
4 Intubation without muscle relaxation—8 ng/mL until patient feels the effect, then reduce to 6–7 ng/mL and induce anaesthesia and intubate.[3]

Advantages
1 Renal and liver disease have **no** effect on remifentanil clearance.
2 Rapidly titratable.
3 Ideal for procedures with intense intraoperative nociceptive stimulation but little postoperative pain.
4 Works synergistically with propofol.

Disadvantages
1 Cannot be used for neuraxial procedures due to glycine content (inhibitory neurotransmitter).
2 For postoperative pain, longer-acting opioids are required to be administered, at least 30 min before cessation of the remifentanil infusion.
3 Possibly causes acute opioid tolerance and hyperalgesia.[4]
4 Remifentanil PCA may cause severe and unpredictable respiratory depression.
5 Can cause hypotension, bradycardia, respiratory depression and muscle rigidity.

⊙ Renal function tests

Urinalysis

May detect proteinuria, which can be indicative of kidney damage. The urine albumin-to-creatine ratio (UACR) is the albumin concentration (mg/L) divided by the creatinine concentration (g/L). Normally it is < 30 mg/g.

1 UACR 30–299 mg/g—moderately increased.
2 UACR > 300 mg/g—severely increased.

Urea

NR 2.5–6.5 mmol/L. Urea is a byproduct of protein metabolism by the liver and is excreted by the kidneys, giving an indication of renal function. Low urea levels may indicate liver disease, low protein diet or overhydration. Elevated urea levels may indicate kidney disease, dehydration, a high protein diet or heart disease.

Creatinine

NR 60–125 µmol/L. It is a breakdown product of creatine phosphate in muscle.
See *Creatine kinase (CK)/creatine phosphokinase (CPK)/phosphocreatine kinase*.
Creatinine is usually produced at a constant rate. It is freely filtered out of the kidneys and the rate of excretion is determined by the glomerular filtration rate (GFR). Elevated creatinine levels can be due to kidney disease, muscle disease, large muscle mass or CCF. Low levels can occur in patients with small stature, the elderly and those with muscle atrophy.

Glomerular filtration rate (GFR) and creatinine clearance (CrCl)

GFR is a measure of the volume of fluid filtered by the kidneys per unit time. Measurement of GFR requires a substance that has a constant level in the blood, is freely filtered by the kidneys and is neither reabsorbed nor secreted by the kidney. GFR would be the clearance rate of the substance under these conditions. Creatinine is not ideal but is used in the calculations. Urine is collected for 24 h and the amount of creatinine collected is measured. If the total creatinine collected is 1440 mg and the serum creatinine is 0.01 mg/mL, then 1 mg/min of creatinine is excreted, therefore 100 mL of fluid is cleared, and so GFR is 100 mL/min. Creatinine clearance can also be calculated from the Cockcroft–Gault equation:

$$\text{CrCl (mL/min) males} = \frac{(140 - \text{age}) \times \text{ideal body weight (kg)}}{0.815 \times \text{serum creatinine micromole/L}}$$

The same formula is used for females but 0.85 is used instead of 0.815 in the denominator.

CrCl can be used to grade renal impairment (see Table R4).

Table R4 Grades of renal disease based on CrCl

Kidney function	Creatinine clearance
Normal	90–100 mL/min
Mild renal disease	60–89 mL/min
Moderate renal disease	30–59 mL/min
Severe renal disease	< 30 mL/min

Estimated GFR (eGFR)

This measurement uses various formulas to take into account factors such as age, sex and race. It can be used to categorise stages of renal failure, as in Table R5. An average body surface area (BSA) of 1.73 m^2 is used in the equation. Small body mass may disguise renal failure by indicating a normal eGFR.

Table R5 Stage of renal failure based on eGFR

Stage of renal failure	eGFR mL/min/1.73 m^2
Stage 1—very mild disease	90 or higher with evidence of kidney damage
Stage 2—mild renal disease	60–89 with evidence of kidney damage
Stage 3—moderate renal disease	30–59
Stage 4—severe renal disease	15–29
Stage 5—renal failure requiring dialysis	< 15

Renal transplant

Preoperative phase

1 Ensure the patient receives preoperative immunosuppressive therapy.
2 Preoperative dialysis is desirable, aiming for a $K^+ < 6$ mmol/L and a pH > 7.25.
3 Do not use the cephalic vein for venous access as this vein may be needed for fistula formation in the future. Do not use an arm with an arteriovenous (AV) fistula for IV access or BP cuff. Pad an AV fistula carefully.
4 An arterial line is not required unless indicated because of other co-morbidities e.g. significant valvular heart disease.
5 A central line is not strictly indicated for the surgery as CVP measurements do not correlate well with intravascular filling. However, some units insist on central venous access for reasons such as reliable IV access and ease of frequent blood sampling postoperatively. A central line may also be indicated if an inotrope is required e.g. dobutamine for heart failure.
6 Be hypervigilant for cardiovascular disease as this is very common in renal failure patients.
7 Treat diabetes mellitus if present, as described in the section ***Diabetes mellitus (DM)***.

Intraoperative phase

1 Insert a 16–18 G cannula into a peripheral arm vein.
2 Induce anaesthesia with appropriate doses of midazolam, fentanyl and propofol. Give prophylactic antibiotic cover e.g. cefazolin 2 g. Consider vancomycin if the patient is penicillin allergic.
3 Maintain anaesthesia with sevoflurane or TCI propofol.
4 Although cisatracurium is traditionally the preferred muscle relaxant, the use of rocuronium with sugammadex reversal is acceptable.[5]
5 Plasma-Lyte may be superior to normal saline in renal transplant surgery due to:[6]
   a) lower incidence of hyperkalaemia
   b) lower incidence of perioperative dialysis
   c) better graft function at 3 months.

QUICK FLICK R

Normal saline may lead to hyperchloraemic metabolic acidosis, which may increase serum potassium levels. Elevated chloride levels may have nephrotoxic effects, although this is unproven.[7]

6 Monitor temperature and keep the patient normothermic.

7 The surgical team will insert a urinary catheter.

8 The patient needs to be 'well filled' to optimise graft function e.g. 4–6 L intraoperatively (60–100 mL/kg). The actual amount required will vary depending on factors such as patient co-morbidities and whether the patient is fluid restricted or not.

9 If a blood transfusion is required, use a leukocyte reduction filter e.g. a Sepacell filter.

10 Treat hyperkalaemia as described in the section *Potassium*.

11 Treat hypotension with IV fluids in the first instance. A vasopressor such as metaraminol may be required, but alpha-adrenoreceptor agonists may reduce graft perfusion and function.[8]

12 As directed by the surgeon and, just prior to kidney reperfusion, administer mannitol 20% solution 0.25 g/kg IV and frusemide 60–80 mg IV.

13 It is essential that the patient does not cough or strain during the implantation of the graft and before the closure of the abdominal wall. Damage to delicate anastomoses and renal pelvic structures may occur. Monitor the depth of paralysis with a nerve stimulator and keep the patient well paralysed.

14 Administer anti-emetic medication such as ondansetron 4–8 mg IV.

15 Do not use morphine or pethidine due to metabolite side effects. Do not use NSAIDs due to nephrotoxic effects. Fentanyl, oxycodone and paracetamol are acceptable.

16 Consider a TAP block for postoperative analgesia. *See Transversus abdominis plane (TAP) block/subcostal TAP block*. The block can be done by the surgeon at the time of wound closure.

Postoperative phase

Prescribe IV fentanyl PCA for pain, plus regular paracetamol.

▶ Renin-angiotensin system

Renin is secreted by the kidneys in response to:

1 decreased blood pressure

2 decreased sodium load delivered to the distal tubules

3 stimulation of beta-1 adrenergic receptors by the sympathetic nervous system.

Renin breaks down angiotensinogen (secreted by the liver) to angiotensin I. Angiotensin I is cleaved by angiotensin-converting enzyme (ACE) in the lungs to form angiotensin II. This substance is a potent vasoconstrictor of all blood vessels, resulting in an increase in blood pressure. By causing increased levels of angiotensin II, renin causes increased secretion of aldosterone from the adrenals. This leads to increased sodium and water retention by the kidneys, increasing intravascular volume and potassium excretion. *See Conn's syndrome*.

▶ Respiratory acidosis

In this condition, blood pH < 7.35 due to excess CO_2 in the blood. This can be acute or chronic. If chronic, blood bicarbonate levels will increase by 3–4 mmol/L per 10 mmHg increase in $PaCO_2$. *See Arterial blood gas (ABG) interpretation for acidosis/alkalosis*.

▶ Respiratory failure

Definition
Respiratory failure is defined as a failure of the lungs to provide adequate gas exchange of oxygen or carbon dioxide, or both.

Types of respiratory failure
- Type 1—hypoxaemic respiratory failure.
- Type 2—hypercapnic respiratory failure.

Diagnosis of respiratory failure
Respiratory failure is suggested by:
1. Maximum negative inspiratory pressure or negative inspiratory force (NIF) < 20 cmH$_2$0. NR 50–100 cm H$_2$0.
2. Vital capacity < 1 L or 15 mL/kg. Normal is 70 mL/kg.
3. TV < 5 mL/kg.
4. pH < 7.25.
5. Respiratory rate > 35 breaths/min.
6. PaCO$_2$ > 55 mmHg.
7. PaO$_2$ < 70 mmHg.
8. PF ratio—ratio of PaO$_2$ to FiO$_2$. This should be greater than 300. A PF < 200 suggests respiratory failure.

▶ Respiratory function tests

See Lung function tests.

▶ Restrictive cardiomyopathy

Description
Restrictive cardiomyopathy is also called infiltrative cardiomyopathy or idiopathic myocardial fibrosis. In this illness, diseases of the heart muscle result in impaired ventricular filling or weakened ventricular contraction or both. Restrictive cardiomyopathy accounts for 5% of all cardiomyopathies. It has a similar presentation to restrictive pericarditis.

Aetiology
1. Cardiac amyloidosis.
2. Haemochromatosis or iron overload from frequent transfusions. *See Haemochromatosis* and *Iron overload*.
3. Cardiac sarcoidosis.
4. Eosinophilic endocarditis.
5. Carcinoid heart disease. *See Carcinoid tumours and carcinoid syndrome.*
6. Diseases of the heart lining such as endomyocardial fibrosis and Loeffler syndrome.
7. Scarring of the heart from an unknown cause.
8. Scarring due to chemotherapy or radiotherapy.
9. Scleroderma.

Pathophysiology
1. Ventricular function may be well preserved initially but the heart does not relax appropriately during diastole, leading to increased LV end-diastolic pressure but decreased end-diastolic volume.

2 Both atria become dilated and mean atrial pressure is increased.

3 As the disease progresses, systolic function becomes affected.

4 The RV is usually more affected than the LV.

Clinical effects

1 Cough.

2 Dyspnoea/orthopnoea.

3 Fatigue.

4 Peripheral oedema.

5 Ascites, enlarged liver.

6 Low volume pulse.

7 Diastolic murmur, third heart sound.

8 Dysrhythmias due to SA or AV node involvement e.g. AF, bradycardia.

9 Chest pain.

10 Pulmonary oedema.

11 Intra-cardiac thrombosis with risk of stroke.

Diagnosis

1 ECG—conduction abnormalities.

2 CXR—pulmonary congestion, pleural effusion. The heart is usually not enlarged.

3 Echocardiography—pronounced biatrial enlargement, regional wall motion abnormalities.

4 Heart MRI/PET scan.

5 Right heart catheterisation.

6 Myocardial biopsy.

Treatment

This depends on the cause. For general treatment of heart failure, **see *Congestive cardiac failure (CCF)—chronic*.** Other treatments may target the cause e.g. phlebotomy for haemochromatosis or steroids for sarcoidosis. A permanent pacemaker or AICD may be required. Anticoagulation may be indicated for AF or intra-cardiac clot. Heart transplantation is the only effective surgical option.

Anaesthesia

These patients are at high risk of morbidity and mortality. GA causes vasodilatation, myocardial depression and reduced venous return. All these effects are deleterious in restrictive cardiomyopathy.

1 Consider invasive blood pressure monitoring.

2 Cardiac output is rate and preload dependent.

3 Bradycardia will decrease CO and tachycardia will also decrease CO by reducing filling time.

4 Preload must be maintained. Preload can be reduced by IPPV, PEEP and hypovolaemia. IPPV can cause cardiac arrest.[q]

5 Maintain SR if possible, treat arrythmias promptly.

6 Maintain SVR.

7 Consider early use of transoesophageal echocardiography if decompensation occurs.

◖ Resuscitation of the newborn

*See **Neonatal resuscitation**.*

▷ Resuscitative hysterotomy

Description

This term describes an emergency Caesarean section performed during attempted resuscitation of the mother at the time of cardiac arrest or imminent cardiac arrest, with the aim of improving the chances of survival of the mother and the baby. The incidence of cardiac arrest in pregnancy is about 1:30 000. It was previously called perimortem Caesarean section.

Causes of maternal cardiac arrest

These are many and include:

1 obstetric causes—amniotic fluid embolus, preeclampsia/eclampsia, obstetric haemorrhage, pulmonary embolus
2 chronic illness exacerbated by pregnancy e.g. pulmonary hypertension
3 cause unrelated to pregnancy—trauma, subarachnoid haemorrhage, asthma.

BEAU CHOPS acronym for causes of pregnancy cardiac arrest

The letters stand for:

B – **B**leeding
E – **E**mbolism
A – **A**naesthetic
U – **U**terine atony

C – **C**ardiac disease
H – **H**ypertension
O – **O**ther
P – **P**lacental abruption/praevia
S – **S**epsis

Maternal resuscitation from cardiac arrest

This should follow Australian Resuscitation Council guidelines, with the following caveats:

1 Pregnant women desaturate faster and $PaCO_2$ rises more quickly than in the non-pregnant state. Also, they are at a high aspiration risk. **See *Physiology of term pregnancy*.** Intubate the airway as soon as possible and give 100% O_2.
2 If the patient is more than 20 weeks pregnant, a rescuer should provide manual uterine displacement to the left and towards the patient's left upper quadrant. This is to relieve inferior vena cava compression.
3 Chest compressions should be provided slightly higher on the sternum than in the non-pregnant state due to displacement of the heart cephalad.
4 Note that CPR is relatively ineffective in mid-to-late pregnancy due to the low resistance of the uterine circulation diverting blood away from the brain and heart, IVC compression and the metabolic demands of the uterus, placenta and fetus.

Resuscitative hysterotomy

1 If the patient is 24 weeks pregnant or greater, make preparations for emergency CS at the start of resuscitation (summon instruments, neonatal and obstetric/surgical staff). A 24-week pregnancy correlates with a uterine fundal height about 4 cm above the umbilicus or higher.

2 If return of spontaneous circulation (ROSC) is not achieved by 4 min, perform resuscitative hysterotomy, aiming to deliver the fetus by 5 min after the cardiac arrest is declared.

3 Delivery of the fetus will reduce IVC compression, reduce uterine blood flow, remove O_2 demands of the fetus and placenta and increase FRC. It will give the fetus **and the mother** their best chance of survival.

4 **Do not delay CS.** Do not transport the patient; do not attempt to establish fetal viability; do not wait for anything; do not perform a TOE.

Performance of resuscitative hysterotomy

1 The most qualified person present—obstetrician, surgeon, any doctor—should perform the CS.

2 No attempt to obtain consent should be made. Minimal sterile precautions should be undertaken. Continue resuscitation throughout the procedure, except when this poses an immediate risk to surgical staff.

3 Perform a midline incision from uterine fundus to pubic symphysis, cutting through all layers of muscle.

4 Fingers of the assistants are used as retractors to pull the muscles laterally.

5 Incise the peritoneum with a scalpel or scissors.

6 Make a 2 cm incision into the lower uterine segment with the scalpel.

7 Insert 2 fingers into the uterine cavity, between the body of the fetus and the internal uterine wall. Guard the fetus from injury from sharp instruments.

8 Use scissors to cut the uterus towards the fundus. If the placenta is encountered, use the scalpel to cut sharply through it. Make an incision large enough to deliver the baby.

9 Deliver the infant, clamp the cord in two places and cut the cord between the clamps. Pass the baby off for resuscitation.

10 Deliver the placenta.

11 Pack the uterus with sterile gauze.

12 Close the uterus with a skin stapler if available.

13 Continue resuscitative efforts and transport patient to the operating theatre.

14 Continue the resuscitation as per the section *Cardiac arrest.*

◐ Retained placenta

Description

Retained placenta is defined as a failure of part of the placenta, or the entire placenta, to be delivered within 30–60 minutes of delivery of the baby. This can lead to postpartum haemorrhage. It occurs in 1–3% of vaginal deliveries and is the second most common cause of postpartum haemorrhage. *See Postpartum haemorrhage (PPH).*

Causes

1 Uterine atony.

2 Prolonged oxytocin use in labour.

3 Abnormally adherent placenta—*see Placenta accreta spectrum.*

4 Closure of the cervix prior to placental expulsion.

5 Uterine pathology.

Prevention

Active management of labour (oxytocin, controlled cord traction and uterine massage).

Management

1 Manual extraction of the uterus under anaesthesia—see below.

2 Empty the bladder.

3 GTN may be required—**see Uterine relaxation.**

4 More invasive types of surgery may be required such as curettage of the uterus.

5 Maternal resuscitation—**see Postpartum haemorrhage (PPH).**

Anaesthesia

1 If an epidural is already in situ for labour, top this up, unless significant blood loss.

2 In some situations, sedation and analgesia may be sufficient. Ketamine may be helpful.

3 Low-dose SAB (e.g. 1.5 mL of heavy bupivacaine 0.5% + fentanyl 25 mcg) can be considered if the patient has not had significant blood loss.

4 GA with rapid sequence induction.

◐ Rivaroxaban (Xarelto)

Description

Oral anticoagulant drug that prevents activated factor X from converting prothrombin to thrombin. It is an FXa inhibitor. It is approved for the treatment of DVT, PE, non-valvular AF and prevention of thromboembolic disease after hip or knee joint replacement surgery. It is sold under the trade name Xarelto®.

Dose

1 VTE prevention after hip/knee surgery—10 mg/day.

2 Treatment of DVT—15 mg q 12 h for 3 weeks then 20 mg daily.

3 Stroke prevention in non-valvular AF—20 mg/day.

Advantages

1 No monitoring is required.

2 Lower rate of fatal bleeds compared with warfarin.

3 Onset of action 2.5–4 h.

4 Effects last 8–12 h.

5 Surgery, neuraxial block and deep nerve blocks can be undertaken in the following time frames:

  a) Moderate bleeding risk/normal renal function—24 h.

  b) Moderate bleeding risk/impaired renal function—48 h.

  c) High bleeding risk/normal renal function—48–72 h.

  d) High bleeding risk/impaired renal function—72 h.

Disadvantages

1 Higher rate of GIT bleeds than warfarin.

2 Contraindicated in patients with severe liver or kidney disease.

3 Contraindicated in patients on HIV protease inhibitors or azole antifungals.

Bleeding and Rivaroxaban (adult)

1 Andexanet alfa (Andexxa) reverses the effect of rivaroxaban and apixaban. **See Andexanet alfa (Andexxa).**

2 Tranexamic acid 1 g IV over 15 min, then infusion 1 mg/kg/h.

3 Consider prothrombinex – VF 50 IU/kg.

4 Consider FEIBA 50 IU/kg. **See FEIBA-NF (factor VIII inhibitor bypassing activity).**

▶ Robotic surgery/robot-assisted surgery

Introduction

Robotic surgery allows for extremely precise and relatively fatigueless surgery by a seated non-sterile surgeon helped by a sterile nursing and surgical assistant team. There are many potential patient and surgeon benefits that are beyond the focus of this section.

The main types of surgery are:

1 Urological.
2 Gynaecological.
3 Upper gastrointestinal surgery such as gastric bypass surgery.
4 Cardiothoracic surgery.

For lower abdominal and pelvic surgery, steep Trendelenburg positioning for prolonged periods, combined with laparoscopic surgery. *See Laparoscopic surgery*.

Contraindications to robotic surgery

Absolute contraindications are:

1 intracranial mass lesions and/or cerebral oedema
2 glaucoma
3 carotid and/or basilar artery disease
4 cyanotic congenital heart disease
5 known patent foramen ovale.

Relative contraindications include morbid obesity, severe ischaemic or valvular heart disease and significant respiratory disease.

Anaesthetic considerations

Surgery is often prolonged and there is limited access to the patient. **The patient must not move while the robotic instruments are inside them.**

1 The patient must be paralysed, intubated and ventilated.
2 Secure large-bore IV access. In the event of bleeding, access to the patient is severely limited.
3 Insert a temperature probe and use a warming blanket and calf-compressors. The surgical team will insert a urinary catheter.
4 Many anaesthetists (but not all) feel an arterial line is essential.
5 There is often steep Trendelenburg positioning at 25–45°. Even steeper angles may be needed, which can result in the following:
   a) The patient may slip down the table. Make sure the patient's skin rests on a non-slip mat (with egg-carton foam). Any attempt to restrict slipping by shoulder restraints may cause brachial plexus injury.
   b) Gastric acid may regurgitate and damage the eyes. Insert an orogastric tube and use Tegaderm dressings to securely close the eyes. Pad the eyes with gauze.
   c) Laryngeal and tongue oedema with airway obstruction after extubation may occur.
   d) Eye swelling, conjunctival swelling, orbital oedema and decreased optic nerve perfusion may cause vision impairment/blindness post procedure. Corneal abrasions are the most common injury.[10]
   e) Intracranial and intraocular pressures are increased.

f) Cerebral autoregulation may be impaired, although this may be less likely with propofol anaesthesia compared with sevoflurane anaesthesia.[11]

g) The ET tube must be carefully placed. The tip may enter a bronchus with steep Trendelenburg positioning combined with pneumoperitoneum.

h) Hypoxia may result from basal atelectasis, reduced lung volumes and ventilation/perfusion mismatching, particularly in obese patients.

i) Increased risk of surgical emphysema.

j) Lateral femoral cutaneous nerve injury may result from the lithotomy position.

k) Carefully pad and wrap the arms by the patient's sides.

6 The patient must not move. Use rocuronium at an intubating dose followed by an infusion of 0.6–1 mg/kg/h. This will be roughly the intubating dose per hour. Use a nerve stimulator to ensure there is effective muscle paralysis. A remifentanil infusion will provide added protection against cough/movement.

7 The patient's face may be struck by a robotic arm. Place a right-angle bar over the patient's face at eye level to reduce the risk of facial injury.

8 For patients at significant risk of arrhythmias, place cardioversion/defibrillation/pacing pads at the start of the case. Defibrillation can be done while the robot is docked, if necessary.

9 Consider pressure-controlled ventilation with TV 6–8 mL/kg and PEEP to reduce atelectasis.[10]

10 GFR and urine output may be reduced.

11 Restrict IV fluids to reduce the risk of eye, facial and laryngeal oedema.[10]

12 The table position must not change once the robot is docked and the instruments engaged. Ensure that the table control cannot be accidently activated.

13 Provide anti-emetic medication.

14 Sugammadex is very useful for rocuronium reversal involving profound block.

15 Postoperatively, assess the patient for significant laryngeal oedema. Only extubate the patient if it is safe to do so. Check that there is a leak around the tube when the cuff is deflated.

16 Be aware of the risk of ischaemia-induced lower limb compartment syndrome. *See Well leg compartment syndrome*.

17 Perform a post-procedure eye assessment.

◐ Rocuronium

Description

Quaternary amino-steroid non-depolarising neuromuscular blocking drug (NDNMBD). It is an analogue of vecuronium.

Dose

- For elective surgery use 0.6 mg/kg IV. Effects last 30–40 min.
- For modified rapid sequence induction use 1.2 mg/kg.
- Maintenance dose—0.15 mg/kg IV.
- Infusion dose—0.6–1 mg/kg/h IV.

Advantages

1 Rapid onset of action—can be used for rapid sequence induction.

2 Minimal haemodynamic side effects.

3 Presented as a ready-to-use solution, unlike vecuronium.

4 Can be immediately and fully reversed at any time with sugammadex. *See Sugammadex*.

Disadvantages

1 Cleared principally by uptake in the liver and secretion in the bile. Hepatic disease may prolong effects.
2 Some rocuronium is excreted in the urine. Effects can be prolonged in renal disease.
3 Significant incidence of anaphylaxis, which is greater than for vecuronium. An incidence of 1:2500 is quoted from some sources, which is similar to the incidence of anaphylaxis to suxamethonium.[12,13] Rocuronium is 3 × more likely to cause anaphylaxis than vecuronium.[14] There are conflicting reports as to whether sugammadex is beneficial in treating rocuronium-induced anaphylaxis. *See Sugammadex*. The risk of rocuronium anaphylaxis appears to be increased with pholcodine consumption.[14]

⟶ Ropivacaine (Naropin)

Description

Aminoamide LA drug presented as the pure S enantiomer. Useful for all types of blocks except for intravenous blocks (not discussed in this manual). It is about 25% less potent than bupivacaine and less lipophilic.

Dose[15]

Maximum dose 3–4 mg/kg. Maximum dose in 24 h for epidural infusion 770 mg and for wound infusion 480 mg.

Adult lumbar epidural

- 10–15 mL of 0.75% ropivacaine for surgical anaesthesia.
- For labour analgesia, use 10–20 mL of 0.2% solution to establish the block. The block can be maintained with 0.1% ropivacaine with fentanyl 2 mcg/mL. *See Epidural anaesthesia/analgesia*.
- For postoperative analgesia, use an infusion of 0.2% ropivacaine run at 6–14 mL/h.

Adult thoracic analgesia

- Use 5–15 mL of 0.75% ropivacaine to establish the block intraoperatively.
- Use an infusion of 0.2% ropivacaine run at 6–14 mL/h for postoperative analgesia.

Adult subarachnoid block

Use 0.5% solution—3.5 mL is effective for hip surgery.

Adult infusion for continuous peripheral nerve blockade

5–10 mL/h 0.2% ropivacaine. Use for up to 48 h.

Addition of adrenaline

The addition of adrenaline does not prolong the duration of effect of ropivacaine nerve blocks. However, for cutaneous block, adding adrenaline may decrease bleeding.

Advantages

1 Less cardiotoxic and neurotoxic than bupivacaine, and treatment of toxicity is more likely to be successful compared with bupivacaine toxicity. *See Intralipid for the treatment of ropivacaine/bupivacaine toxicity* and *Local anaesthetic cardiac toxicity/arrest management*.
2 Ropivacaine has some vasoconstrictor properties. It produces a longer duration of cutaneous block than bupivacaine.
3 Causes less motor block than bupivacaine for an equivalent sensory block.

Disadvantages

1 More cardiotoxic than lignocaine.

2 Due to its vasoconstrictor properties, there are concerns with the use of ropivacaine for penile block.[16]

◯ Ross procedure

In this procedure, the patient's stenotic aortic valve is replaced by their pulmonary valve. The pulmonary valve is replaced with a cadaveric valve.

REFERENCES

1 Frerk C, Mitchell VS, McNarry AF et al. Difficult Airway Society 2015 guidelines for management of unanticipated difficult intubation in adults. *BJA* 2015; 115: 827–848.

2 *Flippin' Blood,* Second Edition, June 2012: 17. Accessed online: www.blood.gov.au/flippin-blood, October 2022.

3 Atterton B, Lobaz S. *WFSA Tutorial 342: Remifentanil use in anaesthesia and critical care* 2016. Accessed online: https://resources.wfsahq.org/atotw/remifentanil-use-in-anaesthesia-and-critical-care/#:~:text=Remifentanil%20is%20a%20versatile%20drug%20that%20can%20be,effectively%20for%20awake%20fibre-optic%20intubation%20and%20conscious%20sedation, October 2022.

4 Yu EHY, Tran DHD, Lam SW, Irwin MG. Remifentanil tolerance and hyperalgesia: short-term gain, long-term pain? *Anesthesia* 2016; 7: 1347–1362.

5 Carron M, Andreatta G, Pesenti E et al. Impact on kidney function of rocuronium-sugammadex vs cisatracurium-neostigmine strategy for neuromuscular block management. An Italian single-centre, 2014–2017 retrospective cohort case-control study. *Perioper Med* 2022; 11, article number: 3. Accessed online: https://perioperativemedicinejournal.biomedcentral.com/counter/pdf/10.1186/s13741-021-00231-2.pdf, January 2023.

6 Adwaney A, Randall DW, Blunden MJ et al. Perioperative Plasma-Lyte reduces the incidence of renal replacement therapy and hyperkalaemia following renal transplantation when compared with 0.9% saline: a retrospective cohort study. *Clin Kidney J* 2017; 10: 838–844.

7 Saini V, Samra T, Naik NB et al. Normal saline versus balanced crystalloids in renal transplant surgery: a double-blind randomised controlled study. *Cureus* 2021; 13(9) e18247. Accessed online: https://www.cureus.com/articles/72105-normal-saline-versus-balanced-crystalloids-in-renal-transplant-surgery-a-double-blind-randomized-controlled-study#!/, January 2023.

8 Lemmens HJM. Anesthesia for kidney transplantation. *UpToDate* October 2021. Accessed online: https://www.uptodate.com/contents/anesthesia-for-kidney-transplantation, January 2023.

9 Ibrahim IR, Sharma V. Cardiomyopathy and anaesthesia. *BJA Education* 2017; 17: 363–369.

10 Iqbal H, Gray M, Gowrie-Mohan S. *WFSA Tutorial 408: Anaesthesia for robot-assisted urological surgery* 2019. Accessed online: https://resources.wfsahq.org/atotw/anaesthesia-for-robot-assisted-urological-surgery, October 2022.

11 Robertson TJ, McCulloch TJ, Paleologos MS et al. Effects of sevoflurane versus propofol on cerebral autoregulation during anaesthesia for robot-assisted laparoscopic prostatectomy. *Anaesth Intensive Care* 2022; 50: 361–367.

QUICK FLICK R

12 Reddy J, Cooke P, van Schalkwyk J et al. Anaphylaxis is more common with rocuronium and succinylcholine than with atracurium. *Anesthesiology* 2015; 122: 39–45.

13 Takazawa T, Mitsuhata H, Mertes PM. Sugammadex and rocuronium-induced anaphylaxis. *J Anaesth* 2016; 30: 290–297.

14 Sadleir PH, Clarke RC, Goddard CE et al. Relationship of perioperative anaphylaxis to neuromuscular blocking agents, obesity and pholcodine consumption: a case-control study. *BJA* 2021; 126: 940–948.

15 Fresenius Kabi Australia Pty Limited. *Australian product information - Ropivacaine Kabi (ropivacaine hydrochloride). Date of revision,* December 13, 2022. Accessed online: https://www.fresenius-kabi.com/au/documents/Ropivacaine_PI.pdf, September 2023.

16 Burke D, Joypaul V, Thomson MF. Circumcision supplemented by dorsal penile nerve block with 0.75% ropivacaine: a complication. *Reg Anesth Pain Med* 2000; 25: 424–427.

○ Saddle block

See **Subarachnoid block (SAB)**.

○ Safe apnoea time

This is the time for critical oxygen desaturation to occur in the apnoeic patient. Critical oxygen desaturation is 88–90%. This is the upper inflection point of the oxygen-haemoglobin dissociation curve, beyond which further desaturation will occur very rapidly. Safe apnoea time can be increased from about 1 min breathing air, to as much as 8 min after breathing 100% O_2, in a healthy patient.

○ Salbutamol/albuterol (Ventolin)

Description

A short-acting beta-2 agonist. It is used to:
1 Treat and prevent bronchospasm in conditions such as asthma and COPD. It relaxes the smooth muscle of the airways.
2 Treat hyperkalaemia.
3 Inhibit premature labour.

Presentation

1 Metered inhaler, commonly called a 'puffer' (100 mcg/dose).
2 Salbutamol powder.
3 Nebuliser solution 2.5–5 mg in nebules. A salbutamol puffer, with a spacer, is just as effective as nebulised salbutamol.[1]
4 IV salbutamol. This solution can also be used subcut. **Do not give nebuliser solution IV.**
5. Oral Ventolin syrup 2 mg/5 mL.

Dose

Asthma

1 Metered inhaler—1–2 inhalations up to every 4 h.
2 Nebulised solution—adults and children > 12 yrs 2.5–5 mg q 4–8 h. Can be used up to every 20 min, depending on severity of bronchospasm.
3 IV/subcut salbutamol. In adults/children > 40 kg, give a LD of 200 mcg IV, over 1 minute, then an infusion of 5 mcg/min to a maximum of 20 mcg/min. In children < 40 kg, give a LD of 5–7.5 mcg/kg (maximum 300 mcg) over 10 min then an infusion of 1 mcg/kg/min to a maximum of 5 mcg/kg/min (maximum 80 mcg/h). If only a peripheral line is available, use ≤ 200 mcg/mL dilution of salbutamol.
If giving subcut to adults, use 500 mcg q 4 h as needed. For children, use 8 mcg/kg q 4 h as needed.

Uterine relaxation to halt/delay premature labour

Load 25 mg salbutamol into 1000 mL Hartmann's solution. Infuse 60–100 mL over 10–20 min then run the solution at 0.6 mg/h (24 mL/h), increased at 10 min intervals until there is a response. Then increase rate more slowly until contractions cease. The usual dose is 0.6–2.7 mg/h (24–108 mL/h). Once contractions have stopped for

1 h, reduce the rate by decrements of 50% every 6 h. Maximum treatment duration is 48 h. Oral salbutamol 6 mg q 6 h can be used for maintenance therapy.

Hyperkalaemia

Beta-2 agonists reduce potassium levels by causing potassium to enter skeletal muscle cells. Salbutamol is effective given IV or by nebuliser. Give 10–20 mg via nebuliser over 30 min in the adult.[2]

▶ Saphenous nerve block

See Adductor canal block.

▶ Scalp block

Anatomy

The posterior scalp is innervated by:

1 The greater occipital nerve (C2, 3)—supplies the skin over the occiput and vertex.
2 The lesser occipital nerve (C2)—supplies the skin over the mastoid process and the adjacent area above and behind the mastoid process.
3 The third occipital nerve (C3)—supplies the skin over the lower occiput.
4 The supraorbital and supratrochlear nerves—supply the anterior scalp. These are branches of the frontal nerve, which is, in turn, a branch of the ophthalmic division of the trigeminal nerve.
5 Contributions from the zygomaticotemporal, auriculotemporal and greater auricular nerves.

Indications

1 Awake craniotomy.
2 Trauma/lacerations/abscess drainage.
3 Skin tumour resection.
4 Migraines.
5 Chronic pain.
6 Postoperative analgesia.

Technique

Use 2% lignocaine with 1:200 000 adrenaline.

1 To block the front of the scalp, *see Forehead block.*
2 The zygomaticotemporal nerve can be blocked by finding the junction of the zygomatic and temporal bone, about 2.5 cm lateral to the lateral canthus. Block this nerve by injecting subcutaneously in a fan-shape manner at this site.
3 The auriculotemporal nerve lies 1–1.5 cm anterior to the tragus deep to the temporal artery. Infiltrate in a fan-shape manner subcutaneously with 2 mL of LA under the artery but do not inject into the artery.
4 To block the greater and lesser occipital nerves, identify the greater occipital protuberance and the mastoid process. Draw a line between these two points and divide it into thirds. The junction of the posterior third and anterior two-thirds is where to block the greater occipital nerve but avoid the occipital artery. The junction of the anterior third and posterior two-thirds is where to block the lesser occipital nerve. At both sites, inject 3 mL of LA in a fan-like pattern subcutaneously.

▶ Scalp capillary pH measurement

See Fetal scalp blood sampling.

▷ Sciatic nerve block

Anatomy

1 The sciatic nerve is formed from the L4, L5 and S1–3 nerve roots of the lumbosacral plexus.
2 The nerve leaves the pelvis in the greater sciatic foramen and descends beneath the gluteus maximus, between the greater trochanter and the ischial tuberosity, to enter the thigh behind the adductor magnus.
3 It then travels along the posteromedial aspect of the femur and divides in the apex of the popliteal fossa into the tibial nerve and the common peroneal nerve.
4 The sciatic nerve supplies motor to the hamstring muscles and all the muscles of the leg below the knee.
5 The sensory supply of the sciatic nerve is to the back of the thigh and all the leg and foot below the knee (bone, muscle and skin), except for the medial side of the leg and medial malleolus.

Uses

Anaesthesia/analgesia for surgery below the knee except for the medial side.

Technique for popliteal sciatic nerve block

There are many techniques. The easiest is to block the nerve in the region of the popliteal fossa:

1 Position the patient in the lateral position with the leg to be blocked uppermost on a pillow.
2 Apply sterile prep to the lower lateral thigh and knee area.
3 Place the ultrasound probe in a transverse orientation along the popliteal skin crease. See Figures S1 and S2.

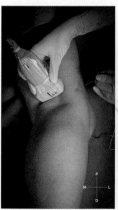 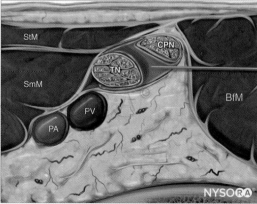

Figure S1 Probe position and anatomy of popliteal sciatic nerve block. TN = tibial nerve, CPN = common peroneal nerve, PV = popliteal vein, PA = popliteal artery, StM = semitendinosus muscle, SmM = semimembranosus muscle, BfM = biceps femoris muscle
Image courtesy of NYSORA

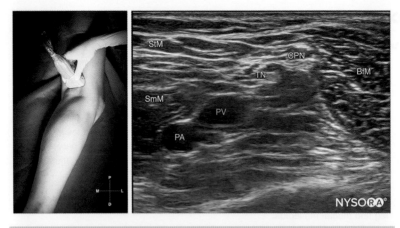

Figure S2 Probe position and sonoanatomy of popliteal sciatic nerve block. TN = tibial nerve, CPN = common peroneal nerve, PV = popliteal vein, PA = popliteal artery, StM = semitendinosus muscle, SmM = semimembranosus muscle, BfM = biceps femoris muscle
Image courtesy of NYSORA

4   Identify (moving from superficial to deep) the common peroneal nerve and tibial nerve, the popliteal vein and the popliteal artery (the 'snowman' at the back of the knee). The vein can be made more obvious by squeezing the calf.
5   Move the probe proximally until the common peroneal and tibial nerves join up, forming the sciatic nerve. Deep to the nerve will be the popliteal vein, and deeper still the popliteal artery. Dorsiflexing and plantar flexing the foot will make the sciatic nerve's medial and lateral side move alternately at the branching point. This is the site at which to perform the block.
6   Anaesthetise the skin and use an in-plane approach with a 10 cm block needle from lateral to medial at the same depth as the nerve.
7   When the needle tip is just deep to the nerve (and after negative aspiration), inject a 0.5 mL test dose. If in good position, inject 10 mL of 1% ropivacaine.
8   Withdraw the needle then reinsert so the tip is just superficial to the nerve and repeat (aspirate, 0.5 mL test dose then 10 mL of LA).
9   It may take up to 30 min for the block to be effective.
10 Alternatively, insert the needle so the tip is between the common peroneal and tibial nerves, at the point where they branch from the sciatic nerve. The needle tip should penetrate the tough, perineural sheath that surrounds the larger tibial nerve and the smaller common peroneal nerve. There is often a big 'give' when the sheath is entered. Attempt aspiration, then inject a 0.5 mL test dose of LA. If the tip is in good position, inject 19.5 mL of 0.5% ropivacaine.

◐ Septic shock

Description
Septic shock is defined as a life-threatening condition, due to an infective process, causing severe hypotension, that can result in organ ischaemia and/or damage. To diagnose septic shock there should be hypotension (SBP ≤ 90 mmHg, MAP ≤ 65 mmHg) plus signs of hypoperfusion such as oliguria and/or altered mental state.

Effects and diagnosis

Sepsis can occur anywhere in the body and affect any organ system.

1 CNS—meningitis, encephalitis, delirium, leukoencephalopathy, impaired blood–brain barrier.
2 CVS—reduced SVR, myocardial depression, hypotension, arrhythmias.
3 Respiratory—pneumonia, ARDS, V/Q mismatch, decreased lung compliance, interstitial oedema.
4 Renal—acute kidney injury, renal failure, oliguria.
5 GIT—vomiting, diarrhoea, hepatic failure, cholestasis, compromised intestinal barrier.
6 Haematological—thrombocytopenia, DIC, high WCC, bone marrow suppression, endotheliopathy.
7 Musculoskeletal—immobility, myopathy, catabolic state.

Management

1 Antibiotic therapy.
2 Organ support with IV fluids, vasopressors, respiratory support and renal replacement therapy. At least 30 mL/kg (ideal body weight) of crystalloid should be given within the first 3 h of resuscitation. Serum lactate levels may provide evidence of response to treatment.
3 Aim for a MAP ≥ 65 mmHg.[3]
4 Control of the source of the infection.

⊙ Serotonin syndrome/toxicity

Description

Serotonin is also known as 5-hydroxytryptamine (5-HT). Serotonin syndrome is a potentially fatal condition due to over-activation of serotonergic receptors in the central nervous system. It is due to the therapeutic use of serotonergic drugs, overdose of these drugs or interaction between different types of serotonergic drugs.

Causes

There are many drugs that increase serotonin levels in the brain. They include:

1 SSRIs—citalopram, escitalopram, fluoxetine
2 SNRIs—desvenlafaxine
3 tricyclic antidepressants—amitriptyline
4 some opioids—methadone, pethidine, tramadol, tapentadol, oxycodone, fentanyl
5 anti-nausea drugs—ondansetron, granisetron, metoclopramide
6 monoamine oxidase inhibitors—phenelzine, selegiline
7 amphetamines
8 cocaine, MDMA (ecstasy), LSD
9 L-Dopa
10 lithium
11 propranolol
12 methylene blue **(patients taking serotonin reuptake inhibitors must not be given methylene blue or fatal serotonin toxicity may occur).**[4]
13 herbal drugs—St John's wort.

Serotonin toxicity is frequently associated with certain combinations of serotonergic drugs including:

1 SSRIs with MAOIs.
2 MAOIs with opioids—*see Monoamine oxidase inhibitor (MAOI) drugs.*
3 Tramadol with mirtazapine/olanzapine.

There are many other combinations.

Clinical effects

Serotonin syndrome can develop over 24 h and resolve within 24 h with treatment. It causes a wide range of mental, neuromuscular and autonomic effects, including:

1 altered mental status—agitation, anxiety, disorientation
2 tremor, clonus, hyperreflexia
3 akathisia (inability to keep still)
4 muscle rigidity
5 hypertension
6 tachycardia
7 hyperthermia
8 dilated pupils
9 horizontal ocular clonus
10 sweating
11 shivering
12 vomiting and diarrhoea.

In severe cases, patients can experience fever > 41.1°C, unstable pulse and blood pressure, muscle rigidity, rhabdomyolysis, renal and respiratory failure, DIC, coma and death. Presentation can be similar to malignant hyperthermia. *See Malignant hyperthermia (MH).*

Diagnosis

1 Clinical picture plus accurate drug history.
2 Medical toxicologist diagnosis.

Treatment

1 Stop the serotonergic drug(s). Usually this is all that is required.
2 Supportive care—airway, ventilation, heart rate and blood pressure optimisation (esmolol, sodium nitroprusside).
3 Sedation with benzodiazepines.
4 Cooling measures for fever.
5 Cyproheptadine (Periactin) is a serotonin antagonist—the PO dose is 12 mg then 2 mg every 2 h if needed. Maintenance if needed is 8 mg q 6 h.
6 In the worst cases, intubation and ventilation may be required.
7 Dantrolene has no role in the treatment of serotonin syndrome.

◐ Serratus anterior plane block

Description

This block is useful for the management of anterior and lateral rib fractures and for chest surgery such as mastectomy. The nerves blocked are the lateral divisions of the thoracic intercostal nerves and the long thoracic and thoracodorsal nerves. The nerves lie between latissimus dorsi and serratus anterior. This block can provide analgesia from T3 to T9. Use 30 mL of ropivacaine 0.5%.

Technique (superficial approach)

1 Position the patient supine with arm adducted to 90°. See Figure S3.
2 Place the probe in a coronal plane, at the level of the nipple in males, in the midaxillary line. The probe should lie over the 5th rib. Aiming towards a rib will improve safety.
3 Identify the plane between latissimus dorsi and serratus anterior. Identify and do not penetrate the thoracodorsal artery.
4 Using a sterile technique, advance the needle in-plane in a ventral to dorsal direction, until the tip is in the plane between serratus anterior and latissimus dorsi.
5 After negative aspiration and a a 2 mL test dose, inject 28 mL of LA.

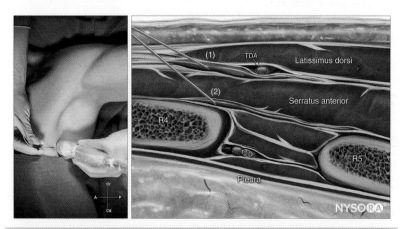

Figure S3 Probe and needle position and anatomy for serratus anterior plane block. R4 = rib 4, R5 = rib 5, TDA = thoracodorsal artery. Needle approach (1) is the approach described above.
Image courtesy of NYSORA

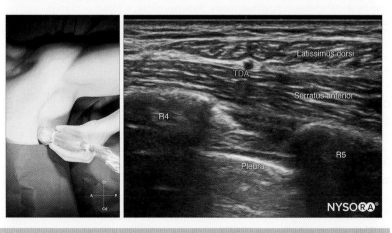

Figure S4 Probe and needle position and sonoanatomy for serratus anterior plane block. R4 = rib 4, R5 = rib 5, TDA = thoracodorsal artery
Image courtesy of NYSORA

▶ Sevoflurane

Description
Volatile inhalational halogenated ether-type anaesthetic agent with a MAC of 2.05. It is currently the most widely used of the volatile anaesthetic agents.

Advantages
1 Pleasant to breathe, can be used for gaseous induction.
2 Low blood gas solubility leading to rapid induction of anaesthesia and rapid emergence.
3 Cerebral autoregulation is preserved up to 1.5 MAC.
4 Causes bronchodilation.
5 Less harmful to the environment than desflurane.

Disadvantages
1 Can cause malignant hyperthermia.
2 Exists in the atmosphere for 1.1 years. Contributes to global warming.
3 Prolongs the QT interval. *See Long QT syndrome (LQTS)* and *Torsades de pointes*.

▶ Sevredol

This is a brand name for a form of immediate-release oral morphine. *See Morphine*.

▶ Shivering

See Postoperative shivering.

▶ Short QT syndrome (SQTS)

Description
This is a very rare autosomal dominant genetic heart disease associated with arrhythmias and sudden cardiac death. There is enhanced potassium channel flow out of the cell or reduced calcium channel flow into the cell, resulting in a shortened cardiac action potential. This results in an increased risk of arrhythmias. SQTS can also be acquired due to hypercalcaemia, hyperkalaemia, acidosis or digoxin.

Clinical effects
1 Arrhythmias such as atrial fibrillation, ventricular fibrillation (VF).
2 Palpitations, dyspnoea, fatigue.
3 Blackouts.
4 Sudden death.

Diagnosis
ECG shows a very short QT interval of $\leq$ 330 milliseconds. However, $\leq$ 360 milliseconds may also be used as a cut-off when considered with other factors e.g. family history. There may be tall, peaked T waves and PR segment depression. Genetic testing can be helpful.

Treatment
1 Implantable defibrillator.
2 Antiarrhythmic drugs e.g. quinidine, sotalol.

▶ Sick sinus syndrome (SSS)

This arrhythmia (also termed sinus node dysfunction) is due to pathology such as fibrosis affecting the SA node. This disease process results in effects such as sinus bradycardia, sinus pauses or sinus arrest. There may be episodes of tachycardia alternating with bradycardia (tachy-brady syndrome). SSS is often associated with AF.

Treatment
Permanent pacemaker if patient is symptomatic.

Points to note
1 Adenosine is contraindicated.
2 Drugs used to treat associated AF such as beta blockers and calcium channel blockers may make the SA node dysfunction worse.

◯ Sickle cell disease (SCD)

Description
This inherited haemoglobinopathy results from a mutant version of the beta haemoglobin gene. It occurs mainly in African and some Mediterranean people. This mutation creates haemoglobin S (HbS). HbSS patients are homozygous for this gene while heterozygotes are HbAS or sickle cell trait (SCT). SCT is a reasonably benign condition and may offer survival advantages if malaria infection occurs. Sickle cell trait may become an issue if there is an extreme physiological challenge e.g. mountain climbing.

Sickle cell disease can also occur in patients with sickle cell trait plus an abnormality of the other beta chain including:
1 Sickle-beta thalassaemia (**see Thalassaemia**).
2 Haemoglobin SC disease—this illness is particularly associated with retinopathy. Avascular necrosis of the femoral head is another complication of HbSC and is most likely to occur during the final months of pregnancy. HbSC disease is less severe than SCD. Vaso-occlusion can still occur but less frequently than in SCD. Lifespan is significantly reduced.

Pathophysiology
Deoxygenation results in the erythrocytes forming a sickle shape, and re-oxgenation reverses the process. The sickle-shaped red cells cause blockages in the microcirculation, slowing blood flow and causing more cells to sickle in a 'vicious cycle'. This can result in infarction of tissue. Attacks can be precipitated by dehydration, exercise, high altitude, temperature changes and stress.

Clinical picture
This disease can affect any organ to any extent of severity. It is a multisystem illness typified by:
1 Chronic haemolytic anaemia. SCD RBCs only have a lifespan/clearance time of 10–20 days, compared with 120 days for normal RBCs.
2 Vaso-occlusive crises. These cause severe pain and organ ischaemia/infarction. These can be induced by stress, over-exertion, dehydration, acidosis, hypothermia, fever, labour and infection. Thrombolysis should not be used in strokes due to SCD—use mechanical thrombectomy.[5]
3 Acute chest syndrome—chest pain, cough, fever and hypoxia. **See Treatment of sickle cell crisis**.
4 Pulmonary hypertension/heart failure.
5 Splenic sequestration crises. A vaso-occlusive episode in the spleen causes a large percentage of the total blood volume to be trapped there.
6 Haemolytic crisis—severe acute haemolysis with anaemia, jaundice and reticulocytosis (increase in the numbers of circulating immature RBCs).

QUICK FLICK S

7 Aplastic crisis—sudden bone marrow failure precipitated by such causes as viral infections.
8 Increased risk of infection due to splenic infarcts causing functional hyposplenism.
9 Increased thromboembolic risk.
10 Any tissue structure/organ can be damaged e.g. kidney, bone.
11 Priapism.

Diagnosis

A SICKLEDEX test will detect HbS but does not identify the type of disease. The genotype can be detected by Hb electrophoresis.

Treatment other than sickle cell crisis

1 Preventative measures include hydroxycarbamide (hydroxyurea) to increase HbF levels and decrease the adhesiveness of sickle cells to the endothelium. Voxelotor may also be helpful. It is a HbS polymerisation inhibitor.
2 Crizanlizumab-tmca—helps prevent sickle cells from clumping together.
3 Folic acid.
4 Niprisan—delays the time period of sickling in deoxygenated HbS, reducing the incidence of sickle cell crises.
5 L-glutamine oral powder (Endari) reduces the incidence of sickle cell crisis events.
6 Bone marrow transplant.

Anaesthetic management

Always seek expert haematologist advice regarding the management of these patients. A multidisciplinary team approach is essential.

1 Depending on the type of surgery being performed and the baseline Hb level, consider a consider a preoperative blood transfusion, aiming for a Hb of 70–100 g/L. This should not be undertaken lightly, as patients with SCD have a high incidence of alloimmunisation. The blood bank should always be informed that the patient has SCD and extra care with cross-matching is required, including C, E and Kell antibodies. An exchange transfusion may be required in high-risk patients having high-risk surgery.
2 These patients should be operated on first on the list to avoid prolonged fasting. Avoid dehydration. Do not perform elective surgery if the patient has acute pain or fever.
3 Antibiotic prophylaxis, if indicated, is extremely important.
4 Surgery under neuraxial block may be less risky than with GA.[5]
5 Avoid hypoxia, acidosis, hypovolaemia, hypothermia, pain and stress.
6 Tourniquet use should be avoided. If it is used, exsanguinate the limb before tourniquet inflation and minimise the duration of tourniquet application.[5]
7 Cell salvage is controversial due to the risk of sickling and haemolysis of the salvaged red cells. If the patient has had an exchange transfusion, then cell salvage is probably acceptable.
8 Caution with drugs that decrease respiration such as opioids.
9 Provide postoperative oxygen therapy, aiming for an oxygen saturation of 96% until mobilising.
10 Monitor in a suitable environment such as a high dependency unit.
11 Use VTE prophylaxis.

Obstetrics and SCD

Women with SCD are at increased risk during pregnancy.
1 Neuraxial anaesthesia is useful for managing labour and Caesarean section.
2 Increased risk of preeclampsia in SCD patients.

3 Cell salvage is not recommended.[6]

4 Postpartum LMWH should be used for 6 weeks.

Treatment of sickle cell crisis

1 Supportive measures—hydration, oxygenation, analgesia.

2 Antibiotics if infection is present.

3 Blood transfusion if pain is refractory to maximum analgesic therapy or patient suffers a stroke or acute chest syndrome. Acute chest syndrome is a new radiodensity on CXR with fever and/or respiratory symptoms in a patient with SCD. It may be due to sickling in the small blood vessels of the lung with pulmonary infarction, emboli or infection. It can rapidly progress and cause death.

○ Single ventricle physiology and anaesthesia

In certain types of congenital heart disease (CHD), there is only 1 functioning ventricle which acts as the systemic circulation pump. Pulmonary blood flow is passive and determined by the pressure gradient between the pulmonary artery and left atrium. Examples include:

1 hypoplastic left heart syndrome

2 tricuspid/mitral/pulmonary atresia

3 double-inlet left ventricle.

Treatment

Management includes staged procedures such as:

1 Blalock–Taussig (BT) shunt—attaching the subclavian artery to the pulmonary artery on the same side. A modified BT shunt involves a prosthetic graft between the subclavian and pulmonary arteries.

2 Another option is to apply a pulmonary artery band. This decreases pulmonary blood flow. It can be used, for example, in transposition of the great arteries prior to repair, to prepare the LV for a higher systemic load.

3 Glenn shunt. This is the connection of the superior vena cava (SVC) to the right pulmonary artery. The BT shunt is removed. Alternatively, a hemi-Fontan procedure can be performed (also called a bidirectional Glenn shunt). In this procedure there is an end to side anastomosis of the SVC and right pulmonary artery. The aim is to reduce the workload of the functioning ventricle, which now only has to pump blood to the systemic circulation.

4 Fontan procedure—the inferior vena cava (IVC) is attached to the pulmonary artery so that the SVC and IVC now bypass the heart.

○ Sinoatrial nodal re-entrant tachycardia (SANRT)

SANRT is defined as a specific focal atrial re-entrant tachycardia involving the SA node. It usually has an abrupt onset and offset. ECG features are identical to sinus tachycardia. The usual heart rate is 100–150 bpm.

Treatment

Treatment is often not required unless the episodes are persistent. Tachycardia-mediated cardiomyopathy may occur. Treatments include:

1 vagal manoeuvres

2 adenosine for acute attacks

3 verapamil for chronic suppressive therapy.

▷ Sodium

Description

Sodium is one of the most important electrolytes in the body and is located mainly in the blood and interstitial fluid. Its concentration in plasma is about 140 mmol/L but it is only 10 mmol/L in the cell. It has many functions, including:

1 regulating extracellular volume
2 control of blood pressure
3 involvement in the action potential of excitable cells.

Only a brief outline of sodium-related metabolic disturbance is discussed in this manual, due the complexity of these abnormalities and space constraints.

Hyponatraemia

Defined as a sodium level < 135 mmol/L (severe if < 120 mmol/L). In simplistic terms, sodium and water are linked. In certain conditions or illnesses (e.g. excessive sweating), sodium and water are lost together. Hyponatraemia will occur if more sodium than water is lost, or more water is replaced than sodium. In other types of conditions excess sodium and water are retained e.g. heart failure. If more water is retained (or consumed) than sodium, hyponatraemia will result. Hyponatraemia will also occur if a substance in the blood draws intracellular fluid into the extracellular space (e.g. glycine or mannitol).

Hypovolaemia with more sodium than water lost

1 Vomiting, diarrhoea.
2 Salt-wasting nephropathy.
3 Burns.
4 Pancreatitis.
5 Trauma.
6 Diuretics.
7 Mineralocorticoid deficiency.
8 Osmotic diuresis without replacement.

Euvolaemia with more water replaced than sodium

1 Vomiting, diarrhoea with IV fluid replacement that is sodium deficient e.g. 5% glucose.
2 Hypotonic fluid replacement post surgery.
3 Excess water intake.

Euvolaemia with more water retained than sodium

1 SIADH.
2 Glucocorticoid deficiency.
3 Hypothyroidism.

Hypervolaemia with more water retained than sodium

1 Renal failure.
2 CCF.
3 Nephrotic syndrome.
4 Cirrhosis.

Effects of hyponatraemia

The NR for serum sodium is 135–145 mmol/L. Hyponatraemia above 125 mmol/L is well tolerated. As sodium and osmolality fall, water enters the cells, causing them to swell.

Na^+ 110–125 mmol/L

1 Lethargy.
2 Nausea.
3 Headaches.
4 Weakness.
5 Confusion.

Na^+ < 110 mmol/L

1 Seizures.
2 Coma.
3 Brain herniation from cerebral oedema.
4 Na^+ < 100 mmol/L may cause intravascular haemolysis.

Treatment of acute hyponatraemia

Identify and treat the cause. Patients who are symptomatic from acute hyponatraemia may rapidly deteriorate and treatment is urgent. Although controversial, hyponatraemia that has developed acutely (< 48 h) can probably be safely treated with rapid correction (about 2 mmol/L/h) in symptomatic patients, to a level where they become asymptomatic. Usually an increase by 6 mmol/L is sufficient. Give 100 mL boluses of 3% sodium chloride over 10 min × 3.

Treatment of chronic hyponatraemia

Identify and treat the cause. Correct by not more than 8 mmol/L per day. Overly rapid correction of hyponatraemia can result in osmotic demyelination syndrome (ODS), also known as central pontine myelinolysis, especially in patients with alcoholism, cirrhosis, malnutrition or hypokalaemia. Brain damage can occur due to acute demyelination.

Treatments include:

1 fluid restriction
2 boluses of hypertonic saline in symptomatic patients.

Hypernatraemia

Causes include:

1 excessive salt intake
2 inadequate water intake
3 loss of sodium and water but more water than sodium
4 Conn's syndrome
5 Cushing's syndrome
6 administration of sodium bicarbonate.

Effects of hypernatraemia

The brain can become acutely and severely dehydrated with shrinkage and tearing of cerebral veins, leading to brain haemorrhage. Demyelination can also occur. Other effects include:

1 Thirst.
2 Lethargy.
3 Twitching.
4 Seizures/coma.

Treatment of hypernatraemia

Rapid correction is not associated with any special risk in adults. A reduction in serum sodium of 10 mmol/L/24 h is suggested.

1 Identify and treat the cause.
2 Replace the water deficit (WD) using the formula: WD (L) = 0.6 × Wt (kg) × 1–140/ measured Na$^+$.
  If the patient is 70 kg and the measured sodium is 160 mmol/L, the WD is 5.25 L. Use 5% glucose IV replacement fluid, aiming for a 10 mmol/L/24 h reduction in serum sodium.
3 If the patient is hypervolaemic, remove excess sodium with loop diuretics or dialysis.

❯ Sodium bicarbonate

Sodium bicarbonate ($NaHCO_3$) is an inorganic salt, presented as an 8.4% solution in 100 mL bottles (100 mmol or 100 mEq or 8.5 g per 100 mL bottle). This contains 100 mmol of sodium bicarbonate, or 100 mEq, or 8.4 g in 100 mL. It is an alkalinising agent that acts by the carbonate combining with acid to produce CO_2 and water.

Indications

1 Severe metabolic acidosis from various causes e.g. diabetic ketoacidosis and shock. It is especially urgent if there is haemodynamic instability. For example, in lactic acidosis consider sodium bicarbonate if the pH < 7.1. If there is (in addition) acute kidney injury, give bicarbonate if pH < 7.2. Aim for a pH > 7.3.
2 Prolonged cardiac arrest (> 15 min).
3 Cardiac arrest associated with hyperkalaemia.
4 Treatment of barbiturate overdose. The sodium bicarbonate increases the alkalinity of the urine, increasing urinary drug excretion.
5 To reduce the amount of free drug in the serum after tricyclic antidepressant overdose.
6 For forced alkaline diuresis to treat salicylate poisoning or rhabdomyolysis.

Dose—adult

1 Give 50–100 mL IV.
2 Give more, depending on arterial acid-base measurements.
3 A sodium bicarbonate infusion can be given at a rate of 100–200 mL/h.

Points to note

1 The CO_2 produced from sodium bicarbonate administration may enter the cells and cause intracellular acidosis—ensure ventilation is adequate.
2 Sodium bicarbonate results in a high IV sodium load.
3 Sodium bicarbonate produces a shift to the left of the oxygen-haemoglobin dissociation curve, inhibiting release of O_2 to the tissues.
4 Do not allow sodium bicarbonate and calcium chloride/calcium gluconate to mix as calcium carbonate (a solid) will form.

❯ Sodium nitroprusside (SNP)

Description

SNP is a direct-acting vasodilator of arteries and veins, administered by IV infusion. It acts by breaking down to nitric oxide (NO). It is 44% cyanide by weight. SNP is used to treat/prevent hypertension in situations such as cerebral aneurysm surgery and phaeochromocytoma surgery. It is also used to produce hypotension and treat some types of heart failure. Onset is within 2 min.

Dose

Mix 50 mg of SNP powder with 100 mL 5% glucose. Protect the SNP from light. If marked degradation of SNP does occur, the solution turns blue. Administer at a dose of 0.3–4 mcg/kg/min, titrating to effect. In a 70 kg patient, this is 2.5–33 mL/h. The maximum permissible rate is 10 mcg/kg/min and this should not be used for longer than 10 min. Boluses can also be given of 1–2 mcg/kg. In a 70 kg patient, this equates to 0.14–0.28 mL.

Advantages

1 Fast onset and offset.
2 Easily titratable.

Disadvantages

1 Can result in cyanide (CN) toxicity. *See Burns and Cyanide (CN) toxicity.*
2 Contraindicated if recent ingestion of PDE V inhibitor such as sildenafil.
3 Can cause fetal cyanide poisoning.
4 Thiocyanate toxicity can occur, especially if prolonged infusions and if renal function is impaired. This can cause tinnitus, abdominal pain, weakness and decreased level of consciousness.
5 May cause methaemoglobinaemia.
6 SNP may increase ICP by dilating cerebral blood vessels.

◑ Sodium thiosulphate

This drug can be used to treat cyanide poisoning. *See Burns and Cyanide (CN) toxicity.* It transfers a sulphur to cyanide to form thiocyanate, which is excreted by the kidneys.

◑ Sotalol (Sotacor)

Description

Non-selective beta-adrenergic receptor blocker drug with marked class III antiarrhythmic properties.

Indications

1 Second-line drug for the prevention/treatment of atrio-ventricular (AV) nodal and AV re-entrant tachycardias. *See Supraventricular tachycardia (SVT).*
2 Termination of sustained VT and for the prevention of recurrent VT/VF.
3 Prevention of recurrent AF after cardioversion.

Dose

Adult

PO 160–640 mg daily in 2 or 3 divided doses. IV dose 0.5–1 mg/kg over 5–20 min.

Points to note

1 Can cause hypotension, bradycardia, AV block, polymorphic VT or torsades de pointes.
2 Contraindicated in asthma and long QT syndrome. *See Long QT syndrome (LQTS).*

◑ Sphenopalatine ganglion (SPG) block

Anatomy and function

The SPG is a small triangular structure located in the pterygopalatine fossa, inferior to the maxillary nerve and posterior to the middle turbinate. It is a parasympathetic ganglion of the trigeminal nerve. It contains autonomic and sensory fibres supplying the lacrimal glands and the inner lining of the nose and sinuses.

SPG block

This is thought to be helpful in treating some kinds of headaches such as migraines and dural puncture headache. *See Post dural puncture headache*. To do the block:

1 Position the patient so they are comfortable and there is good access to the nose.
2 Soak a 10 cm long cotton tip applicator in LA (e.g. lignocaine 2% or ropivacaine 1%).
3 Insert the applicator into the nose on the side of the headache (both sides using 2 applicators if a bilateral headache). The applicator should be inserted along the superior border of the middle turbinate, until resistance is felt.
4 Leave the cotton tip applicator(s) in place for 10 min then remove.

❍ Spina bifida occulta

Description

This condition is common, occurring in up to 20% of the population. It is usually asymptomatic. It is due to failure of fusion of low lumbar or sacral vertebral bodies in the midline. In a small percentage of patients, there is a spinal cord abnormality such as:

1 Tethering of the spinal cord with stretching and damage.
2 The filum terminale can be thickened and fatty.
3 Splitting of the spinal cord.

These abnormalities may be referred to as 'spinal dysraphism' (spina bifida occulta + spinal cord abnormality) and can cause:

1 Pain in the back or legs.
2 Leg weakness, numbness.
3 Bladder and/or bowel problems.

There may be a dimple in the skin or a sinus, fatty lump, discoloration or hair over the defect.

Neuraxial anaesthesia

1 In the asymptomatic patient, epidural anaesthesia should be performed at a level well above the defect.
2 There is an increased risk of dural puncture with epidural insertion as the ligamentum flavum can be deficient.
3 Epidural blocks may be patchy or inadequate.
4 SAB has an increased risk of injury to the stretched spinal cord or filum terminale. An MRI will determine whether the spinal cord is tethered.

❍ Spinal anaesthesia

See Subarachnoid block (SAB).

❍ Spinal anatomy

Bones

There are 33 vertebrae: 7 cervical, 12 thoracic, 5 lumbar, 5 sacral (fused) and 3–5 coccygeal.

Spinal cord

In adults, the spinal cord terminates at L1–2, and in children it terminates at L3–4.

Landmarks

1 A line joining the iliac crests (Tuffier's line) passes through the lower part of the L4 vertebra or the L4–5 disc space.

2 C7 spinous process (vertebra prominens) is the first prominent spinous process when running the fingers down the back of the neck.

3 The angles of the scapulae are at the same level as the T7 spinous process.

Spinal nerves

There are 31 pairs of nerves: 8 cervical, 12 thoracic, 5 lumbar, 5 sacral and 1 coccygeal.

Subarachnoid space

Extends from the top of the inner skull (between the arachnoid and pia layers) to the S2 vertebra. At this level, the dura continues (without a space) as part of the filum terminale that attaches to the coccyx.

Epidural space

Extends from the top of the inner skull to the sacral hiatus.

○ Spinal cord injury (pre-existing) and anaesthesia

The main concerns are:

1 autonomic dysreflexia (AD)
2 respiratory inadequacy
3 muscle spasms.

Autonomic dysreflexia

This is also referred to as autonomic hyperreflexia, hypertensive autonomic crisis or mass reflex. AD is typically associated with lesions above the T6 vertebra and is due to autonomic nervous system dysregulation. AD can also be associated with Guillain–Barré syndrome. Attacks usually begin within 12 months of the injury and consist of episodes of unopposed massive sympathetic activity causing:

1 severe hypertension
2 bradycardia
3 headache
4 blurred vision
5 sweating, skin pallor, piloerection (goose-pimples), facial flushing
6 severe vasoconstriction below the level of injury
7 intracerebral haemorrhage
8 retinal haemorrhage.

Most attacks have a urological source such as bladder distension or a UTI. Attacks can also be due to:

1 surgery
2 bowel distension
3 uterine contractions
4 pressure ulcers.

Treatment

This is a crisis situation. Management steps include:

1 Notify the surgeon, cease surgical stimulation and deepen anaesthesia if under GA.
2 Remove the cause if possible e.g. empty the bladder.

3 Lower BP with glyceryl trinitrate (GTN) IV bolus of 50–100 mcg and an infusion of 10–100 mcg/min. Do not use GTN if the patient is on sildenafil or vardenafil as severe hypotension may occur. Nitrolingual spray or anginine under the tongue can be used while GTN is being prepared. A GTN transdermal patch 5 mg/24 h may also be effective.

4 Other drugs to consider are clevidipine or sodium nitroprusside. **See *Clevidipine*** and ***Sodium nitroprusside (SNP)***.

5 Position patient head up.

6 Monitor BP invasively.

7 Diagnose/treat haemorrhage, myocardial ischaemia, dysrhythmias or seizures. Heart block may occur.

◐ Spinal epidural abscess

See *Epidural abscess, spinal.*

◐ Status epilepticus (SE)

Description

SE describes a seizure lasting more than 5 min or having more than one seizure within a 5 min period, without regaining consciousness between episodes. It is a medical emergency that can result in brain injury or death.

Clinical effects

It can be convulsive (tonic-clonic) or non-convulsive, with the appearance of vacantness, irrational behaviour, difficulty speaking, nystagmus or eye twitching.

Causes

1 Epilepsy (rarely).

2 Infection with fever in children.

3 Low blood sugar—**see *Hypoglycaemia***.

4 Excess alcohol or alcohol withdrawal or other types of drug abuse.

5 Stroke.

6 Brain tumour.

7 Head injury.

8 Kidney or liver failure.

9 Encephalitis.

10 Eclampsia. **See *Preeclampsia/eclampsia.***

11 Dysrhythmia.

12 Genetic causes such as Fragile X syndrome or Angelman syndrome.

13 Electroconvulsive therapy.

Treatment

1 If a convulsive seizure, prevent the patient from injuring themselves.

2 Identify and treat the cause, if possible e.g. hypoglycaemia. **See *Hypoglycaemia***.

3 Lorazepam IV 4–8 mg (adult) or 0.1 mg/kg (child). This dose can be repeated after 10 min if needed.

4 Diazepam IV 10–20 mg (adult) or 0.2 mg/kg (child). If no IV access, consider diazepam PR rectal gel 10 mg (adult) or 0.1 mg/kg (child). Diazepam is faster acting than lorazepam.

5 Midazolam IV 5–10 mg or 0.07–0.3 mg/kg IM in the adult. It is very short acting.

6 Consider a midazolam infusion—0.05–0.4 mg/kg/h.

7 Phenytoin 10–15 mg/kg LD IV. Give 10 mg/kg LD if already on phenytoin. Can give a subsequent bolus of 10 mg/kg if the seizure is not terminated by first LD. Give no faster than 50 mg/min. Fosphenytoin is a phosphate ester prodrug of phenytoin. It can cause severe tissue necrosis if it extravasates. *See Phenytoin (Dilantin) and fosphenytoin*. Maintenance dose of phenytoin 100 mg q 6–8 h (PO or IV).

8 Anaesthetic doses of thiopentone or propofol. It may be necessary to paralyse and intubate the patient. Maintain anaesthesia with a propofol infusion.

9 EEG monitoring will be required, as seizures may continue under GA.

Desperate measures

1 Levetiracetam—inhibits burst firing of neurones.

2 Valproic acid—decreases seizure activity.

○ Stents, cardiac and non-cardiac surgery

See Coronary artery stents (CAS).

○ Steroid cover

See Stress steroids.

○ Steroid equivalents

Table S1 Equivalent doses of different types of steroid drug

Drug	Equivalent dose
Hydrocortisone (IV or PO)	80 mg
Dexamethasone (IV or PO)	3 mg
Methylprednisolone (IV or PO)	16 mg
Prednisone/prednisolone (PO)	20 mg
Betamethasone (IV)	3 mg
Cortisone acetate (PO)	100 mg

For inhaled steroids

750 mcg fluticasone or 1500 mcg beclomethasone/day is equivalent to prednisone 10 mg/day PO.

○ Stress steroids

Description

This is a highly controversial area, and the need for stress steroids has been questioned by several researchers based on small numbers of patients.[7] The following guidelines are based on the best available evidence, which is sparse and inadequate. Patients who take 10 mg of prednisone or more per day for longer than 3 weeks[8] (or equivalent dose of another steroid) may have suppression of their adrenal gland. Cessation of steroid therapy (prednisone $\geq$ 10 mg/day or greater or equivalent other steroid) for < 3 months may also result in adrenal suppression. *See Steroid equivalents*. This may result in an inadequate supply of extra cortisol at times of surgical stress. Normal endogenous cortisol production is 15–20 mg/day, and this can increase to 50 mg/day for minor stress and up to 150 mg/day for major stress.

Clinical effects of suppressed cortisol response to stress

1 Hypotension.
2 Hypoglycaemia.
3 Dehydration.
4 Confusion.

Steroid replacement regimen[9]

Continue usual oral steroid therapy up until the day of surgery and recommence oral therapy the next day or whenever gastrointestinal function allows. For perioperative steroid therapy see Table S2.

Table S2 Perioperative stress steroid therapy using IV hydrocortisone

Type of surgery	Stress steroid dosages
Minor surgery e.g. hernia	25 mg hydrocortisone on induction.
Moderate surgery e.g. gall bladder	50 mg hydrocortisone on induction + 25 mg q 8 h for 24 h.
Major surgery e.g. hemicolectomy	100 mg hydrocortisone on induction + 50 mg q 8 h for 24 h. Taper dose by half each day until on maintenance dose.

Other points

1 Etomidate should be avoided—it inhibits steroid synthesis. **See Etomidate**.
2 In patients with possible adrenal suppression, the presence of nausea, hypotension, deterioration of mental status, hyponatraemia or hyperkalaemia should prompt consideration of additional steroid therapy.

○ Subarachnoid block (SAB)

See also *Ultrasound-assisted neuraxial anaesthesia.*

Description

SAB is a form of neuraxial anaesthesia in which LA and opioids are injected into the CSF to anaesthetise the spinal nerves. It is commonly referred to as a spinal block, spinal anaesthesia or intrathecal anaesthesia. SAB is an excellent technique for surgery in the lower abdomen, pelvis and lower limbs.

Anatomy

An imaginary horizontal line just touching the tops of the iliac crests, crosses the lumbar spine at the L4 (Tuffier's line). The space just above this line is the L3–4 disc space. The structures penetrated by the spinal needle are the same as those described for epidural anaesthesia, but in SAB, the dura and arachnoid layers are also penetrated.

Absolute contraindications

1 Patient refusal.
2 Significant coagulopathy.
3 Infection at the site of insertion.
4 Raised ICP, except for benign intracranial hypertension—**see Benign intracranial hypertension (BIH).**

Technique

1 Explain the procedure to the patient and discuss the risks and benefits.
2 Prepare the patient in the same way as described for epidural block. **See *Epidural anaesthesia/analgesia*.** Use a fully sterile technique.
3 Anaesthetise the skin and deeper structures with 5 mL of 1% lignocaine.
4 Insert the introducer needle that is matched with the selected spinal needle.
5 Insert the spinal needle through the introducer needle into the subarachnoid space as evidenced by return of CSF. A 27G Sprotte needle is preferred because of the low incidence of post subarachnoid block headache.
6 Inject the LA +/− opioid.
7 Place the patient supine and prepare to deal with any side effects such as hypotension.

Spinal needles

The preferred type is a 27 G Sprotte needle. This has a pencil point and a more rounded conical point than a Whitacre needle which is the next best option. The least popular type is the Quincke point, which has a sharp bevelled cutting point and is more likely to produce a spinal headache.

Selection of LA and opioid for SAB in the adult

1 For CS use heavy bupivacaine 0.5% 2–2.4 mL (depending on patient's height) + fentanyl 20–25 mcg + morphine 100 mcg. SAB lasts about 2–3 h. Morphine analgesia lasts about 16 h.
2 For knee replacement (if SAB is the primary anaesthetic) use heavy bupivacaine 0.5% 3–3.5 mL + fentanyl 25 mcg + morphine 100–150 mcg.
3 Pruritis is common when SAB morphine is used, especially for CS. Naloxone is effective at 40 mcg boluses up to 240 mcg.
4 Fentanyl has a rapid onset but a short duration of effect—about 1 h.
5 Intrathecal morphine can cause delayed respiratory depression, and patients must be observed for this.

Combined spinal epidural (CSE) technique

CSE enables a lower dose of spinal anaesthetic to be used and the opportunity to 'top up' the neuraxial anaesthetic via the epidural catheter. In this technique:

1 The epidural space is identified with the CSE kit Tuohy needle, as described in the section ***Epidural anaesthesia/analgesia***. This Tuohy needle has a back 'eye' or hole and a locking system.
2 The CSE kit spinal needle is then inserted through the Tuohy needle and locked in place. The return of CSF identifies that the spinal needle is properly deployed. Inject LA and opioid then remove the spinal needle.
3 An epidural catheter is passed through the Tuohy needle, the Tuohy needle is removed and the catheter secured.

CSE for labour

1 Give 2 mL of bupivacaine 0.125% + fentanyl 5 mcg/mL via the spinal needle.
2 Start epidural anaesthesia when the pain begins to reoccur.

CSE for CS

1 Inject 2 mL of heavy bupivacaine 0.5% + fentanyl 25 mcg + morphine 100 mcg. Use less heavy bupivacaine for high-risk patients e.g. cardiomyopathy.
2 Supplement the SAB with epidural lignocaine 2% + adrenaline 1:200 000 2–5 mL boluses.

Anticoagulant drugs and platelet count considerations for SAB

1   SAB should not be performed within 6 h of prophylactic heparin injection or 12 h of prophylactic LMWH. SAB should not be performed within 24 h of therapeutic LMWH.

2   If the patient is on a heparin infusion, cease for 8 h and check APTT before SAB.

3   For patients on apixaban, dabigatran or rivaroxaban, cease for 3 days before SAB (longer if impaired renal function).

4   If the patient is on warfarin, cease for 5 days and check INR before SAB. INR needs to be < 1.5.

5   A platelet count > 75000/mm³ is generally acceptable. 50–75000/mm³ is a grey area. If the platelet count is < 50000/mm³, SAB is contraindicated.

Saddle block

In this technique, the aim is to only block the sacral nerves, for procedures such as removal of a cervical suture or haemorrhoid surgery. Inject 1.5–1.75 mL of heavy bupivacaine 0.5% intrathecally, with the patient kept in the sitting position for 5–10 min post injection.

Complications of SAB

1   Hypotension—this can be treated with vasopressors such as metaraminol, ephedrine or phenylephrine and IV fluids. A metaraminol or phenylephrine infusion should be initiated immediately after SAB for CS. *See Caesarean section (CS).*

2   Bradycardia—this can progress to profound bradycardia/asystole. It is thought to be due to:

   a) Bezold–Jarisch reflex—bradycardia and decreased contractility in response to reduced ventricular filling. Reduced ventricular filling (preload) is due to sympathetic blockade below the level of the block.

   b) Block of sympathetic supply to the heart (T1–T4).

   c) Young people are possibly more at risk due to high vagal tone.

   d) Pre-procedure hypovolaemia.

   e) Excessive dose of LA.

   Treat with IV atropine and IV fluids. If cardiac arrest occurs, *see Cardiac arrest.*

3   Nausea and vomiting.

4   Dizziness.

5   Transitory deafness—possibly due to middle-ear changes as a result of CSF loss.

6   Post dural puncture headache. *See Post dural puncture headache (PDPH).*

7   Nerve damage.

8   Spinal cord injury, especially the conus medullaris.

9   Epidural or spinal haematoma.

10 Infection at the site of insertion/meningitis.

◗ Subarachnoid haemorrhage

See Cerebral aneurysm and subarachnoid haemorrhage (SAH).

◗ Subclavian vein central venous access

Anatomy

The subclavian vein is the continuation of the axillary vein. It becomes the subclavian vein as it passes over the lateral edge of the first rib. It passes under the clavicle and over the first rib anterior to the scalenus anterior and the subclavian artery.

Landmark technique

This must be done as a fully sterile technique with sterile gown, gloves, sterilisation of the skin around the entry point and sterile drape.

1 Prepare the central line by priming all the lumens with N/S. Attach 3-way taps, in the closed position, to each lumen except the brown one.
2 Position the patient supine with a rolled towel or a 1 L fluid bag between the shoulder blades. Tilt the operating table 10–15° head down.
3 The insertion point is between the midpoint of the clavicle and the first rib. Sterilise this area and cover with a sterile drape.
4 If the patient is awake, anaesthetise the entry point with 1% lignocaine.
5 Pass the Seldinger needle attached to a syringe with the shaft parallel to the floor just under the midpoint of the clavicle, aiming towards the sternal notch. Use a very flat trajectory and aspirate continuously.
6 If the subclavian artery is punctured, the needle needs to be redirected more superficially (i.e. a flatter trajectory).
7 Once the vein is punctured, detach the syringe and pass the wire into the vein.
8 Use the scalpel to nick the skin at the entry point of the wire. Make a cut big enough to allow the dilator to pass over the wire.
9 Dilate the tissues and puncture wound into the subclavian vein.
10 Pass the central line over the wire and into the subclavian vein to a depth of about 12 cm (in the adult). The guidewire's proximal end must be grasped prior to the central line entering the patient.
11 Remove the wire and attach a 3-way tap to the brown lumen. Ensure blood can be aspirated from each lumen and then flush each lumen with N/S. Ensure no lumen is open to air.
12 Perform a post-procedure CXR to check the position of the tip of the central line and to exclude a pneumothorax.

Technique with ultrasound

1 Visualise the axillary vein and artery with the probe covered with a sterile sheath, placed just medial to the axilla on the chest wall in transverse view.
2 The artery is deeper, has a rounder shape and is pulsatile. The pleural line can also be seen.
3 Slide the probe towards the first rib to see the subclavian vein. Rotate the probe to give a longitudinal view of the vein.
4 The Seldinger needle, with syringe attached, is inserted in-plane from lateral to medial, into the subclavian vein.
5 Pass the guidewire and visualise the wire in the vein with the ultrasound.
6 The rest of the process is as described above.
7 An alternative approach is to puncture the axillary vein prior to it becoming the subclavian vein.
8 Place the probe on the chest wall just medial to the axilla. Visualise the axillary vein and artery in the transverse view.
9 Puncture the vein in the short or long axis view, then pass the wire into the vein. The vein will be about 3 cm under the skin. The pleura will be at a depth of about 5 cm.
10 The rest of the process is as described in the landmark technique section.

Complications

1 Pneumothorax.
2 Subclavian artery puncture.
3 Infection.

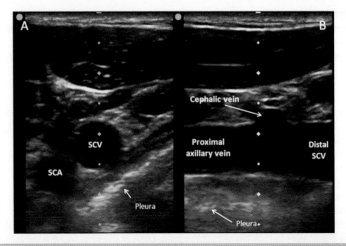

Figure S5 Transverse (A) and longitudinal (B) sonoanatomy of the subclavian and proximal axillary vein. SCA = subclavian artery, SCV = subclavian vein

Source Reproduced with permission Rezayat, Talayeh & Stowell, Jeffrey & Kendall, John & Turner, Elizabeth & Fox, John & Barjaktarevic, Igor. (2016). Ultrasound-Guided Cannulation: Time to Bring Subclavian Central Lines Back. Western Journal of Emergency Medicine. 17. 216–221

▶ Sublimaze

This is a trade name for fentanyl. *See Fentanyl.*

▶ Sublocade

Extended-release formulation of buprenorphine used subcut once per month.

▶ Suboxone

This is a trade name for a drug which is a combination of buprenorphine and naloxone (4:1) and is used to treat opioid addiction. The drug is used sublingually. Naloxone is thought to have little effect unless higher doses of suboxone are used (> 4 mg). If suboxone is injected or snorted, the naloxone will cause withdrawal.

▶ Sub–Tenon's block

See Eye blocks.

▶ Subutex

A trade name for buprenorphine, which is used to treat opioid addiction. It is administered sublingually.

▶ Succinylcholine

See Suxamethonium/succinylcholine.

▶ Sufentanil

Extremely powerful synthetic opioid. It is 5–10 × more potent than fentanyl, and 1000 × more potent than morphine.

◐ Sugammadex

Description

This drug is a modified gamma cyclodextrin which encapsulates rocuronium and, to a lesser extent, vecuronium, preventing the neuromuscular blocking effects of these drugs. Sugammadex has 2.5 × more affinity for rocuronium than vecuronium. It is fast acting and can reverse any level of rocuronium blockade (if sufficient sugammadex is used).

Dose

IV in adult

Shallow block—200 mg or 2 mg/kg.
Deep block—400 mg or 4 mg/kg.
Immediately after rocuronium administration—1200 mg or 16 mg/kg.
The drug works in 2–3 minutes.

Advantages

1 Effective, reliable and rapid reversal of rocuronium, allowing complete control over neuromuscular blockade.
2 There are no haemodynamic effects.
3 Laboratory tests do not support the use of sugammadex to treat rocuronium anaphylaxis.[10] There are conflicting reports from the literature as to whether sugammadex is beneficial in the treatment of anaphylaxis due to rocuronium.[10]

Disadvantages

1 High cost.
2 Incidence of anaphylaxis is about 1:34 500, but with few deaths.[10] Risk of anaphylaxis to neostigmine and glycopyrrolate/atropine is probably zero.
3 Only effective at reversing rocuronium and, to a lesser extent, vecuronium. It has no effect on other neuromuscular blocking drugs.
4 The sugammadex/rocuronium complex is excreted renally. In patients with end-stage renal disease, use of sugammadex is not recommended. However, case reports suggest that this practice is not unsafe.[11]
5 Binding to progesterone—this may reduce the effectiveness of the oral contraceptive pill (OCP). Alternative contraceptive techniques are recommended for 7 days after sugammadex use, in women taking the OCP.

◐ Sulfonamide allergy

Patients with a sulfonamide allergy are allergic to the sulfonamide group in several drugs including sulfamethoxazole, acetazolamide, frusemide and celecoxib. Bactrim contains trimethoprim and sulfamethoxazole and cannot be used in these patients. These patients may report an allergy to 'sulfa'. This does not mean they are allergic to sulphur-containing drugs such as thiopentone. They are also not allergic to sulfates and sulfites contained in such things as preservatives.

◐ Superior vena cava syndrome (SVCS)

Description

SVC obstruction is usually due to malignancy, most commonly bronchial carcinoma or lymphoma. Other causes include:
1 idiopathic fibrosing mediastinitis
2 SVC thrombosis

3 TB

4 other types of mediastinal masses—*see **Mediastinal mass syndrome (MMS)**.*

Clinical effects

1 Oedema of the head, neck, arms and chest.

2 Cerebral venous congestion with headaches, visual disturbance, raised ICP and altered mentation.

3 Venous distension in the neck and chest wall.

4 Dyspnoea, wheezing, stridor.

5 Hoarseness, laryngeal oedema.

6 Dysphagia.

7 Symptoms get worse with coughing, leaning forward or lying flat.

8 Proptosis.

Anaesthetic management

Anaesthesia and surgery may be required to diagnose the cause of the SVCS or the condition may be incidental. Avoidance of GA or GA with spontaneous breathing are preferred options. SVCS is associated with high morbidity and mortality, and anaesthesia should not be undertaken without the utmost care. In general:

1 Manage the patient in the head-up position.

2 Laryngeal oedema due to venous engorgement may make intubation difficult. Consider awake intubation. Also, the bronchial endoscope may help identify a site of tracheal compression, due to the mediastinal mass responsible for the SVCS. The tip of the ET tube can then be manoeuvred past the compression site.

3 Keep the patient well hydrated to maintain preload but avoid overhydration.

4 Obtain IV access in the leg. Use a femoral central line for IV access if significant surgery is planned. IV drugs in the upper extremity will have a long and unpredictable circulation time. Upper limb IV fluids may also exacerbate SVC obstruction effects.

5 There is an increased risk of bleeding for upper body surgery due to venous engorgement.

6 Perioperative steroids may decrease airway oedema and decrease the oedema around a tumour.

7 Patients may experience post-extubation breathing problems.

⊙ Supraventricular tachycardia (SVT)

These tachycardias are usually narrow complex because the pathology is above the bundle of His. The rate is > 100 bpm.

Sinus node re-entry tachycardia

In this tachycardia there is a re-entrant circuit in the area of the SA node. The ECG looks exactly like sinus tachycardia and the P waves are identical. It usually has an abrupt onset and offset.

Focal atrial tachycardia

This is a regular atrial rhythm at a rate > 100 bpm that arises from a single site in either atrium.

Atrial flutter

This is usually due to a re-entrant circuit between the orifice of the IVC and the tricuspid valve (called the cavotricuspid isthmus). Typically, the flutter rate is 300 bpm and the ventricular rate 150 bpm. *See **Atrial flutter**.*

Atrial fibrillation. *See **Atrial fibrillation**.*

Multifocal atrial tachycardia (MAT)

There is variable P wave morphology and a variable PR interval. If the rate is 60–100 bpm, the patient is said to have a 'wandering atrial pacemaker'.

Atrioventricular re-entrant tachycardia (AVRT)

This is a re-entrant (or reciprocating) tachycardia that requires two distinct pathways— the AV node and an accessory pathway (AP). If the antegrade conduction of the electrical impulse is through the AV node, the QRS will be narrow. If it is through the AP, pre-excitation occurs. The ventricle is excited prematurely and from a different position to the AV node, leading to a slurred upstroke of the QRS complex (delta wave).

AV nodal re-entrant tachycardia (AVNRT)

In this SVT, the re-entry circuit is confined to, or near, the AV node. It usually has an abrupt onset and termination and the QRS complexes are narrow. It is the most common form of recurrent paroxysmal SVT (PSVT). On the ECG the P wave is usually buried in the QRS complex. It may be evident just after the QRS complex (double R). P waves may be inverted in the inferior leads. Post arrhythmia T wave inversion may occur.

Treatment

See the entry for each type of arrhythmia.

◖ Suxamethonium/succinylcholine and sux apnoea

Description

Depolarising dicholine ester neuromuscular blocking drug with a rapid onset and short duration of action. Useful for:

1 ultra-short procedures requiring muscle relaxation e.g. ECT
2 rapid-sequence induction required e.g. for full stomach
3 emergency intubation.

Dose

Adult—1.5 mg/kg IV (or 2.5 mg/kg IM if no IV access maximum 150 mg). For ECT use 40–100 mg IV.
Child—2 mg/kg IV (or 4 mg/kg IM if no IV access).

Advantages

1 Rapid onset of profound paralysis (30–60 s).
2 Fasciculations signal that paralysis is soon to follow.
3 Short duration of action (metabolised by pseudocholinesterase). This may also be a disadvantage if intubation is difficult/prolonged.

Disadvantages

1 Causes serum K^+ to rise. This may be dangerous in patients with an elevated K^+ level e.g. renal failure.
2 Massive rise in serum K^+ can occur with many conditions, including significant burns and denervation illnesses such as Guillain–Barré syndrome, paraplegia, tetanus, Duchenne muscular dystrophy and motor neurone disease. This can result in cardiac arrest and these conditions are contraindications to the use of suxamethonium.
3 Can cause malignant hyperthermia—**see *Malignant hyperthermia (MH)*.**
4 Relatively high risk of anaphylaxis (about 1:2000).

5 Contraindicated in patients with myotonic disease such as myotonia congenita and dystrophia myotonica.
6 Suxamethonium can cause prolonged paralysis in patients who are deficient in, or have abnormal, pseudocholinesterase (also called plasma cholinesterase). See sux apnoea below.
7 Can cause moderately severe muscle pains.
8 Can cause bradycardia, especially in children and especially with a second dose of suxamethonium.
9 Causes elevation of intraocular and intracranial pressure.
10 If suxamethonium is given after neostigmine, muscle paralysis may be prolonged due to inhibition of pseudocholinesterase.

Sux apnoea

This condition is due to a deficiency in pseudocholinesterase or abnormal pseudocholinesterase. Abnormal cholinesterase is an inherited condition (autosomal recessive pattern). It results in prolonged paralysis that lasts from minutes to 4 h or longer.
1 In about 4% of people sux will last up to 10 minutes due to a slightly abnormal enzyme.
2 In about 1:2000–3000 patients the paralysing effect may last up to 4 h or longer.

Sux apnoea can also be due to pseudocholinesterase deficiency, due to conditions such as:
1 pregnancy
2 liver disease/renal failure/dialysis
3 cardiac failure, cardiac bypass
4 thyrotoxicosis
5 cancer
6 the use of certain drugs such as lithium, methotrexate, MAOI.

Diagnosis
1 Failure of suxamethonium to wear off in the expected time frame.
2 Evidence of prolonged paralysis using a nerve stimulator.

Treatment
1 Treatment is supportive: anaesthetise and ventilate the patient until sux wears off.
2 FFP will speed up the process but is not recommended.

Investigations
1 Blood tests cannot be done until at least 48 h after sux is administered (6 weeks if FFP used).
2 Order serum/plasma cholinesterase and cholinesterase phenotype in an EDTA tube.
3 A useful test is the dibucaine number. If normal plasma is added to a solution of benzoylcholine, light is emitted at a specific wavelength which can be measured. If dibucaine is also added, no light is emitted. The reaction is **inhibited.** Dibucaine is also called cinchocaine, an amino amide LA.
4 If abnormal plasma is added to benzoylcholine and dibucaine, some light is emitted—dibucaine does not inhibit or fully inhibit the emission of light.
5 The lower the dibucaine number (DN), the more severe the sux apnoea.

6 A dibucaine number of 80 is normal, 40 is associated with prolonged sux effect (minutes) and 20 is associated with sux apnoea for hours.

7 If blood tests do show an inherited form, close relatives may also be affected and should be tested.

◗ Syntocinon (Oxytocin)

Description

Synthetic form of oxytocin. Causes uterine contraction(s). Has an antidiuretic effect.

Uses

1 Induction and/or augmentation of labour 1.5–12 mU/min titrated to response. Mix with Hartmann's solution. Do not mix with 5% glucose because of the risk of water intoxication.

2 Uterine contraction after delivery. Give 3 units IV or 5–10 units IM.

3 For CS give a bolus as above + infusion—40 units in 1000 mL Hartmann's run at 250 mL/h.

4 Second trimester abortion.

Points to note

1 Do not infuse syntocinon in the same line as blood or plasma because the drug will be inactivated by plasma oxytocinase.

2 Syntocinon can cause vasodilation, hypotension and tachycardia. This may cause decompensation in patients with highly significant pathology such as severe mitral stenosis.

◗ Syntometrine

Description

This drug contains oxytocin 5 units and ergometrine 500 mcg in a total volume of 1 mL. Ergometrine is an ergot alkaloid which causes uterine contraction and peripheral vasoconstriction. It is used to treat postpartum haemorrhage (PPH) due to uterine atony. **See** **Postpartum haemorrhage (PPH)**. It is also used to treat haemorrhage associated with incomplete abortion.

Dose

Give 0.5 mL slowly IV and 0.5 mL IM. This drug may cause vomiting, hypertension and coronary artery spasm. It is contraindicated if there is pre-existing hypertension e.g. preeclampsia/eclampsia, occlusive vascular disease or ischaemic heart disease.

◗ Systemic inflammatory response syndrome (SIRS)

SIRS describes a complex pathophysiological whole-body response to a wide variety of severe pathological insults such as infection, burns, ischaemia, pancreatitis, major surgery and trauma. This response has anti-inflammatory and pro-inflammatory components. Manifestations include at least two of:

1 hypothermia ($< 36°C$) or hyperthermia ($> 38°C$)

2 tachycardia > 90 beats/min

3 tachypnoea > 20 breaths/min or $PaCO_2 < 32$ mmHg

4 low ($< 4 \times 10^9$/L) or elevated ($> 12 \times 10^9$/L) white cell count (WCC).
All septic patients have SIRS but not all SIRS patients have sepsis.

REFERENCES

1 National Asthma Council Australia. Accessed online: https://www.nationalasthma.org.au>resources>factsheets, April 2023.

2 Ahee P, Crowe AV. The management of hyperkalaemia in the emergency department. *Emergency Medicine J* 2000; 17: 188–191.

3 Evans L, Rhodes A, Alhazzani W et al. Surviving sepsis campaign: international guidelines for management of sepsis and septic shock 2021. *Intensive Care Med* 2021; 47: 1181–1247.

4 Ng BK, Cameron AJ. The role of methylene blue in serotonin syndrome: a systematic review. *Psychosomatics* 2010; 51: 194–200.

5 Walker I, Trompeter S, Howard J et al. *Guideline on the peri-operative management of sickle cell disease. 2021 Consensus document produced by the working party established by the Association of Anaesthetists approved by the Board of Directors of the Association of Anaesthetists of Great Britain and Ireland.* Published by John Wiley and Sons Ltd.

6 Ezihe-Ejiofor A, Jackson J. Peripartum considerations in sickle cell disease. *Curr Opin Anaesthesiol* 2021; 34: 212–217.

7 Mathis AS, Shah NK, Mulgaonkar S. Stress dose steroids in renal transplant patients undergoing lymphocele surgery. *Transplant Proc* 2004; 36: 3042–3045.

8 Cooper MS, Stewart PM. Corticosteroid insufficiency in acutely ill patients. *N Engl J Med* 2003; 348: 727–734.

9 Hamrahian AH, Roman S, Milan S. The management of the surgical patient taking glucocorticoids. *UpToDate.* Topic last updated October 2019. Accessed online: https://www.uptodate.com/contents/the-management-of-the-surgical-patient-taking-glucocorticoids, October 2022.

10 Takazawa T, Mitsuhata H, Mertes PM. Sugammadex and rocuronium-induced anaphylaxis. *J Anaesth* 2016; 20: 290–297.

11 Pfaff K, Tumin D, Tobias JD. Sugammadex for reversal of neuromuscular blockade in a patient with renal failure. *J Pediatr Pharmacol Ther* 2019; 24: 238–241.

▷ Tachy-brady syndrome

See Sick sinus syndrome (SSS).

▷ Takotsubo cardiomyopathy (broken heart syndrome)

Description

Takotsubo cardiomyopathy is a sudden, transient and life-threatening cardiomyopathy. It usually occurs after severe emotional or physical stress, especially in postmenopausal women. A death of a loved one is an example of the emotional stress which can bring on this syndrome. It is also called transient left ventricular ballooning syndrome or stress cardiomyopathy. It can also occur with sepsis, shock, or be the result of a phaeochromocytoma. *See Phaeochromocytoma.*

Pathophysiology

During the attack, the shape of the LV changes. It becomes enlarged and rounded and resembles a 'takotsubo', a Japanese octopus trap (a chamber with a narrow neck and a round bottom). The cause is unknown, but it is hypothesised that:

1 Severe emotional/physical stress leads to an intense sympathetic discharge.
2 This excess catecholamine surge leads to myocardial stunning.
3 The adrenaline surge suddenly increases SVR, raising blood pressure.
4 Spasm of the coronary arteries may occur.
5 There is sudden congestive heart failure.

Clinical presentation

The presentation is indistinguishable from an acute coronary syndrome. Symptoms and signs include:

1 chest pain
2 dyspnoea
3 hypotension, syncope
4 dysrhythmia/palpitations
5 nausea
6 cardiac arrest.

Diagnosis

1 ECG—may show changes consistent with anterior myocardial infarction.
2 Troponin elevation may occur.
3 Coronary angiography—normal coronary arteries or minimal disease, shape of ventricle as described for echocardiography.
4 Echocardiography—bulging of the LV apex with a hypercontractile base (resembles a rounded container with a narrow, thickened neck).

Treatment

1 Treat this condition as a myocardial infarction until takotsubo cardiomyopathy is diagnosed.
   See Acute coronary syndrome and *Cardiogenic shock.*

2 The use of catecholamines may be problematic as the condition is probably caused by catecholamine excess. Catecholamines may increase the degree of left ventricular outflow obstruction. Optimise fluid therapy and consider vasopressors. Mechanical circulatory support may be required. Seek expert cardiologist referral and management.

3 Beta blocker drugs, or combined alpha and beta receptor blocker drugs e.g. labetalol may be used to prevent the recurrence of attacks.

◑ Tapentadol (Palexia)

Description

Analgesic opioid drug agonist at the mu, delta and kappa opioid receptors used orally. *See Opioid receptors.* Also acts by inhibiting noradrenaline reuptake, which is useful for treating neuropathic pain. Tapentadol was developed from tramadol. It is a much weaker inhibitor of serotonin reuptake than tramadol.

Dose

Adults

Immediate-release (IR) form: 50–100 mg PO up to every 4–6 h. Max 600 mg/day. Extended-release (ER) form: 100 mg q 12 h.

Advantages

1 Effective oral analgesic—50 mg tapentadol is equivalent to 5–7.5 mg oxycodone.
2 Useful for treating neuropathic pain.
3 Less abuse potential than oxycodone.
4 Specifically indicated for controlling the pain of diabetic neuropathy.

Disadvantages

1 Excreted rapidly and completely by the kidneys. Unsuitable for patients with renal impairment/failure.
2 Should be used in reduced dosage in patients with moderate hepatic impairment. If severe hepatic impairment, **do not use**.
3 Cannot be used in patients on MAOIs until these have been ceased for two weeks.
4 Greater abuse potential than tramadol.
5 Increased risk of serotonin syndrome but less than with tramadol. *See Serotonin syndrome/toxicity.*
6 Not recommended for use in children.
7 Raises intracranial pressure and should not be used in patients with raised ICP.
8 Reduces the seizure threshold. It should be used with caution in patients with a history of seizures.
9 Only available in oral form.

◑ Tardive dyskinesia

See Dystonic reaction, acute.

◑ Targin

Description

Targin is a combination of oxycodone (modified-release) and naloxone in a 2:1 ratio (oxycodone/naloxone). It is used orally in tablet strengths ranging from oxycodone 2.5 mg/naloxone 1.25 mg to oxycodone 80 mg/naloxone 40 mg. The naloxone component is poorly absorbed by the gut and offsets the constipating effect of oxycodone. It is indicated for:

1 moderate to severe persistent pain but not acute pain
2 second-line treatment of restless legs syndrome.

Dose

Adult

The usual starting dose for Targin is one 10/5 tablet q 12 h.

Advantages

1 Naloxone component may deter illicit IV use.
2 Reduced risk of opioid-induced constipation.

Disadvantages

1 Contraindicated in patients with moderate to severe hepatic impairment.
2 Cannot be used in patients taking non-selective MAOI drugs.

◗ Terbutaline (Bricanyl)

Description

Short-acting beta-2 agonist drug similar to salbutamol. Used to treat asthma, COPD and as a tocolytic drug.

Dose

Adult

Inhaled—0.5 mg (1 inhalation) prn up to q 5 min. Maximum dose 3 mg/day.
Oral—5 mg q 8 h, maximum dose 15 mg/day.
Subcutaneous—0.25 mg repeat in 15–30 min if needed. Max 0.5 mg within 4 h.
For tocolysis—100–250 mcg subcut or IV infusion—start at 2.5–5 mcg/min. Increase gradually at 20–30 min intervals. Usual effective dose range is 17.5–30 mcg/min.

◗ Tetralogy of Fallot (ToF)

Description

This is one of the commonest types of cyanotic congenital heart disease (CHD). The tetralogy is made up of:

1 Right ventricular outflow tract (RVOT) obstruction. This is a subvalvular obstruction due to infundibular muscle bundles. There may also be a hypoplastic pulmonary valve annulus, and sometimes pulmonary valve stenosis. Narrowing of the pulmonary artery may also be present. The severity of cyanosis is determined by the degree of RVOT obstruction.
2 Ventricular septal defect (VSD)—usually subaortic.
3 Overriding aorta—the aorta is displaced to the right and over the VSD. This means the blood entering the aorta comes mainly from the LV but also from the RV.
4 Concentric right ventricular hypertrophy. This is due to the RVOT obstruction, and the greater the obstruction, the greater the hypertrophy.

It makes up 7–10% of complex CHD cases with an incidence of 4–5:10000 live births. Other cardiac abnormalities are frequently present, such as coronary artery anomalies. There may be a right-sided aortic arch, meaning that the aortic arch is on the right side of the trachea instead of being on the left side. Patients with Down syndrome are at increased risk of having ToF. *See Down syndrome.*

Pathophysiology

Blood flows in the direction of least resistance, so the worse the RVOT obstruction, the more blood transits through the VSD and into the aorta (right-to-left shunt), producing cyanosis. If the RVOT obstruction is more minor, more RV blood can enter the pulmonary circulation and the condition will be acyanotic (pink Fallot). Pulmonary and systemic circulations are said to be balanced.

RVOT obstruction may fluctuate due to spasm of the infundibular ventricular muscle. This can be produced by agitation, crying or beta agonists. Increased RVOT obstruction or a fall in SVR (hypovolaemia, sepsis) can cause increased right-to-left flow through the VSD. This can lead to sudden worsening of hypoxaemia (tet spells). Older children often learn to squat (increasing SVR) to relieve these episodes. Over time, the RVOT obstruction tends to worsen.

If ToF is not corrected:

1 RV hypertrophy develops due to long-standing pressure overload and increased resistance caused by the narrowing of the pulmonary trunk.
2 Paradoxical emboli may occur with strokes.
3 RV failure, followed by LV failure.
4 Dilated cardiomyopathy may occur.
5 Endocarditis.

Mortality for uncorrected ToF is 50% in the first 3 years of life.

Diagnosis

1 RV impulse, systolic thrill.
2 Systolic ejection/pansystolic murmur (primarily due to RVOT obstruction rather than the VSD).
3 Echocardiography.
4 ECG—typically shows RA hypertrophy (tall P waves), RV hypertrophy, right axis deviation, tall R wave in V1, prominent S waves posteriorly and an upright T wave in V1.
5 CXR—boot-shaped heart, right-sided aorta, reduced pulmonary vascular markings.
6 Coronary angiography to detect coronary artery abnormalities. Only required in more complex cases.

Medical treatment

1 Severe or complete RVOT obstruction may benefit by maintaining a patent ductus arteriosus to provide/augment a pulmonary circulation. This can be done with prostaglandin therapy. **See Patent ductus arteriosus (PDA)**.
2 Beta blockers (propranolol) may relieve infundibular muscle spasm.

Cardiac catheter interventions

Can buy time until definitive surgery can be undertaken. Strategies include:

1 pulmonary valvotomy
2 RVOT stenting
3 PDA stenting.

Corrective surgery

Options include:

1 Total corrective surgery with closure of the VSD and reconstruction of the RVOT.
2 A modified Blalock–Taussig shunt is a palliative procedure in which the subclavian artery is joined to the pulmonary artery, enabling systemic blood to enter the pulmonary circulation.

Anaesthesia and corrected ToF

The main issues of concern for the anaesthetist are:

1 Pulmonary regurgitation.
2 RV dysfunction/failure, decreased exercise tolerance, arrhythmias such as VT, AF and atrial flutter. There may also be LV failure due to septal shift and disordered ventricular synchronisation.
3 Pulmonary valve replacement—the valve's function may deteriorate over time.
4 Endocarditis risk.
5 Residual RVOT obstruction.
6 Ascending aortic root dilatation leading to aortic valve dysfunction.
7 An AICD may be present. **See Pacemakers.**
8 Sudden cardiac death.

⊙ Thalassaemia

Description

Thalassaemia is an inherited haemoglobin disorder. It is the most common monogenetic recessive disorder worldwide. There are two main types: alpha and beta thalassaemia. In each type there is a quantitative deficiency in the alpha or beta subunit—too little is produced. This decreases RBC production and destabilises the Hb molecule. The Hb has impaired O_2 carrying capacity and there is increased RBC destruction. This in turn can lead to anaemia, enlarged spleen, pigmented gallstones, jaundice, extra-medullary haematopoiesis and hypertension in pregnancy. The forehead may enlarge due to expansion of the bone marrow in the frontal bone. Definitive diagnosis requires molecular genetic testing. Haemoglobin electrophoresis can also be very helpful.

About 1.7% of the world's population has an alpha or beta thalassaemia trait. It is much more common in people of Mediterranean, African, Pacific Islands, Middle East, India and Southeast Asian ethnicity. These areas also have the highest incidence of malaria.

Alpha thalassaemia (affecting the alpha chains of Hb)

There are two genes for the alpha chains, HBA1 and HBA2. There are two copies of each gene, making four alleles. **See Allele.**

Patients may have one, two, three or four alleles missing (or, less commonly, mutated), leading to four different types of alpha thalassaemia:

1 Alpha thalassaemia carrier/alpha thalassaemia silent carrier (one allele missing)—no symptoms.
2 Alpha thalassaemia trait/alpha thalassaemia carrier (two alleles missing)—mild microcytic hypochromic anaemia. Anencephaly is more common in the fetuses of mothers with this condition.[1] These patients should take preconception folic acid.
3 HbH disease (three alleles missing)—beta chains are in excess and form an unstable tetramer called HbH. There may be mild to moderate anaemia, hepatosplenomegaly and bone changes. RBC transfusion is often needed and this can lead to iron overload. **See Iron overload.**
4 Alpha thalassaemia major/hydrops fetalis/Hb Bart syndrome/Hb Bart's disease (four mutated alleles)—there is usually death in utero or soon after birth. Hb is made up of 4 gamma globulins that bind O_2, but cannot release it to the tissue (Hb Bart's). This causes severe anaemia, microcytosis, hepatosplenomegaly and cardiac and other organ defects. **See Hydrops fetalis/fetal hydrops.**

Beta thalassaemia

There is a deficit of beta subunit production. There are only two genes involved—one from each parent. The types are:

1 Beta thalassaemia minor (beta thalassaemia trait)—one mutated gene. This is asymptomatic.
2 Beta thalassaemia intermedia—two mutated genes that reduce beta subunit synthesis; there is reduced beta chain production.
3 Beta thalassaemia major—there are two mutated genes with no beta chain production. There is an excess of alpha chains in the RBC, leading to RBC inclusions and increased haemolysis. This leads to anaemia, jaundice, hepatosplenomegaly, increased pigmented gall stones and secondary haemochromatosis (iron overload, especially in the liver). Secondary haemochromatosis can lead to cirrhosis, arrhythmias, diabetes mellitus and hypothyroidism. There may be an enlarged forehead and cheek bones. *See Haemochromatosis and Iron overload.*
4 Haemoglobin E. This disease is caused by a specific mutation on a beta subunit gene. Patients who are homozygous have mild haemolytic anaemia. The heterozygous state (HbE trait) is asymptomatic. However, HbE combined with beta thalassaemia intermedia can lead to severe disease, similar to beta thalassaemia major.

Treatment of thalassaemia

1 RBC transfusion.
2 Deferoxamine—to reduce iron overload by binding to free iron in the plasma and enabling its excretion in the urine. *See Iron overload.*
3 Splenectomy, to decrease the rate of RBC destruction.

Haemoglobin C-beta thalassaemia

Haemoglobin C is an inherited abnormality of the beta chain of Hb. HbC trait is a benign condition. *See Haemoglobin C (HbC) disease.* However, a combination of HbC and beta thalassaemia can lead to serious illness with mild to moderately severe anaemia, splenomegaly and bone changes.

Thalassaemia and anaesthesia including obstetric anaesthesia

1 In frequently transfused patients, assess for any evidence of iron overload related organ damage. *See Iron overload.*
2 Patients requiring transfusions may have alloimmunisation so cross-matching may be difficult. Cross-matching for C, E and Kell antigens may reduce the alloantibody rate by 53% and is recommended.
3 These patients tend to be at increased risk of thromboembolic disease.
4 Chronic haemolysis leads to chronic haemoglobinaemia, which scavenges nitric oxide. This can lead to increased PVR, pulmonary hypertension and right heart failure. The incidence of preeclampsia and gestational hypertension may be increased in patients with thalassaemia.
5 Patients requiring transfusions over many years, particularly in developing countries, may have acquired Hep B, Hep C or HIV infections.
6 Aspirin given to pregnant women with thalassaemia, who have also had a splenectomy, have a reduced rate of thromboembolism.[1]
7 Aim for a Hb > 80 g/L during pregnancy. These patients should receive folic acid 5 mg/day. In patients with beta thalassaemia trait, consider iron supplements +/− erythropoietin therapy. Blood transfusion should only be considered as a 'last resort'.
8 The presence of alpha thalassaemia trait is strongly associated with gestational diabetes.

◖ Thiopentone

Description
IV general anaesthetic barbiturate drug with anticonvulsant properties.

Dose for IV anaesthesia

Adult
3–5 mg/kg. Effects last 5–15 min.

Child
5 mg/kg.

Advantages
1 Painless on injection.
2 Inexpensive.
3 Potent anticonvulsant, although favoured for ECT.
4 Reduces intracranial pressure and cerebral O_2 demand.
5 No animal products (unlike propofol).

Disadvantages
1 Produces a hangover effect.
2 No euphoric properties (unlike propofol).
3 Presented as a powder. It has to be mixed with sterile H_2O before use.
4 Higher doses result in accumulation with recovery dependent on metabolism. This may take hours. It is not suitable for total IV anaesthesia.
5 May have some broncho-constrictive effects.
6 Can precipitate neurotoxicity in some forms of porphyria. *See Porphyria.*
7 Intra-arterial thiopentone can cause severe tissue damage and gangrene.
8 Extravasation of thiopentone may cause tissue necrosis.
9 Severe/fatal anaphylaxis may occur (1:20000).

◖ Thrombin time (TT)

Thrombin converts fibrinogen to fibrin in the clotting cascade. *See Clotting pathways.* In the TT test, plasma is anticoagulated and an excess of thrombin is added. The clotting time is then measured. In this way the amount of functional fibrinogen is measured. A normal TT is 14–19 seconds.

◖ Thrombocytopenia

Defined as a platelet count < 150000 per mm^3. Causes include:
1 Pregnancy related causes (see below).
2 Immune thrombocytopenia (ITP).
3 Thrombotic thrombocytopenic purpura (TTP).
4 Inherited thrombocytopenia.
5 Sepsis-induced thrombocytopenia.
6 Autoimmune diseases such as lupus.
7 Disseminated intravascular coagulation (DIC).
8 Heparin-induced thrombocytopenia syndrome (HITS).
9 Von Willebrand disease type IIb. *See Von Willebrand disease (VWD).*
10 Bone marrow disease.
11 Hypersplenism.
12 Vitamin B12/folate deficiency.

Thrombocytopenia due to pregnancy

5% or more of obstetric patients will have thrombocytopenia (platelet count < 150 000 per mm³). Causes include:

1 Gestational thrombocytopenia (70–80% of total). **See Gestational thrombocytopenia (GT).**
2 Hypertensive disorders of pregnancy (about 20% of total cases). **See Preeclampsia/eclampsia.**
3 Acute fatty liver of pregnancy.
   If the platelet count is > 30 000 per mm³, vaginal delivery is considered safe.[2]
CS, under GA, is considered safe if the platelet count is > 50 000 per mm³. However, neuraxial anaesthesia should not be performed if the platelet count is < 70 000 per mm³.[2] Spontaneous bleeding may occur with a platelet count < 10 000 per mm³. Transfuse platelets. **See Platelets.**

◗ Thromboelastography/thromboelastometry

Introduction

Thromboelastography/thromboelastometry are synonymous terms describing the measurement of the viscoelastic properties of a blood sample as it clots. The information is displayed graphically, with the x axis being time and the y axis being amplitude in mm above or below a zero point. Amplitude over time gives an indication of:

1 clot initiation time
2 clot's maximum strength
3 clot's stability over time.

The aims of this test are to:

• Identify whether the clotting process is normal or abnormal (within the limits of the test).
• Identify which component(s) of clotting is/are deficient (clotting factors, platelets or fibrinogen).
• Detect excessive clot lysis (hyperfibrinolysis).

Two types of technology are presented in this manual, ROTEM and TEG.

ROTEM

ROTEM stands for rotational thromboelastometry. The steps in performing the test are:

1 Blood is collected in a citrated (blue top) tube.
2 A sample of the citrated blood is placed in a small cuvette.
3 The blood is mixed with calcium to inactivate the citrate and begin the clotting process.
4 A pin protrudes into the sample and the pin undergoes rotational oscillations.
5 As the blood clots, there are torque effects on the pin.
6 These torque effects are graphed over time.
7 The graph thus formed is called a TEMogram.

The process of blood clotting is sped up by adding clotting initiators, so that meaningful results can be obtained in about 10 min.

The measurements

1 **CT**—clotting time. Time for amplitude to rise 2 mm. NR 43–80 s. If > 80 s, this suggests inadequate clotting factors or fibrinogen.
2 **CFT**—clot formation time. Time from 2 mm to 20 mm. NR 48–127 s.
3 **Alpha (α)**—the alpha angle. Angle of slope between the end of CT and the end of CFT. It gives an indication of the level of fibrinogen or, put another way, the speed

of fibrin mesh formation. A shallow angle suggests fibrinogen deficiency. A normal alpha angle is 50–70°.

4 A5, 10, 15—amplitude at 5, 10, 15 min after CT. An A5 > 35 mm suggests a strong clot. A5 > 35 mm suggests a weak clot, usually due to low platelet numbers or low fibrinogen levels or both. NR for A10 is 40–60 mm.

5 MCF—max clot firmness, max amplitude. NR 50–70 mm (roughly A10 + 10 mm). MCF < 30 mm indicates no effective haemostasis.

6 ML—maximum lysis, describes the percentage of clot destroyed at any time on the x axis. ML 100% means no clot is remaining. A ML < 15% at 1 h suggests a stable clot. ML > 15% at 1 h suggests excessive fibrinolysis.

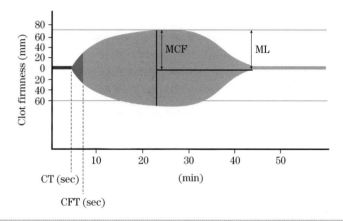

Figure T1 ROTEM graph

There are five types of graph.

EXTEM (similar to PT)

Tests the extrinsic clotting pathway. It assesses factors VII, X, V, II, I, platelets and fibrinolysis. It can be considered a basic clotting screening test.

1 Calcium is added to neutralise the citrate and tissue factor (TF) is added to initiate the clotting process via the extrinsic pathway. *See Clotting pathways.*

2 If the CT > 90 s (NR 43–82 s), this is probably due to low levels of clotting factors but it could be due to low fibrinogen.

3 If the A5 > 35 mm, this suggests a strong clot. If A5 < 35 mm, this suggests a weak clot which could be due to low platelets or low fibrinogen.

4 If the ML ≥ 5% at 20–40 min, this suggests excessive clot lysis.

5 If the EXTEM is normal, the other tests can be ignored.

INTEM (similar to APPT)

Tests the intrinsic clotting pathway. It assesses factors XII, XI, IX, VIII, X, V, II, I, platelets and fibrinolysis.

1 Phospholipid and ellagic acid are added to the sample to initiate the clotting process.

2 An abnormal graph will reflect any deficiency in the clotting factors listed above or the presence of heparin.

APTEM

APTEM is the same as EXTEM except aprotinin or tranexamic acid is added to inhibit fibrinolysis. If the ML on the EXTEM ≥ 5% and on the APTEM < 5%, this suggests excess fibrinolysis and the need for tranexamic acid.

FIBTEM

This test is used to assess for fibrinogen deficiency. If the EXTEM A5 < 35 mm (inadequate clot strength), this could be due to inadequate fibrinogen or platelets or both. FIBTEM helps analyse the contribution of fibrinogen to clot strength. The test is done in the same way as EXTEM, except that cytochalasin D is added to block platelets. The resulting clot is entirely due to the effects of fibrinogen. If the FIBTEM A5 > 10 mm then fibrinogen levels are adequate, and if ≤ 10 mm give fibrinogen.

HEPTEM

Coagulation is activated in the same way as INTEM but heparinase is added to block heparin.

Interpretation of ROTEM in the presence of haemorrhage

If the EXTEM is normal the other tests can be ignored. If abnormal:

1 *Fibrinolysis:* The first step is to determine if excessive fibrinolysis is occurring. If the FIBTEM CT > 600 s (resulting in a flat curve) and the EXTEM A5 < 35 mm, this suggests excessive fibrinolysis and the treatment is tranexamic acid (TXA). *See Tranexamic acid (TXA) (Cyclokapron).* An argument can be made for giving TXA in all cases of major haemorrhage.

2 *Fibrinogen:* Secondly, assess fibrinogen levels as this is the most common abnormality. This will result in an inadequate clot as evidenced by an EXTEM A5 < 35 mm. Look at the FIBTEM. If the FIBTEM A5 < 10 mm, the problem is low fibrinogen levels. Administer fibrinogen.

3 *Platelets:* Next assess platelets. The EXTEM A5 ≤ 35 mm and the FIBTEM A5 > 10 mm—this is evidence of inadequate platelet numbers. Give platelets.

4 *Fibrinogen and platelets:* If the EXTEM A5 ≤ 25 mm and the FIBTEM A5 ≤ 10 mm this suggests both fibrinogen and platelets are inadequate and both require replacement.

5 *Clotting factors:* Finally assess clotting factors. If the EXTEM CT > 80 s and the FIBTEM A5 ≤ 10 mm the prolonged clotting time is likely due to low fibrinogen levels. If the FIBTEM > 10 mm the prolonged clotting time is likely due to low levels of clotting factors. Give FFP.

6 *Clotting factors and fibrinogen:* If the EXTEM CT > 140 s and the FIBTEM A5 ≤ 10 mm, the issue is probably low fibrinogen and low clotting factors, so both need replacing.

Limitations of ROTEM

1 No detection of aspirin or other antiplatelet drugs.
2 Poor sensitivity to LMWH and oral anticoagulants.
3 Von Willebrand Disease effects not detected.

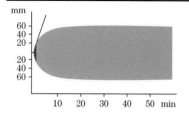

EXTEM, IV
Volunteer nr. 8

RT:	01 : 00 : 21					
CT	:	48	s	[	38 –	79]
CFT	:	75	s	[	34 –	159]
α	:	77	°	[	63 –	83]
A10	:	57	mm	[	43 –	65]
A20	:	64	mm	[	50 –	71]
MCF	:	66	mm	[	50 –	72]
ML	: *	4	%	[	0 –	15]

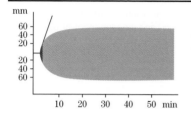

INTEM, IV
Volunteer nr. 8

RT:	01 : 00 : 17					
CT	:	147	s	[	100 –	240]
CFT	:	69	s	[	30 –	110]
α	:	76	°	[	70 –	83]
A10	:	56	mm	[	44 –	66]
A20	:	62	mm	[	50 –	71]
MCF	:	63	mm	[	50 –	72]
ML	: *	4	%	[	0 –	15]

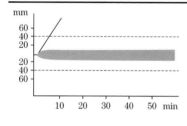

FIBTEM, IV
Volunteer nr. 8

RT:	01 : 00 : 17					
CT	:	58	s	[		
CFT	:		s	[		
α	:	64	°	[		
A10	:	14	mm	[	7 –	23]
A20	:	14	mm	[	8 –	24]
MCF	:	14	mm	[	9 –	25]
ML	: *	3	%	[		

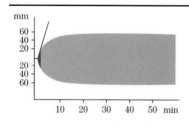

APTEM, IV
Volunteer nr. 8

RT:	01 : 00 : 19		
CT	:	48	s
CFT	:	84	s
α	:	77	°
A10	:	54	mm
A20	:	61	mm
MCF	:	63	mm
ML	: *	4	%

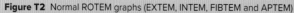

Figure T2 Normal ROTEM graphs (EXTEM, INTEM, FIBTEM and APTEM)

TEG

The steps with TEG are:

1 Blood is collected in a citrated (blue top) tube.
2 A sample of the citrated blood is placed in a small cuvette and mixed with calcium to initiate the clotting process. Kaolin and tissue factor are added to speed up the measurement.
3 A pin is suspended in the cup by a torsion wire.
4 The cup rotates through an angle of 4°45'.
5 As the blood clots there are torque effects on the pin.
6 These torque effects are graphed over time.
7 The graph thus formed is called a thromboelastogram.
8 The latest machines do not use a pin-in-cup method. They use resonance by exposing the blood to a fixed vibrational frequency and measurement of the vertical motion of the blood meniscus.

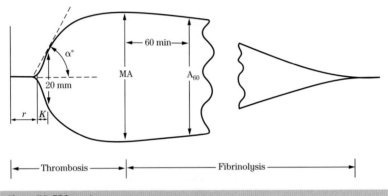

Figure T3 TEG graph

The measurements

1 **R** – **r**eaction time—time for clotting process to begin. Correlates with CT in ROTEM. NR 4–9 min. It is mainly determined by clotting factors and fibrinogen.
2 **K** – **k**inetics—this correlates with CFT in ROTEM (time for clot to go from 2 mm to 20 mm amplitude). This is strongly influenced by fibrinogen. NR 1–3 min.
3 **α** – angle—this is the same measurement as in ROTEM. It gives an indication of the level of fibrinogen or, put another way, the speed of fibrin mesh formation. A shallow angle suggests fibrinogen deficiency. A normal α angle is 59–74°.

4 **MA**—**M**aximum clot **A**mplitude—this correlates with MCF in ROTEM. A reduced MA may be indicative of platelet deficiency. Normal value is 55–74 mm.

5 **TMA**—**T**ime to reach **MA**.

6 **LY30**—this is the percentage of clot lysis 30 min after MA. This correlates with ML at 30 min in ROTEM. A normal value is 0–8%. If > 8% treat with tranexamic acid.

7 **CLT**—**C**lot **L**ysis **T**ime. Time from MA until 100% clot lysis.

TEG graphs

Standard

Kaolin is added to the blood sample. R time is 5–10 min. K time is 1–3 min.

CRT or citrated rapid TEG (r-TEG)

Uses tissue factor (TF) to activate blood coagulation. This speeds up the test. The R value is measured in seconds rather than minutes. This correlates with EXTEM in ROTEM.

Heparinase TEG

Corresponds to HEPTEM in ROTEM.

Platelet mapping TEG

This seeks to determine to what degree platelet function is inhibited by the arachidonic acid (AA) pathway (e.g. aspirin) or the adenosine diphosphate pathway (ADP), as occurs with clopidogrel. The test is run twice, once as a standard TEG and secondly as a TEG with AA or ADP to neutralise the antiplatelet drug effect. The contribution of fibrin to the MA is subtracted using a mathematical formula. There is no ROTEM equivalent.

CKH—citrated kaolin with heparinase TEG

This graph is to determine whether ongoing bleeding is due to heparin (after reversal with protamine). The test is done twice—once as a normal TEG and once with heparinase to neutralise heparin. If the graphs are the same, the bleeding is not due to heparin. Correlates with HEPTEM.

CCF—citrated functional fibrinogen

A shortcoming of TEG is determining the relative contribution of platelets and fibrinogen to clot integrity. In this test, which correlates to the FIBTEM in ROTEM, the effects of platelets on clot strength are neutralised.

Some typical TEG patterns

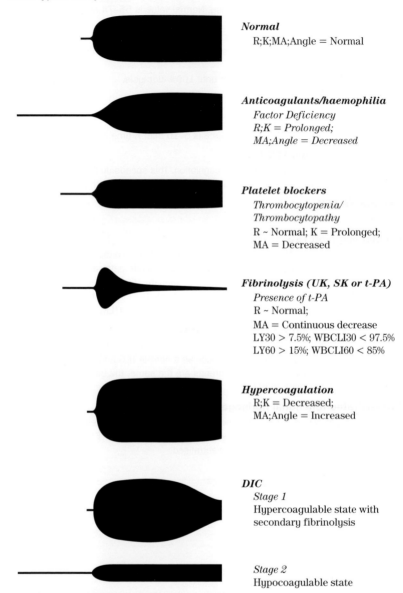

Normal
R;K;MA;Angle = Normal

Anticoagulants/haemophilia
Factor Deficiency
R;K = Prolonged;
MA;Angle = Decreased

Platelet blockers
Thrombocytopenia/
Thrombocytopathy
R ~ Normal; K = Prolonged;
MA = Decreased

Fibrinolysis (UK, SK or t-PA)
Presence of t-PA
R ~ Normal;
MA = Continuous decrease
LY30 > 7.5%; WBCLI30 < 97.5%
LY60 > 15%; WBCLI60 < 85%

Hypercoagulation
R;K = Decreased;
MA;Angle = Increased

DIC
Stage 1
Hypercoagulable state with
secondary fibrinolysis

Stage 2
Hypocoagulable state

Figure T4 Some typical TEG patterns
Source: Whiting D, DiNardo JA. TEG and ROTEM: technology and clinical applications. Am J Hematol. 2014 Feb;89(2):228–232.

Interpretation of TEG

1 Deficiency in clotting factors—long R time, K time increased: give FFP.
2 Low platelets—R time normal, K time increased, MA decreased: give platelets.
3 Low fibrinogen—R time normal, increased K time with reduced α angle: treat with fibrinogen.
4 Fibrinolysis—e.g. massive trauma. Normal R but MA will be continuously decreasing: treat with tranexamic acid.
5 Hypocoagulable state—globally abnormal TEG. Long R and K time and MA decreased. Requires platelets, clotting factors and fibrinogen.
6 Hypercoagulation with fibrinolysis. Short R and K time. Increased MA and LY30. The trace is teardrop shaped—'the teardrop of death'. This type of trace may indicate DIC.

⭗ Thrombolytic therapy

See Alteplase/recombinant tissue plasminogen activator (rtPA) (Activase) and Pulmonary embolism (PE).

⭗ Thrombophilia

Description

Thrombophilia is a disease in which there is an increased tendency for blood to clot, leading to thromboembolic disease. This can be due to excess procoagulant factors or deficiency in anticoagulant factors. Conditions causing thrombophilia include:

1 excess procoagulants—increased FVII, FVIII, FIX, FXI
2 factor V Leiden mutation
3 antithrombin III deficiency
4 lupus anticoagulant
5 abnormal prothrombin
6 dysfibrinogenaemia
7 deficiency of anticoagulants such as antithrombin, protein C or protein S
8 abnormal fibrinolysis due to a deficiency of tissue plasminogen activator, plasminogen or increased plasminogen activator inhibitor
9 hyperhomocysteinaemia.

Treatment

Anticoagulants are the mainstay of therapy. Fractionated and unfractionated heparin and warfarin are the main drugs used. An IVC filter may be required. More specific treatments include:

1 Protein C for protein C deficiency.
2 Antithrombin.
3 Cryoprecipitate.
4 FFP can be used to treat FV deficiency. Plasma exchange may be effective in treating patients with thrombotic thrombocytopenic purpura.[3] *See Thrombotic thrombocytopenic purpura (TTP).*

⭗ Thrombotic thrombocytopenic purpura (TTP)

Description

TTP is a thrombotic microangiopathy, caused by severely reduced activity of von Willebrand factor-cleaving protease (ADAMTS13). There are small vessel platelet rich clots that can cause organ damage, with associated thrombocytopenia and haemolytic anaemia. It is a medical emergency and fatal if not treated.

Causes

1 Immune mediated, due to antibodies against ADAMTS13.
2 Hereditary, due to abnormalities of the ADAMTS13 gene.
3 Drug induced e.g. clopidogrel.

Treatment

1 Therapeutic plasma exchange.
2 Steroids.
3 Rituximab.
4 Caplacizumab.

▶ Thyroid storm/thyrotoxic crisis

Description

Thyroid storm is a life-threatening complication of untreated or undertreated hyperthyroidism. It has a mortality of 10–20%.[4] It is a multisystem disorder that presents suddenly.

Causes

It is unknown why thyroid storm occurs. Thyroid hormone levels are elevated, but the degree of elevation is not directly related to the clinical picture. Causes include:

1 Graves' disease
2 toxic multinodular goitre
3 toxic thyroid adenoma
4 abrupt discontinuation of antithyroid medicine
5 surgery (thyroid and non-thyroid)
6 acute medical illnesses such as myocardial infarction, diabetic ketoacidosis and COVID-19
7 trauma such as burns
8 radioiodine therapy
9 pregnancy/hyperemesis gravidarum
10 medication side effect, due to drugs such as amiodarone and alpha interferon.

Clinical presentation

1 Hyperthermia. This is a cardinal sign of thyrotoxicosis. If thyroid storm occurs under GA, it may be misdiagnosed as malignant hyperthermia. *See Malignant hyperthermia (MH)*.
2 Profuse sweating—leading to dehydration and electrolyte loss.
3 Tachycardia, arrhythmias e.g. AF, hypertension.
4 High-output cardiac failure, peripheral oedema, pulmonary oedema, respiratory compromise.
5 Tachypnoea.
6 Hypercarbia.
7 Delirium, psychosis, stupor, coma, seizures.
8 Respiratory and metabolic acidosis.
9 Electrolyte derangements such as hypokalaemia, hypercalcaemia, hypomagnesaemia and hyponatraemia.
10 Nausea, vomiting, diarrhoea, abdominal pain.
11 Liver dysfunction, jaundice.

Diagnosis

1 Elevated FT3 and/or FT4.
2 History of thyroid disease/exophthalmos.
3 High index of suspicion.

Treatment

General measures

1 Ensure adequate airway, breathing and circulation. Intubation and other resuscitative measures may be immediately required.
2 Treat the cause e.g. infection.
3 IV fluid including glucose solution. Severe dehydration may occur. Normalise glucose and electrolytes.
4 Treat hyperthermia with cooling blankets, ice packs, cooled IV fluids, paracetamol and, if an intraoperative event, cold lavage of abdominal cavity.

Specific treatments (adults)

1 Antithyroid drugs e.g. propylthiouracil (PTU) 1 g PO then 250 mg PO q 4–6 h **or** carbimazole 20–30 mg PO q 4–6 h.[4] These drugs can be given by nasogastric tube if necessary. Effects usually begin after 1 h.
2 Potassium iodide or Lugol's solution, to inhibit hormone release. This can be given 1 h after an antithyroid drug. Dose of potassium iodide is 500 mg PO q 8 h or 200 mg in 500 mL N/S over 2 h every 12 h. **Do not give iodine prior to PTU, as this may increase thyroid hormone levels.** If the patient is allergic to iodine, give lithium carbonate 300 mg PO q 6 h.
3 Propranolol or other beta-adrenergic blocker drug. This is to inhibit the peripheral effects of excess thyroid hormone. The dose of propranolol is 40–80 mg PO q 4–6 h. Aim for a heart rate of 90 bpm.
4 Hydrocortisone 100 mg IV q 8 h. This will decrease T4 release and its conversion to T3. Alternatively, administer dexamethasone 2 mg IV q 6 h.
5 Guanethidine or reserpine should be considered for propranolol-resistant thyroid storm or in patients unable to tolerate beta blockers. Administer guanethidine 1–2 mg/kg/day PO in divided doses **or** reserpine 2.5–5 mg/kg q 4–6 h.
6 In refractory cases, remove thyroid hormone from the body using plasmapheresis, plasma exchange, dialysis or charcoal haemoperfusion.
7 Oral cholestyramine 4 g q 6 h can be used in severe cases, to reduce entero-hepatic recycling of thyroid hormone by bile acid sequestration.
8 Consider dantrolene if the above measures are unsuccessful or inadequate.
9 **Do not give aspirin, because it will increase free thyroid hormone levels.** It does this by interfering with thyroid-binding protein.

Prevention of thyroid storm in hyperthyroid patients having ELECTIVE surgery

1 Render patients euthyroid with a 6–8-week course of an antithyroid drug such as propylthiouracil.
2 Give potassium iodide for 1–2 weeks before surgery.
3 Add a beta blocker drug for tachycardia management if required.

Prevention of thyroid storm in hyperthyroid patients having EMERGENCY surgery

1 Start a beta blocker.
2 Give propylthiouracil PO 200–400 mg q 6 h.
3 Hydrocortisone 40 mg IV q 6 h.
4 Potassium iodide 5 drops PO q 6 h or Lugol's solution 30 drops q 6 h. This inhibits release of T3 and T4.

◑ Tibial nerve sheath catheter

Used to provide postoperative analgesia after below-knee amputation. The catheter is positioned by the surgeon intraoperatively.

1　Establish the block with 20 mL bupivacaine 0.25% or 20 mL of ropivacaine 1%.
2　Commence an infusion of bupivacaine 0.25% at 6 mL/h for 72 h. This technique may reduce the incidence of phantom limb pain.[5]

◑ Ticagrelor (Brilinta)

Platelet adenosine diphosphate receptor antagonist (also called a $P2Y_{12}$ receptor antagonist). Used with aspirin to treat acute coronary syndrome. *See Acute coronary syndrome* and *Anticoagulant and antiplatelet drugs and surgery/neuraxial anaesthesia*. It should be stopped for five days before surgery.

◑ Ticlopidine (Ticlid)

Platelet adenosine diphosphate receptor antagonist (also called a $P2Y_{12}$ receptor antagonist). Needs to be ceased for 14 days before surgery/neuraxial anaesthesia. *See Anticoagulant and antiplatelet drugs and surgery/neuraxial anaesthesia*.

◑ Tissue plasminogen activator (tPA)

tPA activates plasminogen to convert it to plasmin. Plasmin lyses clots. A deficiency in tPA is thrombogenic. Alteplase is the first FDA-approved recombinant human tissue plasminogen activator. *See Alteplase/recombinant tissue plasminogen activator (rtPA) (Activase)*.

◑ Torsades de pointes

Description

This is a polymorphic ventricular tachycardia that occurs with long QT syndrome. *See Long QT syndrome (LQTS)*. The amplitude and polarity of the QRS complexes rhythmically change in a sinusoidal pattern. The points appear to twist around the isoelectric baseline.

Treatment

Most episodes are self-limiting so there may be little time for medical management.

1　If cardiac arrest occurs—*see Cardiac arrest*. Avoid amiodarone for shockable rhythm arrest. Use lignocaine instead.[6] Amiodarone has a proarrhythmic effect due to prolongation of the QTc interval.
2　If haemodynamic instability occurs, give sedation and cardiovert the patient with an initial biphasic energy of 50 J. *See Cardioversion, electrical*.
3　Discontinue any QT prolonging medication.
4　Increase serum potassium to high normal levels (4.5–5 mmol/L) and correct hypocalcaemia.
5　Magnesium is the most effective medical management of this condition. Administer a magnesium bolus of 2 g IV over 2 min, then an IV infusion of 1–4 g/h. Aim to keep magnesium levels > 2 mmol/L. *See Preeclampsia/eclampsia* for more details regarding magnesium infusions. The bolus dose can be repeated if needed.
6　Consider using an IV isoprenaline infusion to increase the heart rate, starting at 2 mcg/min. Titrate the infusion to achieve a rate of 100 bpm. *See Isoprenaline/ isoproterenol (Isuprel)*. Alternatively use electrical overdrive pacing to a rate of 100–140 bpm.[6] *See Pacemakers*.
7　Mexiletine may be useful. *See Mexiletine (Mexitil)*.

◉ Tracheal injury

Description

An injury to the trachea can be intrathoracic or extrathoracic. It is an airway emergency. 30–80% of victims die before reaching hospital.[7,8]

Causes

1 Trauma (usually blunt).
2 Iatrogenic—intubation injury due to stylet, overinflation of tracheal cuff, neck/tracheal surgery.
3 Malignancy.
4 Infection.
5 Vigorous coughing, especially if associated with tracheobronchomalacia.

Clinical presentation

1 Subcutaneous emphysema, which can be massive.
2 Pneumothorax.
3 Respiratory compromise.
4 Stridor.
5 Haemoptysis.
6 Pneumothorax that does not drain with a chest tube.
7 Cardiovascular collapse/death.

Diagnosis

1 Clinical findings.
2 Neck, chest X-rays—prevertebral air, subcutaneous and mediastinal emphysema. Pneumoperitoneum and pneumopericardium can also develop.
3 Chest/neck CT—this will help elucidate other injuries as well.
4 Bronchoscopy—this will indicate the site and the extent of injury and also help guide ET tube positioning.

Treatment

Management depends on the severity of the rupture, site of rupture and degree of patient compromise. In virtually all cases, the site of rupture needs to be inspected with a bronchoscope.

1 Small extrathoracic tears with slight air leaks can be treated conservatively with airway humidification, chest physiotherapy and antibiotics.
2 A laceration that is < 1 cm long may heal without surgical intervention, with an ET tube placed across the injury to stent the trachea.
3 If the patient is in extremis with falling oxygen saturation, intubate immediately with extreme caution. Attempt to position the cuff below the injury prior to inflation and ventilation.
4 Stable, cooperative patients should have an awake bronchoscopy, careful inspection of the injury, then gentle intubation. Carefully position the cuff of the ET tube below the injured area, prior to cuff inflation and ventilation.
5 Less cooperative patients can be considered for gaseous induction, maintaining spontaneous ventilation, with bronchoscopy and intubation as described above.
6 Awake emergency tracheostomy under LA may be another option.
7 In extreme circumstances, consider ECMO, cardiopulmonary bypass and cross-field ventilation (intraoperative replacement of an ET tube by the surgeon to allow better access to the injury).

◗ Tracheostomy anaesthesia and tracheostomy-related emergencies

Introduction

Tracheostomy emergencies can occur any time during or after insertion. Short-term complications include:

1 failure of insertion
2 bleeding
3 obstruction.

Longer-term complications include infection, fistula formation e.g. with the oesophagus, and tracheal stenosis or tracheomalacia. Cuffed tracheostomy tubes are used in patients requiring ventilation or who are unable to protect their airway from aspiration. Uncuffed tubes are used for chronic airway obstruction.

Anaesthesia

The procedure is usually semi-elective in an intubated patient.

1 Position the patient with a 1 L fluid bag between the scapulae and use a head ring, ensuring the neck is extended.
2 Ensure that the patient is well paralysed.
3 Just before incision into the trachea, change the inspired gas to air or the lowest FiO_2 tolerated by the patient. This is because of the risk of airway fire if diathermy is used. *See Laser surgery.*
4 If the ET tube cuff ruptures, change to bag-tube ventilation.
5 When the surgeon is ready to insert the tracheostomy tube, deflate the ET tube cuff and pull the ET tube back just enough to make room. The ET tube may have to be reinserted at any time.

Tracheostomy tube obstruction

Patient HAS HAD laryngectomy

There is **no** connection between the mouth and the trachea. The trachea is connected to the neck stoma.

1 Declare an emergency and send for skilled assistance, preferably an ENT surgeon.
2 Remove the internal components of the tracheostomy tube such as the inner cannula and valves. This may relieve the obstruction.
3 Pass a suction catheter down the tracheostomy tube to check for patency. If the tracheostomy tube is patent, consider other causes for the patient's condition. If it is not patent, the tracheostomy tube may be blocked or dislodged—deflate the tracheostomy tube.
4 If all the above measures fail, remove the tracheostomy tube cuff. The patient may be able to breathe through the stoma. Breathing through the stoma can be assisted by attaching the anaesthetic circuit to a LMA and placing the inflated cuff over the stoma.
5 If this fails, pass an ET tube through the stoma, preferably using a fibre-optic or digital bronchoscope, or a Teflon or Frova bougie.

Patient HAS NOT HAD laryngectomy

1 Declare an emergency and send for skilled assistance, preferably an ENT surgeon.
2 Apply high-flow oxygen to the face. Bag mask ventilation may be required.
3 Use the same manoeuvres as described above to detect/clear the tracheostomy tube blockage (steps 2, 3, 4).

4 If these manoeuvres are unsuccessful, intubate the patient orally. If unable to intubate but bag mask or supraglottic ventilation is possible, cover the stoma to prevent a leak.

5 If unsuccessful, intubate the stoma as described above.

Tracheostomy-associated bleeding

This may be due to a tracheostomy-innominate artery fistula. This condition has a very high mortality. Adjustment of a cuffed tracheostomy tube position and/or hyperinflation of the cuff may tamponade the bleeding. Extra-large suction catheters may be required to remove clots from the airway. Urgent surgical intervention will be required.

◗ Tramadol (Tramal)

Description

Tramadol is an analogue of codeine and is an analgesic drug with multimodal actions. It decreases the neuronal reuptake of serotonin and noradrenaline (SNRI) and stimulates mu receptors. It is about one-tenth as potent as morphine. It is presented in both immediate-release and modified-release forms.

Dose

Adult

PO/PR 50–100 mg q 4–6 h max 400 mg/day. IV bolus dose 50–100 mg over 2–3 min q 4–6 h. PCA dose 300 mg in 60 mL N/S, start with a 20 mg bolus with a 5 min lockout.

Child

1–2 mg/kg PO or IV q 4–6 h.

Advantages

1 Lower addiction potential than other opioids.
2 Effective orally and intravenously.
3 Useful for treating postoperative shivering.
4 Low potential for respiratory depression.
5 Does not cause withdrawal effects when used in patients on methadone.
6 Has some anxiolytic and antidepressant effects due to its SNRI activity.
7 Does not cause histamine release.

Disadvantages

1 Less potent than morphine. It is only suitable for moderate pain in conjunction with other painkillers such as paracetamol.
2 There is a risk of serotonin syndrome if tramadol is given with a drug that increases serotonin levels in the CNS such as sertraline, tricyclic antidepressants, moclobemide, venlafaxine or St John's wort. *See Serotonin syndrome/toxicity*.
3 Tramadol can cause dizziness, nausea, vomiting, confusion and headache.
4 Causes dysphoria in some patients.
5 Tramadol's metabolites are active and mainly renally excreted. Tramadol should be avoided or used in a reduced dose in patients with renal impairment/failure.
6 Tramadol is mainly metabolised in the liver so use cautiously in patients with liver impairment.

7 Ondansetron is not effective for nausea induced by tramadol. Ondansetron also decreases the analgesic effects of tramadol.

8 There is a risk of seizures if the patient is receiving drugs that lower the seizure threshold, such as tricyclic antidepressants. Also use with caution if the patient has a history of seizures.

9 Prolongs the QT interval. Should not be used in patients at increased risk of torsades de pointes. *See Long QT syndrome (LQTS)* and *Torsades de pointes*.

◖ Tranexamic acid (TXA) (Cyklokapron)

Description
Anti-fibrinolytic lysine analogue that inhibits the conversion of plasminogen to plasmin, thus inhibiting fibrinolysis and clot breakdown.

Indications
1 Reduce the amount of intraoperative and postoperative bleeding in certain types of surgery e.g. prostate, hip and knee replacement (off-label use).

2 Treatment of major haemorrhage. *See Blood loss—assessment, management and anaesthesia approach*. Off-label use.

3 Orally for menorrhagia/nose bleeds.

4 Mouthwash to reduce bleeding after tooth extraction.

5 Reduce bleeding after tooth extraction in patients with haemophilia. *See Haemophilia*.

6 Prevention of attacks of angioedema in hereditary angioedema through an unknown mechanism. *See Angioedema*.

7 Massive haemoptysis. Used in nebulised form (500 mg in 5 mL N/S q 8 h).

Dose for reducing intraoperative/postoperative bleeding

Adult
1 g in 100 mL N/S over 10 min then repeat dose in 6 h. There are several other protocols.

Dose for major trauma

Adult
1 g in 100 mL N/S over 10 min followed by 1 g in 100 mL N/S over 8 h.[q]

Points to note
1 Should not be used in patients with a history of DVT/PE or patients on the OCP.

2 Convulsions can occur if given too rapidly IV.

3 Renally excreted. Use cautiously in renally impaired patients.

◖ Transposition of the great arteries (TGA)/transposition of the great vessels (TGV)

Description
Only a brief overview of this complex cyanotic congenital heart disease can be provided in this manual. This condition is a heart defect in which the aorta arises from the right ventricle and the pulmonary artery arises from the left ventricle. In malposition of the great arteries, both may arise from the same ventricle. TGA is incompatible with life after birth, unless some other defect allows mixing of the systemic and pulmonary circulations e.g. a VSD, ASD or PDA. Untreated, TGA has a 90% mortality in the first year of life.

Surgical repair

Atrial switch procedure
In this procedure, systemic return to the heart is redirected into the pulmonary circulation and pulmonary venous return is redirected into the systemic circulation at the atrial level. This is achieved by a baffle inserted through the atrial septum which redirects blood flow appropriately. The RV provides the systemic pump and progressive RV failure and tricuspid regurgitation are likely to occur over time.

Arterial switch procedure
The pulmonary artery and aorta are detached from the incorrect ventricles and attached to their correct ventricles. The coronary arteries must be detached from the pulmonary artery and attached to the aorta. This is the most difficult part of the surgery. The pulmonary valve becomes the aortic valve and the aortic valve becomes the pulmonary valve. Any ASD, VSD and/or PDA are also repaired at the same surgery.

Complications of arterial switch repair
1 The pulmonary valve may leak.
2 Supravalvular pulmonary artery stenosis may occur.
3 The aorta may become dilated above its anastomotic connection.
4 Coronary artery stenosis may occur.

◗ Trans-urethral resection of prostate (TURP)

Introduction
TURP is used to treat benign prostatic hyperplasia causing urinary voiding problems. Surgical options include:
1 prostate urethral lift
2 resection—monopolar electrocautery resectoscope, bipolar TURP, robotic water jet treatment
3 ablation—water vapour thermal therapy, holmium laser enucleation, microwave therapy
4 compression
5 simple prostatectomy.

Monopolar resectoscope method
A non-conducting irrigation fluid such as glycine or mannitol must be used. Glycine 1.5% is hypo-osmolar (230 mosm/L). The main risks with this type of surgery are:
1 bleeding
2 absorption of the irrigation fluid, causing dilutional hyponatraemia (the TURP syndrome).

Anaesthetic technique
1 SAB or GA. SAB provides postoperative analgesia, early detection of the TURP syndrome and reduced blood loss.[10] Anaesthesia to T9, 10 is required if SAB is used. For most patients use 3 mL of bupivacaine 0.5%.
2 If using hypotonic irrigation fluid, limit the height of the bag to 60–70 cm above the prostate. Use glycine 1.5% or mannitol 0.5% or sorbitol 3.5%. Do not use water. The risk of TURP syndrome (see below) is increased if the duration of surgery is longer than 60 min.
3 Measure how much irrigation fluid is returned—a discrepancy suggests bladder perforation.

4 Give gentamicin 120–240 mg IV.

5 Only use N/S for intravascular fluid replacement.

6 Treat hypotension with vasopressors rather than IV fluid to reduce the risk of fluid overload.

7 Consider tranexamic acid 1 g in 100 mL N/S over 10 min to reduce blood loss. **See Tranexamic acid (TXA) (Cyklokapron).**

8 Thromboembolic prophylaxis postoperatively.

TURP syndrome

This is due to excessive glycine absorption into the circulation resulting in hypervolaemia and hyponatraemia. Effects include:

1 restlessness, headache, vision problems, blindness

2 confusion, convulsions, coma

3 tachypnoea, hypoxia, pulmonary oedema

4 burning sensation in the face and hands

5 nausea and vomiting

6 dysrhythmias, cardiovascular collapse.

Pathophysiology

1 Hyponatraemia occurs due to glycine, which cannot enter the cells, drawing fluid out of the cells into the plasma (like mannitol).

2 Acute fluid overload.

3 Glycine toxicity—can in itself cause transient blindness and elevated serum ammonia levels (ammonia is a metabolite of glycine). Glycine is also toxic to the heart.

4 Glycine inhibits CNS neurotransmission at GABA receptors and potentiates NMDA receptors.

Treatment

1 Warn the surgeon and cease operating if TURP syndrome is detected intraoperatively.

2 Supportive—O_2 therapy, haemodynamic support.

3 Frusemide 1 mg/kg to treat hypervolaemia.

4 Hypertonic saline 3% 100 mL boluses over 10 min. Up to three doses can be given. **See Sodium.** Do not increase serum sodium by more than 12 mmol/L in the first 24 h. If the hyponatraemia is less than 48 h in duration, there is probably no risk of causing osmotic demyelination syndrome.[11]

5 Fluid restriction.

◗ Transversus abdominis plane (TAP) block/subcostal TAP block

Description

The abdominal wall derives its sensory innervation from the anterior division of the spinal segmental nerves T7–T11. The TAP plane lies between the transversus abdominis and internal oblique muscles through which these nerves pass.

Indications

Postoperative analgesia for lower abdominal surgical wounds below the umbilicus e.g. Caesarean section. Bilateral blocks are needed for wounds that cross the midline.

Technique using ultrasound (lateral approach)

When moving the ultrasound probe from above the umbilicus laterally we see (in order) the linea alba, the rectus abdominis, aponeurosis of the internal oblique and transversus abdominis muscle (Figures T5 and T6). We then see two muscle layers (internal oblique and transversus abdominis), then three muscle layers (external oblique comes into view).

1 Obtain IV access and position the patient supine.

2 Use aseptic technique—sterilise the area of the block (lateral abdominal wall) and use sterile gloves and a probe cover.

3 Scan the lateral abdomen between the iliac crest and the rib margin with the probe oriented in the transverse plane in the mid-axillary line.

4 Identify the three abdominal muscle layers—from superficial to deep: the external oblique, internal oblique (the thickest layer) and transversus abdominis.

5 Using a 100 mm block needle and an in-plane approach, place the tip of the needle between the internal oblique and transversus abdominis layers anterior to the mid-axillary line, at a shallow angle. The transversus abdominis muscle comes to an end in the mid-axillary line.

6 For a unilateral block, inject 1% ropivacaine 20 mL + 5 mL of N/S. For a bilateral block, use 0.5% ropivacaine 20 mL + 5 mL of N/S **each** side. Hydro-dissect between the muscle layers towards the mid-axillary line and where the transversus abdominis ends, using a 'stick, inject, move' sequence.

7 The LA should be seen to form an ellipse between the innermost and middle muscle layers.

8 If having trouble identifying the muscle layers, consider the 'tectonic sign'. Because the internal and external oblique fibres are at right angles to each other, fanning the probe in a cephalad/caudad fashion gives the impression that the external and internal obliques are sliding over each other.

Complications

1 Abdominal organ damage.

2 Infection.

3 Bleeding.

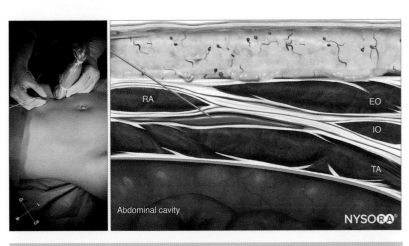

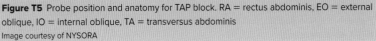

Figure T5 Probe position and anatomy for TAP block. RA = rectus abdominis, EO = external oblique, IO = internal oblique, TA = transversus abdominis
Image courtesy of NYSORA

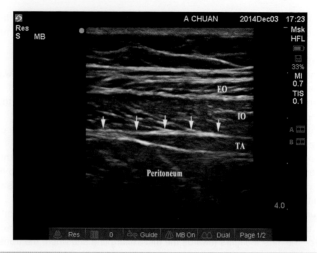

Figure T6 Sonoanatomy of the abdominal wall. EO = external oblique, IO = internal oblique, TA = transversus abdominis. The arrows indicate the plane of the block
Image courtesy of Dr Alwin Chuan

Subcostal TAP block

This block is useful for abdominal wounds above the umbilicus.

1 Moving the probe along the subcostal margin from lateral to medial, the medial edges of the external and internal oblique can be seen.
2 As the probe moves medially, the lateral edge of the rectus abdominis is seen. Between the rectus and the oblique muscle edges is the aponeurosis of the transversus abdominis.
3 Starting laterally, identify the transversus abdominis and internal oblique.
4 Insert the block needle in-plane from lateral to medial, and inject LA between these layers, hydro-dissecting towards the xiphisternum and under the lateral edge of the rectus abdominis. Use a total of 20 mL ropivacaine 1%.
5 This should anaesthetise the T9–11 dermatomes.

○ Tricuspid regurgitation (TR)/tricuspid incompetence (TI)

Aetiology

Tricuspid incompetence can be caused by:

1 Functional—due to dilatation of the RV (in turn due to causes such as pulmonary hypertension, pulmonary stenosis, mitral stenosis, cardiomyopathy).
2 Rheumatic fever. There is usually tricuspid stenosis as well.
3 Congenital heart disease. **See Ebstein's anomaly.**
4 Carcinoid.
5 Connective tissue diseases such as Marfan syndrome.
6 Endocarditis. Tricuspid valvectomy without replacement may be required to treat endocarditis.
7 Medications e.g. methysergide, pergolide.
8 Papillary muscle dysfunction e.g. after myocardial infarction.
9 Right atrial myxoma.

10 Endomyocardial fibrosis.

11 SLE.

12 Chest trauma.

Pathophysiology

1 Mild-to-moderate TR is usually well tolerated.

2 Severe TR causes RV volume overload, leading to RV failure, hepatomegaly, ascites and peripheral oedema. The RV copes with volume overload much better than pressure overload. Even severe TR may be asymptomatic in some patients.

3 RA overload and distension.

4 Cardiorenal syndrome may occur—cardiac disease causing renal disease and vice versa.

Clinical features

1 Fatigue.

2 Reduced exercise capacity.

3 Right upper quadrant abdominal pain from hepatomegaly.

4 Peripheral oedema.

5 Atrial fibrillation.

6 Pansystolic murmur over the LSE which increases in intensity with inspiration.

Diagnosis

Trivial or mild TR is frequently seen in normal people.

1 CXR—cardiomegaly due to RA and RV enlargement.

2 ECG—RBBB, AF.

3 Cardiac echo reveals the defect.

Treatment

1 Medical therapy—diuretics.

2 Surgical repair/annuloplasty.

3 Valve replacement.

Anaesthetic goals

Think 'fast, full and forward'.

1 Invasive arterial blood pressure monitoring, consider central line.

2 Maintain preload in the high normal range. It is critical to avoid hypovolaemia as this will decrease RV filling.

3 Maintain sinus rhythm.

4 Consider antibiotic prophylaxis for relevant procedures. ***See Bacterial endocarditis (BE) prophylaxis.***

5 Keep heart rate normal-to-high to maintain forward flow.

6 If right-heart failure occurs, provide inotropic support with dobutamine.[12]

7 Maintain afterload—keep systemic blood pressure within 20% of pre-anaesthetic values.[12]

8 Avoid any increase in pulmonary vascular resistance—e.g. avoid hypercarbia, hypoxia, acidosis, N_2O.

9 Avoid high airway pressures.

◐ Tricuspid stenosis (TS)

Description

It is usually a benign lesion and often does not require specific treatment. TS often coexists with mitral stenosis.

Causes

1 Rheumatic fever.
2 Carcinoid.
3 Congenital.

Pathophysiology

1 The RA is initially able to enlarge and compensate for the stenosis.
2 There is back pressure on the venous circulation, causing hepatomegaly and jugular venous distension.
3 The development of AF is less likely than with mitral stenosis.

Clinical features

1 Fluttering discomfort in the neck due to giant A waves.
2 Fatigue.
3 Liver enlargement. This may cause right upper quadrant abdominal pain.
4 Heart murmur. Typically, there is a soft opening snap, then a mid-diastolic rumble with a pre-systolic accentuation. It is best heard at the LSE.
5 AF.

Diagnosis

1 ECG—tall, peaked P waves (RA enlargement).
2 CXR—dilated SVC, RA enlargement.
3 Cardiac echo—mean forward gradient across the valve > 5 mmHg suggests severe disease.

Treatment

1 Diuretics, aldosterone antagonist.
2 Rarely repair/replacement.

Anaesthesia

1 Maintain preload.
2 Maintain HR in the low normal range. Tachycardia will result in less time for RV filling and bradycardia will result in overdistension of the RA.
3 Maintain SVR.

❯ Trigeminal cardiac reflex/trigeminocardiac reflex

Stimulation of trigeminal nerve fibres can cause powerful vagal stimulation with sudden onset of bradycardia leading to asystole, asystole with no preceding bradycardia, hypotension, apnoea and gastric hyper-mobility. This can occur during surgery on the base of the skull. It usually resolves spontaneously when surgical manipulation stops. If bradycardia persists, give atropine or glycopyrrolate. *See Atropine* and *Glycopyrrolate.*

If this is ineffective, start an adrenaline infusion at 2–10 mcg/min. If asystole occurs, start CPR. Do not give 1 mg boluses of adrenaline. Instead use increments of 50–100 mcg. If a dose of 1 mg is reached without a response, subsequent doses should be 1 mg. Consider cardiac pacing.

❯ Trisomy 21

See Down syndrome.

❯ Tropisetron

5-HT_3 antagonist used mainly to treat chemotherapy-related nausea and vomiting.

Dose

Adult

2–5 mg IV.

◗ Troponins

See Acute coronary syndrome.

◗ Turner syndrome

Description

Turner syndrome is a genetic disorder that occurs in about 1:2000 females. It is due to the absence, or partial absence, of a second X chromosome (45, XO). It is associated with:

1 short stature
2 webbed neck
3 hypertension
4 coarctation of the aorta–*see Coarctation of the aorta*
5 aortic stenosis
6 bicuspid aortic valve
7 single kidney/horseshoe kidney
8 skeletal abnormalities such as fused cervical vertebrae
9 increased incidence of cancer
10 micrognathia, high-arched palate
11 shortened trachea, with the carina higher in the chest than normal
12 vision and hearing problems.

Anaesthetic implications

1 Intubation may be difficult due to the abnormalities described above.
2 Endobronchial intubation may occur due to a short trachea.

REFERENCES

1 Leung T, Lao T. Thalassaemia in pregnancy. *Best Pract Res Clin Obstet Gynaecol* 2012; 26: 37–51.

2 Ciobanu AM, Colibaba S, Cimpoca B et al. Thrombocytopenia in pregnancy. *Maedica* 2016; 11: 55–60.

3 Shah U, Narayanan M, Smith J. Anaesthetic considerations in patients with inherited disorders of coagulation. *Cont Edu Anaesth Crit Care & Pain* 2015; 15: 26–31.

4 Carroll R, Matfin G. Endocrine and metabolic emergencies: thyroid storm. *Ther Adv Endcrinol Metab* 2010; 1: 139–145.

5 Fisher A, Meller Y. Continuous postoperative regional analgesia by nerve sheath block for amputation surgery—a pilot study. *Anesth Analg* 1991; 72: 300–303.

6 De Noronha D, Mauricio S, Rodrigues I. *Long QT syndrome and anaesthesia.* WFSA Tutorial 449, 8 June 2021. Accessed online: https://resources.wfsahq.org/wp-content/uploads/atow-449-00.pdf, January 2023.

7 Wei P, Yan D, Huang J et al. Anesthetic management of tracheal laceration from traumatic dislocation of the first rib: a case report and literature review. *BMC Anesthesiol* 2019; 19. Accessed online: https://bmcanesthesiol.biomedcentral.com/articles/10.1186/s12871-019-0812-9, October 2022.

8 Sehgal S, Chance JC, Steliga MA. Thoracic anaesthesia and cross field ventilation for tracheobronchial injuries: a challenge for anesthesiologists. *Case Reports in Anesthesiol* 2014; 2014: 972762. Published online. Accessed online: https://www.hindawi.com/journals/cria/2014/972762/, October 2022.

9 Roberts I. Tranexamic acid in trauma: how should we use it? *J Thromb Haemost* 2015; 13: S195–199.

10 Bhattacharyya S, Bisai S, Biswas H et al. Regional anaesthesia in transurethral resection of prostate (TURP) surgery: a comparative study between saddle block and subarachnoid block. *Saudi J Anaesth* 2015; 9: 268–271.

11 Emmett M, Istre O, Hahn R. Hyponatraemia following transurethral resection, hysteroscopy, or other procedures involving electrolyte-free irrigation. *UpToDate*. Accessed online: https://www.uptodate.com/contents/hyponatremia-following-transurethral-resection-hysteroscopy-or-other-procedures-involving-electrolyte-free-irrigation#!, October 2022. Topic last updated 22 November 2022.

12 Bansal P, Popli S. Anaesthetic management of a case of severe tricuspid regurgitation posted for open cholecystectomy. *Int J Contemp Med Res* 2017; 4: 430–432.

▶ Ultrasound-assisted neuraxial anaesthesia

Introduction

Ultrasound can be useful for determining:

- the midline of the spinal column
- the correct space for insertion
- the depth of the dura.

Use the curvilinear probe because it gives a wider image, deeper penetration and clearer anatomy.

Transverse view

1 When the probe is placed over a spinous process, a shape that looks like a fan is seen with the spinous process as the handle (Figure U1).
2 The fan spreads at the base of the handle. These structures are the vertebral laminae.
3 When the probe is placed between spinous processes, a central blur is visible with a concave white line inferiorly between two small humps.
4 The two small humps are the articular processes and the concave white line is the dura (Figure U2).
5 Measure the depth to the dura.

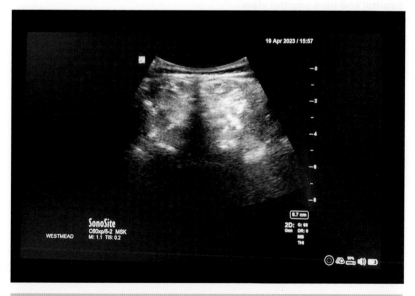

Figure U1 Transverse view through spine with the probe over a lumbar spinous process. Note the fan-like appearance of the vertebral lamina/transverse processes.

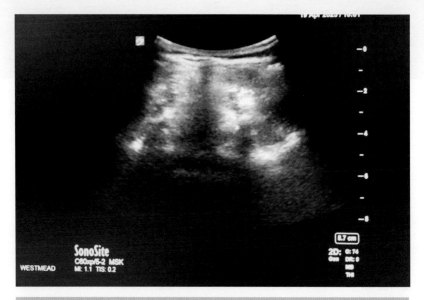

Figure U2 Probe placed transversely over a lumbar interspinous space. The dura can be seen at 5 cm depth in the midline. The dark areas on either side of the midline are the articular processes

Sagittal and para-sagittal view

If the probe is placed in the midline of the spinal column, a series of bumps is seen—the spinous processes. Again, this will confirm where the midline is. Move the probe slightly to one side. This will show a row of triangular smaller humps—the articular processes. Next, tilt the probe inwards (like a paramedian approach to an epidural). This will show the intralaminar view. In this view there is a deeper white line (posterior dura), and a still deeper white line (anterior dura), with saw-tooth humps on either side—the vertebral laminae.

How to find the L3–4 interspace

Place the probe longitudinally at the top of the natal cleft in a para-sagittal position and tilted slightly towards the midline. The sacrum looks like a more or less straight line. See Figure U3.

1 Just cranial to the sacrum triangular humps are seen. These are the articular processes. See Figure U4.

2 The space between the first hump and the sacrum is L5–S1. The space between the second and third humps (counting up from the sacrum) will be the L3–4 interspace.

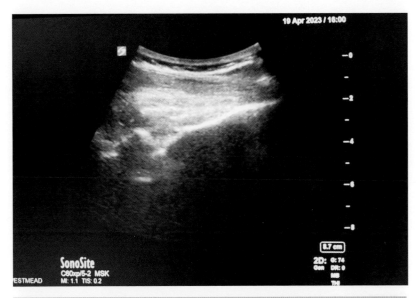

Figure U3 Para-sagittal longitudinal view of sacrum with probe tilted inwards. Note the almost straight-line appearance of the sacrum

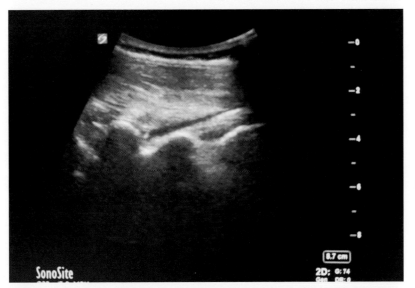

Figure U4 Moving the probe cranially from the sacrum (para-sagittal longitudinal view) the articular processes are clearly seen (L5 and L4)

Putting it together

1 Identify the sacrum and the L3–4 interspace as described above. Draw a horizontal line on the patient that would pass through the centre of the longitudinally orientated probe. This gives the correct level of insertion.
2 Turn the probe through 90° and directly over the L3–4 interspace.
3 Centre the probe over the dura and measure the depth to the dura. Note that this may not be in the exact midline of the patient.
4 Draw a vertical line that would pass through the centre of the probe.
5 Remove the probe and extend the horizontal and vertical lines. Where these lines meet is the target.

○ Umbilical cord prolapse

Description

Umbilical cord prolapse is an acute obstetric emergency endangering the fetus.
It requires immediate Caesarean section (CS) delivery. This is because the cord is in front of the fetal presenting part. Compression of the cord by the presenting part will compromise the oxygen supply to the fetus. The cord may also undergo umbilical vein occlusion or umbilical artery vasospasm, also compromising fetal oxygenation.
The cord may be in the vagina or outside the vagina.

Causes

Most cases of cord prolapse occur in low-risk women at term.[1] Predisposing factors include:
1 Premature rupture of the membranes.
2 Artificial rupture of the membranes (ARM).
3 Preterm labour.
4 Multiple gestation pregnancies—especially a risk for second twin.
5 Polyhydramnios.
6 Malpresentation of the fetus e.g. breech, transverse, oblique and unstable lie.
7 High-presenting part.
8 Abnormal placentation.
9 Abnormally long umbilical cord.
10 Fetal procedures such as manual rotation of the fetal head.

Diagnosis

1 Seeing the umbilical cord protruding from the vagina or feeling it in the vagina.
2 Fetal bradycardia (< 120 bpm).
3 If the cord is alongside the presenting part, this is called occult cord prolapse; if the cord is past the presenting part, this is called overt cord prolapse.
4 Cord presentation is when the cord is between the presenting part and the cervix.

Treatment—first stage of labour

1 Check for umbilical cord pulsation—if the cord is not pulsating, confirm fetal death with ultrasound and aim for a vaginal delivery.
2 If the umbilical cord is pulsating, organise a code critical CS.
3 Cease oxytocin infusion if this is in progress.
4 Administer O_2 to the mother via a non-rebreathing mask at 8 L/min.
5 Monitor CTG continuously
6 Place the mother in the knee-chest position (on knees, face on pillow) or left lateral with the hips elevated. Elevate the foot of the bed if possible.

7 Use fingers to elevate the fetal presenting part off the cord but minimise handling of the cord.

8 Consider tocolysis with glyceryl trinitrate—*see **Glyceryl trinitrate (GTN)**.*

9 Consider filling the bladder with warm N/S to elevate the presenting part. Ensure the bladder is emptied before any birth attempt.

10 If the cord is protruding outside the vagina, place it into the vagina or wrap it gently in a pad soaked in warm saline.

11 Prepare for resuscitation of the newborn.

12 Obtain paired arterial and venous cord samples immediately after birth. This will help determine if possible intrapartum fetal hypoxic brain damage has occurred.

Treatment—second stage of labour

It may be possible to achieve a vaginal birth if the presenting part is below spines. This may involve:

1 Instrumental birth (vacuum, forceps).

2 Vigorous pushing by the mother.

3 If immediate vaginal birth is not feasible, prepare for immediate CS.

4 Prepare for resuscitation of the newborn. ***See Neonatal resuscitation**.*

Anaesthesia and cord prolapse[1]

1 A GA will usually be required.

2 If the woman has a working epidural in place, topping up the epidural on the way to operating suite may be an option to avoid GA.

3 Expeditious SAB in the left lateral position may be possible if the fetal heart rate is acceptable.

❍ Umbilical vein catheterisation

*See **Neonatal resuscitation**.*

❍ Unfractionated heparin

*See **Heparin (unfractionated and low-molecular-weight heparins)**.*

❍ Unstable angina

*See **Acute coronary syndrome**.*

❍ Uterine atonia, postpartum

*See **Postpartum haemorrhage (PPH)**.*

❍ Uterine inversion/puerperal uterine inversion

Description

This is an obstetric emergency that can result in severe haemorrhage, shock, pain and death. It is due to the placenta exiting the vagina while it is still attached to the uterine wall. This results in the uterus being inverted. It can be graded as:

1 Incomplete inversion/first degree—the fundus is within the endometrial cavity.

2 Complete inversion/second degree—the fundus protrudes through the cervical os.

3 Prolapsed inversion/third degree—the fundus protrudes to or beyond the introitus.

4 Total inversion/fourth degree—both the uterus and vagina are inverted (usually associated with a cancer rather than childbirth).

Causes

Inversions are rare and can occur spontaneously. Inversions are associated with:
1 long labour
2 short umbilical cord
3 excessive traction on the umbilical cord
4 placenta accreta—*see Placenta accreta spectrum*
5 use of magnesium infusion
6 retained placenta—*see Retained placenta*.

Pathophysiology

1 Haemorrhage may occur due to the invaginated uterus being unable to properly contract—it can be severe.
2 Shock may be out of all proportion to blood loss due to increased vagal tone from stretching of the pelvic parasympathetic nerves and severe pain. However, both this process and severe haemorrhage may occur at the same time.

Clinical presentation

1 Mild to severe bleeding—due to the inability of the uterus to contract and can lead to hypovolaemic shock.
2 Mild to severe lower abdominal pain.
3 A protruding smooth, round mass.

Treatment

There are two management priorities—resuscitate the patient and correct uterine prolapse.
1 Declare an emergency, summon skilled assistance immediately.
2 Cease oxytocic agents.
3 Establish large-bore IV access and give IV fluids (crystalloid/colloid/blood).
4 Maintain airway and oxygenation.
5 The obstetrician or another rescuer should attempt to push the uterus back into the normal position. This may be difficult due to a contracted cervix.
   The placenta should be left attached as removal at this point may result in massive haemorrhage. However, the placenta may be too big to be pushed back through the cervix.
6 Hydrostatic pressure may be used to correct inversion. A 1000 mL bag of warmed N/S is hung from an IV pole and an infusion line is placed in the vagina, with the patient in a Trendelenburg lithotomy position. The obstetrician can use his hands to squeeze the vagina closed or a vacuum extraction silicone cup can be used to form a seal in the vagina. 2–5 L of fluid may be needed.
7 GTN may be needed to relax the contracted cervix so the uterus can pass through it. *See Uterine relaxation*.
8 Appropriate analgesia e.g. fentanyl.

Anaesthesia for uterine inversion

1 Perform a rapid sequence induction (using sux or rocuronium) and intubation with suitably modified anaesthetic drug dosages.
2 Continue resuscitation with appropriate IV fluids (crystalloid/blood).
3 The obstetrician will continue to try and manually correct the uterine inversion with the assistance of GTN boluses.
4 Rarely, laparotomy may be needed to replace the uterus. Even more rarely, hysterectomy is required.

5 Prophylactic antibiotic cover.
6 Once the uterine position is corrected, give oxytocin to contract the uterus and an oxytocin infusion (40 units in 1000 mL Hartmann's solution).
7 Await separation of the placenta. Manual removal of the placenta may be needed.

◗ Uterine relaxation

Indications
1 Retained placenta.
2 External cephalic version of the second twin.
3 Uterine inversion.
4 Fetal entrapment e.g. entrapment of the after-coming head during breech delivery.

Techniques
1 Increasing volatile concentration of GA.
2 IV glyceryl trinitrate (GTN). *See Glyceryl trinitrate (GTN)*. To prepare GTN remove 1 mL (5 mg) from an ampoule of GTN (which contains 50 mg in 10 mL). Dilute the 5 mg of GTN to a total volume of 10 mL (500 mcg/mL). Remove 1 mL from this syringe and dilute this to a total volume of 10 mL (50 mcg/mL). Give 1 mL boluses as required. 100–200 mcg is usually effective.

◗ Uterine rupture

Description
This is an obstetric emergency with a maternal mortality of about 0.1% for a scarred uterus and about 10% for an unscarred uterus. Fetal mortality is about 6–25%. The incidence is about 1:5000–7000 births and is increasing.[2]

Causes
1 Uterine scar (previous CS, uterine perforation).
2 Use of oxytocics during labour.
3 Prolonged labour.
4 Increasing parity and age.
5 High rotation forceps.
6 Trauma.

Clinical presentation
1 Abdominal pain, which is often atypical. It may have a sudden tearing, ripping quality.
2 Chest pain.
3 Acute fetal bradycardia or sudden profound fetal distress or loss of detectable fetal heart beat.
4 Contractions cease or become less intense.
5 PV blood loss.
6 Maternal tachycardia, hypotension, hypovolaemic shock.
7 Change in abdominal shape.
8 Haematuria.
9 Fetal body parts palpable through the abdominal wall.
10 Abdominal ultrasound, time permitting, will aid in diagnosis.

Anaesthetic management

Prepare for emergency surgery and potential or actual massive blood loss.

1 Stop oxytocin if running.
2 Large-bore IV access × 2—send blood for cross-match.
3 Appropriate resuscitation fluids IV (crystalloid, colloid, blood).
4 Rapid sequence induction with precautions—**see *Caesarean section (CS)***.
5 **See *Blood loss—assessment, management and anaesthetic approach***.

REFERENCES

1 Government of South Australia SA Health. *South Australian Perinatal Practice Guideline: Cord Presentation and Prolapse*. Accessed online: https://www.sahealth.sa.gov.au/wps/wcm/connect/bae906804ee1fea9b28fbfd, September 2022. 150ce4f37/Cord+Presentation+and+Prolpase_PPG_v5_0.pdf?MOD=AJPERES&CACHEID=ROOTWORKSPACE-bae906804ee1fea9b28fbfd150ce4f37-obYKocq, September 2022.

2 Togioka B, Tonismae T. Uterine rupture. *StatPearls Publishing* January 2022. Last updated June 2022. Accessed online: https://pubmed.ncbi.nlm.nih.gov/32644635/, October 2022.

○ Vagal manoeuvres

These are actions to increase the activity of the vagus nerves to treat tachycardia. The increased vagal activity has a negative chronotropic action on the SA node and slows conduction through the AV node. These manoeuvres include:

1 Carotid sinus massage—only perform this on one side of the neck at a time.
2 The Valsalva manoeuvre (attempted forced exhalation against a closed glottis).
3 Putting an ice-cold wet towel or bag of ice on the face, or immersing the face in icy water.
4 Coughing.
5 Squatting.

○ Valdecoxib

Long-acting oral COX-2 selective NSAID. Also available as a parenteral pro-drug, parecoxib. **See Parecoxib.**

○ Vaping

Vaping is the inhalation of aerosols for pleasure or as an aid to reducing/ceasing cigarette smoking. Substances inhaled can be nicotine, vitamin E acetate, propylene glycol, glycerol, cannabinoids, heavy metals and potentially hundreds of other substances. It is felt that vaping has up to 5% of the health risk associated with smoking.[1]

EVALI

EVALI is an acronym for **e**-cigarette, or **v**aping product, use-**a**ssociated **l**ung **i**njury. Vitamin E acetate is particularly harmful. This is a diagnosis of exclusion in patients that vape. It is characterised by:

1 pulmonary infiltrates
2 injury to alveolar epithelial cells and vascular endothelial cells
3 severe acute respiratory distress
4 dyspnoea, chest pain, cough
5 fever
6 nausea and vomiting
7 diarrhoea.

Burns injuries

As the vapour is heated with power from a battery, a malfunction can result in burns to the user or injuries from the device igniting or exploding. Chemical burns may also occur.

Anaesthetic implications

At this stage there is little information in the literature about this issue. Patients who vape may have an increased risk of airway irritability and complications such as bronchospasm. However, the risk is probably less than in patients who smoke cigarettes.

◗ Vasa praevia

Description
In this condition, some fetal umbilical cord blood vessels run across or very close to the internal uterine os. These vessels are at risk of rupturing if their surrounding membranes break, as can occur with labour. This can result in fetal haemorrhage and death.

Causes
The cause is unknown but it may be associated with:
1 placenta praevia
2 in vitro fertilisation technology
3 multiple pregnancy.

Diagnosis
1 Routine obstetric ultrasound may identify placenta praevia.
2 Transvaginal ultrasound is the best test.
3 PV blood loss with severe fetal compromise.
4 Undiagnosed vasa praevia results in a fetal mortality > 50%.

Management
1 Elective CS at 35–37 weeks.
2 Emergency CS for fetal distress.

◗ Vasopressin (Vasostrict, Pitressin)

Description
Vasopressin is a peptide prohormone produced in neurones of the hypothalamus. It is converted to arginine vasopressin (AVP) and secreted from the pituitary gland. It is released in response to increased extracellular fluid hypertonicity, hypovolaemia and hypotension. It has three effects:
1 It acts on the kidneys to increase the amount of solute-free water that is resorbed from nephrons. AVP is also called antidiuretic hormone. In acts on renal V2 receptors in the distal tubule of the nephron.
2 It constricts arterioles by acting on V1 receptors. This increases peripheral vascular resistance (PVR) and blood pressure. Vasopressin diverts blood from non-vital (skin, small bowel, fat) to vital (heart, brain, lung) vascular beds.
3 It inhibits inflammatory mediators, decreasing their vasodilatory effects, and decreases nitric oxide-mediated vasodilation.

Use as a drug
Vasopressin is used for the treatment of:
1 Diabetes insipidus.
2 Low blood pressure due to decreased PVR/vasodilatation (sepsis, anaphylaxis, post-cardiac surgery) resistant to treatment with fluids and noradrenaline.

3 Low blood pressure in carcinoid crisis. *See Carcinoid tumours and carcinoid syndrome.*

4 Bleeding from oesophageal varices.

5 Abdominal distension.

Dose for different types of shock in adults

Mix 20 units in 40 mL 5% glucose. Give preferably through a central line. In an emergency situation, start the infusion at 1–2 units/h (2–4 mL/h).

Post-cardiac surgery shock

Initial dose 0.03 units/min. Titrate up by 0.005 units/min at 10–15 min intervals until desired BP attained. Max rate 0.1 units/min.

Septic shock

Initial dose 0.01 units/min. Titrate up as above, max rate 0.07 units/min.

Anaphylaxis not responsive to adrenaline

Bolus 1–2 units then 2 units/h by continuous infusion IV. *See Anaphylaxis.*

Dose in children

Mix 1 unit/kg in 50 mL 5% glucose. Give a 2 mL bolus then run the infusion at 1–3 mL/h (0.02–0.06 units/kg/h).

◐ Vecuronium

Description

Intermediate duration of action non-depolarising neuromuscular blocking drug. It is a bis-quaternary amino-steroid analogue of pancuronium.

Dose

IV 0.1 mg/kg with recovery in about 30 min. Can also be given by infusion—50–80 mcg/kg/h.

Advantages

1 Incidence of anaphylaxis about 3 × less than rocuronium.

2 Low potential for histamine release.

3 Little haemodynamic impact. Does not cause tachycardia (unlike pancuronium).

Disadvantages

1 Slow onset compared with rocuronium. Unsuitable for rapid sequence induction.

2 Only partially reversed by sugammadex. *See Sugammadex.*

3 Effects prolonged by renal or liver disease. About 25% is excreted unchanged by the kidney. The remaining 75% is metabolised by the liver.

4 It is presented as a powder which must be reconstituted with water before use.

◗ Veins of the upper limb

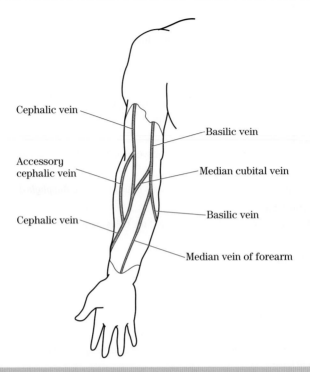

Cephalic vein

Accessory cephalic vein

Cephalic vein

Basilic vein

Median cubital vein

Basilic vein

Median vein of forearm

Figure V1 Veins of the upper limb

◗ Velamentous cord insertion

In this condition, the umbilical vessels diverge as they traverse between the amnion and chorion before reaching the placenta. The umbilical vessels are not protected by Wharton's jelly and are prone to compression and rupture. The cause is unknown.

◗ Venous air embolism

See Gas embolism.

◗ Venous thromboembolism

See Deep venous thrombosis (DVT) prophylaxis and Pulmonary embolism (PE).

◗ Ventilator settings and modes

Introduction
A ventilator is a machine which assists the patient to breathe or takes over breathing from them or both. In its most basic form, the ventilator drives gas into the patient's lungs, which the patient then passively exhales.

1 The volume of gas driven into the patient is the tidal volume (TV) and the number of breaths per minute × TV equals the minute ventilation (MV).

2 The TV as set by the operator is the inspiratory flow rate × time. If the inspiratory flow rate is 0.25 L/s and the inspiratory time is 2 s, the TV is 500 mL.

The operator can manipulate many settings on modern ventilators and anaesthetic machines. These are described below.

Concepts

Dead space

This is the inspired gas that does not take part in gas exchange. Anatomical dead space in the adult is about 150 mL but this can be increased by equipment dead space.

I:E ratio

This is the ratio of inspiratory time to the expiratory time and is normally set to 1:2. For example, if the set respiratory rate is 10 and the I:E ratio is 1:2, 2 s are spent in inspiration and 4 s in expiration.

Inspiratory flow rate

This is the rate at which gas enters the lungs for inspiration. The flow rate equals the volume/time. Thus, volume can be delivered slowly or quickly, depending on the flow rate. The inspiratory flow rate set on the ventilator for a normal patient is 60 L/min or 1 L/s.

Intrinsic positive end-expiratory pressure/intrinsic PEEP/'auto'-PEEP

This is positive pressure in the airways at the end of expiration due to intrinsic resistance to expiration. By definition airflow does not return to zero at end-expiration.

Continuous positive airway pressure (CPAP)

CPAP is typically used with non-invasive ventilation. *See Non-invasive ventilation.* The pressure is set by the operator and is continuous. The range is from 5 cm H_2O to 20 cm H_2O. It is used for illnesses such as obstructive sleep apnoea (OSA) to keep the airway patent. *See Obstructive sleep apnoea (OSA).* It also maintains alveolar recruitment and decreases cardiac afterload.

Minute ventilation (MV)

This is the TV × breaths per minute. MV is usually set at 5–10 L/min.

PEEP

PEEP is used during invasive ventilation (with an ET tube). The range is from 5 cm H_2O to 20 cm H_2O. It keeps the alveoli open at the end of expiration (recruitment). However, PEEP also increases the intrathoracic pressure, which decreases venous return to the heart, leading to reduced cardiac output and lower systemic blood pressure.

Peak inspiratory pressure (PIP)

PIP is determined by the resistance in the airways. A high peak inspiratory pressure can be due to, for example, a kinked tube, mucus plug, bronchospasm. Aim to keep the PIP < 35 cm H_2O to prevent lung injury.

Plateau pressure (Pplat)

This is the pressure applied by the ventilator to the small airways and alveoli during inspiration once the flow of inspiratory gas has stopped. It is determined by the volume of gas that has entered the lungs and the compliance of the lungs. To measure the plateau pressure, a breath-hold in inflation is required and there is zero flow. An increase in plateau pressure suggests a decrease in lung compliance due to such causes as pneumothorax, pulmonary oedema, ARDS, pneumonia. Normal plateau pressure is about 20 cm H_2O. Aim to have a plateau pressure < 30 cm H_2O.

Respiratory rate

In a patient with healthy lungs, this would be set to 6–8 breaths per minute on the ventilator.

Tidal volume (TV)

TV is the volume of gas breathed in or out during respiration/ventilation. The ideal TV for ventilation is about 8 mL/kg of ideal body weight—usually between 500–600 mL for an adult. ***See Ideal body weight***. Set the ventilator TV to 6–8 mL/kg in a patient with healthy lungs.

Ventilator settings and arterial blood O_2 levels

In terms of ventilator settings, the main determinants of arterial blood O_2 levels are:
1 FiO_2—the fractional inspired O_2 concentration. An $FiO_2 < 50\%$ is preferred.
2 PEEP—the higher the PEEP, the more the alveoli are recruited.

Ventilator settings and arterial blood CO_2 levels

The most important ventilator settings affecting arterial blood CO_2 levels are:
1 Respiratory rate (RR). As this increases, $PaCO_2$ decreases.
2 Tidal volume (TV). Increasing TV is more efficient at decreasing the level of $PaCO_2$ than increasing RR.

Breath stacking

This is when a second and subsequent breaths are given before the initial/previous breaths are exhaled. This results in a decrease in MV despite increasing the rate and/ or TV because the air has not had sufficient time to come out of the lung. This can occur with COPD and asthma. Breath stacking is suggested by:
1 rising peak pressure
2 rising plateau pressure (> 30 cm H_2O)
3 intrinsic PEEP > 20 cm H_2O.

Modes of ventilation

These include:
1 assist control (AC)
2 volume controlled ventilation (VCV)
3 pressure controlled ventilation (PCV)
4 synchronous intermittent mandatory ventilation (SIMV).

Assist control (AC)

Assist control is also called assist control ventilation (ACV). It is referred to in some texts as controlled mandatory ventilation (CMV). AC is a volume-cycled mode of ventilation. The operator sets a tidal volume (TV) e.g. 500 mL and a ventilation rate e.g. 12 breaths per min. A TV breath is triggered if the patient attempts to breathe as sensed by the ventilator (either by the patient creating a negative pressure or an inspiratory flow). If the patient does not make any attempt to breathe, the ventilator will provide a breath up to every 5 s (with a ventilation rate of 12 breaths per min). This is called time-triggered control. The operator can set a PEEP but there is no pressure support—when the patient tries to take a breath, the ventilator delivers the set volume. It is not supporting the patient's inspiration; it is triggered by the patient's effort.

Pressure support (PS) ventilation

Pressure support ventilation is a mode in which the ventilator provides a set positive pressure (pressure support) when the patient triggers the ventilator. The amount of pressure support that can be set ranges from 5–20 cm H_2O. The higher the pressure the larger the TV.

Volume controlled ventilation (VCV)

In this mode, the operator sets a desired TV and rate. The operator can also set the maximum flow rate, which will be proportional to the time taken for the set volume to enter the lungs. Increasing the inspiratory time (decreasing the flow rate) decreases the pressure in the lungs. The maximum inspiratory pressure in the lungs is not set. Pressure measurement is required to detect pressures that are too high. This can occur if TV are too large or the lungs become stiff (less compliant).

Pressure controlled ventilation (PCV)

In this mode, the operator sets a maximum peak pressure that the lungs will be inflated to with each inspiration and a ventilation rate. The operator can also set a PEEP level. The TV is not set. Volume measurement is required to detect whether volumes are too low or too high.

Synchronous intermittent mandatory ventilation (SIMV)

This resembles AC ventilation and is also a type of volume control ventilation. The operator can select a TV, respiratory rate and PEEP, and the patient will be ventilated at this rate if they are not attempting to breathe. However, if the patient attempts to breathe, the ventilator will support that breath with a pre-set pressure support. The patient determines the TV. If the patient breathes at a faster rate than the mandatory ventilation rate, the mandatory ventilations do not occur. If they breathe at a slower rate than the mandatory ventilation rate, some ventilations will be from the ventilator. This way the ventilator is not fighting the patient. Patient and ventilator efforts are synchronised—'harmonised' would probably be a better term. SIMV mode is very popular in the ICU.

Pressure-regulated volume control ventilation (PRVC)

PRVC is also called volume-targeted pressure control, volume pre-set pressure-controlled ventilation or pressure-controlled ventilation volume-guaranteed (PCV-VG). This is pressure-controlled ventilation with a volume target, termed a 'dual mode of ventilation'. A volume target is selected by the operator and the ventilator will 'work out' how to achieve this volume at the lowest pressure. To do this, the ventilator will give a test breath and an inspiratory hold to calculate the plateau pressure. The ventilator then gives the next breath at this pressure, optimising inspiratory flow using a decelerating flow pattern. By measuring exhaled volumes and inspiratory pressures, the ventilator calculates the lowest pressure required to achieve the desired VT.

PSV-Pro

This is pressure-support ventilation (meaning when the patient takes a breath, the ventilator provides pressure support for that breath). In addition, if the patient does not breathe for a pre-set period, the machine will revert to a mandatory rate of ventilation. This is similar to SIMV.

Ventilation strategies for particular conditions

ARDS—*see Acute respiratory distress syndrome (ARDS)*.

Chronic obstructive pulmonary disease (COPD)

The compliance of the lungs is usually high but there is also high resistance in the airways. It is hard for air to get out of the lungs.

1 A slow respiratory rate (RR) with a long expiratory time (e.g. I:E ratio 1:3 or 1:4) is needed to allow time for exhalation. A high inspiratory flow rate is required to get the gas in quickly. Use an inspiratory flow rate of 80–100 L/min.
2 Increasing the RR or the TV may make CO_2 levels paradoxically higher due to breath stacking. This will be evident from flow volume loops if the volume is not returning to zero after expiration.
3 If hyperinflation occurs, this increases intrathoracic pressure which will decrease CO.
4 Temporarily disconnecting the patient from the ventilator will allow the hyperinflated lungs to deflate.

CCF

Increasing PEEP can increase lung aeration and decrease venous return to the heart. CPAP and BiPAP in non-invasive ventilation have the same effect. This reduces preload, helping ameliorate CCF.

Hypotension

1 Intubation and ventilation are likely to worsen hypotension. Provide appropriate fluid loading and consider placement of a central venous line for inotropic support prior to intubation. Invasive arterial blood pressure monitoring should also be initiated before intubation.
2 Increasing PEEP may make hypotension worse for the reasons discussed above (by decreasing venous return to the heart).

Metabolic acidosis and ventilation

A patient that has compensated for a metabolic acidosis by tachypnoea should be ventilated with a high MV, otherwise the pH may decrease significantly.

Asthma

See Asthma.

Liberation from ventilation (LFV)/weaning

A patient is unsuitable for LFV if:

1 An FiO_2 > 45% is needed.
2 Patient is on high doses of vasopressors.
3 On a spontaneous breathing trial (SBT) pH < 7.35, $PaCO_2$ > 45 mmHg, PaO_2 < 60–70 mmHg.
4 Rapid shallow breathing index (RSBI) > 105. This is the patient's RR divided by the TV in L. For example an RR of 30 and a TV of 0.3 L gives a RSBI of 100.
5 NIF (negative inspiratory flow) < 30 L/min.
6 MV > 15 L/min. They are working very hard to breathe.
7 Decreased mental status/airway protection capability.
8 Absence of air leak on cuff deflation.

◐ Ventricular fibrillation (VF)

See Cardiac arrest.

○ Ventricular septal defect (VSD)

Description
After bicuspid aortic valve, VSDs are the most common form of congenital heart disease (CHD), accounting for 25–35% of all CHD. They are divided into five types— membranous, muscular, malalignment defects, subpulmonic and atrioventricular (AV) canal or inlet defects.

Membranous defects
These lie just below the aortic valve and behind the septal leaflet of the tricuspid valve. These defects can be associated with left ventricular outflow tract (LVOT) obstruction and coarctation of the aorta.

Muscular defects
These may close spontaneously, especially if central. Multiple defects give rise to what is called 'Swiss cheese' septum.

Malalignment defects
These defects are in a similar location to a membranous defect but there is anterior or posterior malalignment of the conal septum. Anterior malalignment defects are part of the Tetralogy of Fallot complex. *See Tetralogy of Fallot (ToF).*

Subpulmonic
These VSDs are located immediately beneath the aortic and pulmonary valves.

AV canal or inlet defect
These occur posterior and superior, between the annulus of the tricuspid valve and the valve's attachment to the RV wall and septum.

Pathophysiology
The onset and severity of effects depend on the size of the VSD. They are:
1. Volume overload of the left atrium (LA) and left ventricle (LV).
2. LV dilatation and failure. This is high-output LV failure.
3. Increased pulmonary blood flow and increased pulmonary venous return. There may be pulmonary congestion and oedema.
4. Pulmonary vascular changes and pulmonary hypertension.
5. Increased systemic vascular resistance (SVR) to maintain systolic blood pressure (SBP).
6. Patients with some types of VSD may have an associated aortic valve incompetence.

Clinical effects
1. Small VSDs may close spontaneously or produce no significant clinical effects.
2. There is an increased risk of endocarditis, arrhythmia and sudden death.
3. Left-to-right shunt effects. *See Congenital heart disease (CHD) overview.*
4. Irreversible pulmonary vascular disease may occur with RV pressure overload and hypertrophy.
5. If/when pulmonary vascular resistance (PVR) exceeds SVR, right-to-left shunting occurs (Eisenmenger syndrome—*see Eisenmenger syndrome/Eisenmenger complex*). This degree of disease is usually irreversible.
6. Tachypnoea.
7. Tachycardia, systolic ejection murmur, LV 'heave'.

QUICK FLICK **V**

Grading of VSDs[2]

The size of the VSD can be compared with the size of the aortic valve annulus:
- Small: < ⅓ aortic annulus size.
- Moderate: ⅓–⅔ aortic annulus size.
- Large: > ⅔ aortic annulus size.

Another classification is based on the amount of pulmonary blood flow compared with systemic blood flow:
- Small—pulmonary < 1.5 × systemic.
- Moderate—pulmonary 1.5–2 × systemic.
- Severe—pulmonary > 2 × systemic.

   VSDs can be also described as a restrictive or non-restrictive defect. A restrictive defect is small enough to provide resistance to shunting. In a non-restrictive defect there is no resistance to shunting.

Investigations

1 Chest X-ray—may see cardiomegaly and increased pulmonary vascular markings. Pulmonary oedema may occur.
2 ECG—electrical evidence of LA and LV hypertrophy or biventricular hypertrophy.
3 Echocardiography—determines size, location and chamber effects of the VSD.
4 Pulse oximetry—hypoxia suggests right-to-left shunting.

Treatment

1 Medical treatment for CCF. **See Congestive cardiac failure (CCF)—chronic**.
2 Surgical closure of the defect.
3 Pulmonary artery banding.
4 Transcatheter closure.

VSD and anaesthesia

Patients may have a repaired or unrepaired VSD. If unrepaired, the clinical effects of a VSD range from asymptomatic to severely affected, depending on the factors described above (size of VSD, proportion of pulmonary blood flow relative to systemic blood flow etc). The presence of Eisenmenger syndrome is especially concerning. **See Eisenmenger syndrome/Eisenmenger complex**.

   The general principles are:

1 Attempt to keep circulation 'balanced'—avoid factors which increase left-to-right shunt and right-to-left shunt. **See Eisenmenger syndrome/Eisenmenger complex** and **Congenital heart disease (CHD)—overview**.
2 Consider bacterial endocarditis prophylaxis if appropriate. **See Bacterial endocarditis (BE) prophylaxis**.
3 More detailed management guidelines depend on the degree of cardiac decompensation and are covered in other sections of this manual.

◐ Ventricular tachycardia (VT)

Description

Defined as greater than two consecutive ventricular ectopic beats. Termed 'sustained ventricular tachycardia' if the duration of the arrythmia is longer than 30 s. It is a wide-complex tachycardia originating from the ventricles at a rate > 100 bpm. It may be:

1 pulseless—**see Cardiac arrest**
2 monomorphic—all the complexes are the same
3 polymorphic—the QRS complexes have different morphologies.

Monomorphic VT

It is the most common type of a broad complex tachycardia. It may be associated with myocardial infarction. A SVT with LBBB can be confused with monomorphic VT.

Treatment

VT is a medical emergency. Seek urgent expert cardiologist advice.

1 If pulseless—*see Cardiac arrest*.
2 Haemodynamically unstable patient (chest pain, dyspnoea, SBP < 90 mmHg, heart failure or HR > 150 bpm)—provide cardioversion under sedation with **synchronised shocks** 50, 100, 200 J.
3 If shocks are unsuccessful, give amiodarone—*see Amiodarone*.
4 If haemodynamically stable VT, obtain a 12-lead ECG and consider chemical cardioversion—amiodarone or sotalol. Seek urgent cardiologist referral and advice.
5 Identify and treat the cause.

Polymorphic

1 If pulseless—*see Cardiac arrest*.
2 If torsades de pointes—*see Torsades de pointes*. The QRS complexes twist around the isoelectric line.
3 If not torsades, treat as for monomorphic VT.
4 Identify and treat the cause.

◐ Verapamil

Description

This is a non-dihydropyridine calcium channel blocker drug, similar to diltiazem.
See Calcium channel blocker.

Indications

1 Arrhythmias such as paroxysmal supraventricular tachycardia, atrial fibrillation/flutter (**not** in Wolff–Parkinson–White syndrome). *See Wolff-Parkinson-White (WPW) syndrome*.
2 Coronary artery disease.
3 Hypertension.
4 Migraine.

Contraindications

1 Atrial fibrillation/flutter associated with Wolff–Parkinson–White syndrome. *See Wolff-Parkinson-White syndrome (WPW)*.
1 Ventricular tachycardia.
2 Cardiogenic shock unless arrhythmia induced.
3 Second or third degree heart block—*see Heart block (HB)*.
4 Sick sinus syndrome.
5 LVF.
6 Concomitant beta blocker use. Severe bradycardia may occur.
7 Patients who have received dantrolene for malignant hyperthermia. Verapamil in this situation can worsen hyperkalaemia, myocardial depression and hypotension.

Dose

Adult

Slow IV 1–5 mg, repeated after 5–10 min if needed. IV infusion 5–10 mg/h. The usual oral starting dose is 120 mg q 12 h titrated up to 240 mg q 12 h.

◎ Vitamin K₁/konakion/phytomenadione/phylloquinone

One of the important uses of this vitamin is to acutely reverse the effects of warfarin. *See Warfarin*. IV effects take 6–8 h to work but PO and IV vitamin K_1 have similar efficacy at 24 h. The IV dose is 5–10 mg.

◎ Von Willebrand disease (VWD)

Description

This spectrum of diseases is due to a mutation on chromosome 12 resulting in deficiencies in quality and quantity of von Willebrand factor (VWF). The normal level of VWF is a 50–100 IU/100 mL. It is the most common hereditary coagulopathy (1–2% of the population). It is of clinical significance in only 1:10000 patients.[3] VWF is a blood glycoprotein which is important for platelet adhesion during haemostasis. It is produced in megakaryocytes, endothelium and subendothelial connective tissue. It acts as a binder to platelets, FVIII, collagen and other substances. VWD is usually inherited but can occur spontaneously by mutation. It can be acquired in certain conditions such as lymphoproliferative disorders, autoimmune disorders and congenital heart disease.

Classification of VWD

Type 1—VWF has decreased effectiveness and insufficient quantities are present (80% of sufferers).
   In type 1C VWF is cleared abnormally quickly.

Type 2—VWF levels are normal but the factor is defective. Subdivided into:
- *2A*—usually autosomal dominant.
- *2B*—autosomal dominant. Causes platelets to clump together (VWF-induced platelet binding is increased). There is a platelet disease called platelet type VWD (pseudo-VWD) in which there is increased binding of VWF and the platelet, but the fault lies with the platelet.
- *2M*—usually autosomal dominant with reduced binding of platelets.
- *2N*—VWF has a carrier function for FVIII. This is lost in type 2N disease, leading to reduced FVIII levels and a haemophilia A-type clinical picture. *See Haemophilia*.

Type 3—Very severe illness in which there is no or almost no VWF present.

Clinical effects

There is a spectrum of effects ranging from no clinical features to life-threatening haemorrhage. It may only become manifest when there is serious trauma or surgery. VWD may present with:
1 epistaxis
2 easy bruising
3 prolonged bleeding after tooth extraction
4 heavy periods.
   Patients with type 2 VWD tend to have a moderate to severe bleeding tendency. Type 3 is associated with a severe bleeding tendency.

Diagnosis

1 In all types of VWD, APTT may be prolonged due to FVIII deficiency. PT is usually normal.

2 Platelets may be reduced in type 2B disease due to sequestration of VWF/platelet complexes.

3 Microcytic anaemia may result from chronic blood loss.

4 Apparent haemophilia A in a female should raise suspicion of type 2N VWD.

Specific tests include:

1 VWF antigen test—this measures VWF levels.

2 VWF activity—this measures the efficacy of the VWF that is present.

3 FVIII clotting activity—this is reduced in type 2N VWD.

4 VWF multimers—this test helps determine the type of VWD.

Treatment

1 Desmopressin (DDAVP)—stimulates the secretion of endothelial VWF. Useful in mild disease when the patient is having minor surgery. DDAVP can worsen thrombocytopenia in type 2B disease by increasing sequestration. It is contraindicated unless on the advice of a haematologist. Do not use DDAVP if serious or life-threatening bleeding. *See Desmopressin (DDAVP)*.

2 VWF replacement therapy. This can be by plasma derived FVIII/VWF concentrate (*see Biostate*) or recombinant VWF (Vonvendi®).

3 Tranexamic acid.

VWD and anaesthesia/surgery

1 The patient must be carefully assessed by a multidisciplinary team including surgeon, anaesthetist and haematologist. Treatment prior to surgery is determined by the type and severity of VWD.

2 Administration of VWF and/or DDAVP, if required, should occur 30–60 min before surgery. Maintain levels of VWF at 100 IU/100 mL perioperatively and 50 IU/100 mL in the postoperative period.[3]

3 Tranexamic acid may be helpful.

4 In type 3 VWD, 10–15% of patients develop inhibitors. Recombinant-activated FVIIa can be helpful in this situation.

5 If all other treatments fail, consider platelet transfusion and/or cryoprecipitate. Avoid drugs that may cause increased risk of bleeding such as aspirin.

VWD and obstetrics

1 In pregnancy, VWF levels increase by 3–5 × pre-pregnancy levels, but decline precipitously after delivery. This may lead to postpartum haemorrhage up to 15 days postpartum.

2 Pregnant women with VWD should be reviewed by a multidisciplinary team, including a haematologist.

3 A target level of VWF of 40 IU/100 mL is required for safe vaginal delivery.

4 Target levels of 50–150 IU/100 mL are thought to be advisable before CS and neuraxial anaesthesia.[3] Additionally, the platelet count should be > 70 000 per mm³ and PT/APPT tests should be normal, if neuraxial anaesthesia is to be contemplated.

5 Following CS, VWD patients may require ongoing VWF and/or DDAVP as VWF levels decline quickly after delivery.

Type 1 VWD

1 Usually, VWF levels increase sufficiently during pregnancy for neuraxial block to be safely performed, but this must be confirmed by a haematologist.

2 This type of VWD is usually very responsive to DDAVP. The dose is 0.3 mcg/kg IV, which is effective in 30–60 min. It is relatively contraindicated in cardiovascular disease and preeclampsia.[3]

3 Desmopressin should be considered if PPH occurs.

Type 2 VWD

1 DDAVP is usually ineffective because the VWF is defective and inducing increased levels of VWF does not help.

2 In type 2B VWD, giving DDAVP may make matters worse by causing profound thrombocytopenia.

3 These patients may require biostate (VWF and FVIII) or recombinant VWF, prior to neuraxial anaesthesia/surgery or if haemorrhaging. *See Biostate*.

Type 3 VWD

1 There is no augmentation of VWF in pregnancy and no response to DDAVP.

2 VWF replacement therapy is the only option.

REFERENCES

1 Cutts TG, O'Donnell AM. The implications of vaping for the anaesthetist. *BJA Educat* 2021; 21: 243–249.

2 Rolo V, Walker I, Wilson K. *Ventricular septal defects*. WFSA Tutorial 316 June 2015. Accessed online: https://resources.wfsahq.org/atotw/ventricular-septal-defects, January 2023.

3 Reale S, Farber M, Lumbreras-Marquez M et al. Anaesthetic management of Von Willebrand disease in pregnancy: a retrospective analysis of a large case series. *Anesth Analg* 2021; 133: 1244–1250.

W

⚪ Warfarin

Description

Synthetic coumarin derivative oral vitamin K antagonist. Warfarin is an anticoagulant drug, which acts by preventing the synthesis of vitamin K dependent clotting factors (II, VII, IX and X) in the liver. There are four main indications for warfarin:

1. Non-valvular AF.
2. Artificial heart valve.
3. AF associated with diseased heart valve.
4. Thromboembolic disease (prevention or treatment) e.g. DVT, PE, stroke.

Warfarin risk/benefit analysis for patients with non-rheumatic AF

The use of warfarin must balance the risk (bleeding) with the benefit (prevention of stroke) in non-valvular AF. A useful tool is the CHA_2DS_2-VASc score, as demonstrated in Tables W1 and W2.[1]

Table W1 CHA_2DS_2-VASc score

Letter	Condition	Points
C	Congestive heart failure	1
H	Hypertension—BP > 140/90 or treated hypertension	1
A	Age ≥ 75 yrs	2
D	Diabetes mellitus	1
S_2	Prior stroke, TIA or thromboembolism	2
V	Vascular disease (e.g. peripheral artery disease, MI)	1
A	Age 65–74 y	1
Sc	Sex category—female	1

The maximum score is 9.

Annual stroke risk is summarised in Table W2.

Table W2 CHA_2DS_2-VASc score and annual stroke risk

Score	Annual stroke rate risk (approx)
1	0.6%
2	2%
3	3%
4	5%
5	7%
6	10%
7	11%
8	11%
9	12%

A score of zero is possible e.g. a 50-year-old man with non-valvular AF and no other risk factors.

Table W3 CHA$_2$DS$_2$-VASc score and recommended action

Score	Action
0 (male) or 1 (female)	No anticoagulant therapy
1 (male)	Consider anticoagulant therapy
2 or greater	Anticoagulant therapy

The risk of bleeding in non-valvular AF can be calculated from the HAS-BLED score, as demonstrated in Table W4.[2]

Table W4 Calculating the HAS-BLED score

Letter	Clinical characteristic	Points
H	Hypertension	1
A	Abnormal liver or renal function	1–2
S	Stroke	1
B	Bleeding	1
L	Labile INR	1
E	Elderly (age > 65 y)	1
D	Drugs or alcohol	1–2
Maximum score		9

The HAS-BLED score signifies a person's approximate annual risk of major bleeding as a percentage, as demonstrated in Table W5.

Table W5 HAS-BLED score and annual risk rate of major bleeding

Score	Risk (approx)
1	1%
2	2%
3	4%
4	8%
5	12%

A score ≥ 3 is considered high. HAS-BLED is used to help identify factors that can be modified to reduce the risk of bleeding in patients on warfarin.

Dose

Warfarin takes days to exert its effects. Due to its slow onset, it may be necessary to overlap initial warfarin therapy with fractionated or unfractionated

heparin. **See _Heparin (unfractionated and low-molecular-weight heparins)_.**
To 'warfarinise' an adult, give:

1 Day 1—< 70 y 10 mg PO, > 70 y 5 mg PO.
2 Day 2—5 mg PO.
3 Day 3—check INR. If INR < 2 give 5 mg; INR 2–3 give 4 mg; INR > 3 omit.

Continue to titrate dose until INR is stable and in the therapeutic range.

Therapeutic range for INR

1 Mechanical mitral valve or combined mitral and aortic valves—**2.5–3.5.**
2 Other indications including single mechanical valve (not mitral)—**2–3.**

Is bridging therapy required?

The risk of stroke/thromboembolism, if warfarin is stopped, can be classified as:

1 **_Low (no bridging therapy required)_**
   a) Bi-leaflet aortic valve prosthesis without AF and no other risk factors.
   b) AF with CHA_2DS_2-VASc score $\leq$ 2.
   c) VTE > 1 yr ago and no other risk factors.
2 **_Moderate (consider bridging therapy—obtain expert specialist advice)_**
   a) Bi-leaflet mechanical aortic valve plus other risk factors.
   b) VTE 3–12 months ago.
   c) Recurrent VTE.
   d) Active cancer.
   e) Non-severe thrombophilia e.g. factor V Leiden gene mutation.
3 **_Severe (need bridging therapy)_**
   a) Any mitral valve prosthesis, caged ball or tilting disc aortic valve.
   b) Mechanical heart valve and stroke/TIA within 6 months.
   c) AF and stroke/TIA within 3 months, CHA_2DS_2-VASc score > 4, rheumatic heart disease.
   d) VTE within 3 months, severe thrombophilia.

How to provide bridging therapy

1 Give last dose of warfarin 6 days before surgery.
2 Check INR from 4 days before surgery and every subsequent day until INR $\leq$ 2.
3 When INR $\leq$ 2, start clexane 1 mg/kg subcut 12 h or 1.5 mg/kg daily. Give the last dose 24 h before surgery. Alternatively, start a heparin infusion. **See _Heparin (unfractionated and low-molecular-weight heparins)_.** Aim for an APTT of 50–90 s. Cease the infusion at least 6 h before surgery.

Anticoagulation after surgery

Seek expert specialist advice. Patients who are at low to moderate risk of stroke/thromboembolism can restart their warfarin on the night after surgery at their usual maintenance dose. Consider clexane at a prophylactic dose until warfarin is therapeutic. For patients at high risk, restart heparin infusion 6–48 h postoperatively, depending on the perceived risk of postoperative bleeding. Alternatively, give clexane at a therapeutic dose, 48–72 h after surgery, depending on the perceived risk of postoperative bleeding.

Advantages of warfarin

1 Highly effective anticoagulant suitable for any condition requiring long-term anticoagulation.
2 Long history of safe use.

3 Monitoring indicates compliance or non-compliance.

4 Can be used in patients with moderate to severe renal impairment.

Disadvantages of warfarin

1 Takes days to exert its effects.

2 Requires blood test monitoring of INR. However, battery powered, easy to use, home INR monitoring devices are available e.g. the CoaguChek INRange meter.

3 Warfarin takes days to wear off, but it can be rapidly reversed. See below.

4 Effects may be unstable due to dietary changes e.g. eating foods rich in vitamin K such as kale.

5 Bleeding is more likely with warfarin than with alternative drugs (non-vitamin K antagonist oral anticoagulants—NOACs).

6 Many drug interactions e.g. Bactrim, statins and amiodarone.

7 Some herbal medicines interact with warfarin such as St John's wort.

8 Only 60% of patients have an INR in the therapeutic range at any given time of treatment.[3]

Warfarin and surgery/neuraxial block

*See **Anticoagulant and antiplatelet drugs and surgery/neuraxial anaesthesia**.*

Warfarin overdose

If INR is elevated (4.5–10) and there is no bleeding, withhold warfarin and restart at a lower dose when INR is therapeutic. If bleeding, treat as for warfarin and emergency surgery/haemorrhage.

Warfarin and emergency surgery/haemorrhage

To reverse warfarin emergently use:

1 Vitamin K 5–10 mg IV over 20 min. There is a risk of anaphylaxis/anaphylactoid reaction. INR begins to decrease after 1–2 h, with a peak effect in 4–6 h.

2 Prothrombinex-VF. *See **Prothrombinex-VF*** for dose. Vitamin K is essential to maintain the effect of prothrombinex-VF.

3 Fresh frozen plasma (FFP). Use if prothrombinex-VF is not available or is ineffective. Give 15 mL/kg.

◖ Well leg compartment syndrome

Description

This condition is due to prolonged surgery in the lithotomy position or steep head-down laparoscopic surgery (or both) causing lower limb ischaemia. When the patient is returned to the supine position, reperfusion injury can occur, with tissue oedema and swelling, leading to impaired blood supply to the lower limbs. It is probably due to the combination of prolonged reduced arterial blood supply and impaired venous drainage. Other risk factors may be:

- muscular legs
- obesity
- hypotension
- peripheral vascular disease.

This can result in rhabdomyolysis, leg pain and myoglobin-related renal failure. Absent peripheral lower limb pulses may be noted.

Prevention[4]

1 Return the patient to the horizontal position every 2 h for 10 min.
2 During this time, massage the patient's lower limbs.
3 Pulse oximetry on the patient's toe intraoperatively may help detect decreased foot perfusion.

Treatment

Immediate fasciotomies to release all four leg compartments.

○ Wilson's disease/hepatolenticular degeneration

Description

This is a rare inherited autosomal recessive disease of copper metabolism. There is a reduction in the synthesis of the copper transporter protein ceruloplasmin, preventing the elimination of copper in bile. Copper builds up in the body and damages organs, especially the brain, liver, kidneys and cornea.

Clinical effects

1 Tremor.
2 Dysarthria.
3 Rigid dystonia.
4 Seizures.
5 Psychiatric disorders.
6 Cirrhosis/liver failure/chronic hepatitis.
7 Renal involvement—haematuria.
8 Cardiac involvement—arrhythmias.
9 Kayser–Fleischer corneal rings (due to copper deposition).

Diagnosis

1 24 h urinary copper levels (usually elevated).
2 Blood ceruloplasmin levels (usually decreased).
3 Slit-lamp corneal examination for Kayser–Fleischer rings.
4 Liver biopsy.

Treatment

1 Zinc sulphate—this reduces/prevents copper absorption from food.
2 D-penicillamine.
3 Minimise copper intake in food, avoiding foods such as shellfish, mushrooms.
4 Vitamin B6.
5 Liver transplant.

Anaesthesia

1 NDNMBDs that rely on liver metabolism (e.g. rocuronium) may have a prolonged effect. Cisatracurium is a suitable alternative.
2 Check for coagulopathy.

○ Wolff–Parkinson–White syndrome (WPW)

Description

WPW is a rare congenital conduction disorder, due to the presence of an aberrant electrical pathway (bundle of Kent) between the atria and ventricles. It is a pre-excitation syndrome and results in tachycardias. *See Pre-excitation*. The accessory pathway (AP) relies on fast sodium channels for depolarisation, whereas the AV node relies on slow calcium channels. In most cases, electricity can flow in either direction through the AP. 'Antegrade conduction' means from atria to ventricles and 'retrograde conduction' means from ventricles to atria.

Diagnosis

Patients may be asymptomatic or suffer from palpitations, syncope, dyspnoea, angina and death. The tachycardias tend to start and stop abruptly. When the patient is **not** having a tachycardia, the ECG may show pre-excitation—short PR interval, delta waves and ST and T wave changes as described in *Pre-excitation*. This means there is antegrade conduction through the AP and the AV node.

The AP can result in atrioventricular re-entrant tachycardias (AVRT). **See** *Atrioventricular re-entrant tachycardia (AVRT)*. These can be:

1 Narrow complex—the electricity in the circuit travels in an antegrade direction through the AV node into the ventricles, then in a retrograde direction through the AP into the atria.

2 Wide complex—the electricity in the circuit travels in a retrograde direction through the AV node, into the atria then in an antegrade direction through the AP into the ventricles.

Atrial fibrillation can also occur. The QRS complexes are typically wide, bizarre and irregular. Very fast heart rates may occur and VF may eventuate. This condition is therefore potentially fatal.

Patients may have a normal ECG preoperatively and then develop a typical WPR ECG intra- or postoperatively. Other patients may have WPW pattern ECG without arrhythmias. WPW usually exists in isolation. Associated conditions are Ebstein's anomaly and, possibly, mitral valve prolapse. **See** *Ebstein's anomaly*. Asymptomatic patients are at very low risk of a life-threatening arrhythmia.

Treatment

Asymptomatic patients with a WPW-type ECG should be considered for electrophysiological studies (EPS) and ablation. Patients with symptomatic WPW should undergo electrophysiological studies and radiofrequency ablation of the AP. Patients may require chronic antiarrhythmic therapy such as calcium channel blockers or beta blockers.

Anaesthetic management

Discuss the patient's management with their cardiologist. Find out what treatments have been successful in the past. In general:

1 Avoid any drugs that may slow AV nodal conduction time such as neostigmine.

2 Avoid drugs that increase AV nodal conduction time such as desflurane.

3 Avoid drugs that increase heart rate such as atropine, glycopyrrolate and ketamine.

4 Increased sympathetic activity (e.g. from pain, light anaesthesia, intubation) may increase the risk of arrhythmias. Therefore, avoid sympathetic activation.

5 Consider the use of an arterial line to monitor the haemodynamic effects of any arrhythmia that may occur.

Management of dysrhythmias

If the patient has haemodynamic instability, perform DC cardioversion with sedation. **See** *Haemodynamic instability*. Medical management for stable patients depends on the arrhythmia.

Atrial fibrillation (AF), atrial flutter

The QRS complexes will be wide and irregular as the AF is being conducted down the AP.

1 Do **not** give any drugs that slow AV conduction such as adenosine, calcium channel blockers, beta blockers or digoxin. Carotid sinus massage should **not** be performed. If these drugs are given, conduction through the AP will be enhanced, promoting degeneration of the AF into VF.

2 Cardioversion may be effective.

3 Procainamide is a Na^+ channel blocker and can be of benefit by blocking the AP. *See Procainamide*. Ibutilide is an alternative.

Narrow complex tachycardias

The HR is fast and regular. These are atrioventricular re-entrant tachycardias with orthodromic conduction. *See Atrioventricular re-entrant tachycardia (AVRT)*. The aim is to reduce the AV node conduction rate.

1 Vagal manoeuvres such as carotid sinus massage can be attempted. *See Vagal manoeuvres*.

2 Nodal blockers such as adenosine, beta blockers and/or calcium channel blockers. Some patients given adenosine may develop AF, so have a defibrillator/cardioverter available.

Wide complex tachycardias

The HR is fast and regular. These can be due to AVRT with antidromic conduction or AVRT with orthodromic conduction and bundle branch conduction abnormalities. Treatment is the same as for narrow complex regular tachycardias.

◐ Wound infusion catheters

Wound infusion catheters are useful for the treatment of postoperative pain, especially after abdominal surgery. The positioning of the catheter is at the discretion of the surgeon and may be in the rectus sheath space or in the pre-peritoneal space or other sites. In general, ropivacaine 0.2% can be safely infused at a dose rate of 5–10 mL/h.

Intermittent bolus infusion (programmable pump) dosage regime

One catheter

Establish the block with 40 mL ropivacaine 0.2%. Set the pump to infuse 20 mL of ropivacaine 0.2% every 4 h with the first bolus given in 2 h.

Two catheters

Establish the block with 20 mL ropivacaine 0.2% each side. Use 2 infusion pumps, labelled 'left' and 'right'. Program each pump to infuse 10 mL boluses of ropivacaine 0.2% every 2 h, with the first bolus to be given in 2 h.

◐ Wrist blocks

The median, ulnar and radial nerves can all be blocked at the wrist. For the distribution of these nerves in the hand, *see Arm blocks in the elbow region*. Also see Figure W1.

Technique

Median nerve

The median nerve lies between the tendon of palmaris longus (roughly the middle of the wrist) and flexor carpi radialis (just lateral to the palmaris longus). The nerve is deep to both tendons and closer to the palmaris longus.

1 Mark the point 2 cm proximal from the most distal wrist crease (proximal to the carpal tunnel).
2 Insert a 25 G needle through the deep fascia at this point between the tendons described above. Insert the needle about 4–5 mm at an angle of 45° towards the hand.
3 Inject 5 mL of 1% lignocaine as the needle is withdrawn.

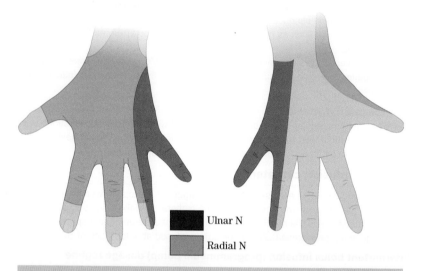

Figure W1 Innervation of the hand

Reproduced with permission from Tintinalli JE, Ma O, Yealy DM, Meckler GD, Stapczynski J, Cline DM, Thomas SH, eds. Tintinalli's Emergency Medicine: A Comprehensive Study Guide, 9e. McGraw Hill; 2020.

Ulnar nerve

1 Identify the ulnar artery and ulnar styloid.
2 Two finger breadths proximal to the ulnar styloid, inject a wheal of LA parallel to the wrist crease.
3 Make sure you do not inject into the artery.
4 Use 3–5 mL of 1% lignocaine.

Radial nerve

1 Insert the needle just lateral to the radial artery (thumb side) 2.5 cm proximal to the wrist joint.
2 Aim to make a wheal of LA over the distal forearm in line with the anatomical snuff box.
3 Use 3–5 mL of 1% lignocaine.

REFERENCES

1 Lip G, Nieuwlaat R, Pisters R et al. Refining clinical risk stratification for predicting stroke and thromboembolism in atrial fibrillation using a novel risk-factor based approach: the Euro Heart Survey on atrial fibrillation. *Chest* 2010; 137: 263–272.

2 Pisters R, Lane DA, Nieuwlaat R et al. A novel user-friendly score (HAS-BLED) to assess 1-year risk of major bleeding in patients with atrial fibrillation: the Euro Heart Survey. *Chest* 2010; 138: 1093–1010.

3 Del Zoppo GJ, Eliasziw M. New options in anticoagulation for atrial fibrillation. *N Engl J Med* 2011; 11 Supp 1: 122–128.

4 Hayden P, Cowman S. Anaesthesia for *laparoscopic surgery. Cont Educ in Anaesth, Crit Care Pain* 2011; 11: 177–180.

X

Xarelto

See *Rivaroxaban*.

Xenon

Description

Inert noble gas with potent anaesthetic properties. The inhaled concentration required for GA is 60–70%. The lungs must be denitrogenated by breathing 100% O_2 for 15–20 min prior to anaesthesia.

Advantages

1 No negative inotropic effects.
2 Does not trigger MH.
3 Environmentally safe.
4 Non-toxic.
5 Not teratogenic.
6 Rapid induction and recovery.
7 Profoundly analgesic.

Disadvantages

1 Very expensive.
2 Weak agent with a MAC of 63.
3 Can cause diffusion hypoxia—use 100% O_2 at end of case.

⬤ Zydol

This is a trade name for tramadol. ***See Tramadol***.

Appendix 1

▶ **Adult emergency IV drug infusion regimens—a quick reference guide**

Please note that, for the sake of accuracy, the volume of the carrier solution that is removed from the container prior to mixing should match the volume of the drug ampoule(s).

Adrenaline

Mix 6 mg adrenaline with 100 mL of 5% glucose (60 mcg/mL). Start the infusion at 5 mL/h and titrate to effect. Can be commenced through a peripheral IV cannula in an emergency until central venous access is established.

Clevidipine

This drug is administered undiluted (0.5 mg/mL), starting with an initial dose of 1–2 mg/h. Double the dose every 90 s until the desired MAP is achieved, to a maximum of 32 mg/h.

Dobutamine

Mix 250 mg with 100 mL 5% glucose (2.5 mg/mL). Initial dose is 0.5–1 mcg/kg/min. In a 70 kg patient this equals 0.8–1.6 mL/hr. Maintenance dose is 2–20 mcg/kg/min (70 kg patient 3.2–32 mL/h). The maximum dose is 40 mcg/kg/min. It can be given peripherally through a large-bore cannula. Titrate to heart rate and blood pressure.

Esmolol

Administer undiluted. Esmolol ampoules contain 100 mg of drug in 10 mL. The LD is 500 mcg/kg over 1 min (70 kg patient = 3.5 mL). Commence the infusion at 20 mL/h and titrate to effect to a maximum of 60 mL/h.

Glyceryl trinitrate (GTN)

Mix 50 mg GTN with 500 mL 5% glucose in a glass bottle (100 mcg/mL). Administer at an initial rate of 3–5 mL/h. Titrate to effect to a maximum of 120 mL/h. Administer via an approved giving set (blue) to reduce absorption into plastics.

Isoprenaline

Mix 2 mg of isoprenaline with 50 mL of 5% glucose (40 mcg/mL). Administer through a central venous line only. For complete heart block, give 10–20 mcg then an infusion of 0.5–8 mcg/min (1–12 mL/h).

Levosimendan

Mix 12.5 mg levosimendan with 250 mL 5% glucose (50 mcg/mL). Administer a LD of 6–24 mcg/kg over 10 min–1 h (70 kg patient = 8.4–33.6 mL), then commence an infusion of 0.1 mcg/kg/min (70 kg patient = 8.4 mL/h). If after 30–60 min there is excessive hypotension or tachycardia, reduce the rate by half. If the initial infusion is well tolerated, double the infusion rate.

Milrinone

Mix 20 mg of milrinone with 100 mL 5% glucose (200 mcg/mL). Infuse preferably through a central line. Start the infusion at 0.5 mcg/kg/min and assess response in 2 h. Increase or decrease dose by increments of 0.125 mcg/kg/min. The usual dose range is 0.125–0.5 mcg/kg/min and the maximum dose 0.75 mcg/kg/min.

Noradrenaline

Mix 6 mg NA with 100 mL 5% glucose (60 mcg/mL). Administer by a central line (or a large peripheral vein in an emergency). Start at 2–10 mL/h and titrate by 1 mL/h every 15 min, depending on response. In terms of mcg/min, start the infusion at 2–10 mcg/min = 2–10 mL/h. Titrate to desired blood pressure. The usual dose range is 0.5–30 mcg/min = 0.5–30 mL/h.

Sodium nitroprusside (SNP)

Mix 50 mg of SNP with 100 mL 5% glucose (500 mcg/mL). Protect the SNP from light. Administer at a dose of 0.3–4 mcg/kg/min, titrating to effect. In a 70 kg patient this is 2.5–33 mL/h.

Vasopressin

Mix 20 units of vasopressin with 40 mL 5% glucose (0.5 units/mL). Administer preferably through a central line. Start the infusion at 1–2 units per h (2–4 mL/h). For severe hypotension e.g. anaphylaxis, consider a bolus of 1–2 units.

Appendix 2

▶ Some important blood/serum reference ranges

Sodium	136–146 mmol/L
Potassium	3.2–5.5 mmol/L
Chloride	94–107 mmol/L
Urea	2.5–6.5 mmol/L
Creatinine	60–125 micromol/L
Creatinine clearance	90–100 mL/min
Estimated glomerular filtration rate (eGFR)	> 90 mL/min/1.73 m^2
Total bilirubin	2–21 micromol/L
Total protein	63–84 g/L
Albumin	35–53 g/L
Alkaline phosphatase	44–147 IU/L
Gamma-glutamyl transferase (GGT)	8–43 IU/L
Alanine aminotransferase	10–47 IU/L
Lactate	0.3–1.3 mmol/L
Prothrombin time	11–18 s
Activated partial thromboplastin time	25–36 s
Fibrinogen	2–4 g/L
White cell count	$4–11 \times 10^9$/L
Haemoglobin	130–180 g/L
Platelets	150 000–400 000/mm^3
Blood glucose level	3.9–6.2 mmoL/L
Haemoglobin A1c	NR 4–5.6%
	Diabetes $\geq$ 6.5%
Cardiac enzymes	Troponin I > 0.04 ng/mL indicates cardiac damage
	Troponin I > 0.4 ng/mL indicates severe cardiac damage
	Troponin T > 22 ng/mL (males) or > 14 ng/mL (females) indicates myocardial damage
B-type natriuretic peptide	BNP < 100 pg/mL indicates no heart failure
	BNP > 100 pg/mL **may** be a sign of heart failure
	BNP > 450 pg/mL in a patient > 50 y indicates acute heart failure